TORSO, PELVIS, AND LOWER EXTREMITIES

Grabb's Encyclopedia of Flaps

THIRD EDITION

Volume III

TORSO, PELVIS, AND LOWER EXTREMITIES
Grabb's Encyclopedia of Flaps

THIRD EDITION

Editors

Berish Strauch, MD
Professor of Plastic Surgery
Albert Einstein College of Medicine
Bronx, New York

Luis O. Vasconez, MD
Professor of Surgery and Director
Division of Plastic Surgery
University of Alabama Medical Center, Birmingham
Chief Plastic Surgeon
University of Alabama Hospital
Birmingham, Alabama

Elizabeth J. Hall-Findlay, MD
Plastic Surgeon
Banff Mineral Springs Hospital
Banff, Alberta, Canada

Bernard T. Lee, MD
Instructor in Surgery
Harvard Medical School
Division of Plastic and Reconstructive Surgery
Beth Israel Deaconess Medical Center
Boston, Massachusetts

Wolters Kluwer | Lippincott Williams & Wilkins
Health
Philadelphia • Baltimore • New York • London
Buenos Aires • Hong Kong • Sydney • Tokyo

Acquisitions Editor: Brian Brown
Managing Editor: Michelle La Plante
Marketing Manager: Lisa Parry
Project Manager: Bridgett Dougherty
Senior Manufacturing Manager: Benjamin Rivera
Creative Director: Doug Smock
Production Service: Nesbitt Graphics, Inc.

Library of Congress Cataloging-in-Publication Data

Grabb's encyclopedia of flaps / editors, Berish Strauch ... [et al.]. -- 3rd ed.
    p. ; cm.
Includes bibliographical references and index.
ISBN 978-0-7817-6432-2
ISBN 978-0-7817-7492-5
1. Flaps (Surgery) I. Grabb, William C. II. Strauch, Berish, 1933- III.
Title: Encylopedia of flaps.
[DNLM: 1. Surgical Flaps. 2. Reconstructive Surgical Procedures. WO 610G727 2009]
RD120.8.G78 2009
617.9'5--dc22

                                                                2008024234

Care has been taken to confirm the accuracy of the information presented and to
describe generally accepted practices. However, the authors, editors, and publisher are not
responsible for errors or omissions or for any consequences from application of the
information in this book and make no warranty, expressed or implied, with respect to the
currency, completeness, or accuracy of the contents of the publication. Application of the
information in a particular situation remains the professional responsibility of the
practitioner.

The authors, editors, and publisher have exerted every effort to ensure that drug
selection and dosage set forth in this text are in accordance with current recommendations
and practice at the time of publication. However, in view of ongoing research, changes in
government regulations, and the constant flow of information relating to drug therapy and
drug reactions, the reader is urged to check the package insert for each drug for any change
in indications and dosage and for added warnings and precautions. This is particularly
important when the recommended agent is a new or infrequently employed drug.

Some drugs and medical devices presented in the publication have Food and Drug
Administration (FDA) clearance for limited use in restricted research settings. It is the
responsibility of the health care provider to ascertain the FDA status of each drug or device
planned for use in their clinical practice.

To purchase additional copies of this book, call our customer service department at (800)
638-3030 or fax orders to (301) 223-2320. International customers should call (301) 223-
2300.

Visit Lippincott Williams & Wilkins on the Internet: at LWW.com. Lippincott Williams &
Wilkins customer service representatives are available from 8:30 am to 6 pm, EST.

10 9 8 7 6 5 4 3 2 1

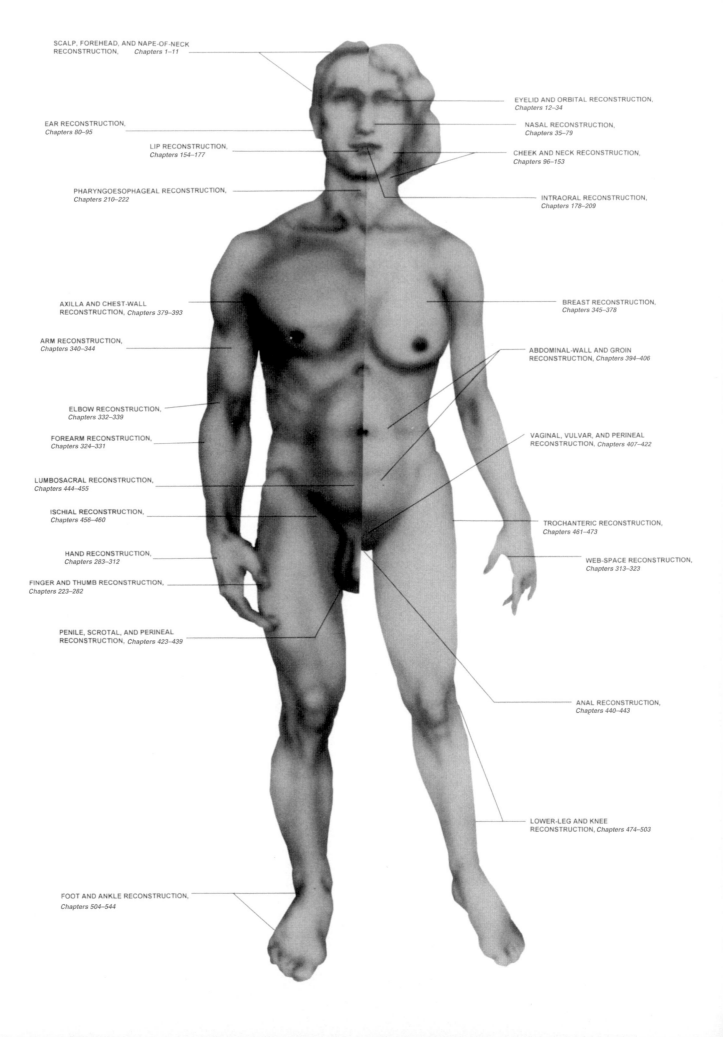

SCALP, FOREHEAD, AND NAPE-OF-NECK
RECONSTRUCTION, *Chapters 1–11*

EYELID AND ORBITAL RECONSTRUCTION,
Chapters 12–34

EAR RECONSTRUCTION,
Chapters 80–95

NASAL RECONSTRUCTION,
Chapters 35–79

LIP RECONSTRUCTION,
Chapters 154–177

CHEEK AND NECK RECONSTRUCTION,
Chapters 96–153

PHARYNGOESOPHAGEAL RECONSTRUCTION,
Chapters 210–222

INTRAORAL RECONSTRUCTION,
Chapters 178–209

AXILLA AND CHEST-WALL
RECONSTRUCTION, *Chapters 379–393*

BREAST RECONSTRUCTION,
Chapters 345–378

ARM RECONSTRUCTION,
Chapters 340–344

ABDOMINAL-WALL AND GROIN
RECONSTRUCTION, *Chapters 394–406*

ELBOW RECONSTRUCTION,
Chapters 332–339

FOREARM RECONSTRUCTION,
Chapters 324–331

VAGINAL, VULVAR, AND PERINEAL
RECONSTRUCTION, *Chapters 407–422*

LUMBOSACRAL RECONSTRUCTION,
Chapters 444–455

ISCHIAL RECONSTRUCTION,
Chapters 456–460

TROCHANTERIC RECONSTRUCTION,
Chapters 461–473

HAND RECONSTRUCTION,
Chapters 283–312

WEB-SPACE RECONSTRUCTION,
Chapters 313–323

FINGER AND THUMB RECONSTRUCTION,
Chapters 223–282

PENILE, SCROTAL, AND PERINEAL
RECONSTRUCTION, *Chapters 423–439*

ANAL RECONSTRUCTION,
Chapters 440–443

LOWER-LEG AND KNEE
RECONSTRUCTION, *Chapters 474–503*

FOOT AND ANKLE RECONSTRUCTION,
Chapters 504–544

To my wife, and children, and especially to my grandchildren, David Michael,
Kimberly Ann, Carolyn Beth, Alexandra Rae, and Matthew Jost.

BERISH STRAUCH, MD

To my wife, Diane, my daughters, Cristina, Nessa and Rachel, and to
my grandchildren, Francesca and Elisa, for their continued support
and joy they have given me throughout the years.

LUIS VASCONEZ, MD

To my mother, Betty Hall, who has been an inspiration to all her children;
and to my own three children, Jamie, David and Elise,
who have become very enjoyable young adults.

ELIZABETH J. HALL-FINDLAY, MD

To my wife, Britt, for her unwavering love, support, and sacrifice.
I am truly fortunate to be married to such an amazing woman.
To my sons, Brodie and Teddy, for the never-ending joy they bring.
Finally, to my parents, who share a contagious thirst for knowledge.

BERNARD T. LEE, MD

D. L. Abramson, MD
42A East 74th Street,
New York, New York 10021

W. P. Adams, Jr., MD
Children's Medical Center
Parkland Memorial Hospital
Veteran's Administration Medical Center
Zale Lipshy University Hospital
Baylor Medical Center
5323 Harry Hines Boulevard
Dallas, Texas 75235-9132

J. E. Adamson, MD, FACS (Retired)
P. O. Box 695
Linville, North Carolina 28646

J. Aftimos, MD
Centre Hospitalier D'Agen
Rue des Héros de la Résistance
F-47000 Agen, France

Galip Agaoglu, MD
Department of Plastic Surgery
The Cleveland Clinic Foundation
Cleveland, Ohio

F. C. Akpuaka, MBBS (Ibadan), FRCS (Ed), FRCS (Glasgow), FWACS, FICS
Professor of Plastic Surgery, College of Medicine, Abia State
University, Uturu, Nigeria
Director of Plastic Surgery
Plastic Surgery Unit
St. Francis Hospital
2 Richard Street
Asata-Enugu, Nigeria

R. S. Ali, MD
Department of Plastic and Reconstructive Surgery
Castle Hill Hospital
Castle Road
Cottingham, United Kingdom

R. J. Allen, MD
Division of Plastic Surgery
Medical University of South Carolina
Charleston, South Carolina

E. C. Almaguer, MD
Chief of Plastic Surgery, Santa Rosa Medical Center,
San Antonio
Baptist Hospital System
343 West Houston, #211
San Antonio, Texas 78205

C. Angrigiani
Posadas 1528 PB
Buenos Aires
Argentina

P. Andrades, MD
Assistant Professor
Division of Plastic Surgery and
Division of Maxillofacial Surgery
University of Chile Clinical Hospital
Hospital del Trabajador
Santiago, Chile

N. H. Antia, FRCSEng, FACSHon (Deceased)

S. Arena, MD (Retired)
125 Greenwood Road
Fox Chapel
Pittsburgh, Pennsylvania 15238

R. V. Argamaso, MD, FACS (Deceased)

L. C. Argenta, MD
North Carolina Baptist Hospital
Bowman-Gray Plastic Surgery
Medical Center Boulevard
Winston-Salem, North Carolina 27157

S. Ariyan, FACS
Yale-New Haven Hospital
Connecticut Center for Plastic Surgery
60 Temple Street, Suite 7C
New Haven, Connecticut 06510

D. P. Armstrong, MD, FACS
Community Memorial Hospital of San Buenaventura
Clinical Faculty, UCLA, Division of Plastic Surgery
168 North Brent Street, Suite 403
Ventura, California 93003

C. Arrunátegui, MD
Department of Plastic Surgery
Hospital da Santa Casa de Misericordia
Belo Horizonte, Brazil

H. Asato, MD
Assistant Professor
Department of Plastic and Reconstructive Surgery
University of Tokyo Hospital
7–3–1 Hongo Bunkyo-ku
Tokyo 113, Japan

E. Atasoy, MD
University of Louisville
Christine M. Kleinert Institute for Hand and Microsurgery
225 Abraham Flexner Way, Suite 700
Louisville, Kentucky 40202–1817

C. Augustin, MD
Centre Hospitalier D'Agen
29, Bd. de la République
F-47000 Agen, France

J. M. Avelar, MD
Albert Einstein Hospital, São Paulo
Al Gabriel Monteiro
Da Silva 620
01442–000 São Paulo-SP, Brazil

K. Azari, MD
Assistant Professor
Division of Plastic Surgery
University of Pittsburgh Medical Center
Pittsburgh, Pennsylvania

H. A. Badran, MB, BCh, FRCS, FRCSEd
Head, Department of Plastic Surgery
Ain Shams University
98 Mohamed Farid Street
Cairo 11111, Egypt

G. J. Baibak, FACS
3634 West Bancroft Street
Toledo, Ohio 43606

B. N. Bailey, MD, FRCS
Oxford Regional Health Authority
Stoke Mandeville Hospital
Mandeville Road
Aylesbury, Buckinghamshire, HP21 8AL
United Kingdom

V. Y. Bakamjian, MD (Retired)
Roswell Park Cancer Institute
Department of Head and Neck Surgery
Elm and Carlton Streets
Buffalo, New York 14263

C. R. Balch, MD
Naples Community Hospital
201 Eight Street, South, Suite 102
Naples, Florida 34102

T. Barfred, MD, PhD
Assistant Professor of Surgery, Odense University
Head of Hand Surgery, Department of Orthopaedic Surgery,
Odense University Hospital, Odense, Sweden
Head of Hand Surgery
Section of Orthopaedic Surgery
Odense University Hospital
500 Odense, Denmark

Marguerite P. Barnett, FACS
530 South Nokomis Avenue, Suite 6
Venice, Florida 34285

R. L. Baroudi, MD
Rua Bahia 969
São Paulo, SP 01244–001
Brazil

J. N. Barron, MS, FRCSEd, FRCSEng (Deceased)

F. E. Barton, Jr., MD
Baylor University Medical Center
Parkland Hospital
Presbyterian Hospital
Mary Shiels Hospital
411 North Washington Avenue, #6000 LB 13
Dallas, Texas 75246–1774

R. M. Barton, FACS
Vanderbilt University Hospital
Nashville Virginia Hospital
Baptist Hospital
Vanderbilt University Hospital
Medical Center South, Room 230
Nashville, Tennessee 37232

J. Baudet, MD
Professor of Plastic and Reconstructive Surgery
University of Bordeaux
Chief of Department of Plastic and Reconstructive Surgery
C.H.U.-Hôpital du Tondu
Groupe Pellegrin-Tondu
Place Amélie Raba-Léon
F-33076 Bordeaux, France

C. Beard, MD (Retired)
University of California, San Francisco
400 Parnassus Avenue, Suite 750-A
San Francisco, California 94143

R. W. Beasly, MD
Professor at NYU Medical Center
Director of Hand Surgery at Bellevue Hospital Center
Hand Surgery Associates
310 East 30th Street
New York, New York 10016–8303

Col. D. W. Becker, Jr., MD
Wilford Hall USAF Medical Center, San Antonio, Texas
2200 Bergquist Drive, Suite 1
Lackland AFB, Texas 78236–5300

H. Becker, MD, FACS
Boca Raton Community Hospital
5458 Town Center Road
Boca Raton, Florida 33486–1009

Professeur T. Bégué, MD
Chirurgie Orthopédique-Traumatologique et Réparatrice de
l'Appareil Locomoteur
Hôpital Avicenne
125, route de Stalingrad
F-93009 Bobigny Cedex, France

F. C. Behan, FRACS, FRCS
91 Royal Parade
Parkville 3052
Melbourne, Victoria
Australia

M. S. G. Bell, MD
Suite 306
340 McLeod Street, South
Ottawa, Ontario, Canada, K2P 1A4

T. Benacquista, MD
Einstein Weiler Hospital
Department of Plastic and Reconstructive Surgery
Albert Einstein College of Medicine and
Montefiore Medical Center
3331 Bainbridge Avenue
Bronx, New York 10467

M. Ben-Bassat, MD
Deputy-Chief
Department of Plastic Surgery
Beilinson Hospital
Tel Aviv, Israel

S. P. Bhagia, MD
Baugh Farzana Plastic Surgery Centre, Agra, India
4/14 Baugh Farzana
Agra 282 002, India

S. K. Bhatnagar, MD
Professor in Plastic Surgery
Department of Plastic Surgery
King George's Medical College
Lucknow 226 003, India

S. Bhattacharya, MS, MCh, FICS
Awadh Hospital, Lucknow
Neera Hospital, Lucknow
Star Hospital, Gorahpur
Consultant Plastic Surgeon and Oncologist
C-907 Mahanagar
Lucknow 226 006, India

S. L. Biddulph, MD
Chief Hand Surgeon, Johannesburg Hospital
Houghton 2050, South Africa

E. Biemer, MD
Department of Plastic Surgery
Technical University of München
Ismaningerstrasse 22
D-81675 München, Germany

J. H. Binns, MD
Wayne State University
540 East Canfield
Detroit, Michigan 48201

R. J. Bloch, MD
R. Sampaio Viana 628
Paraiso-São Paulo 04004–002
Brazil

J. G. Boorman, MD
Queen Victoria Hospital
East Grinstead
West Sussex, RH19 3DZ United Kingdom

L.J. Borud, MD
Instructor in Surgery
Department of Surgery
Harvard Medical School
110 Francis Street, Suite 5A
Boston, Massachusetts 02215

J.-L. Bovet, MD
Unité de Chirurgie de la Main
Clinique Jean-Villar
F-33520 Burges, France

J. B. Boyd, MD, FRCS, FRCS(C), FACS
Cleveland Clinic Hospital, Ft. Lauderdale
Broward General Hospital, Ft. Lauderdale
Holy Cross Hospital, Ft. Lauderdale
Imperial Point Hospital, Ft. Lauderdale
North Ridge Hospital, Ft. Lauderdale
Department of Plastic and Reconstructive Surgery
Cleveland Clinic Florida
3000 West Cypress Creek Road
Ft. Lauderdale, Florida 33309

R. J. Brauer, MD
Greenwich Hospital, Connecticut
49 Lake Avenue
Greenwich, Connecticut 06830–4519

N. K. Breach, MB, FRCS, FDSRCS
Department of Surgery
Royal Marsden Hospital
Downs Road
Sutton SM2 5PT, United Kingdom

T. D. R. Briant, MD, FRCS(C), FACS
Honorary Consultant, St. Michael's Hospital
32 Dale Avenue
Toronto, Ontario, Canada, M4W 1K5

T. R. Broadbent, MD (Retired)
2635 St. Mary's Way
Salt Lake City, Utah 84108

M. Brones, MD, FACS
Grossman Burn Center at Sherman Oaks Hospital,
California
Suite 102
4849 Van Nuys Boulevard
Sherman Oaks, California 91403

M. D. Brough, MD
University College London Hospitals
Royal Free Hospital
The Consulting Suite
82 Portland Place
London W1N 3DH, United Kingdom

E. Z. Browne, Jr., MD, FACS
Cleveland Clinic
Department of Plastic and Reconstructive Surgery
Cleveland Clinic Foundation
9500 Euclid Avenue
Cleveland, Ohio 44195

C. D. Bucko, MD, FACS
Scripps Memorial Hospital, La Jolla, California
Panerodo Hospital
University of San Diego Medical Center
Sheerp Memorial Hospital
Mission Bay, Columbia
Suite B
9900 Genesee Avenue
La Jolla, California 92037

J. Bunkis, MD, FACS
4165 Blackhawk Plaza Circle, Suite 150
Danville, California 94506–4691

G. C. Burget, MD, FACS
Clinical Assistant Professor, Section of Plastic Surgery,
The University of Chicago Hospitals
2913 North Commonwealth Avenue, Suite 400
Chicago, Illinois 60657

J. A. Butler, MD, FACS
Wausau Hospital
Saint Michael's Hospital, Stevens Point, WI
North Central Wisconsin Plastic Surgery, SC
425 Pine Ridge Boulevard, Suite 202
Wausau, Wisconsin 54401

H. S. Byrd, MD, FACS
Baylor University Medical Center
Children's Medical Center
Zale Lipshy University Medical Center
Suite 6000 LB 13
411 North Washington Avenue
Dallas, Texas 75246

D. Calderón, MD
Hospital del Trabajador
Ramon Carnicer, 185-5 Piso
Providencia
Santiago, Chile

W. Calderón, MD
Professor of Surgery
University of Chile
Chief of Plastic Surgery
Service Hospital del Trabajador
Santiago, Chile

M. A. Callahan, MD, FACS
Eye Foundation Hospital
St. Vincent's Hospital
Medical Center East Outpatient Surgery
700 South 18th Street, Suite 511
Birmingham, Alabama 35233

R. R. Cameron, MD (Retired)
38330 Sweetwater Drive
Palm Desert, California 92211–7048

G. W. Carlson, MD
Wadley R. Glenn Professor of Surgery
Department of Surgery
Associate Program Director
Division of Plastic Surgery
Emory University School of Medicine
Atlanta, Georgia

C. E. Carriquiry, MD
Associate Professor, Plastic Surgery, School of Medicine,
Universidad de la República Montevideo-Uruguay
21 de Setiembre 2353 Ap. 201
Montevideo 11200, Uruguay

N. Carver, MS, FRCS, FRCS(Plast)
Department of Plastic and Reconstructive Surgery
Royal London Hospital
St. Bartholomew's Hospital
London, E1 1BB United Kingdom

V. M. Casoli, MD
Department of Plastic and Reconstructive Surgery
C.H.U.-Hôpital Du Tondu
Groupe Pellegrin-Tondu
Place Amélie Raba-Léon
F-33076 Bordeaux, France

P. C. Cavadas, MD, PhD
Head of the Reconstructive Surgery and Microsurgery Unit
Hospital Vírgen del Consuelo
Hand Transplant Surgery Unit
"La Fe" University Hospital
Valencia, Spain

A. Cerejo, MD
Consultant Neurosurgeon
Hospital S. Joao Medical School
Oporto, Portugal
Avenida Vasco Da Gama
Ed. Silva porto, BL.C, 9B
4490 Povoa de Varzim, Portugal

L. A. Chait, MD
Johannesburg Group of Teaching Hospitals
211 Parkland Clinic
Junction Avenue Park
Johannesburg, South Africa

R. Chandra, MS, MCh
Professor, Plastic Surgery
King George's Medical College
Lucknow 226 003, India

R. A. Chase, MD
Professor, Stanford University School of Medicine
Department of Surgery
Stanford, CA 94305

P. Chhajlani, MD
"Ganga Jamuna Apartments"
South Tukoganj, Near Nath Mandir
Indore 452 001, India

D. R. H. Christie, MBChB, FRACR
John Flynn Hopital, Tugun, Australia
Eastcoast Cancer Centre
Inland Drive
Tugun, QLD 4224, Australia

Y. K. Chung, MD
Yonsei University Wonju College of Medicine
Wonju Christian Hospital
Ilsandong
Wonju, Korea

M. E. Ciaravino, MD
Attending Plastic Surgeon
St. Joseph's Hospital
Houston, Texas
3805 West Alabama, #3105
Houston, Texas 77027

B. E. Cohen, MD, FACS
Academic Chief and Director, Plastic Surgery Residency
Program, Cohen and Cronin Clinic
Director, Microsurgical Research and Training Laboratory,
St. Joseph Hospital, Houston
Plastic and Reconstructive Surgery
Cohen and Cronin Clinic
1315 Calhoun, Suite 920
Houston, Texas 77002

C. C. Coleman, Jr., MD, FACS (Retired)
Consultant Plastic Surgeon, Clinical Professor of Surgery,
University of Virginia, Charlottesville, Virginia
Visiting Professor, University of Virginia
P. O. Box 558
Irvington, Virginia 22480–0558

J. J. Coleman III, MD, FACS
University Hospital
Riley Hospital
Wishad Hospital
VA Medical Center
Professor of Surgery
Director, Division of Plastic Surgery
Indiana University
Emerson Hall 235, 545 Barnhill Drive
Indianapolis, Indiana 46202

P. Colson, MD
Head Surgeon
Burn Unit
Saint Luke's Hospital
34, Place Bellecour
F-69002 Lyons, France

M. B. Constantian, MD, FACS
Adjunct Assistant Professor of Surgery, Dartmouth
Medical School
Active Staff, Department of Surgery (Plastic Surgery),
St. Joseph Hospital and Southern New Hampshire
Regional Medical Center
Nashua, New Hampshire
19 Tyler Street, Suite 302
Nashua, New Hampshire 03060

L. M. Cordero, MD (Deceased)

R. J. Corlett, MD
Royal Melbourne Hospital
Preston and North Gate Community Hospital
766 Elizabeth Street
Melbourne 3000, Australia

H. Monteiro Da Costa, MD
Professor and Consultant Plastic Surgeon,
Plastic and Reconstructive Unit, S. Joao Hospital,
Medical School, Oporto
Consultant Plastic Surgeon, Matosinhos and Vila Nova Eaia
Hospitals, Oporto
Professor in Plastic Surgery
Rua do Corvo, 323
Pr. da Granja
4405 Arcozelo VNG, Portugal

E. D. Cronin, MD, FACS
Chief of Plastic Surgery Section, St. Joseph Hospital
Plastic and Reconstructive Surgery
Cohen and Cronin Clinic
1315 Calhoun, Suite 920
Houston, Texas 77002

T. D. Cronin, MD (Deceased)

J. W. Curtin, MD
Rush-Presbyterian-St. Luke's Medical Center,
Chicago, Illinois
1180 Hill Road
Winnetka, Illinois 60093

R. K. Daniel, MD, FACS
Hoag Memorial Hospital/Presbyterian Hospital, California
1441 Avocado Avenue, Suite 308
Newport Beach, California 92660–7704

S. K. Das, MD, FACS, FRCS
St. Dominic's Hospital
River Oaks Hospital
River Oaks East Hospital
University of Mississippi Medical Center
Mississippi Methodist Medical Center
Parkview Hospital, Vicksburg
Division of Plastic Surgery
University of Mississippi Medical Center
2500 North State Street
Jackson, Mississippi 39211

J. E. Davis, MD
Matricula No. 7101
Vincente Lopez 2653, Argentina

R. De la Plaza, MD
Director, Plastic Surgery Department, La Luz Clinic,
Madrid
Clínica de Cirugía Plástica y Estética
Salou, 28
E-28034 Madrid, Spain

A. L. Dellon, MD, FACS
Professor, Plastic and Neurosurgery,
The Johns Hopkins University School of Medicine
2328 West Joppa Road, Suite 325
Lutherville, Maryland 21093

G. H. Derman, MD
Attending Staff, Rush-Presbyterian-St. Luke's
Medical Center
Attending Staff, Evanston Hospital
Assistant Professor, Rush Medical College, Chicago, Illinois
4709 Golf Road, Suite 806
Skokie, Illinois 60076–1258

B. Devauchelle, MD, PhD
Department of Maxillofacial Surgery
Centre Hospitalier Universitaire
Amiens, France

C. J. Devine, Jr., MD
400 West Brambleton Avenue, Suite 100
Norfolk, Virginia 23510–1115

I. K. Dhawan, MD
Department of Surgery
Al Mafraq Hospital
Abu Dhabi, India

Dr. A. D. Dias, MS
Professor Emeritus, L.T.M.G. Hospital, Sion, Mumbai
St. Thereza Hospital, Agashi, Virar
"Shanti Sadan"
157-B Perry Road
Bandra, Mumbai 400 050, India

R. O. Dingman, MD (Deceased)

T. A. Dinh, MD
Division of Plastic Surgery
Baylor College of Medicine
6560 Fannin, Suite 1034
Houston, Texas 77030

M. I. Dinner, MD, FACS
Meridia Hillcrest Hospital
Assistant Clinical Professor
Case Western Reserve Medical School
3755 Orange Plaza
Cleveland, Ohio 44122–4455

B. H. Dolich, MD
Albert Einstein College Hospital and Montefiore
Medical Center
New York Eye & Ear Hospital
1578 Williamsbridge Road
Bronx, New York 10461

R. V. Dowden, MD, FACS
Meridia Hillcrest, Mt. Sinai, University Hospital
6770 Mayfield Road, Suite 410
Mayfield Heights, Ohio 44124

G. A. Drabyn, MD, FACS
Riverside Methodist Hospital
3545 Olentangy River Road, Suite 130
Columbus, Ohio 43214

J. M. Drever, MD, FRCS
Etobicoke General Hospital
Cosmetic Surgery Hospital
135 Queens Plate Drive, Fifth Floor
Toronto, Ontario, Canada, M9W 6V1

J.-L. Ducours, MD
Centre Hospitalier D'Agen
Service de Chirurgie Maxillo-faciale
Centre Hospitalier
86 boulevard Sylvain Dumon
F-47000 Agen, France

G. M. Duncan, MChB, FRACS
Plastic Surgical Unit
Hutt Hospital
Private Bag
Lower Hutt, New Zealand

E. C. Duus, MD
Comanche County Memorial Hospital
Southwest Medical Center
5604 Southwest Lee Boulevard, Suite 310
Lawton, Oklahoma 73505–9663

W. Dzwierzynski, MD
Professor of Plastic Surgery
Medical College of Wisconsin
Milwaukee, Wisconsin

A. S. Earle, MD, FACS
Professor (Emeritus) of Plastic Surgery
Case Western University School of Medicine
1656 Emerald Green Court
Deltona, Florida 32725

D. S. Eastwood, MD (Retired)
St. Kames's University Hospital, Leeds, United Kingdom
Leeds University Hospital
11, North Park Road
Roundhay
Leeds LS8 1JD, United Kingdom

B. W. Edgerton, MD
Kaiser Permanente, West Los Angeles
Plastic Surgery Department
6041 Cadillac Avenue
Los Angeles, California 90034

M. T. Edgerton, MD
University of Virginia Health Sciences Center
Department of Plastic Surgery
Charlottesville, Virginia 22908

P. Egyedi, MD, DMD, PhD
Department of Oral and Maxillofacial Surgery
Utrecht University Hospital
P.O. Box 85500
NL-3508 GA Utrecht, The Netherlands

L. Eisenbaum, MD, PC
Colorado Medical Center of Aurora
Longmont United Hospital
Plastic and Reconstructive Surgery
Esthetic and Hand Surgery
Presbyterian Aurora Medical Center
750 Potomac Street, Suite 201
Aurora, Colorado 80011

M. M. El-Saadi, MD
Assistant Professor of Plastic Surgery
Zagazig University Hospital
Zagazig, Egypt

D. Elliot, MA
Woodlands
Woodham Walter
Essex
United Kingdom

R. A. Elliott, Jr., MD, FACS
P.O. Box 39
Slingerlands, New York 12159

L. F. Elliott, MD
Northside Hospital
St. Joseph's Hospital
Piedmont Hospital
Scottish-Rite Children's Hospital
975 Jonson Ferry, Suite 500
Atlanta, Georgia 30342

N. I. Elsahy, MD, PC, FRCS(C), FACS, FICS
Southern Regional Medical Center, Riverdale, Georgia
6524 Professional Place, Suite A
P.O. Box 1318
Riverdale, Georgia 30274

A. J. J. Emmett, MB, BS, FRCS, FRACS
Honorary Consultant, Princess Alexandra Hospital,
Brisbane, Australia
Woodgreen
128 Osborne Road
Bowral NSW 2576, Australia

D. N. F. Fairbanks, MD
Clinical Professor of Otolaryngology, George Washington
University School of Medicine, Washington, DC
Sibley Memorial Hospital, Washington, DC
3 Washington Circle, Northwest, Suite 305
Washington, DC 20037–2356

G. R. Fairbanks, MD
St. Mark's Hospital
Cottonwood Hospital, Primary Children's Medical Center
Bonneville Surgical Center
1151 East 3900 South, B110
Salt Lake City, Utah 84124

R. S. Feingold, MD
Assistant Clinical Professor in Plastic and Reconstructive
Surgery, Albert Einstein College of Medicine
Long Island Jewish Medical Center
Montefiore Medical Center
New York Hospital Medical Center of Queens
North Shore University Hospital
Winthrop-University Hospital
900 Northern Boulevard
Great Neck, New York 11021

M. Feldman, MD, FACS
Shore Memorial, Somers Point, New Jersey
Feldman Plastic Surgery, P. A.
222 New Road, Suite 6
Linwood, New Jersey 08221

A.-M. Feller, Prof. Dr. med.
Chairman, Department of Plastic Surgery
Behandlungszentrum Vogtareuth
Krankenhausstrasse 20
D-83569 Vogtareuth, Germany

R. J. Fix, MD, FACS
University of Alabama at Birmingham
The Children's Hospital of Alabama
Veterans Administration Medical Center
University of Alabama, Plastic Surgery MEB 524
1813 Sixth Avenue, South
Birmingham, Alabama 35294

A. E. Flatt, MD, FRCS
Baylor University Medical Center, Dallas, Texas
Clinical Professor, SW Medical School, Dallas, Texas
Consultant Emeritus in Hand Surgery,
U.S. Air Force
Director of Education
George Truett James Orthopaedic Institute
Baylor University Medical Center
3500 Gaston Avenue
Dallas, Texas 75246-9990

L. Fonseca Dos Santos, MD
Service d'Orthopedie
Hôpital Trousseau
26 Avenue de Dr. A Netter
F-75012 Paris, France

G. Foucher, MD
Head of SOS Main, Strasbourg
4 Bd. du President
F-67000 Strasbourg, France

M. Fox, MD, FACS
4001 Kresge Way, Suite 320
Louisville, Kentucky 40207-4640

J. D. Franklin, MD, FACS
Erlanger Health System, Memorial Hospital
Hutcheson Medical Center
Plaza Ambulatory Care Center
979 East Third Street, Suite 4002
Chattanooga, Tennessee 37403

A. Freiberg, MD, FRCS(C), FACS
Division of Plastic Surgery
Toronto Western Hospital
399 Bathurst Street
Edith Cavell Wing, 4-304
Toronto, Ontario MST 2S8, Canada

R. Fujimori, MD
Department of Plastic Surgery
Kyoto University
465 Kajii-cho Kawar
Kyoto 602, Japan

T. Fujino, MD, FACS, DrMedSci
Professor and Chairman
Department of Plastic Surgery
Keio University School of Medicine
35 Shinanomachi Shinjukuku
Tokyo 160, Japan

L. T. Furlow, Jr., MD, FACS
Clinical Professor, University of Florida College of Medicine,
Gainesville, Florida
3001 Northwest 28th Terrace
Gainesville, Florida 32605

D. W. Furnas, MD, FACS
University of California, Irvine Medical Center
St. Joseph Hospital, Orange
Childrens Hospital of Orange County
VA Hospital, Long Beach
University of California Irvine Medical Center
Division of Plastic Surgery
101 City Drive
Orange, California 92868–2901

F. N. Gahhos, MD
Venice Hospital
135 San Marco Drive
Venice, Florida 34285

A. Gardetto, MD
Professor of Plastic and Reconstructive Surgery
General Hospital of Brixen
Brixen, Italy

P. M. Gardner, MD
Assistant Professor, Department of Surgery,
Division of Plastic Surgery
University of Alabama at Birmingham
1600 7th Avenue South, ACC 322
Birmingham, Alabama 35233

N. W. Garrigues, MD
Scripps Memorial Hospital
Assistant Professor, University of California, San Diego
3405 Kenyon Street, Ste. 401
San Diego, California 92110–5007

J. S. Gaul, MD (Retired)
Charlotte, North Carolina

K. E. Georgeson, MD
University of Alabama Hospitals
The Children's Hospital of Alabama
1600 7th Avenue, South, ACC 300
Birmingham, Alabama 35233

G. S. Georgiade, MD
Duke University Medical Center—Surgery
P.O. Box 3960
Durham, North Carolina 27710

R. Ger, MD, FRCS
Albert Einstein College of Medicine
1300 Morris Park Avenue
Bronx, New York 10461

V. C. Giampapa, MD, FACS
89 Valley Road
Montclair, New Jersey 07042–2212

A. Gilbert, MD
15 rue Franklin
F-75016 Paris, France

D. A. Gilbert, MD, FRCS(C), FACS
Norfolk General Hospital
Children's Hospital of the King's Daughters
De Paul Hospital
Maryview Hospital
Plastic Surgery Associates, Inc.
400 West Brambleton Avenue, Suite 300
Norfolk, Virginia 23510

R. P. Gingrass, MD, SC
Elmbrook Hospital, Brokfield, Wisconsin
St. Joseph's Hospital, Milwaukee, Wisconsin
Plastic and Reconstructive Surgery
9800 West Bluemound
Milwaukee, Wisconsin 53226

F. Giraldo, MD, PhD
Plastic and Reconstructive Unit, University of Málaga
Regional Hospital "Harlos Haya," Málaga, Spain
Plastic and Reconstructive Unit
Regional Hospital "Carlos Haya"
E-29010 Málaga, Spain

D. W. Glasson, MD, FRACS
Wellington Hospital, Wellington, NZ
Hutt Hospital, Lower Hutt, NZ
Bowen Hospital, Wellington, NZ
Plastic Surgery Specialists
140 Ghuznee Street
Wellington 1, New Zealand

A. M. Godfrey, MB, BCh
Consultant Plastic Surgeon
Nuffield Acland Hospital and Nuffield Orthopaedic Centre, Oxford
The Paddocks Hospital, Bucks, and
The Ridgeway Hospital, Wilts
Felstead House
23 Banbury Road
Oxford OX2 6NX, United Kingdom

R. D. Goldstein, MD, FACS
Assistant Clinical Professor
Albert Einstein College of Medicine
Montefiore Medical Center
Bronx, New York 10461

R. M. Goldwyn, MD, FACS
Clinical Professor of Surgery, Harvard Medical School
Division of Plastic Surgery, Beth Israel Deaconess
Medical Center, Boston, MA
1101 Beacon Street
Brookline, Massachusetts 02146

D. J. Goodkind, MD
Yale-New Haven Hospital
Clinical Instructor of Surgery, Yale University
136 Sherman Avenue, South, Suite 205
New Haven, Connecticut 06511–5236

B. Gorowitz, MD
Department of Plastic and Reconstructive Surgery
C.H.U.-Hôpital Du Tondu
Groupe Pellegrin-Tondu
Place Amélie Raba-Léon
F-33076 Bordeaux, France

L. J. Gottlieb, MD, FACS
Professor of Clinical Surgery, Plastic and
Reconstructive Surgery
Department of Surgery
University of Chicago, Illinois
5841 South Maryland Avenue, MC 6035
Chicago, Illinois 60637

D. P. Green, MD
9150 Huebner Road, Suite 290
San Antonio, Texas 78229

B. M. Greenberg, MD, FACS
833 Northern Boulevard, Suite 115
Great Neck, New York 11021

J. M. Griffin, MD, FACS
Piedmont Hospital
Associate Clinical Professor, Department of Surgery
Emory University School of Medicine
Northside Hospital
Scottish Rite Children's Medical Center
Center for Plastic Surgery
365 East Paces Ferry Road
Atlanta, Georgia 30305–2351

B. H. Griffith, MD, FACS
Northwestern Memorial Hospital
Children's Memorial Hospital
Rehabilitation Institute of Chicago
Chief of Plastic Surgery, Shriners Hospital for Crippled Children
Northwestern University Medical Center
251 East Chicago Avenue, Suite 1026
Chicago, Illinois 6061–2641

A. R. Grossman, MD, FACS
The Grossman Burn Center
Sherman Oaks Hospital, California
4910 Van Nuys Boulevard, Suite 306
Sherman Oaks, California 91403–1728

P. H. Grossman, MD
Grossman Burn Center
Sherman Oaks Hospital, California
4910 Van Nuys Boulevard, Suite 306
Sherman Oaks, California 91403

J. C. Grotting, MD, FACS
Children's Hospital of Alabama
Baptist Medical Center-Montclair
The Eye Foundation
Baptist Medical Center-Princeton
Health South Medical Center
Brookwood Medical Center
Outpatient CareCenter
McCollough, Grotting & Associates Plastic Surgery
Clinic P. C.
1600 20th Street, South
Birmingham, Alabama 35205

B. K. Grunert, PhD
Medical College of Wisconsin
Froedtert Memorial Lutheran Hospital
Children's Hospital of Wisconsin
9200 W. Wisconsin Avenue
Milwaukee, Wisconsin 53226

C. R. Gschwind, MD
The Centre for Bone and Joint Diseases
Royal North Shore Hospital, St. Leonards
Department of Hand Surgery
Hand and Microsurgery Unit
Royal North Shore Hospital
St. Leonards, NSW 2065, Australia

J. Guerrerosantos, MD
Chairman and Plastic Surgeon-In-Charge
Jalisco Institute for Reconstructive Surgery
Chairman and Professor, Division of Plastic and
Reconstructive Surgery, University of Guadalajara, Mexico
Garibaldi 1793
Col. L de Guevara
Guadalajara, Jalisco, 44680, Mexico

P. J. Gullane, MD
Otolaryngologist-in-Chief, Toronto Hospital, Toronto
Site Leader, Head and Neck Surgery, Princess Margaret
Hospital and Toronto Hospital
Staff Otolaryngologist, Mount Sinai Hospital, Toronto
Consultant Otolaryngologist
North York General Hospital, Toronto
200 Elizabeth Street, East
Toronto, Ontario, Canada, M5G 2C4

J. P. Gunter, MD, FACS
Presbyterian Hospital of Dallas
Parkland Memorial Hospital
Baylor University Medical Center
8315 Walnut Hill Lane, Suite 125
Dallas, Texas 75231–4211

B. Guyuron, MD, FACS
Medical Director of Zeeba Clinic
Clinical Professor of Plastic Surgery
Case Western Reserve University
29017 Cedar Road
Lyndhurst, Ohio 44124

K. F. Hagan, MD, FACS
Vanderbilt University Hospital, Baptist Hospital,
Columbia Centennial, The Atrium
Nashville Surgery Center
Vanderbilt University Medical Center
2100 Pierce Avenue
230, MCS
Nashville, Tennessee 37232–3631

E. J. Hall-Findlay, MD, FRCS
Plastic Surgeon
Banff Mineral Springs Hospital
Suite 340, Cascade Plaza
317 Banff Avenue
Banff, AT TOL 0C0, Canada

G. G. Hallock, MD, FACS
Consultant in Plastic Surgery, The Lehigh Valley and Sacred
Heart Hospitals, Allentown, Pennsylvania
St. Luke's Hospital, Bethlehem, Pennsylvania
1230 South Cedar Crest Boulevard, Suite 306
Allentown, Pennsylvania 18103

S. K. Han, MD, PhD
Professor of Plastic Surgery
Korea University College of Medicine
Seoul, Korea

R. Happle, MD
Department of Dermatology
University of Münster
Schlossplatz 2
D-4400 Münster, Germany

K. Harii, MD
Graduate School of Medicine, The University of Tokyo
Department of Plastic and Reconstructive Surgery
University of Tokyo Hospital
7–3–1 Hongo Bunkyo-ku
Tokyo 113, Japan

D. H. Harrison, MD
Regional Plastic Surgery Centre, Mount Vernon,
Northwood, UK
Flat 33, Harmont House
20 Harley Street
London WIN 1AA, United Kingdom

S. H. Harrison, MD, FCRS (Retired)
The Plastic Surgery
Mount Vernon Hospital
Rickmansworth Road
Northwood HA6 2RN, United Kingdom

C. R. Hartrampf, Jr., MD, FACS
St. Joseph's Hospital
Atlanta Plastic Surgery
Suite 500, 975 Johnson Ferry
Atlanta, Georgia 30342–1619

S. W. Hartwell, Jr., MD
Emeritus Staff, The Cleveland Clinic Foundation
9500 Euclid Avenue, E48
Cleveland, Ohio 44195–5257

A. Hayashi, MD
Assistant Professor, Department of Plastic and
Reconstructive Surgery, Toho University Hospital
Department of Plastic and Reconstructive Surgery
Toho University School of Medicine
6–11–1 Ohmorinishi, Ohta-ku
Tokyo 143, Japan

F. R. Heckler, MD, FACS
Director, Division of Plastic Surgery
Allegheny General Hospital, Pittsburgh, Pennsylvania
Clinical Associate Professor of Plastic Surgery, University of
Pittsburgh, School of Medicine, Allegheny General Hospital
320 East North Avenue
Pittsburgh, Pennsylvania 15212

T. R. Heinz, MD
University of Alabama Hospitals
The Children's Hospital of Alabama
Veteran's Administration Medical Center
University of Alabama at Birmingham
Plastic Surgery
1813 6th Avenue, South (MEB-524)
Birmingham, Alabama 35294–3295

C. Heitmann, MD, PhD
Department of Plastic, Reconstructive and Hand Surgery
Markuskrankenhaus
Frankfurt am Main
Germany

V. R. Hentz, MD
Stanford University Hospital
900 Welch Road, Suite 15
Palo Alto, California 94304

C. K. Herman, MD
Medical Director of Plastic Surgery
Pocono Health Systems
100 Plaza Court, Suite C
East Stroudsburg, PA 18301
Assistant Clinical Professor of Surgery (Plastic Surgery)
Albert Einstein College of Medicine, New York, NY 10467
Private practice, 988 Fifth Avenue, New York, NY 10021

H. L. Hill, Jr., MD
Tallahassee Memorial Medical Center, Florida
Tallahassee Single Day Surgical Hospital
Tallahassee Plastic Surgery
1704 Riggins Road
Tallahassee, Florida 32308

B. Hirshowitz, FRCS
Emeritus Professor of Plastic and Reconstructive Surgery
Faculty of Medicine
Technion-Israel Institute of Technology, Haifa
55 Margalit Street
Mount Carmel
Haifa 34464, Israel

J. G. Hoehn, MD, FACS
St. Peter's Hospital
Samuel Straton Veterans Administration
Albany Medical Center
The Child's Hospital
Albany Memorial Hospital
Albany Plastic and Reconstructive Surgery Center
Four Executive Park Drive
Albany, New York 12203

W. Y. Hoffman, MD, FACS
University of California, San Francisco Medical Center
Associate Professor of Plastic Surgery
University of California, San Francisco
350 Parnassus, Suite 509
San Francisco, California 94117–3608

J. Holle, MD
Institute of Anatomy
Medical University of Vienna
Department of Plastic and Reconstructive Surgery
Wilhelminen Hospital
Vienna, Austria
Krapfenwald G 9
Vienna, A1190, Austria

T. Honda, MD
Department of Plastic and Reconstructive Surgery
Tokyo Women's Medical University
8-1 Kawada-cho, Shinjuku-ku, 162-0054
Tokyo, Japan

C. E. Horton, MD
Sentara Norfolk General Hospital
Bon Secours DePaul Hospital
Children's Hospital of The King's Daughters
229 West Bute Street, Suite 900
Norfolk, Virginia 23510

A. S. Hoschander, MD
Resident
Department of Surgery
Long Island Jewish Medical Center/North Shore University
Hospital
Manhasset, New York

W. Hu, MD
Centre Hopitalier Universitaire de Brest
Hôpital de la Cavale Blanche
F-29200 Brest, France

T. Huang, MD
Clinical Professor of Surgery
University of Texas Medical Branch
326 Market Street
Galveston, Texas 77550-5664

D. J. Hurwitz, MD
University of Pittsburgh Medical Center
Children's Hospital of Pittsburgh
Plastic and Reconstructive Surgery
Aesthetic and Craniofacial Surgery
University of Pittsburgh Medical Center
3471 Fifth Avenue
Pittsburgh, Pennsylvania 15213

J. J. Hurwitz, MD, FRCS(C)
Ophthalmological Executive Committee,
University of Toronto
Opthalmologist-in-Chief, Mount Sinai Hospital
Professor of Ophthalmology, University of Toronto
Director of Oculoplastics Programme
University of Toronto
600 University Avenue, Suite 408
Toronto, Ontario, Canada, M5G 1X5

Y. Ikuta, MD
Department of Orthopedic Surgery
Hiroshima School of Medicine
Kasumi 1–2–3
Hiroshima 734, Japan

O. Iribarren, MD
Department of Surgery
Surgery Service and Office of Nosocomial Infections Control
Saint Paul Hospital, School of Medicine
Universidad Catolica del Norte
Larrondo 1080
Videla s/n
Coquimbo. IV Region, Chile

F. Iselin, MD
Director of Hand Service
Department of Surgery, Centre de Chirugie de la
Main-Urgences Mains
Hôpital Nanterre
Paris, France

T. I. A. Ismail, MD
29 Nawal Street
Aguiza-Giza
Cairo, Egypt

Y. Itoh, MD, PhD
National Defense Medical College
Division of Plastic and Reconstructive Surgery
Department of Dermatology
3–2 Namiki
Tokorozawa, Saitama 359, Japan

Y. Iwahira, MD
Department of Plastic Surgery
Toho University Hospital
6–11–1 Ohmorinishi, Ohta-ku
Tokyo 143, Japan

H. Izawa, MD
Associate Professor
Department of Plastic and Reconstructive Surgery
St. Marianna University School of Medicine
2–16–1 Sugao
Myamae-ku, Kawasaki 216, Japan

Z. H. Jabourian, MD
Clinch Valley Medical Center, #2300
Richlands, Virginia 24641

I. T. Jackson, MD, DSc(Hon), FACS, FRCS, FRACS(Hon)
Institute for Craniofacial and Reconstructive
Surgery
Diplomate of the American Board of
Plastic Surgery
Institute for Craniofacial and Reconstructive
Surgery
3rd Floor, Fisher Center
16001 West 9 Mile Road
Southfield, Michigan 48075

R. V. Janevicius, MD, PC
Elmhurst Memorial Hospital, Elmhurst, Illinois
Plastic and Reconstructive Surgery
360 West Butterfield Road, Suite 230
Elmhurst, Illinois 60126

H. Janvier, MD
St. Luke's Hospital
34, Place Bellecour
69002 Lyons, France

V.T. Joseph, MBBS, FRCSEd, FRACS, MMED(Surgery), FAMS
Chairman, Division of Pediatric Surgery
KK Woman's & Children's Hospital
100 Bukit Timah Road
Singapore 229899

B. B. Joshi, MS
Mahatma Gandhi Hospital
Parel
Mumbai 400 012, India

J. Juri, MD
National University
Calle Viamonte 430
Buenos Aires, Argentina 1053

M. J. Jurkiewicz, MD, FACS, FRCS
Emory Affiliated Hospitals
25 Prescott Street, Northeast
Atlanta, Georgia 30308

J. B. Kahl, MD, FACS
Director of Plastic Surgery Residency & Department Head,
Christ Hospital
Head of Department of Plastic Surgery, Mercy Hospital
Active Staff, Bethesda Hospitals
Children's Hospital of Cincinnati
Jewish Hospital and
Deaconess Hospital
President, Montgomery North Plastic Surgery Center
Staffs of Providence, St. Luke, Good Samaritan
Clinical Instructor, University of Cincinnati
10545 Montgomery Rd., #100
Cincinnati, Ohio 45242

W. J. Kane, MD
Mayo Clinic
905 14th Avenue, Southwest
200 1st Street, Southwest
Rochester, Minnesota 55905

E. N. Kaplan, MD
1515 El Camino Real, Suite D
Palo Alto, California 94306

I. Kaplan, MB, ChB
Professor of Surgery and Incumbent of Chilewich Chair of
Plastic Surgery
University of Tel Aviv
Head, Department of Plastic Surgery
Belinson Medical Center
Petah-Tiqva 76 100, Israel

I. B. Kaplan, MD
Plastic Surgery Associates, Inc.
400 West Brambleton Avenue, Suite 300
Norfolk, Virginia 23510–1115

M. R. Karapandžić, MD
Belgrade University
Studenski Trg 1
1101 Belgrade 6, Yugoslavia

A. Karev, MD
Head, Department of Hand Surgery, Kaplan Hospital
Rehovot POBA 76100 Israel

R. B. Karp, MD
Courtesy Staff, Suburban Hospital, Bethesda, MD
11510 Old Georgetown Road
Rockville, Maryland 20852

R. G. Katz, MD
3500 Fifth Avenue
Pittsburgh, Pennsylvania 15213

J. C. Kelleher, MD, FACS
Microsurgery Fellow
Division of Plastic Surgery
Department of Surgery
University of Mississippi Medical Center
Jackson, Missouri

A. F. Kells, MD, PhD
Microsurgery Fellow
Division of Plastic Surgery
Department of Surgery
University of Mississippi Medical Center
Jackson, Mississippi

J. M. Kenkel, MD
University of Texas, Southwestern, Dallas, Texas
5323 Harry Hines Boulevard
Dallas, Texas 75235–9132

C. L. Kerrigan, MD, FRCS
Mary Hitchcock Memorial Medical Center
Lebanon, New Hampshire
Veteran Affairs Medical Center, White River Junction, VT
Dartmouth-Hitchcock Medical Center
One Medical Center Drive
Lebanon, New Hampshire 03756

M. Keyes-Ford, PAC (Deceased)

A. A. Khashaba, MD
Assistant Professor of Plastic Surgery
Zagazig University
4 Dr Ahmed Nada Street

Heliopolis, Cairo, Egypt

R. K. Khouri, MD, FACS
Baptist Hospital, Miami, FL
Doctors Hospital, Miami, FL
Cedars Hospital, Miami, FL
Dermatology and Plastic Surgery Center
328 Crandon Blvd., Suite 227
Key Biscayne, Florida 33149

Y. Kikuchi, MD
Department of Plastic and Reconstructive Surgery
Tokyo Women's Medical University
8-1 Kawada-cho, Shimjuku-ku, 162-0054
Tokyo, Japan

S. K. Kim, MD, PhD
Professor
Department of Plastic and Reconstructive Surgery
Dong-A University School of Medicine
Dong-A University Hospital
Seo-Gu
Busan, Korea

K. S. Kim, MD, PhD
Department of Plastic and Reconstructive Surgery
Chonnam National University Medical School
Dong-gu, Gwangju, Korea

Y. Kimata, MD
Professor
Department of Plastic and Reconstructive Surgery
Okayama University
Graduate School of Medicine, Dentistry and
Pharmaceutical Sciences
Shikata-cho, Okayama, Japan

B. Kirkby, MD
Associate Professor
The Royal Dental College
Copenhagen, Denmark

H. W. Klein, MD, FACS
Mercy Hospitals, Sacramento
Sutter Affiliated Hospitals
University of California, Davis
Suite 202
8120 Timberlake Way
Sacramento, California 95823–5412

S. Kobayashi, MD
Head and Professor of Department of Plastic and
Reconstructive Surgery, Iwate Medical University
19–1 Uchimaru Morioka-shi, Iwate 020
Japan

R. Kolachalam, MD
6848 Tiffany Circle
Canton, Michigan 48187

H. Koncilia, MD
Department of Plastic and Reconstructive Surgery
Wilhelminen Hospital, Vienna, Austria

I. Koshima, MD
Associate Professor of Plastic and Reconstructive Surgery
Plastic and Reconstructive Surgery
Kawasaki Medical School
577 Matsushima, Kurashiki City
Okayama 701–01, Japan

S. S. Kroll, MD, FACS (Deceased)

G. Kronen, MD
1115 Mallard Creek Road
Saint Matthews, Kentucky 40207-2489

J. E. Kutz, MD
Clinical Professor of Surgery (Hand)
University of Louisville School of Medicine
Christine M. Kleinert Institute for Hand and
Micro Surgery
225 Abraham Flexner Way, Suite 850
Louisville, Kentucky 40202

R. Kuzbari, MD
Associate Professor of Plastic Surgery
Wilhelminenspital
Montleartstrasse 37, A-1160
Vienna, Austria

S. Kwei, MD
North Shore Plastic Surgery
4 Centennial Drive, Suite 102
Peabody, Massachusetts 01960

H. P. Labandter, MD, FRCS
Herzlia Medical Center
7 Ramot Yam
Herzlia Pituach, Israel

L. Landín, MD
Assistant Surgeon
Reconstructive Surgery and Microsurgery Unit
Hand Transplant Surgery Unit
"La Fe" University Hospital
Valencia, Spain

V. C. Lanier, Jr., MD
300 Crutchfield Street
Durham, North Carolina 27704

N. Laud, MD
Lokmaya Tilak Municipal General Hospital
and Medical College
Saraswati Nilayam
Hindu Colony, Dadar
Mubai (Mumbai) 14, 400 014 India

S. A. Lauer, MD
Department of Ophthalmology
Albert Einstein College of Medicine and
Montefiore Medical Center
111 East 210th Steet
Bronx, New York 10467

D. Le Nen, MD
Centre Hopitalier Universitaire de Brest, France
Hôpital de la Cavale Blanche
F-29200 Brest, France

B. T. Lee, MD
Instructor in Surgery
Department of Surgery
Harvard Medical School;
Division of Plastic and Reconstructive Surgery
Beth Israel Deaconess Medical Center
Boston, Massachusetts

C. Lefevre, MD
Service d'Orthopedie, C.H.U.
Hôpital de la Cavale Blanche
F-29200 Brest, France

P. Leniz, MD
Burn and Plastic Surgery Unit
Hospital del Trabajador de Santiago
Santiago, Chile

A. G. Leonard, FRCS
Northern Ireland Plastic & Maxillofacial Service
The Upper Ulster Hospital
Dundonald, Belfast BT16 ORH
Northern Ireland, United Kingdom

M. A. Lesavoy, MD, FACS
UCLA Medical Center
Harbor-UCLA Medical Center
Santa Lionica-UCLA Medical Center
VA Medical Center-West Los Angeles
Division of Plastic and Reconstructive Surgery
UCLA School of Medicine
64–128 CHS, Box 951665
Los Angeles, California 90095–1665

M. Lester, MD
Assistant Professor
Department of Plastic and Reconstructive Surgery
University of Florida
Gainesville, Florida;
2 Council Street
Charleston, South Carolina 29401

L. A. Levine, MD
Lake Forest Hospital
Department of Urology
Rush-Presbyterian-St. Luke's Medical Center
1725 W. Harrison Street, Suite 917
Chicago, Illinois 60612

M. L. Lewin, MD (Deceased)

J. R. Lewis, Jr., MD, FACS (Deceased)

V. L. Lewis, Jr., MD
Professor of Clinical Surgery
Northwestern University Medical School
707 North Fairbanks Court
Suite 1210, Chicago, Illinois 60611

R. W. Liebling, MD
Associate Professor
Albert Einstein College of Medicine and
Montefiore Medical Center
Department of Plastic and Reconstructive Surgery
Jacobi Medical Center
1825 Eastchester Road
Bronx, New York 10461

B.-L. Lim, MD
Department of Hand Surgery
Singapore General Hospital
Outram Road
Singapore 0316

Chi-hung Lin, MD
Chang Gung Memorial Hospital
Kweishan
Taoyuan, Taiwan

W. C. Lineaweaver, MD
Professor and Chief, Division of Plastic Surgery
University of Mississippi Medical Center
Jackson, Mississippi

P. C. Linton, MD, FACS
Emeritus Professor of Plastic Surgery
University of Vermont College of Medicine
30 Main Street
Burlington, Vermont 05401

G. D. Lister, MD
Division of Plastic Surgery
University of Utah Medical Center
50 Medical Drive
Salt Lake City, Utah 84132

J. W. Little, III, MD, FACS
1145 19th Street, Northwest, Suite 802
Washington, DC 20036

J. W. Littler, MD (Deceased)

S. Llanos, MD
Burn and Plastic Surgery Unit
Hospital del Trabajador de Santiago
Centre for Health Research and Development
Universidad de los Andes
Chile

P. Lorea, MD
SOS MAIN Strasbourg
Strasbourg, France

M. M. LoTempio, MD
Fellow
Division of Plastic Surgery
Medical University of South Carolina

E. A. Luce, MD, FACS
Chief, Division of Plastic Surgery and Kiehn-DesPrez
Professor at University Hospitals of Cleveland/Case Western
Reserve University
Division of Plastic Surgery
11100 Euclid Avenue
Cleveland, Ohio 44106–5044

H. W. Lueders (Retired)
Community Hospital, Monterey, California
4007 Costado Road
Pebble Beach, California 93953

J. R. Lyons, MD
Yale-New Haven Hospital
Hospital St. Raphael
New Haven, Connecticut
330 Orchard Street
New Haven, Connecticut 06511–4417

S. E. MacKinnon, MD, FACS
Shoenberg Professor and Chief, Division of Plastic and
Reconstructive Surgery, Department of Surgery
Washington University School of Medicine
Division of Plastic Surgery and Reconstructive Surgery
One Barnes-Jewish Hospital Plaza, Suite #17424
St. Louis, Missouri 63110

W. B. Macomber, MD
Albany Medical College
1465 Western Avenue
Albany, New York 12203

N. C. Madan, MD
Associate Professor of Surgery
All India Institute of Medical Sciences
New Delhi, India

K. T. Mahan, DPM
Presbyterian Medical Center of University of Pennsylvania
St. Cigner Medical Center
Bethesda National Naval Medical Center
Pennsylvania College of Podiatric Medicine
The Foot and Ankle Institute
810 Race Street
Philadelphia, Pennsylvania 19107–2496

A. M. Majidian, MD
Grossman Burn Center at Sherman Oaks Hospital, California
2080 Century Park East, Ste 501
Los Angeles, California 90067

S. Malekzadeh, MD
Resident, University of Maryland Medical System,
Baltimore, MD
University of Maryland Medical System
22 S. Greene Street
Baltimore, Maryland 21201

R. T. Manktelow, MD
The Toronto Hospital
Mount Sinai Hospital
Hospital for Sick Children
Etobreske General Hospital
St. Michael's Hospital
The Toronto Hospital
Western Division
399 Bathurst Street 5WW835
Toronto, Ontario, Canada M5T 2S8

C. H. Manstein, MD
Chief, Division of Plastic Surgery, Jeans Hospital,
Philadelphia
Assistant Professor of Surgery, Temple University
School of Medicine, Philadelphia
Manstein Plastic Surgery Associates
7500 Central Avenue, Suite 210
Philadelphia, Pennsylvania 19111–2434

B. Maraud, MD
Centre Hospitalier D'Agen
17, Rue de Strasbourg
F-47000 Agen, France

D. Marchac, MD
Hôpital Necker Enfants Malades, Paris, France
130 rue de la Pompe
F-75116 Paris, France

J. M. Markley, MD, FACS
St. Joseph Mercy Hospital, Ann Arbor
University of Michigan Medical Center, Ann Arbor
Suite 5001–5008
5333 McAulery Drive
Ann Arbor, Michigan 48106

D. R. Marshall, FRACS
Monash University
Wellington Road
Melbourne
Victoria 3618, Australia

D. Martin, MD
Department of Plastic and Reconstructive Surgery
C.H.U.-Hôpital Du Tondu
Groupe Pellegrin-Tondu
Place Amélie Raba-Léon
F-33076 Bordeaux, France

Y. Maruyama, MD
Department of Plastic and Reconstructive Surgery
Toho University School of Medicine
6–11–1 Ohmorinishi, Ohta-ku
Tokyo 143, Japan

Professeur A. C. Masquelet
Chirurgie Orthopédique-Tramatologique et
Réparatrice de l'Appareil Locomoteur
Hôpital Avicenne
125, route de Stalingrad
F- 93009 Bobigny Cedex, France

J. K. Masson, MD
Mayo Clinic
102 Southwest Second Avenue
Rochester, Minnesota 55905–0008

A. Matarasso, MD, FACS, PC
Manhattan Eye, Ear, & Throat Hospital
Albert Einstein College of Medicine and Montefiore Medical
Center
Plastic and Reconstructive Surgery
1009 Park Avenue
New York, New York 10028

S. J. Mathes, MD
University of California, San Francisco Hospitals
and Clinics
Department of Surgery
San Francisco, California 94143–0932

H. S. Matloub, MD, FACS
Professor of Plastic Surgery and Director of Hand Fellowship
Program, Froedtert Hospital
Children's Hospital of Wisconsin
Veteran's Administration Hospital
Department of Plastic and Reconstructive Surgery
Medical College of Wisconsin
9200 West Wisconsin Avenue
Milwaukee, Wisconsin 53226

K. Matsuo, MD
Department of Plastic and Reconstructive Surgery
Shinshu University School of Medicine
3-1-1 Asahi, Matsumoto 390, Japan

J. W. May, Jr., MD, FACS
Chief of Division of Plastic Surgery
Massachusetts General Hospital
Massachusetts General Hospital, Rm. 353
Ambulatory Care Center, Ste. 453
15 Parkman Street
Boston, Massachusetts 02214–3139

J. G. McCarthy, MD, FACS
New York University Medical Center
Bellevue Hospital Center
Manhattan Eye, Ear & Throat Hospital
NYU Medical Center
550 First Avenue
New York, New York 10016

J. B. McCraw, MD, FACS
Professor of Plastic Surgery
University of Mississippi
2500 North State Street
Jackson, Mississippi 39216-3600

I. A. McGregor, MD
7 Ledcameroch Road
Bearsden,
Glasgow G61 4AB, Scotland
United Kingdom

S. Medgyesi, MD
Consultant Plastic Surgeon
Rigshospitalet
Copenhagen, Denmark

J. Medina, MD
Hand surgeon
Department of Orthopedics
Las Palmas
Gran Canaria
Spain

B. C. Mendelson, FRCSE, FRACS, FACS
The Avenue Hospital, Melbourne, Australia
109 Mathoura Road
Toorak, Victoria 3142
Australia

N. Menon, MD
Microsurgery Fellow
Stanford University Medical Center
Division of Plastic Surgery
Palo Alto, California

R. Meyer, MD
Postgraduate Professor ISAPS (IPRAS)
Centre de Chirurgie Plastique
4-Avenue Marc-Dufour
CH-1007 Lausanne, Switzerland

D. R. Millard, Jr., MD, FACS
Jackson Memorial Hospital
Miami Children's Hospital
1444 Northwest Fourteenth Avenue
Miami, Florida 33125

R. L. Mills, MD
751 South Bascom Avenue
San Jose, California 95128–2604

T. Miura, MD
Chukyo University
101 Tokodate, Kaizu-cho
Toyota, Aichi, 470–03, Japan

J. R. Moore, MD
Associate Professor of Orthopedic Surgery
The Johns Hopkins University School of Medicine
1400 Front Avenue, Suite 100
Lutherville, MD 21093–5355

S. C. Morgan, MD
Huntington Memorial Hospital
Arcadia Methodist Hospital
USC-LA County Medical Center
10 Congress Street, Suite 407
Pasadena, California 91105–3023

K. Morioka, MD
Department of Plastic and Reconstructive Surgery
Tokyo Women's Medical University
Tokyo, Japan

A. M. Morris, MD
Dundee University
Dundee, DD1 9SV, Scotland
United Kingdom

W. A. Morrison, MD
Plastic Surgeon and Deputy Director
Microsurgery Research Centre
St. Vincent's Hospital
Melbourne, Australia

H. Müller, MD, DMD (Deceased)

W. R. Mullin, MD, FACS
Jackson Memorial
Cedar Medical Center
Children's Medical Center
Plastic Surgery Centre
1444 Northwest 14th Avenue
Miami, Florida 33125

J. C. Mustardé, MD
90 Longhill Avenue
Ayr, Scotland, KA7 4DF, United Kingdom

F. Nahai, MD
Professor of Plastic Surgery, Emory University
Emory University Clinic
1365 Clifton Road, Northeast
Atlanta, Georgia 30322

J. E. Nappi, MD
Riverside Methodist Hospital
3400 Olentauey River Road
Columbus, Ohio 43214

M. Narayanan, MD
Medical Advisor
Ramalingam Medical Relief Centre
Madras, India

T. M. Nassif, MD
Hospital dos Servidores do Estado
Chief, Department of Reconstructive Microsurgery
Hospital dos Sevidores do Estado
22281 Rio de Janeiro RJ, Brazil

Vu Nguyen, MD
Assistant Professor
Division of Plastic Surgery
University of Pittsburgh Medical Center
Pittsburgh, Pennsylvania

J. M. Noe, MD
Harvard Medical School
25 Shattuck Street
Boston, Massachusetts 02115

K. Nohira, MD
Hokkaido University, Department of Plastic and
Reconstructive Surgery
Keiyukai Sapporo Hospital, Division of Plastic Surgery
Chief of Soshundo Plastic Surgery
Otemachi Building 2F
Minami-1, Nishi-4, Chuo-ku
Sapporo 060, Japan

J. D. Noonan, MD, FACS
Albany Medical Center
St. Peter's Hospital, Children's Hospital
1465 Western Avenue
Albany, New York 12203–3512

M. Nozaki, MD
Department of Plastic and Reconstructive Surgery
Tokyo Women's Medical University
8-1 Kawada-cho, Shimjuku-ku, 162-0054
Tokyo, Japan

K. Ohmori, MD
Department of Plastic and Restorative Surgery
Tokyo Metropolitan Police Hospital
2-10-41 Fujima Chiyoda-ku
Tokyo 102, Japan

S. Ohmori, MD (Deceased)

H. Ohtsuka, MD
Associate Professor
Ehime University Hospital
Surgical Division
Section of Plastic and Reconstructive Surgery
Shitsukawa, Shigenobu-cho,
Onsen-gun, Ehime 791–0295, Japan

C. Orreteguy, MD
Centre Hospitalier-Villeneuve Sur Lot
19, Bd. de la Marine
F-47300 Villeneuve Sur Lot, France

M. Orticochea, MD
Montevideo University School of Medicine
Montevideo, Uruguay

A. I. Pakiam, MD, FACS
Hospital of Saint John and St. Elizabeth
London, United Kingdom

C. E. Paletta, MD, FACS
Associate Professor, Division of Plastic and
Reconstructive Surgery, St. Louis University Hospital
Cardinal Glennon Children's Hospital
Veterans Administration–St. Louis
St. Mary's Health Center
St. Louis University
Associate Professor, Division of Plastic Surgery
3635 Vista at Grand
St. Louis, Missouri 63110–0250

F. X. Paletta, MD, FACS (Retired)
3635 Vista at Grand
St. Louis, Missouri 63110–0250

B. Panconi, MD
Department of Plastic and Reconstructive Surgery
of the Hand
Hôpital Pellegrin-Tondu
Place Amélie Raba-Léon
F-33076 Bordeaux, France

S. D. Pandey, MS, MCh
Professor, Hand Surgery
King George's Medical College
Lucknow 226 003, India

W. R. Panje, MD
Rush-Presbyterian-St. Luke's Medical Center, Chicago, Illinois
1725 Harrison Street, Suite 340
Chicago, Illinois 60612

G. S. Pap, MD, DDS, FACS (Retired)
Plastic and Reconstructive Maxillo-Facial Surgery
2403 Spring Creek Road
Rockford, Illinois 61107

C. Papp, MD
Head, Department of Plastic and Reconstructive Surgery
Hospital of Barmherzige Brüder
Salzburg, Austria

A. M. Pardue, MD, FACS
Los Robles Regional Medical Center
Thousand Oaks, California
1993 West Potrero Road
Thousand Oaks, California 91361

K.J. Park, MD, PhD
Assistant Professor
Department of Surgery
Dong-A University Medical Center
3 go 1, Dongdaesin-dong, Seo-Gu, Busan 602-716
South Korea

S. W. Parry, MD
Tulane Medical Center
Professor of Surgery, Tulane University
Tulane Medical Center Hospital and Clinic
1415 Tulane Avenue
New Orleans, Louisiana 70112–2605

A. Patel, MD
Resident
Department of Otolaryngology
The New York Eye & Ear Infirmary
New York, New York

R. M. Pearl, MD, FACS
Stanford University Hospital
Kaiser Hospital, Santa Clara
Physician-in-Chief
The Permanente Medical Group
900 Kiely Boulevard
Santa Clara, California 95051–5386

James M. Pearson, MD
Chief Resident
Department of Otolaryngology
The New York Eye & Ear Infirmary
New York, New York

I. J. Peled, MD
Chairman, Department of Plastic Surgery
Rambam Medical Center
Technion Institute of Technology, Medical School
Department of Plastic Surgery
Rambam Medical Center
Haifa, Israel

P. Pelissier, MD
Chef de Clinique
Service de Chirurgie Plastique et Reconstructrice
Hôpital du Tondu-Pellegrin
F-33076 Bordeaux, France

A. D. Pelly, MD
Plastic Surgery Unit
The Prince of Wales Hospital
195 Macquarie Street
Sydney 2000, Australia

Y. P. Peng, RWH Pho, FRCS
Consultant
Department of Hand and Reconstructive
Microsurgery
National University Hospital, Singapore;
Emeritus Professor of Orthopaedic Surgery
National University of Singapore

J. O. Penix, MD
Sentard Norfolk General Hospital
Surgical Director of Neurological Surgery
Children's Hospital of the King's Daughters
Neurosurgical Associates
607 Medical Tower
Norfolk, Virginia 23507

J. M. Peres, MD
Department of Plastic and Reconstructive Surgery
C.H.U.-Hôpital Du Tondu
Groupe Pellegrin-Tondu
Place Amélie Raba-Léon
F-33076 Bordeaux, France

M. Pers, DrMed
Head, Department of Plastic Surgery
University of Copenhagen
Rigshospitalet
Copenhagen, Denmark

J. Perssonelli, MD
St. Paul Hay Hospital
Av. Moema 170/111
04082-002 São Paulo SP, Brazil

V. Petrovici, MD
Department of Surgery, University of Cologne
Merheim Hospital
Bachemerstrasse 267
D-50935 Köln, Germany

R. W. H. Pho, MBBS, FRCS
Professor in Orthopaedic Surgery
National University of Singapore
Chief, Department of Hand and Reconstructive Microsurgery
National University Hospital
5 Lower Kent Ridge Road
Singapore 119074

K. L. Pickrell, MD (Deceased)

M. J. Pidala, MD
Western Reserve Medical Center
1930 State Route 59
Kent, Ohio 44240

J. L. Piñeros, MD
President of the Chilean Society of Burns
Burn and Plastic Surgery Unit
Hospital del Trabajador de Santiago
Santiago, Chile

P. Poizac, MD
Centre Hospitalier D'Agen
17, rue de Strasbourg
F-47000 Agen, France

B. Pontén, MD
Department of Plastic Surgery
University of Uppsala
750 14 Uppsala, Sweden

L. Pontes, MC
Plastic Surgery Unit
Department of Surgical Oncology
Portuguese Institute of Oncology
Porto, Portugal

J. A. Porter, MD
Clinical Professor of Surgery
Northeastern Ohio Universities College of Medicine
Summa Health Systems
55 Arch Street, Suite 3D
Akron, Ohio 44304

M. A. Posner, MD
Clinical Professor of Orthopaedics
New York University School of Medicine
Chief of Hand Services, Hospital for Joint Diseases
Chief of Hand Services, Lenox Hill Hospital
2 East 88th Street
New York, New York 10128

Z. Potparic, MD
University of Miami School of Medicine
Division of Plastic Surgery
Miami, Florida 33136

N. G. Poy, MD (Retired)
Scarborough General Hospital, Scarborough, Ont, Canada
4151 Sheppard Avenue, East
Scarborough, Ontario, Canada M1S 1T4

J. N. Pozner, MD
Assistant Clinical Professor of Plastic Surgery
The Johns Hopkins Hospital, Baltimore, MD
Plastic and Aesthetic Surgery
1212 York Road, Suite B101
Lutherville, Maryland 21093

G. Pradet, MD
Centre de Chirugie de la Main-Urgences Mains
Hôpital Nanterre
Paris, France

F. E. Pratt, MD (Retired)
P.O. Box 417880
Sacramento, California 95841

J. J. Pribaz, MD
Brigham & Women's Hospital, Boston
Children's Hospital, Boston
Associate Professor/Chief, Hand and Microsurgery
Department of Surgery/Division of Plastic Surgery
Brigham and Women's Hospital
75 Francis Street
Boston, Massachusetts 02115

J. M. Psillakis, MD
Professor of Plastic and Reconstructive Surgery
University of Sao Paulo, Brazil
Av. Cauaxi 222
Ed. San Martin 703
Barueri 06454-020, Brazil

C. L. Puckett, MD, FACS
University of Missouri Hospital and Clinics
Professor and Head
Division of Plastic and Reconstructive Surgery
University of Missouri
One Hospital Drive
Columbia, Michigan 65212

C. Radovan, MD (Deceased)

S. S. Ramasastry, MD
University of Illinois at Chicago Medical Center
Cook County Hospital, Chicago, Illinois
Mount Sinai Hospital, Chicago, Illinois
820 South Wood Street, (M/C 958) 515 CSN
Chicago, Illinois 60612

O. M. Ramirez, MD, FACS
Greater Baltimore Medical Center
Professor, The Johns Hopkins University
School of Medicine
Franklin Square Hospital, Baltimore
Plastic and Aesthetic Surgery
1212 York Road Suite, B-101
Lutherville-Timonium, Maryland 21093–6240

Y. Ramon, MD
Department of Plastic Surgery
Rambam Medical Center, Haifa
4A Mapu Avenue
Haifa, 34361 Israel

V. K. Rao, MD, MBA
University of Wisconsin Hospital and Clinic
University of Wisconsin Medical School
600 Highland Avenue
Madison, Wisconsin 53792

D. A. Campbell Reid, MD, FRCS
Consultant Plastic Surgeon
Plastic and Jaw Department
Fulwood Hospital
Fulwood
Sheffield, S10 3TD, United Kingdom

R. S. Reiffel, MD, PC, FACS
White Plains Hospital
St. Agnes Hospital
Westchester Medical Center
12 Greenridge Avenue, Suite 203
White Plains, New York 10605

J. F. Reinisch, MD, FACS
Head, Division of Plastic Surgery
Childrens Hospital Los Angeles
University Hospital
Associate Professor of Clinical Surgery, University of
Southern California School of Medicine
Division of Plastic Surgery
Childrens Hospital Los Angeles
4650 Sunset Boulevard, MS #96
Los Angeles, California 90027

A. J. Renard, MD, FACS
3845 Bee Ridge Road
Sarasota, Florida 34233–1160

J. E. Restrepo, MD
Clínica Soma
Medellin, Columbia

C. A. Rhee, MD
2879 Hempstead Turnpike, Suite 204
Levittown, New York 11756

M. Ribeiro, MD
Plastic Surgery Unit
Department of Surgical Oncology I
Portuguese Institute of Oncology
Porto, Portugal

D. Richard, MD
Centre Hospitalier D'Agen
Rue Lamennais
F-47000 Agen, France

R. A. Rieger, MBBS, FRCS, FRACS
327 S. Terrace
Adelaide 5001, Australia

R. Roa, MD
President of the Chilean Burn Association;
Assistant Professor
Medical School, Universidad de los Andes
Santiago, Chile

G. A. Robertson, MD
Victoria Hospital, Winnipeg, Manitoba
Manitoba Clinic
790 Sherbrook Street
Winnipeg R3A 1M3, Canada

J. F. R. Rocha, MD
Laboratoire d'Anatomie de l'UER
Biomedicale de Saint Peres
Hôpital Trousseau
Paris, France

C. Rodgers, MD, FACS
Rose Medical Center
Swedish Hospital
Porter Hospital
Littleton Hospital
4600 Hale Parkway, Suite 430
Denver, Colorado 80220

E. Roggendorf, Dr.sc.med. (Deceased)

M. C. Romaña, MD
Hôpital d'Enfants Armand-Trousseau, Paris
Consultant Surgeon
Department of Orthopaedic and Reconstructive Surgery
for Children
Hôpital Trousseau
26 Avenue A. Netter
F-75012 Paris, France

T. Romo III, MD
Director of Facial Plastic and Reconstructive Surgery
Department of Otolaryngology Head and Neck Surgery
Lenox Hill Hospital
The Manhattan Eye, Ear and Throat Hospital
New York, New York

E. H. Rose, MD
Assistant Clinical Professor (Plastic Surgery)
The Mount Sinai Medical School, New York, NY
Attending Staff, The Mount Sinai Medical Center and
Lenox Hill Hospital, New York, NY
Founder and Director, The Aesthetic Surgery Center,
New York, NY
The Aesthetic Surgery Center
895 Park Avenue
New York, New York 10021

M. Rousso, MD
Senior Lecturer of Surgery
Hadassah Hebrew University, Jerusalem
Head of Hand Surgery and Day Care Surgery
Misgav Ladach General Hospital
POB 90
Jerusalem 91000, Israel

R. T. Routledge, MD, FRCS (Retired)
Chief of Plastic Surgery Department
Frenchay Hospital
Bristol, United Kingdom

R. C. Russell, MD, FACS, FRCS
Memorial Hospital, Springfield, IL
St. John's Hospital, Springfield, IL
Illini Hospital, Pittsfield, IL
Southern Illinois University School of Medicine
Plastic Surgery 1511, P.O. Box 19230
Springfield, Illinois 62794

R. F. Ryan, MD, FACS (Retired)
Emeritus Professor of Surgery (Plastic Reconstructive),
Tulane Medical School, New Orleans, LA
Perido Bay Country Club
5068 Shoshone Drive
Pensacola, Florida 32507

F. J. Rybka, MD, FACS
Mercy Hospital
Sutter Hospital
Professor of Plastic Surgery, University of California, Davis
San Juan Medical Plaza, Suite 350
6660 Coyle Avenue
Carmichael, California 95608–6312

M. N. Saad, MD
Honorary Consultant Plastic Surgeon
Wexham Park Hospital, Slough
Consultant Plastic Surgeon
The Thames Valley Nuffield Hospital, Slough and
The Princess Margaret Hospital
Osborne Road, Windsor
Berks SL4 3SJ, United Kingdom

H. Saito, MD, PhD
Fukui Medical University
Matsuoka-cho, Yoshida-gun
Fukui, Japan

S. Sakai, MD
Associate Professor
Department of Plastic and Reconstructive Surgery
St. Marianna University School of Medicine
2-16-1 Sugao
Myamae-ku, Kawasaki 216, Japan

R. H. Samson, MD
Sarasota Memorial Hospital
Columbia Doctors Hospital
Vascular Associates of Sarasota
4044 Sawer Road
Sarasota, Florida 34233

J. R. Sanger, MD, FACS
Medical College of Wisconsin
9200 West Wisconsin Avenue
Milwaukee, Wisconsin 53226

J.R. Ramón Sanz, MD
Head of Department of Plastic and Reconstructive Surgery
"Marqués de Valdecilla" University Hospital
Santander, Spain

G. H. Sasaki, MD, FACS
St. Luke Medical Center
Huntington Memorial Hospital
Arcadia Methodist Hospital
Plastic and Reconstructive Surgery
800 South Fairmount Avenue, Suite 319
Pasadena, California 91105

K. Sasaki, MD
Chief Professor of Nihon University School of Medicine
Department of Plastic and Reconstructive Surgery
Nihon University School of Medicine, Oyaguchi
Itabashi-ku, Tokyo Japan

R. C. Savage, MD, FACS
Assistant Clinical Professor, Division of Plastic Surgery,
Harvard Medical School
Needham Medical Building
111 Lincoln Street, Suite 3
Needham, Massachusetts 02192

H. Schaupp, MD (Retired)
University ENT Hospital
Frankfurt-am-Main, Germany

L. R. Scheker, MD
Christine M. Kleinert Institute for Hand and Microsurgery
Assistant Clinical Professor of Plastic and
Reconstructive Surgery
University of Louisville
225 Abraham Flexner Way, Suite 700
Louisville, Kentucky 40202–3806

R. R. Schenck, MD, FACS
Associate Professor and Director
Section of Hand Surgery
Senior Attending, Departments of Plastic and
Orthopaedic Surgery
Rush-Presbyterian-St. Luke's Medical Center
1725 Harrison Street, Rm 263
Chicago, Illinois 60612–3828

J. D. Schlenker, MD
Christ
Little Co. of Mary
Palos Community
Holy Cross
Illinois Valley Community Hospital
6311 West 95th Street
Chicago, Illinois 60453

J. Schrudde, MD
University of Köln
Osterriethwed 17
D-50996 Köln, Germany

M. A. Schusterman, MD, FACS
Clinical Associate Professor of Plastic and
Reconstructive Surgery
Baylor College of Medicine, Houston, TX
7505 South Main Street, Suite 200
Houston, Texas 77030

S. P. Seidel, MD
Cullman Regional Medical Center
Woodland Community Hospital
Walker Baptist Medical Center
Seidel Plastic Surgery
2035 Alabama Highway #157
Cullman, Alabama 35055

D. Serafin, MD, FACS
Professor, Chief of Plastic Reconstructive
Maxillary Oral Surgery
Duke University Medical Center
P.O. Box 3372
Durham, North Carolina 27710–0001

R. E. Shanahan, MD, FACS
Emeritus Staff, The Toledo Hospital
Emeritus Clinical Associate Professor of Surgery
Medical College of Ohio at JOCTPC
5945 Barkwood Lane
Toledo, Ohio 43560

L. A. Sharzer, MD, FACS
Albert Einstein College of Medicine and
Montefiore Medical Center
Westchester Square Hospital, NY
Beth Israel Hospital, NY
212 East 69th Street
New York, New York 10021

W. W. Shaw, MD, FACS
Professor, Chief, Division of Plastic Surgery
UCLA School of Medicine
Room 64-140 CHS
10833 LeConte Avenue
Los Angeles, California 90095

R. W. Sheffield, MD, FACS
Cottage Hospital, Santa Barbara, CA
1110 Coast Village Circle
Santa Barbara, California 93108

A. Shektman, MD
332 Washington Street
Suite 355
Wellesley, Massachusetts 02181

S. M. Shenaq, MD, FACS
The Methodist Hospital, Texas Medical Center
St. Luke's Episcopal Hospital, Texas Medical Center
Texas Children's Hospital, Texas Medical Center
Ben Taub General Hospital, Texas Medical Center
Veteran's Administration Hospital, Texas Medical Center
Institute for Rehabilitation and Research, Texas
Medical Center
Diagnostic Center Hospital, Texas Medical Center
Poly Ryan Memorial, Richmond, Texas
Northeast Medical Center Hospital, Humble, Texas
Professor of Surgery, Division of Plastic Surgery
Baylor College of Medicine
6560 Fannin Street, Suite 800
Houston, Texas 77030

G. H. Shepard, MD
Riverside Regional Hospital Medical Center
Newport News, Virginia
Mary Immaculate Hospital
Newport News, Virginia
895 Middle Ground Boulevard, Suite 300
Newport News, Virginia 23606

M. M. Sherif, MD
Associate Professor
Department of Plastic and Reconstructive Surgery
Aim Shams University, Cairo, Egypt
2(A) Al Sayed Abou Shady Street, Flat 606
Heliopolis, Cairo 11361, Egypt

K. C. Shestak, MD
Division of Plastic Surgery
University of Pittsburgh
Pittsburgh, Pennsylvania

Y. J. Shin, MD
Department of Plastic Surgery
College of Medicine
Chungnam National University
640 Taesa-Dong, Jung-ku, Taejeon
301-040 Korea

Y. Shintomi, MD
Soshundo Plastic Surgery Hospital
Director of Soshundo Plastic Surgery
Otemachi Building
Minami-1, Nishi-4, Chuo-ku
Sapporo 060, Japan

G. F. Shubailat, MD, FRCS, FACS
Member of the Senate, Jordan Parliament
CEO and Chairman of the Board, Chief of Plastic Surgery,
Amman Surgical Hospital
P. O. Box 5180
Amman 11183, Jordan

M. Siemionow, MD, PhD, DSc
Professor of Surgery
Director of Plastic Surgery Research
Department of Plastic Surgery
Cleveland Clinic
Cleveland, Ohio

C. E. Silver, MD
Professor of Surgery
Albert Einstein College of Medicne
Chief of Head and Neck Surgery
Montefiore Medical Center
111 East 210th Street
Bronx, New York 10467–2401

R. P. Silverman, MD
Chief, Division of Plastic Surgery
University of Maryland Medical Center
Baltimore, Maryland

F. A. Slezak, MD
Professor of Surgery, Northeastern Ohio Universities
College of Medicine, Department of Surgery
Summa Health Systems, Akron, Ohio
55 Arch Street, Suite 3D
Akron, Ohio 44304

C. J. Smith, MD
Swedish Hospital
Providence Hospital
Northwest Hospital
1221 Madison Street, Suite 1102
Seattle, Washington 98104–1360

E. Durham Smith, MD, FRACS
Senior Associate, University of Melbourne
Melbourne, 3052
Victoria, Australia

R. J. Smith, MD (Deceased)

J. W. Snow, MD
St. Vincent's Hospital
1820 Barrs Street, Suite 701
Jacksonville, Florida 32204

B. C. Sommerland, FRCS
Great Ormond St. Hospital for Children, London
St. Andrew's Hospital, Billeriay, Essex
Consultant Plastic Surgery
The Old Vicarage
17 Lodge Road
Writtle
Chelmsford, CMI 3H4, United Kingdom

J. T. Soper, MD
Professor, Department of Gynecological Oncology
Duke University
Division of Gynecologic Oncology
Duke University Medical Center
Durham, North Carolina 27715–3079

M. Soussaline, MD
Institut Gustave Roussy Villefrief
Clinique Ste. Genevieve
Plastic and Cosmetic Surgery Department
American Hospital
46, Boulevard Saint-Jacques
F-75014 Paris, France

D. Soutar, MD
Clinical Director, Consultant Plastic Surgeon
Honorary Senior Lecturer, University of Glasgow
Plastic Surgery Unit
Canniesburn Hospital
Bearsden
Glasgow, G61 1QL, Scotland, United Kingdom

M. Spinner, MD
557 Central Avenue
Cedarhurst, New York 11516–2136

M. Spira, MD, FACS
Chief of Plastic Surgery, St. Luke's Episcopal Hospital,
Houston, Texas
Baylor College of Medicine
6560 Fannin, Suite 800
Houston, Texas 77030

R. K. Srivastava, MD
Athens Regional Medical Center, Athens, Georgia
180 St. George Place
Athens, Georgia 30606

D. A. Staffenberg, MD, DSc (Honoris Causa)
Chief, Plastic Surgery
Surgical Director, Center for Craniofacial Disorders
Montefiore Medical Center
The Children's Hospital at Montefiore
Associate Professor
Clinical Plastic Surgery, Neurological
Surgery, Pediatrics
Albert Einstein College of Medicine
Bronx, New York

W. R. Staggers, MD
Thomas Hospital, Fairhope, AZ
South Bladwin Hospital, Foley, AZ
188 Hospital Drive, Suite 203
Thomas Hospital Medical Office Center
Fairhope, Arizona 36532

R. S. Stahl, MD, MBA
Associate Chief, Department of Surgery, Yale-New Haven
Hospital
Clinical Professor of Surgery, Yale University School of
Medicine
Yale New Haven Hospital, CB228
20 York Street
New Haven, Connecticut 06504

R. B. Stark, MD, FACS (Retired)
35 East 75th Street, 12C
New York, New York 10021

D. N. Steffanoff, MD (Retired)
114 Via Valverde
Cathedral City, California 92234

H.-U. Steinau, MD
BG-Universitätsklinik Bergmannsheil
Department of Plastic Surgery, Burn Center
Bürkle de la Camp Platz 1
D-44789 Bochum, Germany

M. Steiner, MD
Burn and Plastic Surgery Unit
Hospital del Trabajador de Santiago
Santiago, Chile

H. R. Sterman, MD
Albert Einstein College of Medicine and
Montefiore Medical Center
Holy Name Hospital
870 Palisade Avenue, Suite 203
Teaneck, New Jersey 07666

T. R. Stevenson, MD
Professor and Chief
Division of Plastic Surgery
University of California Davis Medical Center
2315 Stockton Boulevard
Sacramento, California 95817

W. Stock, MD
Ltd. Arzt f. Plast. Chirugie
Chirurgische Klinik
Nussbaumstrasse 2
D-80336 München 2, Germany

M. F. Stranc, MD
Head of Plastic Surgery Section, Health Sciences Center,
Winnipeg, Manitoba
Victoria Hospital, Winnipeg, Manitoba
Manitoba Clinic
790 Sherbrook Street
Winnipeg, Canada, R3A 1M3

W. E. Stranc, MD
Victoria Hospital
Winnipeg, Manitoba, R3A 1M3, Canada

B. Strauch, MD, FACS
Professor
Albert Einstein College of Medicine
5 Flagler Drive Bainbridge Avenue
Rye, New York 10580

V. V. Strelzow, MD, FACS, FRCS(C)
16300 Sand Canyon Avenue, Suite 704
Irvine, California 92618–3707

J. H. Sullivan, MD
Clinical Professor, University of California
San Francisco, California
220 Meridian Avenue
San Jose, California 95126–2903

I. Suzuki, MD
Associate Professor
Department of Plastic and Reconstructive Surgery
St. Marianna University School of Medicine
2-16-1 Sugao
Myamae-ku, Kawasaki 216, Japan

W. M. Swartz, MD, FACS
University of Pittsburgh Medical Center
5750 Centre Avenue, Suite 180
Pittsburgh, Pennsylvania 15206

E.-P. Tan, FRCS(Ed), FRACS
2 St. John's Avenue
Gordon, New South Wales 2072, Australia

M. J. Tavis, MD, FACS (Deceased)

G. Allan Taylor, MD, FRCS(C)
Assistant Professor of Surgery
University of Ottawa Medical School
Chief, Division of Plastic Surgery
Ottawa Civic Hospital
737 Parkdale Avenue
Ottawa, Ontario, Canada K1Y 4E9

G. I. Taylor, MD
Royal Melbourne Hospital
766 Elizabeth Street
Melbourne 3000, Australia

H.O.B. Taylor, MD
Plastic Surgery Resident
Harvard Plastic Surgery Program
Boston, Massachusetts

B. Teimourian, MD, FACS
Attending Surgeon, Suburban Hospital, Bethesda, MD
5402 McKinley Street
Bethesda, Maryland 20817

S. Terkonda, MD
University of Alabama at Birmingham, University Hospital
Instructor, Division of Plastic Surgery
University of Alabama at Birmingham, MEB-524
1813 Sixth Avenue, South
Birmingham, Alabama 35294

J. K. Terzis, MD
Sentara Hospitals
International Institute of Microsurgical Research
Eastern Virginia Medical School
330 West Brambleton Avenue
Norfolk, Virginia 23510

M. R. Thatte, MS, MCh (Plastic)
Mumbai Hospital Institute of Medical Sciences
Shushrusha Citizen's Co-Operative Hospital
Consultant Plastic Surgeon
167-F, Dr. Ambedkar Road
Dadar, Mumbai 400 014, India

R. L. Thatte, MD
Consultant Plastic Surgeon, Bhatia Hospital, Mumbai, India
Apartment 46
Shirish Co-op Housing Society
187 Veer Savarkar Marg
Mumbai 400 016, India

H. G. Thomson, MD, FACS
555 University Avenue, Suite 180
Toronto, Ontario, Canada M5G 1X8

G. R. Tobin, MD, FACS
Professor and Director, Division of Plastic Surgery
University of Louisville Hospitals
Department of Surgery
University of Louisville
Louisville, Kentucky 40292

M. A. Tonkin, MD
Clinical Associate Professor and Head, Hand and Peripheral
Nerve Surgery, Royal North Shore Hospital of Sydney
Department of Hand Surgery
The Royal North Shore Hospital of Sydney
Block 4, Level 4
St. Leonards, New South Wales, 2065, Australia

B. A. Toth, MD
Pacific-Presbyterian Medical Center
Assistant Clinical Professor, University of California, San
Francisco
2100 Webster Street, Suite 424
San Francisco, California 94115–2380

H. Tramier, MD
Service d'Orthopedie - Traumatologie - Chirurgie Pediaturgie
Centre Hospitalier, Aubogne Cedex
41, rue Saint-Jacques
F-13006 Marseille, France

G. Trengove-Jones, MD
Sentara Norfolk General Hospital
Sentara Leigh Hospital
De Paul Hospital
Childrens Hospital of the King's Daughters
Department of Plastic Surgery
Eastern Virginia Medical School
Norfolk, Virginia 23501–2401

W. C. Trier, MD, FACS (Retired)
6321 Seaview Avenue, NW, #20
Seattle, Washington 98107–2671

T.-M. Tsai, MD
Jewish Hospital
Suburban Hospital
Alliant Hospitals
University Hospital
Clark County Hospital, Indiana
Shriners Hospital, Lexington, Kentucky
Audubon Hospital
Caritas Hospital
Christine M. Kleinert Institute for Hand and Micro Surgery
225 Abraham Flexner Way, Suite 850
Louisville, Kentucky 40202

M. Tschabitscher, MD
Department of Microsurgical and
Endoscopic Anatomy
Medical University of Vienna
Vienna, Austria

Y. Ullmann, MD
Deputy Head, Department of Plastic and
Reconstructive Surgery, Rambam Medical Center
Faculty of Medicine (Bruce), Hatechnion, Haifa
Department of Plastic Surgery
Rambam Medical Center
Haifa 31096, Israel

S. Unal, MD
Department of Plastic Surgery
The Cleveland Clinic Foundation
Cleveland, Ohio

J. Unanue, MD
Centre Hospitalier Ter de Villeneuve Sur Lot
19 Bd. de la Marine
F-47300 Villeneuve Sur Lot, France

J. Upton, MD, FACS
Beth Israel Deaconess Medical Center, Boston, MA
Children's Hospital, Boston, MA
830 Boylston Street, Suite 212
Chestnut Hill, Massachusetts 02167

M. L. Urken, MD, FACS
Professor and Chairman, Department of Otolaryngology
Mt. Sinai Medical Center
Box 1189, One Gustave L. Levy Place
New York, New York 10029–6574

E. J. Van Dorpe, MD
Plastic Surgery Department
Onze Lieve Vrouw
Kortrijk, Belgium

F. Van Genechten, MD
Saint Augustinus-Saint Camillus Hospital, Antwerp, Belgium
Virga Jesse Hospital, Masself, Belgium
Oude Maasstraat. 1
B-3500 Hasselt, Belgium

L. O. Vasconez, MD, FACS
Chief Plastic Surgeon
University of Alabama at Birmingham Medical Center
Professor of Surgery and Chief
Division of Plastic Surgery
University of Alabama, Birmingham
1813 6th Avenue, South (MEB-524)
Birmingham, Alabama 35294-3295

T. R. Vecchione, MD
Associate Clinical Professor of Surgery, Division of Plastic
Surgery USSD, San Diego, CA
Senior and Past Chief of Staff, Children's Hospital of San Diego
Senior and Past Chief of Plastic Surgery, Morcy Hospital,
San Diego, CA
Senior and Past Chief of Plastic Surgery, Sharp Memorial
Hospital, San Diego, CA
306 Walnut Avenue, Suite 212
San Diego, California 92103

Professor R. Venkataswami, MS, MCh, FAMS, FRCS (EDIN), DSC (Hon)
Emeritus Professor, Dr M.G.R. Medical University
Chennai, Tamilnadv India
99 Dr. Algappa Chettiar Road
Chennai 600 084, India

R. J. J. Versluis, MD
Department of Otorhinolaryngology and
Head and Neck Surgery
Kennemer Gasthuis Deo
Velserstraat 19
NL-2023 EA Haarlem, The Netherlands

L. Vidal, MD
Department of Plastic and Reconstructive Surgery
C.H.U.-Hôpital Du Tondu
Groupe Pellegrin-Tondu
Place Amélie Raba-Léon
F-33076 Bordeaux, France

C. Vlastou, MD
Director, Department of Plastic and Reconstructive Surgery,
Diagnostic and Therapeutic Center of Athens "HYGEIA"
105-7 Vas Sovias Avenue
Athens 11521, Greece

V. E. Voci, MD, FACS
Presbyterian Hospital, Charlotte, NC
McRoy Hospital, Charlotte, NC
Gaston Memorial Hospital, Gastonia, NC
Voci Center Cosmetic Plastic Surgery, P.A.
2027 Randolph Road
Charlotte, North Carolina 28207–1215

H. D. Vuyk, MD
Gooi-Nord Hospital, Department of Otolaryngology,
Head and Neck Surgery
Rijksstraatweg 1
NL-1261 AN Blaricum, The Netherlands

S. C. Vyas, MD
Oakwood Hospital, Dearborn, MI
22260 Garrison
Dearborn, Michigan 48124

M. Wada, MD
Higasishinagawa Clinic
Higasishinagawa 3-18-8
Shinagawaku, Tokyo, Japan

M. S. Wagh, MS, MCh
Lecturer in Plastic Surgery, LTMG Hospital
Sion, Mumbai 400 022, India
601-602, B-Wing
Shantiwar
Shantivan Housing Complex
Borivali Suite 212(E), Mumbai 400 066, India

R. L. Walton, MD, FACS
University of Chicago Hospitals
University of Chicago - MC 6035
Plastic Surgery
5841 South Maryland Avenue
Chicago, Illinois 60637

A. Wangermez, MD
Centre Hospitalier D'Agen
Rue Lamennais
F-47000 Agen, France

P. H. Warnke, MD
Department of Oral and Maxillofacial Surgery
University of Kiel
Kiel, Germany

H. Washio, MD, FACS
Attending Staff, Plastic Surgery, St. Luke's–Roosevelt
Hospital Center, New York, New York
580 Park Avenue
New York, New York 10021

J. T. K. Wee, MD (Deceased)

F-C. Wei, MD
Professor and Chairman
Department of Plastic and Reconstructive Surgery
Chang Gung Memorial Hospital
199 Tung Hwa North Road
Taipei 10591, Taiwan

A. J. Weiland, MD
The Hospital for Special Surgery, New York, New York
The Hospital for Special Surgery
535 East 70th Street
New York, New York 10021–4872

N. Weinzweig, MD, FACS
Associate Professor of Plastic Surgery and Orthopaedic
Surgery, University of Illinois
Cook County Hospital
Associate Professor of Plastic Surgery and Orthopaedic
Surgery
University of Illinois
Division of Plastic Surgery M/C 958
820 South Wood Street, 515 CSN
Chicago, Illinois 60612–7316

A. W. Weiss, Jr., MD
St. Luke's Hospital
Associate Professor of Surgery, Michigan State University
College of Human Medicine
800 Cooper Street, Suite 1
Saginow, Michigan 48602–5371

M. R. Wexler, MD
Head, Department of Plastic and Aesthetic Surgery, Hand
Surgery and the Burn Unit, and Professor of Plastic Surgery,
Hebron
University, Hadassah Medical Center
Department of Plastic and Aesthetic Surgery
Hadassah University Hospital
Jerusalem 91120, Israel

W. White, MD (Deceased)

J. S. P. Wilson, FRCS
The Cromwell Hospital
London, United Kingdom

C. Windhofer, MD
Department of Plastic and Reconstructive Surgery
Hospital of Barmherzige Brüder
Salzburg, Austria

M. S. Wong, MD
Assistant Professor
Division of Plastic Surgery
University of California, Davis
Sacramento, California

J. E. Woods, MD, PhD, FACS
Mayo Medical Center, Rochester, MN
Emeritus Staff
Division of Plastic and Reconstructive Surgery
Mayo Clinic
200 First Street, Southwest
Rochester, Minnesota 55905

A. P. Worseg, MD
Department of Plastic and Reconstructive Surgery
Wilhelminenhospital
Vienna, Austria

E. F. Worthen, MD (Retired)
3504 Forsythe Avenue
Monroe, Louisiana 71201

Y. Yamamoto, MD, PhD
Assistant Professor, Department of Plastic and
Reconstructive Surgery
Hokkaido University School of Medicine
Kita 15, Nishi 7, Kitaku
Sapporo 060, Japan

N.W. Yii, MD
Division of Plastic Surgery
Wexham Park Hospital
Slough, Berkshire SL2 4HL,
United Kingdom

M. Young, MD
Grossman Burn Center at Sherman Oaks Hospital,
California
4929 Van Nuys Boulevard
Sherman Oaks, California 91403

N. J. Yousif, MD
Froedtert and Memorial Lutheran Hospital
9200 West Wisconsin Avenue
Milwaukee, Wisconsin 53226

P. Yugueros, MD
Mayo Medical Center, Rochester, MN
Division of Plastic and Reconstructive Surgery
Mayo Clinic
200 First Street, Southwest
Rochester, Minnesota 55905

L. S. Zachary, MD, FACS
University of Chicago, Division of Plastic Surgery
5841 South Maryland Ave. P.O. Box MC 6035
Chicago, Illinois 60637–1463

S. Zenteno Alanis, MD
Chief of Service
Department of Plastic and Reconstructive Surgery
Hospital General de Mexico
Providence 400 Penthouse
Mexico 12, D.F.

F. Zhang, MD, PhD
Professor
Division of Plastic Surgery
University of Mississippi Medical Center
Jackson, Mississippi

E. G. Zook, MD, FACS
Memorial Medical Center and St. John's Hospital
Southern Illinois University School of Medicine
Institute for Plastic Surgery
PO Box 19230
747 North Rutlidge Street
Springfield, Illinois 62794–1511

R. M. Zuker, MD, FRCS(C), FACS
Head, Division of Plastic Surgery
The Hospital for Sick Children
Professor of Surgery, Department of Surgery
University of Toronto
Head, Division of Plastic Surgery
The Hospital for Sick Children
555 University Avenue, Suite 1524B
Toronto, Ontario, Canada M5G 1X8

Since our last edition of *Grabb's Encyclopedia of Flaps*, major evolutionary changes have occurred in the field of reconstructive plastic surgery. The explosion of perforator flap sites and the techniques of harvesting the pedicle without extensive sacrifice of the underlying muscles are well represented in this new edition.

In the last ten years, the field of transplantation has also been further advanced by plastic surgeons. Face and hand allotransplantation represents some of the most exciting advances in all of medicine, and we have tried to provide a glimpse of this emerging field with the inclusion of two articles on facial transplantation. What was once science fiction has now become reality and may one day even become commonplace.

The changes in the reconstructive ladder are evident in all arenas. With the widespread success of microsurgery, many defects are currently reconstructed with the most complex free tissue transfers as the primary option, jumping straight to the top of the ladder. On the other hand, negative pressure devices have revolutionized wound care management and, in many cases, has supplanted tissue coverage, moving many potential defects rapidly down the ladder.

More than 12,000 citations in the literature on flaps were reviewed, and 43 new chapters were added to this third edition. Many of the older chapters were revised or brought up to date. The new edition includes flaps, both pedicle and microvascular, for reconstruction of the face, orbits, lips, and nose. The latest techniques in nasal reconstruction, including local mucosal flaps as well as providing total reconstruction of the nasal support and lining with microvascular forearm flaps, have been added. Use of innervated muscle for tongue reconstruction is presented. In the hand volume, many new flaps have been added for reconstruction of the palm, the fingers, and the metacarpals. Breast surgery articles, including the use of medial and lateral pedicles, are new to this edition. A major inclusion has been the addition of the multiple perforator flaps used for breast reconstruction. Articles on reconstruction of the chest and abdomen have been chosen, as have the latest techniques for lower extremity reconstruction.

In adding all of these new choices, the editors were faced with a dilemma. How do we keep the concept of an encyclopedic atlas, while still staying within the confines of hard copy pages and costs of printing? The decision was made to keep all of the previous articles but to list some of the lesser used flaps by chapter title and author only in the printed text so that the reader is aware of these choices. In the online edition, all of the articles, new and old, are presented with full text and illustrations. Of course, editorial opinions at the beginning of the chapters have been maintained to help the reader make prudent reconstructive decisions. To access these complete aricles, go to www.encyclopediaofflaps.com.

The third edition of this encyclopedia would not have been possible without the dedication provided by Dr. R.D. (Lee) Landres. In addition, we would like to thank the editorial staff at Lippincott Williams & Wilkins. To all the authors who contributed new chapters or provided revisions of their original chapters in a timely fashion, we extend our thanks, as we are deeply indebted to them.

Berish Strauch, MD
Luis O. Vasconez, MD
Elizabeth J. Hall-Findlay, MD
Bernard T. Lee, MD

PREFACE TO THE SECOND EDITION

In the last ten years, evolutionary changes in the use of flaps in reconstructive plastic surgery have resulted in increased flap reliability, as well as in more definitive reconstruction of particular defects. Currently, there is much less dependence on the use of flap delays and on random skin flaps. The reconstructive surgeon is now provided with a choice not only of skin flaps, but also of composite flaps which may contain skin and muscle, muscle alone or, in cases where bony defects are also involved, associated bone flaps. There is no longer a requirement for empirical questions about whether or not a particular flap will have an adequate blood supply. We presently think in terms of reliable flaps with a known blood supply and a determinate reliability. Where this is not yet possible, the reconstructive surgeon is likely to consider a free microvascular flap.

Another important change is our independence from the so-called reconstructive ladder, according to which surgeons followed the precept of using the simplest method and then advancing to a more complex one. Nowadays, the objective should always be to utilize the best method first, the one that will fulfill the requirements of the reconstruction, even though it may be the most complex, for example, a microvascular composite flap.

It was impossible for the authors to have included every flap that has been described since the first edition. In fact, considerable care has been taken in choosing proven and reliable flaps. Over 10,000 citations in the literature on flaps were reviewed and 120 new and revised chapters were added to the second edition. A considerable number of chapters describing procedures that have not been proven clinically reliable have been deleted. The editors have also added appropriate editorial comments that should be helpful to the reader wherever these seemed indicated.

Undertaking publication of the second edition of the encyclopedia would not have been possible, had it not been for the dedication and immense help provided by the editorial assistance of Dr. R. D. (Lee) Landres. We would also like to thank the editorial staff at Little, Brown and Company, whose work on this second edition has been taken over by Lippincott-Raven Publishers. Additionally, our sincere thanks to all the authors who contributed new chapters or revision of the original chapters in a timely fashion. We are indebted to them.

B. S.
L. O. V.
E. J. H.-F.

An important and very broad area of plastic surgery entails the coverage of defects throughout the body. These defects are usually covered by flaps, of which we now have a great variety. For approximately 50 years, from the introduction of the tubed flap until the middle 1960s, most flaps were tubed. Although we realized that blood supply was important for survival of the tubed flap, it was not until the end of the 1960s that we began to pay attention to the distinct arterial and venous supplies of different flaps. Axial flaps, musculocutaneous flaps, fasciocutaneous flaps, and microvascular free flaps were introduced in the decade of the 1970s. These were rapidly used in great numbers, with clinical applications throughout the body. The concept of "delay" of flaps has just about been abandoned. It is extremely advantageous that we now have a multitude of flaps that can be applied for the coverage of particular defects.

A flap can be designed and made with an adequate dimension with the knowledge of its exact blood supply; one needs only proper execution to be assured of a consistent, satisfactory, and acceptable result. This great number and variety of the flaps that differ not only in their design, but also in their type, as far as the blood supply is concerned, is "wonderful" for the experienced surgeon, but it also may present a quandary for the student plastic surgeon. The young surgeon may not have the clinical experience of having performed many and different flaps for a similar defect. There is usually no problem with execution of the procedure, but the clinical judgment that some learn by previous clinical errors may be supported by consideration and proper description of available options.

This *Encyclopedia* attempts to provide choices for the closure of particular defects throughout the body. Recognized experts described how to execute a particular flap, and each flap is presented in a uniform format, emphasizing the indications and anatomy, including the blood supply, surgical technique, complications, and safeguards. Selected editorial comments are included as a guide to the reader.

The multiauthored format has been chosen to give each author, often the originator of the flap, an opportunity to explain the procedure, and in each chapter the editors have rewritten only to maintain the uniform format, always attempting to keep the authors' information unchanged.

This *Encyclopedia* is intended to serve as a stimulus to experienced surgeons to refresh their memories about a multitude of options for particular defects so that they may choose what, in their judgment, will give a safe, predictable, and acceptable result. This work also will show the student of plastic surgery the numerous options and will teach him or her to choose the most appropriate one and to consider a great many factors that can play a role in what we call "clinical judgment." Once the proper choice is made, this *Encyclopedia* will refresh knowledge of the clinical aspects of flap execution, as well as the blood supply and the safeguards.

This *Encyclopedia* tends to encompass defects throughout the body and is divided into three volumes. For the reader who wants an increased knowledge of a particular flap, selected references are included at the end of each chapter.

We hope that this work will be helpful to all, including the most experienced surgeons, reinforcing with certainty that a good number of options have been considered and that the best were chosen.

Dr. William Grabb dreamed of a sequel to his book on skin flaps. He had organized and outlined the book and had chosen an initial group of contributors. His foresight encompassed the tremendous influence that microvascular and musculocutaneous flaps would have on the availability of usable flaps. He asked Berish Strauch and Luis O. Vasconez to join him as associate editors, to guide the sections on microvascular and musculocutaneous flaps, respectively. The decision to go forward with the *Encyclopedia* was made in 1981 during the annual meeting of the American Society of Plastic and Reconstructive Surgeons in New York.

Dr. Grabb's untimely death in 1982 halted progress on the work for over nine months. The two associate editors finally decided that the concept of the *Encyclopedia* was too important to plastic surgery for the project not to be completed.

Advice was sought from Lauralee Lutz in Ann Arbor. Lauralee had served as Dr. Grabb's administrative secretary and in-house editor. Her advice resulted in bringing aboard Dr. R. D. (Lee) Landres in New York to help with the editing of the *Encyclopedia*. All the contributors were contacted, and the chapters began to be produced.

The enormity of the task soon became apparent, and Dr. Elizabeth Hall-Findlay, who had worked previously with Drs. Strauch and Vasconez, was asked to join the two editors.

Multiauthored textbooks are often disorganized and repetitive. Faced with well over 400 chapters written in several languages and with various styles, we made a decision: Each chapter was to be reorganized into a similar format—with an introduction, a section on anatomy, and a section on flap design and dimensions, followed by operative technique and clinical results. In general, line drawings were to be the main figures, with some case illustrations. Details of history and research results were to be be omitted. Interested readers would be encouraged to refer to original publications, with each chapter followed by a relevant but not overbearing list of references. We knew we were into at least three volumes and did not want the work to be burdened with unnecessary detail. Despite the rewriting and uniform organization, there was a serious attempt to keep the authors' information unchanged.

This work has already traveled extensively. It has originated from all over the world. The chapters were initially rough-edited and placed on computer disks by Dr. Landres. The disks were sent to Dr. Hall-Findlay in Banff, Alberta, in the Canadian Rocky Mountains. There they were edited directly off the disks, and appropriate illustrations and references were chosen. Most of the chapters spent some time deep in the mountains at one of the most beautiful sites in the world—Lake O'Hara Lodge. There, care had to be taken not to lose any of the text or "work in progress" if the electric generator failed. Further work and refinements always seemed to take ten times longer than expected.

Drs. Vasconez and Strauch reviewed the editorial changes as they progressed and, as well, solicited and received new chapters as delays became prolonged. Meetings were held in Banff, where we closeted ourselves away with "the book," reviewing text and illustrations and discussing editorial comments.

The editors at Little, Brown and Company in Boston have been invaluable in seeing the project to completion. Fred Belliveau had organized and supervised the project from its inception. Curtis Vouwie helped during the seemingly never-ending delays, and Susan Pioli has both encouraged and prodded the work to completion.

Although the delays resulted in criticisms of being out of date, we felt that many of these chapters have stood and will stand the test of time. We tried to keep up with the chapters, without adopting the unproven. Of necessity, we stopped inclusions of new chapters in 1987. We hope that the book will not only be comprehensive, but also useful to surgeons in reviewing options when faced with routine or unusual problems or defects.

We can never thank everyone who has been involved in helping, directly or indirectly, with the *Encyclopedia*. Drs. Strauch, Vasconez, and Hall-Findlay wish to express in common their appreciation to Dr. Lee Landres, who has worked tirelessly for the past seven years on this work. Dr. Hall-Findlay wishes to recognize and thank Cheryl Low and Lynn Enderwick, who helped with many endless secretarial chores while, at the same time, handling patients and managing the office. Checking references accurately would not have been possible without the help of Merle Duncan, librarian at the medical library of the University of Calgary. Patricia Velasquez, Elke Berthold, Doris Freytag, Liesbeth Heynen, and Vickilynn Norton have all helped by being loving and devoted nannies to Jamie, David, and Elise. Dr. Hall-Findlay's mother, Betty Hall, and her in-laws, Jim and Edith Findlay, helped immeasurably with child care during their many visits to Banff, so that work on the *Encyclopedia* could go on. Don Findlay cannot be thanked enough for his understanding and patience.

B. S.
L. O. V.
E. J. H.-F.

INTRODUCTION:
THE HISTORY OF VASCULARIZED
COMPOSITE-TISSUE TRANSFERS

R. A. CHASE

The compelling drive of human beings to reconstruct deficient or missing parts and the desire of victims to undergo such reconstruction are best appreciated by recognizing the early development and use of pedicle-flap transfers long before the advent of anesthesia. Imagine the tolerance a patient must have had to undergo nasal reconstruction using a forehead pedicle flap without anesthesia. The seminal work of Sushruta (1) in the pre-Christian era must have resulted in meager success; however, the basic principle behind the "Indian flap" is so sound that the procedure is still used in contemporary surgery.

From those early developments, at first slowly, and then like a wild fire in the last four decades, the world has witnessed enormous progress in tissue-transfer surgery. The latter-day developments in anesthesia, antibiotics, hematology, instrumentation, and wound-healing research have given surgeons devoted to reconstruction the opportunity to achieve results that would have been considered miraculous only four decades ago. When immunologic barriers to risk-free transplantation are breached, a whole new wave of applications of existing and developing reconstructive strategies will break upon the world.

PEDICLE TRANSFERS

It is interesting to note, at least from what can be gleaned from recorded history (2), that the first successful transfer of human tissues to heterotopic sites was done by what we now call pedicle techniques. Such transfers are never even transiently, deprived of blood supply. Thus, on a trial-and-error basis, it should not be a surprise that the success of the Hindu Sushruta (1) during the pre-Christian era depended on the use of pedicle flaps of tissue in the face and forehead.

The designation of "Indian flap" for nasal reconstruction has survived, and its use in contemporary surgery testifies to its practicality. It appears to have taken centuries for the principle and procedure itself to travel from its origin in India to Europe—first to the Brancas in Italy, who became known in the fifteenth century for use of the technique and the principle to develop new and imaginative reconstructive procedures. Tagliacozzi in the sixteenth century made use of the printing press to disseminate knowledge of the techniques abroad through his celebrated *De Curtorum Chirurgia* (3) published in 1597.

Nonetheless, the procedures lay dormant for about 200 years until a newspaper, the *Madras Gazette,* and the *Gentleman's Magazine* (4) reported the Indian method for nose reconstruction in 1794. Among others, Carpue (5) in England and von Graefe (6) in Germany further developed the technique in Europe. Zeis, in his 1830 description of the procedure (7), displayed illustrations suggesting the dusky appearance of the flap early after surgery. Warren was the first in the United States to publish this technique in 1837 (8). It appeared in the *Boston Medical and Surgical Journal* (now the *New England Journal of Medicine*).

The pedicle flap principle, initiated by trial and error in pre-Christian history, was established and refined in the nineteenth century and formed the fundamental basis for the spectacular developments in the modern decades of surgery.

I shall mention a few landmarks in the development of tissue transfers during the nineteenth and twentieth centuries. In 1829, Fricke of Hamburg published a book describing many alternate facial flaps (9). Shortly thereafter, Tripier, Malgaigne (10), Burrow, Estlander, von Graefe (6), Abby, Denonvilliere, Rosenthal, Dieffenbach, and Zeis (2)—to name the principals—added further innovations in the shift of tissues to adjacent areas within the face for reconstruction.

Hamilton of Buffalo reported the first successful cross-leg flap in 1854 (12). He also was the first to apply the principle of delay to flap transfer. In 1868, Prince published *A New Classification and a Brief Exposition of Plastic Surgery* (12) with examples of applications of pedicle-flap techniques in plastic surgery. At the Practitioner's Society of New York in 1891, Shrady used an open jump flap cut from one arm and carried after vascularization by the contralateral index finger to fill a cheek contour defect (13). Shortly thereafter, in 1896, the renowned William Stewart Halsted (14) first "waltzed," by end-over-end transfer, a flap from the abdomen up to the neck of a burn victim. He was the first to use the term *waltzed.*

In pedicle-transfer surgery, aside from studies of the delay phenomenon (11,15,16), effects of drugs and radiation (17), and thinning of the flap (18), the refinements during this era were confined largely to the carrying pedicle itself. In 1849, Jobert of Paris, in his two-volume textbook *Chirurgie Plastique* (19), described "the temperature changes in skin flaps and the reinnervation of flaps" and noted that "the size of the pedicle should be proportional to the size of the flap."

The renowned Sir Harold Gillies stated, "In general, a flap should not be larger than the width of its carrying pedicle." In 1920, he added a rider: "A longer flap could be raised if the flap contained in its base a larger vascular pedicle such as the superficial temporal artery" (20).

Gillies' book, *Plastic Surgery of the Face* (21), is a classic in the field and, together with that of John Staige Davis, ushered in the modern era of plastic surgery. Both were based on lessons learned from current works and publications early in the twentieth century, such as those of Vilray Blair (22), and experiences during World War I. Gillies himself had been stimulated and influenced by Morestin, whom he had visited in France. The war experience was very influential on many great contributors to plastic surgery—V. H. Kazanjian, Ferris Smith, R. H. Ivy, Eastman Sheehan, and Sterling Bunnell, to name a few.

As noted by Khoo Boo-Chai (23), John Wood in 1863 had described a flap that, in 1869 (24), he called a "groin flap." He commented on the importance of incorporating known vessels—in his patients, the superficial epigastric vessels.

John Staige Davis, reporting World War I experiences, expanded the uses of pedicle flaps (2,25) and later with William German et al. (26) explored the vascular anatomy of the skin and subcutaneous tissues important in designing such flaps.

John Roberts of Philadelphia pointed to lessons learned in the war and applicable to reparative surgery using pedicle flaps on the hand (27). In 1919, Albee described the surgical construction of an osteoplastic finger substitute using a pedicle flap and a bone graft (28). Also in 1919, at the clinic day of the American Orthopaedic Association at Jefferson Hospital in Philadelphia, P. G. Skillern presented a patient from Polyclinic Hospital in whom a double-pedicle "strap" flap was used for coverage of the dorsum of the right hand (29). Steinler's books appeared in 1923 and 1925 (30,31), at the same time Allen Kanavel's book (32) was published, and later Marc Iselin's *Atlas* (33,34) and Cutler's *The Hand* (35).

In 1931, Jacques Joseph, using illustrations of Manchot from 1889, justified and published illustrations of deltopectoral flaps as vascular-pattern flaps (36,37). The deltopectoral flap was later popularized and used imaginatively by V. Y. Bakamjian, as described in his papers starting in 1965 (38,39). McGregor and Jackson showed its use in hand surgery (40).

A debate between S. H. Milton (41) and P. M. Stell (42) raged in the early seventies on the appropriate base for random flaps. By then, the classification of flaps according to the nature of the pedicle had begun to crystallize. McGregor and Morgan had hinted at it in 1960 (43). Ten years later, McGregor and Jackson proposed that one could outline self-contained vascular territories (44). They referred to work by Shaw, who, together with Payne, had described such a flap based on the superficial epigastric arterial and venous system (45). The technique was developed for care of the wounded during World War II. Other developments in tissue transfer in hand surgery were described in the volumes on hand surgery in World War II (see below).

General plastic surgery as a discipline made enormous strides during this war. For example, at the beginning of the war, there were only four fully experienced plastic surgeons in Great Britain: Gillies, McIndoe, Mowlem, and Kilner. This nucleus of surgeons and their trainees established plastic surgical centers throughout Great Britain, and each made major contributions to the field.

In the United States, Fomon's 1939 *The Surgery of Injury and Plastic Repair* (46) and Barsky's *Principles and Practice of Plastic Surgery* (47) appeared at the beginning of World War II. During the war, Ivy and a group of plastic surgical luminaries wrote two manuals on plastic and maxillofacial surgery for use by military surgeons (48). Plastic surgical centers such as the one at Valley Forge General Hospital were spawning grounds for consolidation of reconstructive strategies. James Barrett Brown, Sheehan, McDowell, Tanzer, Littler, and Cannon exemplify what could be an enormous list of contributors. Books by Sheehan (49), Ivy (50), Kazanjian and Converse (51), May (52), New and Erich (53), Padgett and Stephenson (54), Pick (55), and Smith (56), among others, were published after experiences during the war.

McGregor et al. described the anatomic basis for a flap based on the superficial circumflex iliac vessels (57), the classic McGregor or groin flap. The groin flap has been a mainstay in reconstructive hand surgery (58,59). The terms *random* and *axial* were applied to flaps in McGregor and Morgan's paper in 1973 (60,61).

Early in the twentieth century, the carrying pedicle for random or chance axial pedicle flaps was large and flat. It was refined to a closed tube independently by the Russian Filatov in 1917 (62) and by Gillies at about the same time (20,63,64). Pedicle flaps with identifiable blood vessels had become the rule wherever possible.

Sterling Bunnell's second edition of *Surgery of the Hand* (65) drew heavily from experiences in hand centers during World War II. It was filled with a variety of types of pedicle flaps, as well as his additional technical modifications of the tubed-pedicle flap technique.

William L. White put together an organized review of flap grafts (66) for a meeting that he organized and chaired in Pittsburgh in 1959.

With waltzing, jumping, and tubing, the transfer of tissues from place to place in endless combinations (67), including composites of skin, fascia, muscle (68), and bone, was firmly established (69).

ISLAND PEDICLE FLAP

Since the turn of this century, further refinement of the carrying pedicle had reached the point where flaps are transferred regularly on vascular and neurovascular bundles. The principle of transfer without an intact epithelialized skin pedicle was initiated by Robert Gersuny, of Vienna. In 1887, he published a description of the transfer of a composite flap of soft tissue from the neck to the oral lining of the cheeks (70) carried on a very narrow pedicle of dermis and subdermal vessels from the periosteum of the mandible. This was a one-stage transfer of a pedicle flap without an intact skin pedicle and without specifically identifiable blood vessels.

In August of 1882, Theodore Dunham, of New York, excised a large epidermoid cancer of the cheek and eyelid. He raised a flap from the forehead, and in his publication (71) said, "This flap was so cut as to contain traversing its pedicle and ramifying in it, the anterior temporal artery." Three days after the first procedure, Dunham dissected out the vascular pedicle and buried it beneath the skin of the cheek. The skin pedicle was returned to its donor site. This was the first recorded two-stage island pedicle flap preserving the transferred blood supply intact.

However, it was Monks in 1898 who repaired the defect resulting from an excision of a lower eyelid epithelioma and who first reported a one-stage island pedicle flap (72). He illustrated the procedure that same year in the *Boston Medical and Surgical Journal*. Shelton Horsely beautifully illustrated the use of a forehead flap carried on temporal vessels in a paper in the *Journal of the American Medical Association* in 1915 (73).

J. F. S. Esser, publishing in the *New York Journal of Medicine* in 1917 (74), pointed out that during his care of wounded soldiers in Austria, he often used flaps from the neck directly under the jawline near the external maxillary artery. These flaps had no skin pedicle, but a carrying arm consisting of soft tissue that contained the external maxillary artery. Said Esser, "I called them 'island flaps' because after being placed in the facial defect resulting when scars are removed, they give the effect of a free transplantation."

There was renewed interest in the island pedicle flap for a variety of uses in the sixties (75–80). For example, temporal arterial island flaps found a place in eyebrow reconstruction and for coverage of difficult areas requiring a permanently transferred blood supply.

In this contemporary period of hand surgery, the biologic or island pedicle flap described earlier was first applied to the hand. Erik Moberg (81), discussing a paper by Donal Brooks on nerve grafting (82) at the annual meeting of the American Orthopaedic Association at Bretton Woods, New Hampshire, in 1954, suggested that neurovascular flap techniques were useful in restoring stereognosis to the hand. He showed some exemplary cases. Littler discussed uses of the neurovascular island 2 years later, and Tubiana et al. (79,80), Frackelton and Teasley (83), Holevich (84), Hueston (85), O'Brien (86), Lewin (87), Peacock (78), Winsten (88), and many, many others (89) published ingenious applications of the versatile techniques. Littler reviewed the development in detail during his Monk's Lecture delivered in Boston in 1982 (90).

The versatile island flap (91) could be used as part of a carrier for a nerve transfer to innervate an intact but anesthetic digit tip. It could be used to bring cover and blood supply to a badly damaged devascularized finger. It was useful in transferring composite parts of useless digits to restore others, including whole joints. Many hand surgeons have pointed to its efficacy in the restoration of protective and useful sensibility and blood supply in osteoplastic thumb reconstruction (92–100).

MUSCLE AND MUSCULOCUTANEOUS FLAPS

The first published, planned muscle flap was that of Louis Ombredanne of Paris in 1906 (101). He described a pectoralis minor flap for breast reconstruction, turning down the humeral insertion of the pectoralis minor to recreate a breast mound following mastectomy.

Tanzini introduced a latissimus dorsi muscle flap for breast reconstruction in 1906 (102). The first true musculocutaneous flap was that described in detail in 1912 by Professor Stefano d'Este and published in a monumental paper on chest-wall reconstruction after mastectomy (103). He used the latissimus dorsi and showed the anatomy of both a musculocutaneous flap and an axial flap of skin alone from the same area. Illustrated examples were shown.

The roots, then, were well set at the beginning of the century for refinement of the principles of the modern muscular and musculocutaneous flaps that have become so popular and important in the current era. The interest in muscle and musculocutaneous flaps was renewed when Neal Owens in 1955 suggested the use of a compound neck pedicle composed of the sternocleidomastoid muscle overlying platysma, subcutaneous tissue, and skin in the reconstruction of major facial defects (104).

Ralph Ger, of Capetown, showed the virtue of muscle transfer for coverage of difficult areas in the distal lower limb in a seminal paper in 1966 (105). Shortly thereafter, Miguel Orticochea, of Bogota, Columbia, described the musculocutaneous flap method (106). He presented the technique, using a gracilis musculocutaneous flap as a cross-leg flap with success.

Typically, the empirical but logical use of muscle alone (107) and muscle with overlying skin led to possible application of that principle throughout the body (108–113). For example, after sporadic reports of muscle flaps and musculocutaneous flaps, McCraw and Dibbell outlined possible independent myocutaneous flaps (114); then, fasciocutaneous flaps (115,116) were launched (117–119). Muscles with nutrient vessels are usable as pedicles to carry substantial skin and soft tissue. As an example, the rectus abdominis muscle with its superior epigastric vascular leash may be used to carry a large transverse segment of soft tissue (120), that is axial on its ipsilateral and random on its contralateral side, from the lower abdomen to the breast area.

Credit goes to Elliott and Hartrampf for championing this remarkable transfer of tissue (121). Muscle and musculocutaneous flaps have found multiple uses in upper limb surgery, and even intrinsic muscles are useful as muscle or musculocutaneous carriers (122). Hentz et al. (123) showed the use of the abductor digiti minimi as a musculocutaneous flap within the hand.

FREE COMPOSITE-TISSUE TRANSFER WITH IMMEDIATE REVASCULARIZATION

Once the pedicle for transfer was refined to require only blood vessels with or without sensory nerves, the only remaining deterrent to unlimited anatomic transfer of composite tissues was the length of vascular tether. It followed predictably that the next advance would be an assault on that deterrent. The answer would come from refinements of techniques described by Carrell at the turn of the century (124,125), made possible by the advent of the operating microscope.

Stimulated by the possibilities offered by microsurgery reported by Jacobson and Suarez from Burlington, Vermont (126), Buncke and Schultz (127) worked tirelessly with methods to improve sutures and instruments. Their influence on Berish Strauch, Avron Daniller, Donald Murray, and others in our Stanford laboratories resulted in rat renal transplant developments and rat limb replants.

Clinically, Komatsu and Tamai's thumb replantation in 1968 (128) ushered in the new era of digit replantation (129–132). Buncke et al. reported their one-stage Nicoladoni thumb reconstruction, transferring a big toe to the thumb position in monkeys (133), and Cobbett soon thereafter reported a successful clinical case of such a free digital toe-to-hand transfer (134). The procedure is now well established in hand surgery (135–137).

Berish Strauch and Donald Murray (138), stimulated by the work of Harry Buncke, worked out and reported the transfer of groin skin flaps to the neck in rats.

With that background, and with knowledge of Goldwyn, Lamb, and White's experiments (139) and the vascularized island experiments of Krizek et al. (140), Kaplan, Buncke, and Murray attempted and reported a free flap from the groin to an intraoral site in 1971 (141). The flap survived for 2½ weeks, but it failed to heal to the poorly vascularized recipient bed. Rollin Daniel, after hearing the paper reporting the case, was stimulated to persevere. When the opportunity arose, he and Ian Taylor tried again and reported the first successful free-flap transfer in 1971 (142).

There followed a rash of reports of free groin flap transfers in hand surgery (143–149). The clear advantages of such free flaps are that they supply skin and soft-tissue cover with permanent arterial blood supply and sometimes sensibility in a single stage. Subsequent tendon grafts then may restore extension function. The flap may be a composite of skin and soft tissue with tendons to eliminate the need for later tendon grafting, or it may carry bone as well (150). Morrison et al. have introduced us to the wraparound free composite flap in thumb reconstruction (151)—a modification that Lister, Steichen, and others have used to restore a thumb tip and nail. Free microvascular transfers apply to any part or composite of parts whose viability may be maintained by isolated vessels (152–154).

FREE FUNCTIONAL MUSCLE AND MUSCULOCUTANEOUS FLAPS WITH IMMEDIATE REVASCULARIZATION

The first reported attempts to free transfer skeletal muscle were those of Noel Thompson (155), who startled those attending the Fifth International Congress of Plastic and Reconstructive Surgery in Melbourne in 1971 by showing a technique of free transfer of the palmeris longus or intrinsic foot muscles (the extensor digitorum brevis) to the face (156) without surgical revascularization. After transfer, the patients regained function through muscular neurotization. In 1975, Gerhard Freilinger, of Vienna, did similar free muscle grafts (157), innervating them with nerve grafts from the contralateral facial nerve.

Meanwhile, Tamai and colleagues had been experimenting with free muscle transfers with microvascular and microneural anatomoses in dog rectus femoris muscles (158). They showed survival of the transferred muscles with an interval of denervation atrophy followed by recovery of innervation at about 3 months. They suggested the use of such transfers in humans.

Harii et al. reported free gracilis muscle transfers to the face using microvascular and microneural revascularization and innervation techniques with success (159). They suggested that the principle of free revascularized and reinnervated muscle transfers "would find broad use in reconstructive surgery."

Ralph Manktelow, of Canada, having seen some examples of free vascularized muscle transfers at the Sixth People's Hospital in Shanghai and having carried out some animal experiments in his laboratory, started to build a series of free, revascularized, and reinnervated muscle transfers in the upper limb of selected patients. In 1978, at the annual meeting of the American Society for Surgery of the Hand, Manktelow and McKee reported their experience with free musculocutaneous transfers, using a gracilis muscle in one patient and a pectoralis muscle in another, transferred to restore finger flexion (160). The feasibility and growing reliability of these free muscle and musculocutaneous transfers (161–163), as prophetically stated by Harii et al. (159), obviously will have a "wide range of applications in reconstructive surgery."

It has taken the perseverance and faith of a Harry Buncke (164), the energetic aggressiveness of a Bernie O'Brien (165), the patience and technical expertise of Tamai and Harii (166), the organization of the Kleinert (167), Kutz (168), and Lister groups, and the ever-growing list of young microsurgeons (169) to take the early work of Jacobson and Suarez and to place it firmly in the armamentarium of reconstructive surgeons. These pioneers found their greatest pleasure in doing what people said could not be done (170).

Work with venous flaps and arteriovenous flaps is moving from the laboratory to clinical application, one more step toward broadening the armamentarium of the reconstructive surgeon.

There appear to be inexhaustible imaginations among surgeons developing new and innovative flaps for use in every part of the body. Progressive liberation from the large carrying pedicle to the refined vascularized and innervated island flaps to vascularized free flaps has opened the way for near-infinite variations in flap design. New additions to these volumes cover the broad spectrum of composite-tissue transfers in reconstructive surgery. The elders in the field look with a mixture of amazement and envy at surgeons active in the development of new strategies to deal with old problems. In facial, neck, intraoral, esophageal, breast, upper and lower limb, abdominal-wall, genital, and anal reconstruction, there have been new reconstructive techniques added to those in the first edition of this encyclopedia.

The advent of anesthesia opened the way for a flood of new operative procedures in the second half of the 19th century. The evolution of microsurgery in this century has been responsible for the current plethora of new techniques. It is my firm belief that the next wave of innovations will emerge as a result of progress in the related field of transplantation. Solutions for the residual immunologic problems in transplantation will prepare the way for a torrent of procedures based on knowledge of techniques developed by surgeons devoted to the field of composite-tissue transfer.

Meanwhile, exhaustive studies of gross and microscopic vascular anatomy, exemplified by Taylor's mapping of neurovascular territories (171), coupled with anatomic studies to clarify the spectacular advances in imaging, feed into the growing armamentarium available to today's reconstructive surgeons.

References

1. Wallace AF. History of plastic surgery. *J R Soc Med* 1978;71:834.
2. Zies E. *The Zeiss index and history of plastic surgery, 900 B.C. to 1863 A.D.,* Vol. 1. Baltimore: Williams & Wilkins, 1977.
3. Tagliacozzi G. *De curtorum chirurgia per institione,* Vol. 2. Venice: 1597.
4. *Gentleman's Magazine.* London, October 1974;891.
5. Carpue JC. An account of two successful operations for restoring a lost nose from the integuments of the forehead. London: 1816.
6. von Graefe CF. *Rhinoplastik.* Berlin: 1818.
7. Zeis E. *Handbuch der Plastischen Chirurgie.* Berlin: 1818.
8. Warren JM. *Boston Med Surg J* 1837.
9. Fricke JCG. *Die Bildung neuer Augenlider (Blepharoplastik) nach Zerstorungen und dadurch hervorge-brachten Auswartswendungen derselben.* Hamburg: 1829.
10. Malgaigne JF. *Manuel de médecine operatoire.* Brusells: 1834.
11. Hamilton FH. Elkoplasty: on ulcers treated by anaplasty. *NY J Med* 1854.
12. Prince D. *Plastics: a new classification and a brief exposition of plastic surgery.* Philadelphia: Lindsay and Blakiston, 1868.
13. Shrady G. The finger as a medium for transplanting skin flaps. *Med Rec* 1891.
14. Halsted W. Plastic operation for extensive burn of neck. *Johns Hopkins Hosp Bull* 1896.
15. Blair VP. The delayed transfer of long pedical flaps in plastic surgery. *Surg Gynecol Obstet* 1921;3:261.
16. Hoffmeister FS. Studies on timing of tissue transfer in reconstructive surgery. *Plast Reconstr Surg* 1957;19:283.
17. Patterson TIS, Berry RJ, Wiernik G. The effect of x-radiation on the survival of skin flaps in the pig. *Br J Plast Surg* 1972;25:17.
18. Colson P, Houot R, Gangolphe M, et al. Utilisation des lambeaux degraisses (lambeaux-greffes) en chirurgie reparatrice de la main. *Ann Chir Plast* 1967;12:298.
19. Jobert AJ. (de Lamballe). *Traité de chirurgie plastique.* Paris: Bailliere, 1849.
20. Gillies HD. Present-day plastic operation of the face. *J Natl Dent Assoc* 1920;1:3.
21. Gillies HD. *Plastic surgery of the face.* London: Frowde, 1920.
22. Blair VP. *Surgery and diseases of the mouth and jaws.* St. Louis: Mosby, 1912.
23. Boo-Chai K. John Wood and his contributions to plastic surgery: the first groin flap. *Br J Plast Surg* 1977;30:9.
24. Wood J. Fission and extroversion of the bladder with epispadias with the results of 8 cases treated by plastic operations. *Med Chir Trans* 1869;2:85.
25. Davis JS. The use of the pedunculated flap in reconstructive surgery. *Ann Surg* 1918;68:221.
26. Germany W, Finesilver EM, Davis JS. Establishment of circulation in tubed skin flaps. *Arch Surg* 1933;26:27.
27. Roberts JB. Salvage of the hand by timely reparative surgery. *Ann Surg* 1919;70:627.
28. Albee FH. Synthetic transplantation of tissues to form a new finger. *Ann Surg* 1919;69:379.
29. Skillern PG Jr. A surgical clinic at Polyclinic Hospital. *Int Clin* 1919;3:75.
30. Steindler A. *Reconstructive surgery of the upper extremity.* New York: Appleton, 1923.
31. Steindler A. *A textbook of operative orthopedics.* New York: Appleton, 1925.
32. Kanavel AB. *Infections of the hand,* 5th ed. Philadelphia: Lea & Febiger, 1925.
33. Iselin M. *Chirurgie de la main: plaies, infections, chirurgie reparatrice.* Paris: Masson, 1933.
34. Iselin M. *Surgery of the hand, wounds, infections and closed tramata.* Philadelphia: Blakiston, 1940.
35. Cutler CW Jr. *The hand: its disabilities and diseases.* Philadelphia: Saunders, 1942.
36. Gibson T, Robinson DW. The mammary artery pectoral flaps of Jacques Joseph. *Br J Plast Surg* 1976;29:370.
37. Joseph J. *Nasenplastik und sonstige Gesichtsplastik nebst einem Anhang ueber Mammaplastik und einige weitere Operationem aus dem Gebiete der ausseren Korper Plastik.* Leipzig: Verlag von Curt Kapitzsch, 1931.
38. Bakamjian VY. A two-stage method for pharyngoesophageal reconstruction with a primary pectoral skin flap. *Plast Reconstr Sutg* 1965;36:173.
39. Bakamjian VY, Long M, Rigg B. Experience with the medially based deltopectoral flap in reconstructive surgery of the head and neck. *Br J Plast Surg* 1971;24:174.
40. McGregor IA, Jackson IT. The extended role of the deltopectoral flap. *Br J Plast Surg* 1970;23:173.
41. Milton SH. Pedicled skin flaps: the fallacy of the length-width ratio. *Br J Surg* 1970;57:502.
42. Stell PM. The viability of skin flaps. *Ann R Coll Surg Engl* 1977;59:236.
43. McGregor I. Flap reconstruction in hand surgery: the evolution of presently used methods. *J Hand Surg* 1979;4B:1.
44. McGregor IA, Jackson IT. The groin flap. *Br J Plast Surg* 1972;25:3.
45. Shaw DT, Payne RL. One-stage tubed abdominal flaps: single-pedicle tubes. *Surg Gynecol Obstet* 1946;83:205.
46. Fomon S. *The surgery of injury and plastic repair.* Baltimore: Williams & Wilkins, 1939.
47. Barsky AI. *Principles and practice of plastic surgery.* Philadelphia: Saunders, 1938.
48. Ivy RH. *Manual of standard practice of plastic and maxillofacial surgery.* Philadelphia: Saunders. 1942.
49. Sheehan JE. *General and plastic surgery with emphasis on war injuries.* New York: Hoeber and Harper, 1945.

50. Ivy RH, Curtis L. *Fractures of the jaws*. Philadelphia: Lea & Febiger, 1945.
51. Kazanjian VH, Converse JM. *The surgical treatment of facial injuries*. Baltimore: Williams & Wilkins, 1949.
52. May H. *Reconstructive and reparative surgery*. Philadelphia: Davis, 1947, 1958.
53. New GB, Erich JB. *The use of pedicle flaps of skin in plastic surgery of the head and neck*. Springfield, Ill.: Charles C. Thomas, 1950.
54. Padgett EC, Stephenson KL. *Plastic and reconstructive surgery*. Springfield, Ill.: Charles C. Thomas, 1948.
55. Pick JF. *Surgery of repair: principles, problems, procedures*, Vols. 1 and 2. Philadelphia: Lippincott, 1949.
56. Smith F. *Plastic and reconstructive surgery*. Philadelphia: Saunders, 1950.
57. Smith PJ, Foley B, McGregor IA, et al. The anatomical basis of the groin flap. *Plast Reconstr Surg* 1972;49:41.
58. Heath PM, Jackson IT, Cooney WP, et al. Simultaneous bilateral staged groin flaps for coverage of mutilating injuries of the hand. *Ann Plast Surg* 1983;11:462.
59. Lister GD, McGregor IA, Jackson IT. The groin flap in hand injuries. *Injury* 1973;4:229.
60. McGregor IA, Morgan G. Axial and random pattern flaps. *Br J Plast Surg* 1973;26:202.
61. Smith PJ. The vascular basis of axial pattern flaps. *Br J Plast Surg* 1973;26:150.
62. Filatov VP. Plastic procedure using a round pedicle. *Surg Clin North Am* 1959;39:277.
63. Gillies HD. The tubed pedicle in plastic surgery. *NY Med J* 1920;11:1.
64. Webster JP. The early history of the tubed pedicle flap. *Surg Clin North Am* 1959;39:261.
65. Bunnell S. *Surgery of the hand*, 2d ed. Philadelphia: Lippincott, 1948.
66. White WL. Flap grafts to the upper extremity. *Surg Clin North Am* 1960;40:389.
67. Holevich J. Our technique of pedicle skin flaps and its use in the surgery of the hand and fingers. *Acta Chir Plast* 1960;24:271.
68. Hokin JAB. Mastectomy reconstruction without a prosthetic implant. *Plast Reconstr Surg* 1983;72:810.
69. Gilles H. Autograft of amputated digit. *Lancet* 1940;1:1002.
70. Gersuny R. Plastischer Ersatz der Wangenschleimhaut. *Zentralbl Chir* 1887;14:706.
71. Dunham T. A method for obtaining a skin flap from the scalp and a permanent buried vascular pedicle for covering defects of the face. *Ann Surg* 1893;17:677.
72. Monks GH. The restoration of a lower eyelid by a new method. *Boston Med Surg J* 1898;139:385.
73. Horsley JS. Transplantation of the anterior temporal artery. *JAMA* 1915;64:408.
74. Esser JFS. Island flaps. *NY Med J* 1917;106:264.
75. Chase RA. Expanded clinical and research uses of composite tissue transfers on isolated vascular pedicles. *Am J Surg* 1967;114:222.
76. Kuei SJ, Chen EC, Li SY. The use of temporal artery pedicle skin flaps in the repair of facial burns and other deformities. *Chin Med J* 1964;83:65.
77. Murray JF, Ord JVR, Gavelin GE. The neurovascular island pedicle flap: an assessment of late results in sixteen cases. *J Bone Joint Surg* 1967;49A:1285.
78. Peacock EE. Reconstruction of the hand by the local transfer of composite-tissue island flaps. *Plast Reconstr Surg* 1960;25:298.
79. Tubiana R, DuParc J. Restoration of sensibility in the hand by neurovascular skin island transfer. *J Bone Joint Surg* 1961;43B:474.
80. Tubiana R, DuParc J, Moreau C. Restauration de la sensibilité au niveau de la main par transfert d'un transplant cutané heterodigital muni de son pedicule vasculo-nerveux. *Rev Chir Orthop* 1960;46:163.
81. Moberg E. Nerve-grafting in orthopedic surgery. *J Bone Joint Surg* 1955;37A:305.
82. Brooks DM, Seddon HJ. Pectoral transplantation for paralysis of the flexors of the elbow. *J Bone Joint Surg* 1959;41B:36.
83. Frackelton WH, Teasley JL. Neurovascular island pedicle: extension in usage. *J Bone Joint Surg* 1962;44A:1069.
84. Holevich J. A new method of restoring sensibility to the thumb. *J Bone Joint Surg* 1973;45B:496.
85. Hueston J. The extended neurovascular island flap. *Br J Plast Surg* 1965;18:304.
86. O'Brien B. Neurovascular pedicle transfers in the hand. *Aust NZ J Surg* 1965;35:1.
87. Lewin ML. Sensory island flap in osteoplastic reconstruction of the thumb. *Am J Surg* 1965;109:226.
88. Winsten J. Island pedicle to restore stereognosis in hand injuries. *N Engl J Med* 1963;268:124.
89. Rose EH. Local arterialized island flap coverage of difficult hand defects preserving donor digit sensibility. *Plast Reconstr Surg* 1983;72:848.
90. Littler JW, George H. Monks lecture: man's thumb, nature's special endowment. Harvard Medical School, October 2, 1982.
91. Chase RA. *Atlas of hand surgery*, Vol. 1. Philadelphia: Saunders, 1973.
92. Chase RA. An alternate to pollicization in subtotal thumb reconstruction. *Plast Reconstr Surg* 1969;44:412.
93. Dykes ER. Reconstruction of the thumb. *Hawaii Med J* 1967;27:33.
94. Floyd WE. Reconstruction of the thumb. *J Med Assoc Ga* 1968;57:425.
95. Greeley PW. Reconstruction of the thumb. *Ann Surg* 1946;124:60.
96. McGregor IA, Simonetta C. Reconstruction of the thumb by composite bone-skin flap. *Br J Plast Surg* 1964;17:37.
97. Reid DAC. The neurovascular island flap in thumb reconstruction. *Br J Plast Surg* 1966;19:234.
98. Suzuki T, Takahashi T, Chang S, et al. Reconstruction of the thumb. *Jpn Med J* 1967;41:1013.
99. Woudstra ST. Reconstruction of the thumb. *Arch Chir Med* 1967;19:29.
100. Murray JF, Ord JVR, Gavelin GE. The neurovascular island pedicle flap: an assessment of late results in sixteen cases. *J Bone Joint Surg* 1967; 49A:1285.
101. Teimourian B, Adham MN. Louis Ombredanne and the origin of muscle flap use for immediate breast mound reconstruction. *Plast Reconstr Surg* 1983;72:905.
102. Tanzini. Sporo il nito nuova processo di aupertozione della menuelle. *Riforma Med* 1906;22:757.
103. d'Este S. La technique de l'amputation de la mamelle pour carcinome mammaire. *Rev Chir* 1912;45:164.
104. Owens N. A compound neck pedicle designed for the repair of massive facial defects: formation, development and application. *Plast Reconstr Surg* 1955;15:369.
105. Ger R. The operative treatment of the advanced stasis ulcer. *Am J Surg* 1966;111:659.
106. Orticochea M. The musculocutaneous flap method: an immediate and heroic substitute for the method of delay. *Br J Plast Surg* 1972;25:106.
107. Minami RT, Hentz VR, Vistnes LM. Use of vastus lateralis muscle flap for repair of trochanteric pressure sores. *Plast Reconstr Surg* 1977;60:364.
108. Carroll RE, Kleinman WB. Pectoralis major transplantation to restore elbow flexion to the paralytic limb. *J Hand Surg* 1979;4A:501.
109. Chase RA, Nage DA. Cosmetic incisions and skin, bone, and composite grafts to restore function of the hand. In: *American academy of orthopaedic surgeons instructional course lectures*. Chap. 6. St. Louis: Mosby, 1974.
110. Hovnanian AP. Latissimus dorsi transplantation for loss of flexion or extension of the elbow. *Ann Surg* 1956;143:493.
111. Jackson IT, Pellett C, Smith, JM. The skull as a bone graft donor site. *Ann Plast Surg* 1983;11:527.
112. Stern PJ, Neale HW, Gregory RO, et al. Latissimus dorsi musculocutaneous flap for elbow flexion. *J Hand Surg* 1982;7:25.
113. Zancolli E, Mitre H. Latissimus dorsi transfer to restore elbow flexion. *J Bone Joint Surg* 1973;55A:1265.
114. McCraw JB, Dibbell DG. Experimental definition of independent myocutaneous vascular territories. *Plast Reconstr Surg* 1977;60:212.
115. Barclay TL, Sharpe DT, Chisholm EM. Cross-leg fasciocutaneous flaps. *Plast Reconstr Surg* 1983;72:843.
116. Fonseca JLS. Use of pericranial flap in scalp wounds with exposed bone. *Plast Reconstr Surg* 1983;72:786.
117. Grabb WC, Myers MB, eds. *Skin flaps*. Boston: Little, Brown, 1975.
118. Mathes SJ, Nahai F. *Clinical atlas of muscle and musculocutaneous flaps*. St. Louis: Mosby, 1979.
119. McCraw JB, Dibbell DG, Carraway JH. Clinical definition of independent myocutaneous vascular territories. *Plast Reconstr Surg* 1977;60:341.
120. Bunkis J, Walton RL, Mathes SJ, et al. Experience with the transverse lower rectus abdominis operation for breast reconstruction. *Plast Reconstr Surg* 1983;72:819.
121. Elliott LF, Hartrampf CR. Tailoring of the new breast using the transverse abdominal island flap. *Plast Reconstr Surg* 1983;72:887.
122. Reisman NR, Dellon AL. The abductor digiti minimi muscle flap: a salvage technique for palmar wrist pain. *Plast Reconstr Surg* 1983;72:859.
123. Chase RA, Hentz VR, Apfelberg D. A dynamic myocutaneous flap for hand reconstruction. *J Hand Surg* 1980;5A:594.
124. Carrel A. La technique operatoire des anastomoses vasculaires et la transplantation des viscere. *Lyon Med* 1920;98:859.
125. Carrel A. Results of the transplantation of blood vessels, organs and limbs. *JAMA* 1908;51:1662.
126. Jacobson JH, Suarez EL. Microsurgery in the anastomosis of small vessels. *Surg Forum* 1960;11:243.
127. Buncke HJ, Schulz WP. Total ear reimplantation in the rabbit utilizing microminiature vascular anastomoses. *Br J Plast Surg* 1966;19:15.
128. Komatsu S, Tamai S. Successful replantation of a completely cut-off thumb. *Plast Reconstr Surg* 1968;42:374.
129. Chen ZW, Meyer VE, Kleinert HE, et al. Present indications for replantation as reflected by long-term functional results. *Orthop Clin North Am* 1981;12:849.
130. Gelberman RH, Urbaniak JR, Bright DS, et al. Digital sensibility following replantation. *J Hand Surg* 1978;3A:313.
131. Weiland AJ, Daniel RK, Riley LH. Application of the free vascularized bone graft in the treatment of malignant or aggressive bone tumor. *Johns Hopkins Med J* 1977;140:85.
132. Vilkki S. Replantation studies on clinical replantation surgery with reference to patient selection, operative techniques and postoperative control. *Acta Univ Tamperensis (A)* 1983;156.
133. Buncke HJ, Buncke CM, Schulz WP. Immediate Nicoladoni procedures in the rhesus monkey, or hallux-to-hand transplantation, utilising microminiature vascular anastomoses. *Br J Plast Surg* 1966;19:332.
134. Cobbett JR. Free digital transfer: report of a case of transfer of a great toe to replace an amputated thumb. *J Bone Joint Surg* 1969;51B:677.

135. Buncke HJ, McLean DH, Geroge PT, et al. Thumb replacement: great toe transplantation by microvascular anastomosis. *Br J Plast Surg* 1973;26:194.

136. O'Brien BM, MacLeod AM, Sykes PJ, et al. Microvascular second toe transfer for digital reconstruction. *J Hand Surg* 1978;3A:123.

137. Ohtsuka H, Torigai K, Shioya N. Two toe-to-finger transplants in one hand. *Plast Reconstr Surg* 1977;60:51.

138. Strauch B, Murray DE. Transfer of composite graft with immediate suture anastomosis of its vascular pedicle measuring less than 1 mm in external diameter using microsurgical techniques. *Plast Reconstr Surg* 1967;40:325.

139. Goldwyn RM, Lamb DL, White WL. An experimental study of large island flaps in dogs. *Plast Reconstr Surg* 1963;31:528.

140. Krizek TJ, Tani R, Desprez JD, et al. Experimental transplantation of composite grafts by microsurgical vascular techniques. *Plast Reconstr Surg* 1965;36:538.

141. Kaplan EN, Buncke HJ, Murray DE. Distant transfer of cutaneous island flaps in humans by microvascular anastomoses. *Plast Reconstr Surg* 1973;52:301.

142. Taylor GI, Daniel RK. The free flap: composite tissue transfer by vascular anastomosis. *Aust NZJ Surg* 1973;43:1.

143. Ohmori K, Harii K, Sekiguchi J, et al. The youngest free groin flap yet? *Br J Plast Surg* 1977;30:273.

144. Daniel RK, Terzis JK. *Reconstructive microsurgery*. Boston: Little, Brown, 1977.

145. Daniel RK, Weiland AJ. Free tissue transfers from upper extremity reconstruction. *J Hand Surg* 1982;7A:66.

146. Taylor GI, Townsend P, Corlett R. Superiority of the deep circumflex iliac vessels as the supply for free groin flaps: experimental work. *Plast Reconstr Surg* 1979;64:595.

147. Taylor GI, Townsend P, Corlett R. Superiority of the deep circumflex iliac vessels as the supply for free groin flaps: clinical work. *Plast Reconstr Surg* 1979;64:45.

148. Baudet J, LeMaire JM, Guimberteau JC. Ten free groin flaps. *Plast Reconstr Surg* 1976;57:577.

149. Brent B, Byrd HS. Secondary ear reconstruction with cartilage grafts covered by axial, random, and free flaps of temporoparietal fascia. *Plast Reconstr Surg* 1983;72:141.

150. Swartz WM. Immediate reconstruction of the wrist and dorsum of the hand with a free osteocutaneous groin flap. *J Hand Surg* 1984;9A:18.

151. Morrison WA, O'Brien BM, MacLeod, AM. Thumb reconstruction with a free neurovascular wrap-around flap from the big toe. *J Hand Surg* 1980;5A:575.

152. Van Genechten F, Townsend PLG. Free composite-tissue transfer in a compound hand injury. *Hand* 1983;15:325.

153. Taylor GI, Corlett R, Boyd JB. The extended deep inferior epigastric flap: a clinical technique. *Plast Reconstr Surg* 1983;72:751.

154. Fisher J, Cooney WP. Designing the latissimus dorsi free flap for knee coverage. *Ann Plast Surg* 1983;11:554.

155. Thompson N. Treatment of facial paralysis by free skeletal muscle grafts. In: *Transactions of the fifth international congress of plastic and reconstructive surgery*. Melbourne: Butterworth, 1971.

156. Smith JW. A new technique of facial animation. In: *Transactions of the fifth international congress of plastic and reconstructive surgery*. Melbourne: Butterworth, 1971.

157. Freilinger G. A new technique to correct facial paralysis. *Plast Reconstr Surg* 1975;56:44.

158. Tamai S, Komatsu S, Sakamoto H, et al. Free muscle transplants in dogs with microsurgical neurovascular anastomoses. *Plast Reconstr Surg* 1970;46:219.

159. Harii K, Ohmori K, Torii S. Free gracilis muscle transplantation with microvascular anastomoses for the treatment of facial paralysis. *Plast Reconstr Surg* 1976;57:133.

160. Manktelow RT, McKee NH. Free muscle transplantation to provide active finger flexion. *J Hand Surg* 1978;3A:416.

161. Ikuta Y, Kubo T, Tsuge K. Free muscle transplantation by microsurgical technique to treat severe Volkmann's contracture. *Plast Reconstr Surg* 1976;58:407.

162. Manktelow RT, Zuker RM, McKee NH. Functioning free muscle transplantation. *J Hand Surg* 1984;9A:32.

163. Terzis JK, Dykos RW, Williams HB. Recovery of function in free muscle transplants using microneurovascular anastomoses. *J Hand Surg* 1978;3A:37.

164. Bunke HJ. Cobbett JR, Smith JW, et al. *Techniques of microsurgery*. Sommerville, NJ: Ethicon, 1969.

165. O'Brien BM, Miller GDH. Digital reattachment and revascularization. *J Bone Joint Surg* 1973;55A:714.

166. Tamai S, Hori Y, Tatsumi Y, et al. Hallux-to-thumb transfer with microsurgical technique: a case report in a 45-year-old woman. *J Hand Surg* 1977;2A:152.

167. Kleinert HE, Kasdan ML, Romero JL. Small blood vessel anastomosis for salvage of severely injured upper extremity. *J Bone Joint Surg* 1963;45A:788.

168. Kutz JE, Dimond M. Replantation in the upper extremity. *Surg Rounds* 1982;14:9.

169. Strauch B. Microsurgical approach to thumb reconstruction. *Orthop Clin North Am* 1977;8:319.

170. Ikuta Y. Free flap transfer: historical review, surgical procedures and some clinical cases. *Hiroshima J Med Sci* 1976;25:29.

171. Taylor GI, Gianoutsos MP, Morris SF. The neurovascular territories of the skin and muscles: anatomic study and clinical implications. *Plast Reconstr Surg* 1994;94:1.

CONTENTS

VOLUME I: HEAD AND NECK

SECTION 1: HEAD AND NECK RECONSTRUCTION

PART A ▪ SCALP, FOREHEAD, AND NAPE OF NECK RECONSTRUCTION

PART B ▪ EYELID AND ORBITAL RECONSTRUCTION

Lower Eyelid

Upper Eyelid

Medial Canthus

Total Eyelid and Socket

PART C ■ NASAL RECONSTRUCTION

Nasal Tip, Dorsum, and Alae

Nasal Columella

PART E ▪ CHEEK AND NECK RECONSTRUCTION

Cheek and Neck

PART F ■ LIP RECONSTRUCTION

PART G ■ INTRAORAL RECONSTRUCTION

Online Chapter

PART H ▪ PHARYNGOESOPHAGEAL

VOLUME II: UPPER EXTREMITIES

SECTION II: UPPER EXTREMITY RECONSTRUCTION

PART A ■ FINGER AND THUMB RECONSTRUCTION

Fingertip

Finger

Thumb Tip

Thumb

PART B ▪ HAND

PART E ■ ELBOW

PART F ■ ARM

VOLUME III: TORSO, PELVIS, AND LOWER EXTREMITIES

SECTION III: BREAST, CHEST WALL, AND TRUNK RECONSTRUCTION

PART A ■ BREAST RECONSTRUCTION

Breast Mound

SECTION IV: ABDOMINAL WALL AND PELVIC-REGION RECONSTRUCTION

PART A ▪ ABDOMINAL WALL AND GROIN RECONSTRUCTION

PART B ▪ VAGINAL, VULVAR, AND PERINEAL RECONSTRUCTION

PART C ▪ PENILE, SCROTAL, AND PERINEAL RECONSTRUCTION

PART D ■ ANAL RECONSTRUCTION

PART E ■ LUMBOSACRAL RECONSTRUCTION

PART F ■ ISCHIAL RECONSTRUCTION

PART G ■ TROCHANTERIC RECONSTRUCTION

SECTION V: LOWER EXTREMITY RECONSTRUCTION

PART A ■ LOWER LEG AND KNEE RECONSTRUCTION

PART B ■ FOOT AND ANKLE RECONSTRUCTION

BREAST, CHEST WALL, AND TRUNK RECONSTRUCTION

CHAPTER 345 ■ SKIN EXPANSION

C. RADOVAN*

Skin expansion is a significant development in plastic surgery and expanders have been used clinically since 1976 (1–4). The postmastectomy chest skin and scar are intermittently and gradually expanded, providing the skin envelope needed for the new breast.

After skin expansion, the temporary expander is replaced by a smaller mammary implant, creating a smaller breast mound within the larger skin envelope. This tends to mimic a natural breast, with forward teardrop projection.

INDICATIONS

The most applicable defect for tissue expansion is the deformity following modified radical mastectomy. However, various postmastectomy deformities can be reconstructed regardless of the thickness of the skin flap or the shape of the scar.

The procedure is attractive to patients, even though it is performed in two stages; neither stage is considered a major surgical procedure.

OPERATIVE TECHNIQUE

First Stage

All breasts are reconstructed subcutaneously through a small 5-cm subaxillary incision, either through the lateral tail of the old mastectomy scar or through a new oblique incision. It is

important to position the inframammary border of the pocket at the same horizontal level as the opposite breast. Preserving the inframammary line and expanding the skin into a larger envelope give the breast a natural fold when the implant is finally placed in the pocket.

The pocket is developed mainly by blunt scissor or finger dissection and is preferably about 3 cm wider in circumference than the base of the expander. A small subcutaneous pocket is developed posterior to the incision for placement of the reservoir dome.

The round, extra-large expander is initially filled with 50 to 100 cc of normal saline through the connecting tube. The tube should be shortened to the appropriate length, and the expander should then be attached to the reservoir dome by the connecting tube. It is important to approximate the subcutaneous tissue between the expander and the reservoir to prevent sliding of the reservoir toward the expander (Figs. 1 and 2).

Subsequent normal saline injections of approximately 50 cc or more are given in the office until the skin becomes tight, at a minimum of 5-day intervals, with minor discomfort to the patient. By palpating the reservoir dome and then holding it between the fingers, a no. 22 or 25 needle is inserted through the skin and into the dome. The expanded breast should be 200 to 300 cc larger than the projected size of the permanent prosthesis.

Patients are encouraged to maintain their normal physical activities during the expansion process. After initial insertion of the expander, the chest skin is expanded every 5 to 7 days, and it is capable of doubling its size in an average of 6 weeks (Fig. 3).

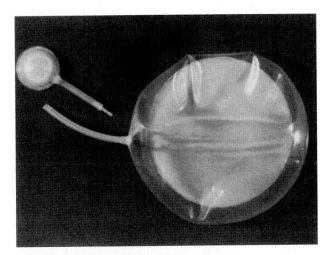

FIG. 1. The temporary expander and reservoir dome. The connecting tube may **be** shortened, as needed, prior to connection.

---

* Deceased.

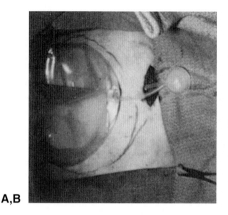
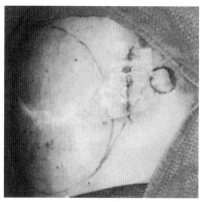

A,B

FIG. 2. A: Position of the expander and reservoir dome on the chest wall, with a small subaxillary incision. B: The reservoir dome is placed in the smaller posterior subcutaneous pocket, and the incision is closed in two layers. A few subcutaneous sutures should be placed around the connecting tube to prevent possible sliding of the reservoir dome toward the expander.

The average starting volume of the expander is 100 to 150 cc normal saline, with additional saline injections of 50 to 100 cc during each office visit. The average expanded breast up to 600 to 650 cc is replaced by a 400- to 450-cc mammary implant.

Second Stage

Through the same subaxillary approach, the expander and the reservoir are removed. Electrocautery should be used for cutting through the subcutaneous planes to remove the expander and reservoir dome, since the silicone envelope is resistant to heat. The amount of normal saline in the expander should be calculated, and a smaller implant should be placed in the pocket to allow mobility and flexibility of the reconstructed breast.

Symmetry and Management of the Opposite Breast

Contralateral round dermal mastopexy with two circumferential periareolar and midbreast incisions has proved satisfactory to match the hemispheric appearance of the reconstructed breast (5). The mastopexy, by reducing the skin around the nipple, simultaneously enlarges the areola, and the outer areolar ring is subsequently used as a graft for reconstruction of the nipple-areola complex of the reconstructed breast (Fig. 4). When indicated, contralateral subcutaneous mastectomy is performed through a similar round dermal pedicle approach with immediate insertion of an implant.

CLINICAL RESULTS

If a hematoma occurs, flap necrosis may occur. The expander should be removed, the hematoma evacuated, and hemostasis established.

A great advantage of this form of reconstruction is that the expander can be deflated if necrosis seems imminent. If the expanded skin changes color or blisters develop, fluid should be withdrawn immediately. The needle should be inserted into the reservoir dome until the skin assumes normal color and tension is relieved. Reexpansion may be resumed 2 to 3 weeks later.

The rate of contracture in these reconstructed breasts is low, a contributing factor being that the initial pocket is 200 to 300 cc larger than the size of the permanent implant.

SUMMARY

The main goal of this form of breast reconstruction is the recovery of lost tissue by expansion of the remaining chest skin. This skin is expanded to large proportions, and the breast envelope is then filled with a small permanent mammary prosthesis.

Because relatively large breasts can be reconstructed using this method, less needs to be done to the opposite breast to achieve symmetry.

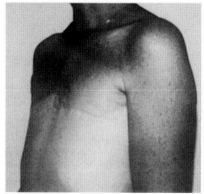
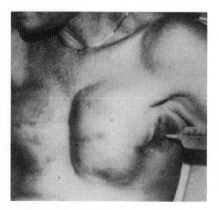
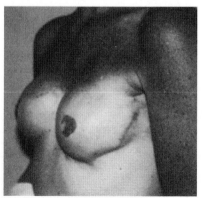

A–C

FIG. 3. A: A 54-year-old woman 7 years after a bilateral modified radical mastectomy. B: At the time of insertion of the expander, extremely tight chest skin would allow injection of only 50 cc normal saline. Expanders were subsequently injected with up to 450 cc normal saline in eight office visits. C: Both expanders were replaced with 300-cc mammary implants. Labial grafts were used for nipple reconstruction.

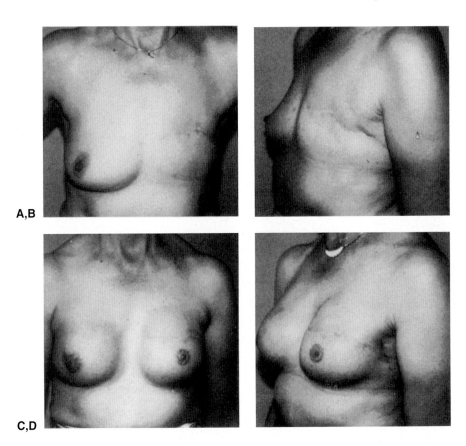

A,B

C,D

FIG. 4. **A,B:** Preoperative views of a 52-year-old woman 2 years after left modified radical mastectomy. **C,D:** The temporary expander was filled with 650 cc normal saline and then replaced with a 450-cc gel-filled implant. The right breast subcutaneous mastectomy was performed through the round dermal mastopexy with immediate reconstruction. Subsequently, the outer ring of the right areola was used for the left areolar reconstruction. Part of the right nipple was used for the left nipple reconstruction.

References

1. Radovan C. Reconstruction of the breast after radical mastectomy using the temporary expander. *Plast Surg Forum* 1978;1:41.
2. Radovan C. Advantages and complications of breast reconstruction using the temporary expander. *Plast Surg Forum* 1980;3:63.
3. Radovan C. Breast reconstruction after mastectomy using the temporary expander. *Plast Reconstr Surg* 1982;69:195.
4. Austad ED, Rose GL. A self-inflating tissue expander. *Plast Reconstr Surg* 1982;70:588.
5. Radovan C, Keunen H. Periareolar breast surgery. Presented at the annual meeting of the American Society of Plastic and Reconstructive Surgeons, Toronto, Canada, 1975.

CHAPTER 346 ■ SUPEROLATERAL PEDICLE FOR BREAST SURGERY

C. K. HERMAN AND B. STRAUCH

The evolution of procedures for reduction of breast volume and improvement of breast shape has been ongoing, based on the rich blood supply that has allowed a plethora of pedicle types. In searching for a technique that could be tailored for use in almost any breast procedure, including both reduction and mastopexy, the following goals have been used as guidelines: (a) an adequate and safe reduction of breast volume or modification of breast shape; (b) correction of ptosis; (c) a lasting and aesthetically pleasing shape with superior pole fullness; and (d) a nipple–areola complex with retained sensibility and vascularity. The superolateral dermoparenchymal pedicle has been adapted for surgery on myriad breast types, using differing skin excisions. It has been used in reduction mammaplasty, mastopexy, and augmentation mastopexy cases.

INDICATIONS

With particular consideration given to the importance of the lateral branch of the fourth intercostal nerve in supplying sensation to the nipple–areola complex (1–3), authors have described and used the superolateral dermoparenchymal pedicle as a basis for surgery on a variety of presenting breast shapes (4). The technique integrates elements from several other procedures. Strombeck (5) developed a horizontal bipedicled dermoparenchymal flap in 1960. Skoog (6) is credited with describing the first lateral pedicle. In 1982, Nicolle (7) presented his experience with the lateral dermoparenchymal pedicle for breast reduction. Cardenas-Camerana and Vergara (8) described their successful use of the superolateral dermoglandular pedicle.

A simple classification system that reflects the versatility of the superolateral pedicle operation has been developed (Figs. 1 and 2), as follows (4): *type I,* superolateral dermoparenchymal pedicle using the modified Wise pattern (9); *type Ia,* reduction mammaplasty of 1,200 g per patient or more; *type Ib,* mastopexy for ptosis, with minimal-to-no reduction of breast parenchyma; *type Ic,* reduction mammaplasty with free nipple grafts; *type II,* superolateral dermoparenchymal pedicle using the vertical pattern; *type IIa,* reduction mammaplasty of 1,200 g per patient or less; *type IIb.i,* mastopexy for ptosis; *type IIb.ii,* mastopexy for ptosis, with mammary prosthetic implant.

ANATOMY

The flap receives its blood supply from its superolateral dermoparenchymal base. Blood supply includes perforators from the internal mammary artery, lateral thoracic artery, multiple

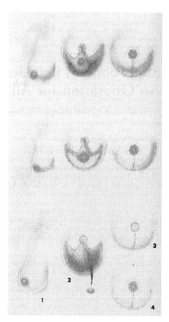

FIG. 1. Wise-type pattern variations (**above**). Superolateral dermoparenchymal resection reserved for larger reductions (type Ia). The pedicle is well vascularized and contains the main innervation to the nipple–areola complex. It provides superior-pole fullness and projection (**center***).* Wise-type pattern resection with superolateral dermoparenchymal resection for mastopexy for correction of ptosis (type Ib) (**below**). Wise-type pattern resection with superolateral dermoparenchymal procedure tailored for very large-breasted women with nipple–areola complexes longer than 40 cm from the sternal notch (type Ic). A free nipple–areola graft is placed on a dermal bed of the superolateral dermoparenchymal pedicle.

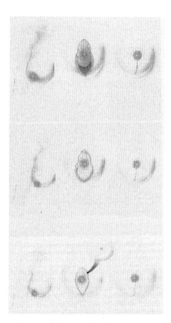

FIG. 2. Vertical pattern variations (**above**). Vertical reduction by using a superolateral dermoparenchymal pedicle for moderate to small reductions (type IIa) (**center**) Vertical mastopexy (type IIb.i). All tissue is used, except for the skin covering of the tissue between the vertical pillars. The superolateral dermoparenchymal pedicle and all the attached deskinned tissues are rotated superiorly. (**below**) Vertical mastopexy with simultaneous augmentation (type IIb.ii). The vertical pillars are redrawn after placement of the inflated prosthesis.

intercostal perforators, thoracoacromial artery, and thoracodorsal artery. Preservation of a parenchymal attachment of the flap to the chest wall along its base enhances the nourishment of the flap and nipple–areola complex. Anatomic innervation to the nipple–areola complex is largely preserved by incorporation of the lateral branch of the fourth intercostal nerve, which is included in the lateral base of the flap.

FLAP DESIGN AND DIMENSIONS

Modified Wise pattern or vertical mammaplasty markings are drawn on the breast. Markings for nipple placement are made along the breast meridian at a level that accounts for the patient's breast size and shape, height, and degree of nipple ptosis. Nipple placement is generally located between 21 and 25 cm from the sternal notch. In designing the superolateral dermoparenchymal pedicle, the areola is first traced with a 42-mm-diameter washer, centering the nipple in the hole of the washer. The superolateral flap is then drawn with a 10- to 12-cm width, starting 2 cm lateral to the meridian and ending 2 to 3 cm lateral to the lower edge of the lateral point of the vertical marking. Depending on the length of the nipple–areola complex, and extending 1 to 2 cm beyond the new 42-mm areolar border, determine the length of the pedicle (Figs. 1 and 2). A 1:1 ratio of length to width is the result.

OPERATIVE TECHNIQUE

The operative procedure involves superior rotation of a superolaterally based dermoparenchymal pedicle, resulting in a "periwinkle" effect, which provides desirable superior pole fullness and increased projection to the breast. The superolaterally based flap is created by incising at the borders of the pedicle perpendicularly down to the level of the pectoralis major fascia.

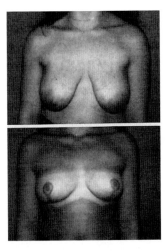

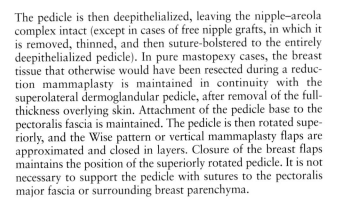

FIG. 3. Wise pattern reduction type Ia. Preoperative (**above**). Postoperative (**below**).

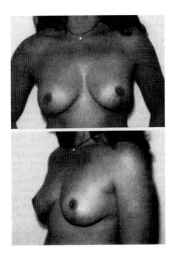

FIG. 4. Same patient as in Fig. 3 at 10 years after operation.

The pedicle is then deepithelialized, leaving the nipple–areola complex intact (except in cases of free nipple grafts, in which it is removed, thinned, and then suture-bolstered to the entirely deepithelialized pedicle). In pure mastopexy cases, the breast tissue that otherwise would have been resected during a reduction mammaplasty is maintained in continuity with the superolateral dermoglandular pedicle, after removal of the full-thickness overlying skin. Attachment of the pedicle base to the pectoralis fascia is maintained. The pedicle is then rotated superiorly, and the Wise pattern or vertical mammaplasty flaps are approximated and closed in layers. Closure of the breast flaps maintains the position of the superiorly rotated pedicle. It is not necessary to support the pedicle with sutures to the pectoralis major fascia or surrounding breast parenchyma.

CLINICAL RESULTS

The superolateral pedicle has been used by the authors in more than 1,500 breast operations. Patients have been followed up for as many as 15 years. Total nipple–areola necrosis was observed in four patients, two patients with bilateral loss and two with unilateral loss (0.2%). Epidermolysis associated with partial areolar loss was seen in three cases (0.2%). Nipple–areola sensitivity was evaluated as normal, or slightly reduced, at 1-year follow-up in 1,440 patients (96%), with only 60 patients reporting significantly diminished or absent sensitivity (4%). Long-term follow-up to 15 years has demonstrated that the results of breast procedures using the superolateral pedicle are maintained well with time (Figs. 3 and 4).

SUMMARY

The superolateral dermoparenchymal pedicle has fulfilled the goals of successful breast surgery. It is a safe and effective technique that has provided long-lasting results for patients. The flap design incorporates both a hearty blood supply and a significant source of innervation to the nipple–areola complex: the lateral branch of the fourth intercostal nerve. It is a reproducible procedure that can be adapted to a variety of skin-excision patterns and breast morphologies.

References

1. Cooper A. *The anatomy of the breast*. London: Longman, 1840.
2. Craig RDP, Sykes PA. Nipple sensitivity following reduction mammaplasty. *Br J Plast Surg* 1970;23:165.
3. Courtiss EH, Goldwyn RM. Breast sensation before and after plastic surgery. *Plast Reconstr Surg* 1976;58:1.
4. Strauch B, Elkowitz M, Baum T, Herman C. Superolateral pedicle for breast surgery: an operation for all reasons. *Plast Reconstr Surg* 2005; 115:1269.
5. Strombeck JO. Mammaplasty: report of a new technique based on the two pedicle procedure. *Br J Plast Surg* 1960;13:79.
6. Skoog TA. technique of breast reduction: transposition of the nipple of a cutaneous vascular pedicle. *Acta Chir Scand* 1953;126:453.
7. Nicolle F. Improved standards in reduction mammoplasty and mastopexy. *Plast Reconstr Surg* 1982;69:453.
8. Cardenas-Camarena L, Vergara R. Reduction mammaplasty with superiorlateral dermoglandular pedicle: another alternative. *Plast Reconstr Surg* 2001;107:693.
9. Wise RJ. A preliminary report on a method of planning the mammaplasty. *Plast Reconstr Surg* 1956;17:367.

CHAPTER 347 ■ MEDIAL PEDICLE FLAP FOR BREAST-REDUCTION SURGERY

E. J. HALL-FINDLAY

Breast surgical techniques have focused on altering the size and shape of the breast while preserving and mobilizing the nipple–areolar complex. Various flaps (or pedicles) have been designed to preserve circulation to the nipple and areola. These flaps should also preserve sensation and breast-feeding potential when possible.

The medial flap for the nipple and areola provides versatility, when contemplating breast reduction or mastopexy procedures.

INDICATIONS

The flap was originally described and used by both Strombeck (1) and Skoog (2). Strombeck initially described the flap as part of a horizontal bipedicle flap, but he would often use it alone in breast surgery. Skoog would use either the lateral or medial pedicle, and the description in this chapter follows his design for orientation in breast-reduction surgery. Asplund and Davies (3) used a similar flap, but they used a dermal flap, rather than a dermal–glandular flap.

ANATOMY

Both dermal and dermoglandular flaps have a good blood supply. As pointed out by Reid and Taylor (4), the blood supply to the breast is superficial.

Arterial

The main arterial input is from the internal thoracic (mammary) system. The superficial branch of the lateral thoracic artery supplies a lateral pedicle. The thoracoacromial system is relatively unimportant.

The second or third intercostal branch of the internal mammary artery passes laterally (supplying a deltopectoral flap), and a strong descending branch supplies a superior pedicle. The intercostal branches come out from under the lateral border of the sternum, quickly penetrate the breast tissue, and become superficial. The branch that supplies a superior pedicle passes just medial to the breast meridian, and about 1 cm deep to the skin surface as it approaches the areola.

The medial pedicle is supplied by the third or fourth intercostal branches of the internal mammary artery. These branches appear above the pectoralis muscle, just lateral to the sternal border. They immediately enter the breast parenchyma and become superficial. A medial pedicle can be thinned, as long as the deep tissue close to the sternal border is preserved. Because these vessels are sometimes damaged in breast-augmentation procedures, a medial pedicle may not be a good choice in a subsequent mastopexy procedure. In those cases, a superior pedicle is more likely to still have an intact arterial supply.

The fourth or fifth branches of the internal mammary artery actually run beneath the pectoralis muscle and perforate the muscle just medial to the breast meridian, about 4 to 6 cm above the inframammary fold. This artery supplies an inferior or central pedicle. It is the only artery that is accompanied by venae comitantes.

Venous

Taylor has pointed out that the veins do not accompany the arteries, except for the perforator, which supplies an inferior pedicle. The veins can often be easily seen just beneath the dermis. They should be noted, and an attempt should be made to include at least one vein in the base of the pedicle (Fig. 1).

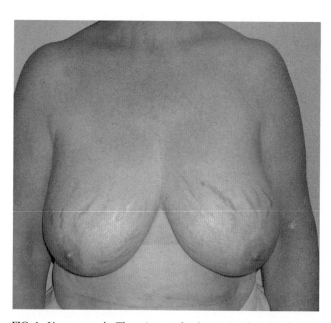

FIG. 1. Venous supply. The veins are clearly seen just beneath the dermis. It is important to try to include a vein in the base of the pedicle. This is best seen on the left breast.

Because the veins are superficial, it is not a good idea to infiltrate the incisions for hemostasis, because these veins can be damaged.

Innervation

It is commonly accepted that the lateral branch of the fourth intercostal nerve supplies sensation to the nipple. Experience with the medial pedicle shows that this nerve is not exclusive. Schlenz et al. (5) showed that both medial and superior nerves also supply the breast.

The lateral fourth intercostal nerve has both a superficial and a deep branch. The deep branch passes just above the pectoralis fascia and then turns immediately upward into the breast parenchyma at the level of the breast meridian. A full-thickness medial pedicle should be able to preserve this deep branch. An analysis of the author's patients has shown that the superior, lateral, and medial pedicles all have equivalent sensation.

FLAP DESIGN AND DIMENSIONS

The medial pedicle is often described as "superomedial" because it does seem to take that direction when the patient is standing. However, the pedicle is technically completely "medial," because the blood supply comes from a medial direction. This is more obvious when the patient is lying down. When a patient stands, the breast sags, but so do the blood vessels.

Designing the base of the pedicle, as Skoog did, with half the base in the areolar opening and half the base in the vertical aspect of the skin-resection pattern, makes the pedicle easy to rotate into position. The dermis can be left attached superiorly, to include either arterial input or venous drainage. In this situation, the deep tissue will have to be resected superiorly, to allow easy inset, but this will not damage the superficial blood supply.

A centimeter cuff of dermis is left around the areola in the pedicle for safety. This is called the Schwartzmann (6) maneuver and is helpful because the pedicle often appears to be undermined, even when it is carefully created as a full-thickness pedicle.

There is no scientific basis for knowing how wide to create the base of the pedicle. It should be wide enough that it is likely to include at least one of the medial intercostal branches of the internal mammary artery. In a small breast reduction, the base may be only 6 to 8 cm, and in larger reductions, the base may be 8 to 10 cm.

No definite numbers are known as to how long a medial pedicle can be for viability. Theoretically, the blood vessels stretch as the pedicle itself stretches with enlargement and sagging of the breast. Conversely, a very long pedicle will be bulky, and the weight of an overlying large medial pedicle can lead to bottoming out. The author warns those patients who have long pedicles that a decision will be made intraoperatively as to whether it would be wise to convert to free nipple grafts.

OPERATIVE TECHNIQUE

A medial flap for the nipple areolar complex can be used with various skin-resection patterns. The medial flap is based on the keyhole pattern, so it is equally applicable to vertical and inverted-T techniques.

Although the inferior pedicle became the standard after the introduction of the vertical bipedicle approach to breast reduction by Paul McKissock, using the inferior pedicle means that the heavy inferior breast tissue is left behind. The medial pedicle allows complete removal of the inferior excess, and the breast tissue that remains is left attached to the superior, superomedial, and superolateral skin. The author believes that this will lead to fewer cases of bottoming out.

The pedicle is deepithelialized (Fig. 2A) and then created as a full-thickness flap, by using either the scalpel or cutting cautery (Fig. 2B and C). It will be noticed during the dissection that most of the bleeding will be superficial.

The excess parenchyma is removed en bloc (Fig. 2D), and the perforator to the inferior pedicle will be encountered. If tumescent-type infiltration is used in the base of the breast, the surgeon must carefully seek out this artery and its venae comitantes to prevent later bleeding and the development of a hematoma. A lateral pillar of approximately 2 cm of

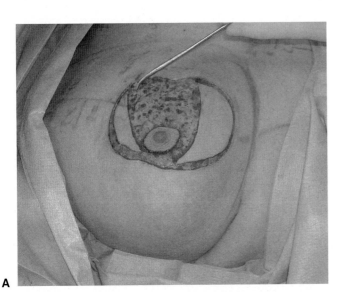

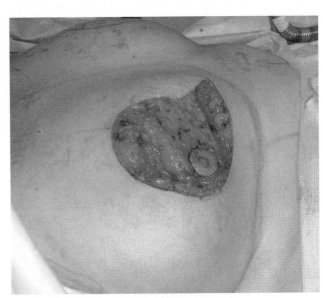

A   B

FIG. 2. Operative technique. A: The medial pedicle is deepithelialized. The hemostat is pointing to a vein preserved just below the dermis. B: The medial pedicle is created as a full-thickness flap. *(continued)*

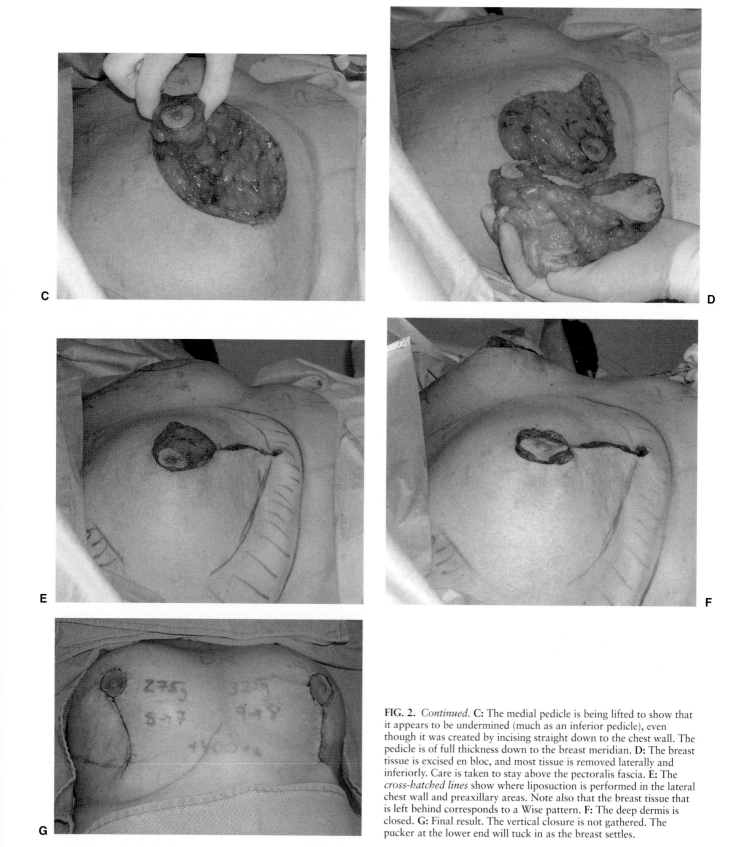

FIG. 2. *Continued.* **C:** The medial pedicle is being lifted to show that it appears to be undermined (much as an inferior pedicle), even though it was created by incising straight down to the chest wall. The pedicle is of full thickness down to the breast meridian. **D:** The breast tissue is excised en bloc, and most tissue is removed laterally and inferiorly. Care is taken to stay above the pectoralis fascia. **E:** The *cross-hatched lines* show where liposuction is performed in the lateral chest wall and preaxillary areas. Note also that the breast tissue that is left behind corresponds to a Wise pattern. **F:** The deep dermis is closed. **G:** Final result. The vertical closure is not gathered. The pucker at the lower end will tuck in as the breast settles.

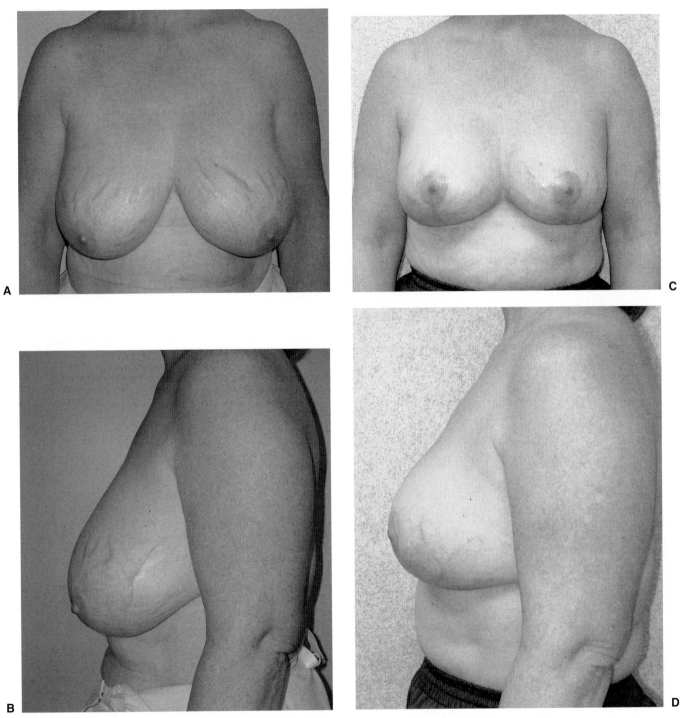

FIG. 3. Results in the same patient as shown in Figs. 1 and 2. **A:** Preoperative frontal view. **B:** Preoperative lateral view; 275 g was removed from the right breast and 325 g from the left breast; 400 cc of fat was removed with liposuction. **C:** Frontal view at 2.5 months. **D:** Lateral view at 2.5 months.

AU1

thickness should be left [following the Wise pattern (Fig. 2F) attached to the lateral skin flap]. Excess breast tissue parallel to the chest wall can be removed from under the flap by beveling out laterally. Some tissue is beveled out medially, as well, just above the inframammary fold. This direct excision can be followed by liposuction peripherally for final tailoring.

The pillars are brought together and sutured. It is important not to place too much tension on the pillar closure. Sutures should be placed in the fibrous tissue on either side

only sufficiently to approximate the pillars so that they can heal together.

The dermis is then closed with deep dermal sutures. At this point, liposuction (Fig. 2E) is performed to tailor the shape of the breast, to leave the tissue behind that resembles a Wise pattern (Fig. 2F). Liposuction is also performed for the excess tissue that is often present in the lateral chest wall and the preaxillary areas.

At this stage, it must be determined whether there is sufficient excess skin that needs to be removed in an inverted

T pattern. This will be more likely in patients with extremely large breasts or in patients with poor skin elasticity. Adding a T is not required as often as surgeons think when they are first learning the vertical approach. Conversely, if it becomes evident that the skin will not redrape, it may be necessary to excise the excess.

The skin is then closed (Fig. 2G). Drains and dressing are used, as preferred by the surgeon. The author rarely uses drains. The incisions are covered by paper tape, and a surgical brassiere is applied, not for compression, but to hold the bandages in place. Patients are encouraged to shower the next day.

CLINICAL RESULTS

Many choices exist for flaps to carry the nipple–areolar complex. The medial pedicle has excellent blood supply and surprisingly good innervation. It is ideal for breast reduction, because it allows easy access to the lateral breast tissue where much of the excess lies (7–9).

Nipple and areolar necrosis can occur with any of the flaps. It is important to include both arterial input and venous drainage, if at all possible. Unfortunately, Doppler examination is not particularly useful, and surgeons must rely on the fact that the blood supply is usually fairly reliable. Four main pedicles and four main blood-supply patterns are found. As often occurs, some variability is seen from one person to another, and often only three of the main blood supplies may be dominant, with the fourth being absent. Nipple necrosis may be based more on anatomic variation, rather than on surgeon error.

SUMMARY

The author believes that the medial flap allows the surgeon to resect (in a breast reduction) or rearrange (as in a mastopexy) parenchyma, as desired. The medial pedicle can be used with various skin-resection patterns and is not exclusive to vertical approaches. The pedicle also allows the surgeon to remove the heavy inferior breast tissue and to leave behind the more superior breast tissue. An understanding of the blood supply is essential in designing and creating the medial flap for breast surgery.

References

1. Strombeck JO. Mammaplasty: report of a new technique based on the two-pedicle procedure. *Br J Plast Surg* 1960;13:79.
2. Skoog T. A technique of breast reduction: transposition of the nipple on a cutaneous vascular pedicle. *Acta Chir Scand* 1963;126:453.
3. Asplund O, Davies DM. Vertical scar breast reduction with medial flap or glandular transposition of the nipple-areola. *Br J Plast Surg* 1996;49:507.
4. Reid CR, Taylor GI. The vascular territory of the acromiothoracic axis. *Br J Plast Surg* 1984;37:194.
5. Schlenz I, Kuzbari R, Gruber H, Holle J. The sensitivity of the nipple-areola complex: an anatomic study. *Plast Reconstr Surg* 2000;105:905.
6. Schwartzmann E. Beitrag zur Vermeidung von Mammillennekrose beieinzeitiger Mammaplastik schwerer Fälle. (Avoidance of nipple necrosis by preservation of corium in one-stage plastic surgery of the breast.) *Rev Chir Struct* 1937;7:206.
7. Hall-Findlay EJ. A simplified vertical reduction mammaplasty: shortening the learning curve. *Plast Reconstr Surg* 1999;104:748.
8. Hall-Findlay EJ. Vertical breast reduction with a medially based pedicle: operative strategies. *Aesthet Surg J* 2002;22:185.
9. Hall-Findlay EJ. Pedicles in vertical reduction and mastopexy. *Clin Plast Surg* 2002;20:379.

CHAPTER 348 ■ SLIDING SKIN FLAP FROM THE ABDOMEN

J. R. LEWIS, JR.*

The sliding flap from the abdomen is a method of transferring tissue from the abdomen, where tissue is plentiful, to the chest when tissue there is insufficient, scarred, and/or damaged (1–4).

INDICATIONS

I have used this method successfully since 1955 for replacing scar tissue of the anterior chest and for replacing tissue following mastectomy (see Fig. 3) (1,5–8). An implant is often utilized in conjunction with this flap.

* Deceased.

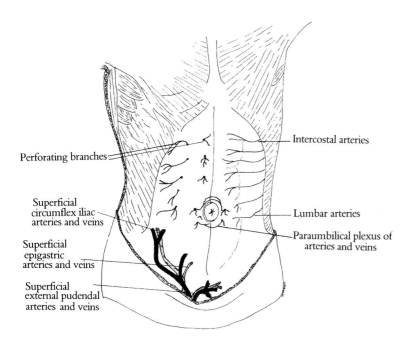

FIG. 1. Superficial abdominal wall circulation. About the umbilicus is the paraumbilical network of vessels, with communications between the right and left sides and between the superficial and deep vessels.

ANATOMY

The abdominal sliding flap is a widely based, thick flap of skin and fat that depends on a broad blood supply, not on a single vessel or even a few discrete vessels. There are two intricate networks of arteries that supply the anterior abdominal wall.

The deep network of vessels runs deep to the rectus muscle and consists of the deep superior and inferior epigastric arteries (Fig. 1). The superficial network includes both the intercostal and lumbar arteries, as well as the superficial inferior epigastric,

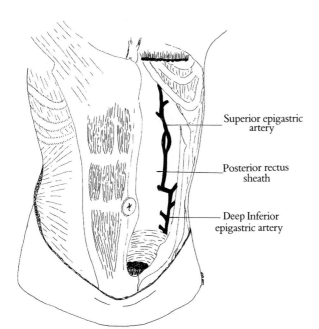

FIG. 2. Deep circulation of abdominal wall. Although shown here with only their major branches, there are numerous branches that pass across the midline to the opposite vessels in the deep plane and perforating branches that pass through the rectus muscle and sheath anteriorly into the subcutaneous tissue to communicate with the superficial vessels. There are further communications with branches of the intercostal and lumbar vessels and a rich network about the umbilicus.

superficial circumflex iliac, and superficial external pudendal vessels (Fig. 2).

There are numerous anastomoses between the deep and superficial systems by means of the perforators. There are a considerable number of cross-anastomoses within and between each system. The anastomoses connecting all levels are particularly rich about the umbilicus.

Obviously, when an incision is made across the upper abdomen to slide the whole width of the abdominal skin upward onto the chest wall, it is necessary to sever most of the upper perforators (see Fig. 3C). However, it is possible to stretch these perforators up at the umbilical level and below this level to preserve more circulation into the flap.

In breast reconstruction, an incision across the upper abdomen is generally not required unless a bilateral reconstruction is planned. In such a case, the circulation into the flap is quite adequate, because of the superficial network in the thick skin-fat flap, which is further supplied by the ascending superficial vessels and deep vessels of the previously described circulation.

Nerve supply in the flap generally is adequate in the lower portion and most frequently will recover to a great extent, even in the upper portion of the flap, except when the flap is thin and pulled more tightly than is usual.

FLAP DESIGN AND DIMENSIONS

The flap may be based inferiorly at a level that allows the tissue to be brought upward onto the chest wall according to the need. The degree of undermining inferiorly depends on the quality and mobility of the skin and subcutaneous tissue and on the degree of shift required for the chest-wall defect.

An upper abdominoplasty, with tightening of the whole abdominal skin, will require a degree of undermining well below the umbilicus level, while most sliding flaps, simply to furnish soft tissue to the chest wall, require undermining only down to the level of the umbilicus or slightly below (Fig. 3).

OPERATIVE TECHNIQUE

The sliding abdominal flap is undermined in the deep subcutaneous plane by a sliding motion using curved, blunt-tipped

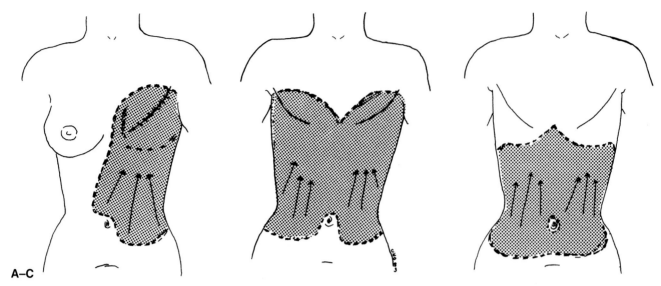

A–C

FIG. 3. A: Outline of undermining in the subcutaneous plane of the abdomen to slide the abdominal flap of skin and fat upward onto the chest for unilateral reconstruction of the breast. The flap slides upward onto the chest wall and is secured along the proposed submammary crease. B: Undermining bilaterally for bilateral breast reconstructions. Undermining is generally through two separate scars of the chest wall, one on each side following bilateral mastectomies. However, the undermining here is shown above the line of the scar (as in part A), because some undermining beneath the flap superiorly is carried out as well for the breast pocket. Undermining inferiorly is generally carried out to the level of the umbilicus or slightly below, leaving the umbilicus in position. C: An incision across the upper abdomen allows for more free sliding of the abdominal skin upward onto the chest wall. This also accomplishes an abdominoplasty. An incision about the umbilicus allows pulling of the abdominal skin upward and reinsertion of the umbilicus into a new opening at a lower level of skin while closing the skin defect as a vertical incision in the midline.

scissors. The incision of access for undermining is generally by resection of a scar on the chest wall present from injury or surgery (see Fig. 3A). If scars are present only high on the chest wall, it is better to make the incision along the estimated submammary fold line. This makes both undermining and hemostasis easier to achieve.

If relaxation is not adequate, further undermining and stretching upward of the perforating vessels are carried out to allow the flap to be moved upward onto the chest. There it is secured by deep buried sutures between the flap and the deep fascia of the chest wall in a semicircular manner to emulate the submammary fold.

Obviously, some superior undermining is generally required to give a contour simulating the opposite breast. After the implant is inserted and the wound is closed, a light pressure dressing is applied across the lower chest to help maintain the flap upward onto the chest wall and to decrease the tension, but excessive pressure may endanger the venous return from the flap.

CLINICAL RESULTS

Complications from the abdominal sliding flap have been rare. A few patients have had some degree of loosening of the support in the submammary fold area, so that the implant tended to slide downward beneath the flap. These patients were corrected quite easily by secondary suture support through a small incision securing the flap to the fascia of the chest wall.

The patient is temporarily aware of some increased tightness on one side or the other, depending on unilateral or bilateral use of the flap. Unilateral advancement is more frequent, but undermining is carried out across the midline to allow a smoother upward movement without kinking the skin.

The only other problem that has occurred is the general one of tightening about the breast implant. To my surprise, the

degree of tightening about the breast implant with breast reconstruction has been less than that which follows subcutaneous mastectomy. Such tightening is more frequent than that following simple augmentation mammaplasty, but it has been a relatively infrequent occurrence, especially to a degree that has required secondary surgery.

Patients have generally been quite happy with breast reconstruction by this method. Patients with burns of the chest and breast have been pleased with the relaxation of the tight burned skin and the degree of breast reconstruction required.

SUMMARY

I feel that this is the simplest method of breast reconstruction of all those I have tried and that the great majority of patients with radical or modified radical mastectomies can be corrected primarily or secondarily without more extensive surgery.

References

1. Lewis JR Jr. Use of a sliding flap from the abdomen to provide cover in breast reconstruction. *Plast Reconstr Surg* 1979;64:4.
2. Pennisi VR. Making a definite inframammary fold under a reconstructed breast. *Plast Reconstr Surg* 1977;60:523.
3. Ryan H. A lower thoracic advancement flap in breast reconstruction after mastectomy. *Plast Reconstr Surg* 1982;70:153.
4. Ryan JJ. The lower advancement technique in breast reconstruction. *Clin Plast Surg* 1984;11:277.
5. Lewis JR Jr. Reconstruction of the breast. Proceedings of International College of Surgeons, Vienna, 1964.
6. Lewis JR Jr. Reconstruction of the breast. *Surg Clin North Am* 1971;51:429.
7. Lewis JR Jr. Presentation and discussion of problem cases in breast surgery. In: Goldwyn RM, ed. *Plastic and reconstructive surgery of the breast.* Boston: Little, Brown, 1976;431–440.
8. Lewis JR Jr. Reconstruction of the breasts. In: Lewis JR Jr., ed. *The art of aesthetic plastic surgery,* Boston: Little, Brown, 1989;941.

CHAPTER 349 ■ TRANSVERSE THORACOEPIGASTRIC SKIN FLAP

T. D. CRONIN* AND E. D. CRONIN

EDITORIAL COMMENT

There is a shortage of skin at the site of the mastectomy. To provide additional skin, the thoracoepigastric flap would have to extend beyond the posterior axillary line, thus making it more risky and requiring delay, as indicated by the authors.

The transverse thoracoepigastric flap may be the procedure of choice in certain patients in whom additional skin is needed for breast reconstruction after mastectomy. This might be the case where, for some reason, a transverse rectus abdominis myocutaneous flap or a latissimus dorsi myocutaneous flap was unsuitable. This flap is of particular value when the mastectomy scar is oblique or vertical and when the skin flaps are tight but not excessively thin and adherent to the chest wall (Fig. 1).

INDICATIONS

The thoracoepigastric flap has the advantages of technical ease, a local donor area, and the possibility of closing the donor wound primarily after wide undermining inferiorly. The flap is usually quite thick, and the scar is usually covered by a bra. The flap can be raised and transposed in one stage if it is not extended past the midaxillary line (Fig. 2). When a modified radical mastectomy has been done, the presence of the pectoralis major muscle permits subpectoral implantation, with the thoracoepigastric flap supplying additional skin and permitting better projection.

When the mastectomy scar extends below the inframammary crease, it may indicate that the perforating branches of the superior epigastric vessels have been taken, and therefore, another method should be used. If a long flap is required, delay procedures may be necessary.

There are certain disadvantages to the flap. It does not correct the absent anterior axillary fold in a radical mastectomy (Fig. 2), and it usually does not completely correct the infraclavicular hollow, even with deepithelialization and burying of the tip of a long delayed flap in the infraclavicular area. Sometimes a later procedure is required to cut across the pedicle of the flap to establish a better inframammary fold.

Although a fairly large thoracoepigastric flap may be raised and inset, it cannot supply additional thickness to the thin skin flaps on each side of the flap, as can be done when the latissimus dorsi muscle is used.

ANATOMY

The transverse thoracoepigastric flap has an axial blood supply by means of the lateral branch of the superior epigastric artery (1,2). The extent of the axial territory, however, is controversial. If the flap includes skin up to the midaxillary line, the portion between the anterior and midaxillary lines may have a random-pattern blood supply (3). This flap is also supplied by several intercostal muscular perforators.

FLAP DESIGN AND DIMENSIONS

With the patient in a sitting position, a piece of cloth 8 × 10 cm is placed with its upper edge at the inframammary crease and its medial end at the lateral border of the rectus abdominis, which will serve as the base or pivoting area. The lateral end of the cloth is swung up along the scar as far as needed. It is then swung back to the horizontal position, and the flap is marked. If the length ends at the midaxillary line, the flap can be moved in one stage, since this is an arterialized flap (1,4,5). Flaps beyond this have a random blood supply and require delaying procedures (6,7).

OPERATIVE TECHNIQUE

With the patient half turned to her opposite side and the table flat or slightly extended at its middle, the flap is raised, beginning laterally, deep to the fascia (7,8). The more proximal portion of the flap overlies the serratus anterior. The medial extent of the elevation is to the lateral edge of the rectus abdominis, where several intercostal muscular perforators are found and must be preserved.

For closure of the donor site, the table is flexed with the table back raised somewhat. Wide undermining of the lower edge, even to the crest of the ilium, may be necessary (8). The patient is then turned on her back.

If there is any question about the viability of the flap, fluorescein is used to test the adequacy of the circulation. Most areas of mottled yellow-blue will survive (5).

Subcutaneous Implantation

If a radical mastectomy has been done, or if the prosthesis will be placed on top of the pectoralis major muscle, the scar is excised. The skin flaps are carefully dissected off the pectoralis major muscle or ribs and intercostal muscles to the sternal border medially, the midaxillary line laterally, almost to the clavicle superiorly, and to the proposed inframammary fold inferiorly.

---

* Deceased.

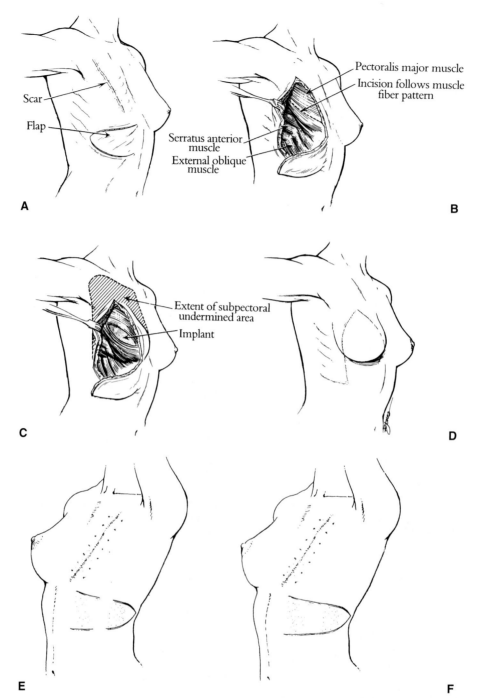

FIG. 1. A: Out to the midaxillary line, the thoracoepigastric flap is arterialized by perforators from the superior epigastric artery. Longer flaps need to be delayed. The donor site is closed primarily after undermining inferiorly toward the iliac crest. B: The flap is elevated deep to the fascia and transposed after opening the old scar. It is most suitable when the mastectomy scar is oblique or vertical. Although many of our patients had subcutaneous placement of the implant, we would prefer the submuscular position. Access to the submuscular pocket is either by incision along the fibers of the pectoralis major or its lateral edge. Alternatively, the incision is made through the serratus anterior at the seventh rib with dissection upward. C: An implant is then placed in the subpectoral subserratus space and the muscle incision is closed. D: The flap is then sutured in place. E: When the flap extends beyond the midaxillary line, it must be delayed. The initial delay consists of incising and undermining the flap but leaving the central bridge undisturbed. F: The second delay consists of incising and undermining the central bridge only. Finally, 1 or 2 weeks later, the entire flap is raised, transposed, and inset, with or without placement of the prosthesis at that time. (From Cronin, ref. 7, with permission.)

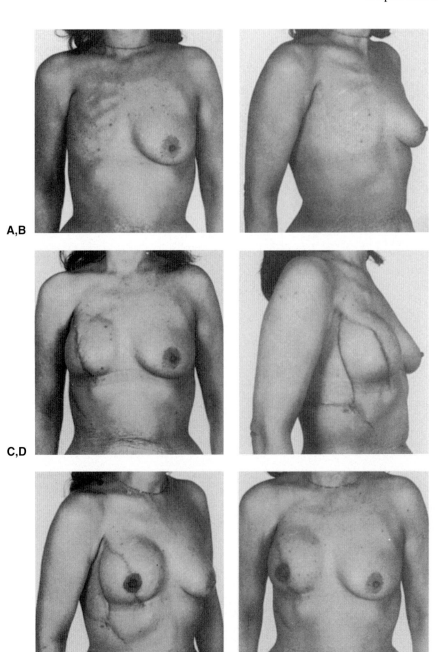

A,B

C,D

E,F

FIG. 2. **A,B:** A 44-year-old woman 9 years after right radical mastectomy. The patient has circumferential tightness, necessitating additional tissue. Note that the mastectomy scar extends below the inframammary crease, and therefore, the flap base will be more caudal than would be ideal. **C,D:** The 10 × 24 cm thoracoepigastric flap was delayed in two procedures and transferred as a third procedure. At a fourth procedure, a 235-cc low-profile round gel implant was inserted subcutaneously. **E,F:** The nipple-areola was reconstructed with full-thickness inner thigh skin for the areola and full-thickness labium minus for the nipple. Two months later, conchal cartilage was used to obtain more nipple projection.

The thoracoepigastric flap is then sutured into place, except for one area large enough to insert the implant. If the circulation of the flap is at all questionable, however, insertion of the prosthesis is delayed for a few days or weeks.

Subpectoral Implantation

If the pectoralis major muscle is present, we usually prefer to place the prosthesis submuscularly for additional cover. The mastectomy scar is excised, but the skin edges need not be undermined as widely as previously described. The submuscular plane may be reached by incising the serratus anterior muscle at the level of the seventh rib and then dissecting superiorly to lift the serratus and pectoralis major muscles off the ribs and intercostal muscles.

The pectoralis major muscle is separated from the minor muscle, leaving the latter attached to the ribs laterally. To relax the pectoralis major muscle further, its attachment to the sternum is released from 3 o'clock to 7 o'clock on the right side.

An alternate subpectoral method is to split through the fibers of the pectoralis major muscle. A large space is easily separated superiorly, while below, the origin of the pectoralis major muscle and serratus anterior muscle is separated down to the sixth rib. The pectoralis major muscle is also separated from the sternum from 3 o'clock to 7 o'clock on the right side.

This is followed by placement of a prosthesis of appropriate size in the cavity: Most often we use a textured saline implant; either round or teardrop shaped.

CLINICAL RESULTS

The most important and serious complication relates to the blood supply of the flap. Out of a total of 40 flaps, there was some circulatory problem with 14. Of these, 5 showed only superficial impairment, as indicated by irregular partial small losses of skin. Observation for several weeks permitted recovery and full use of the flap.

On the other hand, full-thickness losses have occurred in nine patients and have required debridement. It was possible to salvage five such flaps by advancement of the flap near its base. If the thoracoepigastric flap overlies the pectoralis major muscle, a split-thickness skin graft can be applied directly to the muscle after the debridement with satisfactory results. When these methods are unsuccessful, recourse to another method may be tried, such as a free flap.

What can be done to minimize disasters? First, if the scar of the mastectomy, by its location, strongly suggests that the superior epigastric perforating circulation has been destroyed, it would be advisable to use another method. If the flap extends beyond the midaxillary line, delaying procedures are indicated. Even with multiple delays, long flaps tend to be unreliable.

Other complications include malposition of the implant. It may be too low or too high and thus require reoperation to enlarge the pocket and adjust the position as necessary. The same applies to fibrous contracture around the implant. Rarely, extrusion of the implant may occur secondary to contracture and thinning of the tissues, as noted in one patient 5 years later.

A nipple placed at the time of transposition and implantation is likely to be disastrously out of place, since the contour of the breast changes with healing. Hence, delay placement of the nipple for 2 to 3 months. There is no satisfactory way to change the position of a misplaced nipple.

SUMMARY

The thoracoepigastric flap is a useful method of supplying additional cover for breast reconstruction, especially when the mastectomy scar is vertical or oblique. It is best used after a modified radical mastectomy when the pectoralis major muscle remains.

References

1. Bohmert H. Personal method for reconstruction of the female breast following radical mastectomy. In: Marchac D, Hueston J, eds. *Transactions of the Sixth International Congress of Plastic and Reconstructive Surgery.* Paris: Masson, 1976;542.
2. Bohmert H. Personal communication, 1979.
3. Davis AM, McCraw JB, Carraway JH. Use of a direct transverse thoracoabdominal flap to close difficult wounds of the thorax and upper extremity. *Plast Reconstr Surg* 1977;60:526.
4. Becker D, McCraw JB, Horton C. Immediate and delayed use of the thoracoepigastric flap for reconstruction of the total mastectomy defect. Presented at the annual meeting of the American Society for Aesthetic Plastic Surgery, Atlanta, Georgia, 1976.
5. McCraw JB, Myers B, Shanklin K. The value of fluorescein in predicting the viability of arterialized flaps. *Plast Reconstr Surg* 1977;60:710.
6. Cronin TD, Upton J, McDonough JM. Reconstruction of the breast after mastectomy. *Plast Reconstr Surg* 1977;59:1.
7. Cronin TD, Cronin ED. The thoracoepigastric flap in breast reconstruction. In: Gant T, Vasconez L, eds. *Post-mastectomy reconstruction.* Baltimore: Williams & Wilkins, 1980;238.
8. Tai Y, Hasegawa H. A transverse abdominal flap for reconstruction after radical operations for recurrent breast cancer. *Plast Reconstr Surg* 1974; 53:52.

CHAPTER 350 ■ COMPOSITE CONE FLAP

A. J. J. EMMETT

EDITORIAL COMMENT

More important than concentrating on the location of the nipple are the author's efforts to cone the breast. This is accomplished by partly folding the flap in a U-shape.

This is a lateral thoracic flap based on a pedicle of deep fascia and muscle with a variable-width cutaneous pedicle. It is taken from the side of the chest, brought around to the front, and shortened, turning the flap on itself to produce a skin cone (1,2). The deeper muscular tethering laterally facilitates this deliberate shortening and coning.

The design of the flap is such that the cone produces good breast projection and the tip of the cone lies at a site comparable to the opposite nipple-areola complex.

INDICATIONS

I have selected this flap particularly for use in the patient who has a larger opposite breast that she wishes to have matched and is anxious not to have reduced.

ANATOMY

The deeper muscular pedicle is designed according to the muscles that are present (Fig. 1A). It commonly involves the pectoralis major, external oblique, and serratus anterior muscles. Where these muscles are considered to be deficient or there has been heavy irradiation of the area, the anterior half of latissimus dorsi may be hinged with the flap (Fig. 1B). I usually take the deep fascia of the latissimus dorsi with the fat flap anyway and, if necessary, can hinge forward the anterior half of the muscle as a secondary muscular pedicle (3).

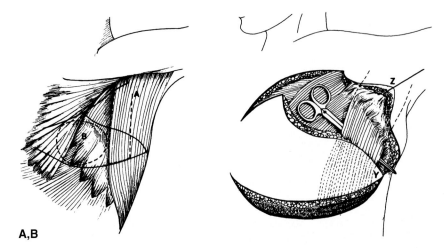

A,B

FIG. 1. **A:** The muscular pedicles on which the flap is based are shown. Where possible, serratus anterior, external oblique, and pectoralis major muscles are used (*B*). The dissection is deep to the muscle pedicle or in the muscle. Where these muscles are deficient from surgery or irradiation, I add in the anterior half of latissimus dorsi (*A*), hinged from the axilia with its nerve and blood supply. **B:** When the latissimus dorsi is used, it is left attached to the distal half of the flap. Deep fascia and the other three muscles are used also in the proximal half of the pedicle. When fibrotic, these latter muscles need more division for the flap to turn adequately.

FLAP DESIGN AND DIMENSIONS

The flap is designed so that the tip of the cone lies at the same level as the opposite nipple-areola complex. As the flap is folded on itself, the surgeon attempts to emphasize the coning. The deeper muscular pedicle shortens the flap on its long axis as it is transposed. By turning the flap on itself, I am able to convert the stress lines in the skin to more of the semicircular pattern of the normal breast, a practice that gives better projection.

Marking the flap preoperatively is important. This is done with the patient in the sitting position (Fig. 2A and B), so that the vertical line of the nipple position is marked on each side. The horizontal level of the nipple and the submammary fold are also marked.

The flap is then drawn around the side of the chest so that the closure will fit the scar line into the line of the brassiere strap. The flap is taken as long and as wide as is reasonable for the patient's size and looseness of chest tissue (Fig. 2B).

The flap is intended to turn through 60 to 80 degrees to fit into the line of the preexisting scar, whether that be horizontal, vertical, or oblique. In Figure 2B, the oblique scar needs only a 60-degree shift. The tip of flap Y is intended to fit into the scar

when opened. Points X in Figure 2B come together at point X in Figure 2C as the flap shortens. The secondary triangular flap M advances as far as necessary into the angle left by turning the flap to assist in closure of the donor site.

OPERATIVE TECHNIQUE

The incision along the flap margins is taken down through the deep fascia into and through muscle, depending on which muscle is to be moved along with the flap. The muscle pedicle of serratus anterior, external oblique, and pectoralis major is dissected, stretched, and divided as much as is necessary to move the flap into a position that will balance the cone of the flap with the nipple prominence of the opposite side. Dissection is deep to the muscle, which moves with the flap.

The original mastectomy scar is then excised and opened out down to muscle, mobilizing flap M, which opens out the chest wound to receive the cone flap.

The implant is put in at a second stage. A larger breast can be produced using a two-stage procedure. This is an advantage for the patient with a large breast who wishes to retain the nor-

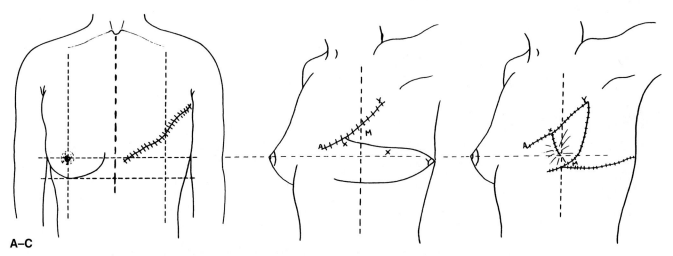

A–C

FIG. 2. **A:** The nipple level is marked in vertical and horizontal planes with the patient sitting upright and arms hanging freely by the sides. The submammary fold level and midline are noted. **B:** The flap is marked on the side of the chest. The tip of flap Y is intended to move to position Y on the anterior chest scar when it is excised and opened out. As the flap shortens, points X on the flap come together to form a prominent cone, as in part **C.** Flap M is mobilized and is advanced into the angle, and the tension along this line further emphasizes the breast coning, making what will later be the lateral fold of the breast. **C:** The flap is shortened and the cone is produced. Both donor site and flap are closed. (Figures 1 and 2 from Emmett, ref. 2, with permission.)

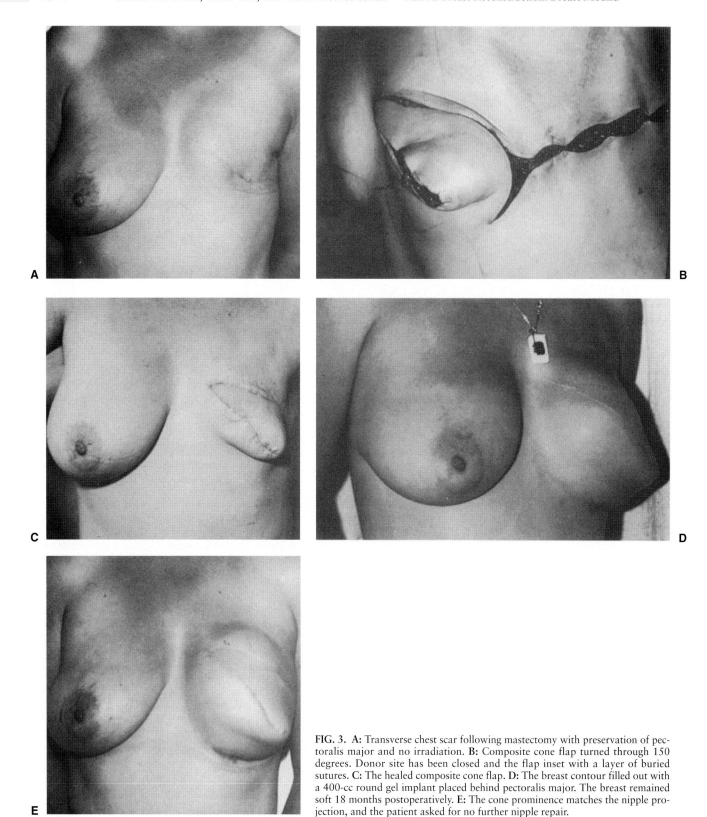

FIG. 3. A: Transverse chest scar following mastectomy with preservation of pectoralis major and no irradiation. **B:** Composite cone flap turned through 150 degrees. Donor site has been closed and the flap inset with a layer of buried sutures. **C:** The healed composite cone flap. **D:** The breast contour filled out with a 400-cc round gel implant placed behind pectoralis major. The breast remained soft 18 months postoperatively. **E:** The cone prominence matches the nipple projection, and the patient asked for no further nipple repair.

mal side unaltered. The use of a two-stage procedure also gives a greater advancement of skin, since the adjacent skin is mobilized in the secondary procedure. In addition, a thicker cone of tissue is kept in front of the implant from the first stage.

The second stage of the repair is carried out 6 months later, when the implant is inserted beneath the available skin and muscle to build the contour to that of the opposite side (Figs. 3 and 4). Usually a standard gel- or saline-filled implant is used, but I have used a composite implant with a thicker silicone

upper part to replace the pectoral muscle contour in four patients (Fig. 5).

CLINICAL RESULTS

In a series of 35 breast reconstructions, the composite cone technique was used in 17 patients. Patients who have had a satisfactory cone prominence established by this method have

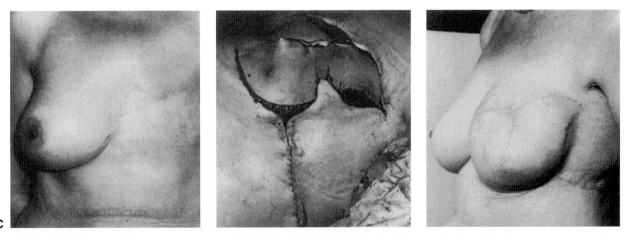

A–C

FIG. 4. **A:** Oblique mastectomy scar. **B:** Flap has been turned on itself and inset to the line of the chest-wall scar. Lateral donor site is closed. Lateral flap tip did not reach the angle and will be trimmed and inset. The cone prominence can be seen. **C:** Flap filled out with implant. Level of cone matched nipple prominence. Note lateral breast fold along line of the secondary triangular flap.

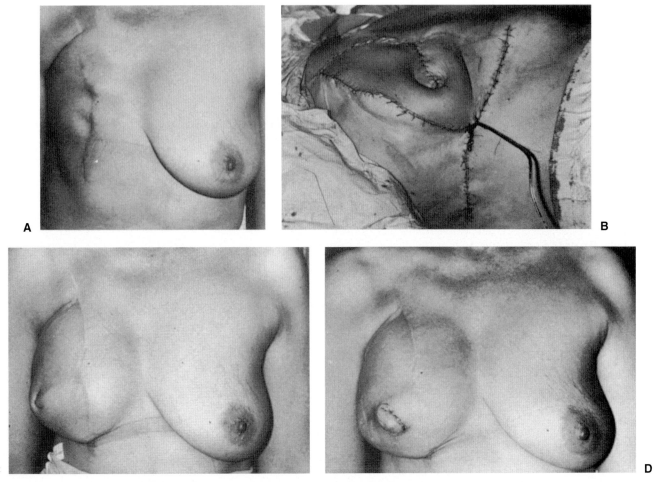

FIG. 5. **A:** Vertical mastectomy scar with absence of pectoralis major. **B:** Cone flap has been turned 90 degrees to create the excess skin that will later project with an implant at the second stage. Some lateral muscle tethering is holding it. The secondary triangular flap is inset to the angle of the turn of the cone flap. **C:** Breast cone is a little high and lateral. The implant used had an extension to fill out pectoral contour and was 400 cc in volume. **D:** Cone prominence has been turned medially and down to correct its position as a secondary transposed flap. I have done this in four patients in whom the cone did not loosen down in the 6 months after inserting the implant.

usually not asked for a separate nipple reconstruction. In 4 patients, the cone prominence was sitting laterally and too high. This was adjusted with a small transposed flap (Fig. 5D).

SUMMARY

A chest-wall flap consisting of skin and muscle is used to create a cone shape for postmastectomy reconstruction.

References

1. Emmett AJJ. The dog-ear flap for reconstruction of the breast cone following mastectomy. *Aus NZ J Surg* 1979;49:526.
2. Emmett AJJ. Composite cone breast reconstruction: two-stage repair after mastectomy. *Br J Plast Surg* 1981;34:272.
3. McCraw JB, Bostwick J, Horton CE. Methods of soft-tissue coverage for the mastectomy defect. *Clin Plast Surg* 1979;6:1.

CHAPTER 351 ■ LATERAL ABDOMINAL SKIN FLAP

J. M. DREVER

The lateral abdominal skin flap was designed primarily for breast reconstruction (1). It is raised mainly from an area of loose skin. The flap has both a good vascular supply and good sensation.

INDICATIONS

I have used this flap only for breast reconstruction. It is particularly useful when there is considerable redundancy of tissue around the midabdominal area. It must be noted that a considerable amount of skin and subcutaneous fat can be transferred with this type of reconstruction, and therefore, the use of silicone implants can be avoided. Use of this flap will leave the patient with an obvious diagonal scar across the abdomen, but the new breast mound, without implants or functional disabilities, usually outweighs this disadvantage (2).

ANATOMY

This is an arterial flap (axial pattern) that carries direct cutaneous arteries (3). These are the lateral cutaneous branches of the posterior intercostal and subcostal arteries, accompanied by venae comitantes and the corresponding cutaneous nerves. Coming from the axillary region, the flap also receives the superficial thoracic and long thoracic arteries, and it is drained by the thoracoepigastric vein (4). This good vascularity enables one to lift and transpose the flap without a delay procedure.

FLAP DESIGN AND DIMENSIONS

The design of the flap is a spearhead shape. It must have a wide base from the midclavicular to the posterior axillary line at a height just above the costal margin. Its medial edge goes toward the umbilicus and then straight down the midline. The lateral edge is placed according to the width of the breast to be reconstructed, usually 20 to 25 cm from its base then tapering downward until it meets the medial edge of the pubis.

OPERATIVE TECHNIQUE

First Stage

The flap is lifted quite easily from the external oblique, but it is slightly more adherent to the rectus abdominis fascia. The lower end is deepithelialized and tapered to what will form the uppermost part of the new mound. This area is tucked under an undermined upper edge of the thoracic incision. It is a horseshoe design, and trapdoor skin is used to line part of the undersurface of the rotated abdominal flap. This arc of rotation has about 100 degrees (Fig. 1B to D).

Closure of the abdominal defect is like a "lipectomy done sideways." After cutting around the umbilicus, the opposite side of the abdomen is undermined at the fascial level up to the flank. The edges are then sutured under some tension, and the umbilicus is brought out through a new opening at the corresponding site.

Second Stage

The pedicle is divided 30 to 40 days later. The lower end is defatted slightly and sutured to the horizontal portion of the T incision. The upper part is marked across what will be the submammary fold, and that portion distal to this line is deepithelialized. The previous trapdoor is excised and discarded. The cone shape of the breast is obtained by excising a central

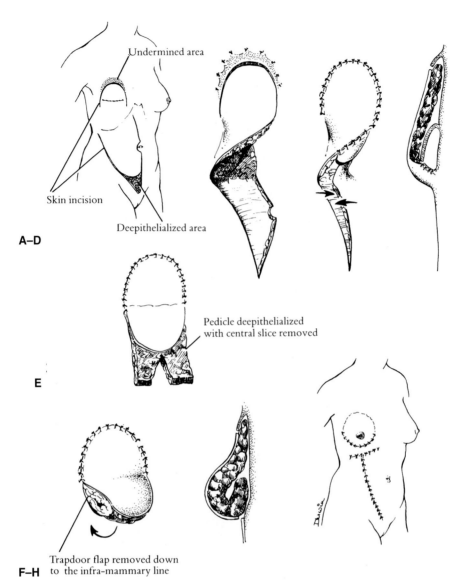

FIG. 1. A: Note the preparation of the breast area with an inferiorly based, hinged trapdoor flap and the undermining above it. The lateral abdominal flap is based at the costal margin, and its end is deepithelialized. **B,C:** Flap has been rotated into place with its upper end set into the undermined upper edge. **D:** Cross section shows the lining provided by the trapdoor flap. **E:** Pedicle is sectioned and deepithelialized from the submammary fold, and a central wedge is removed. **F:** Trapdoor flap is removed, and the deepithelialized pedicle is tucked under the rest of the flap. **G:** Cross section of the same. **H:** The remaining scars.

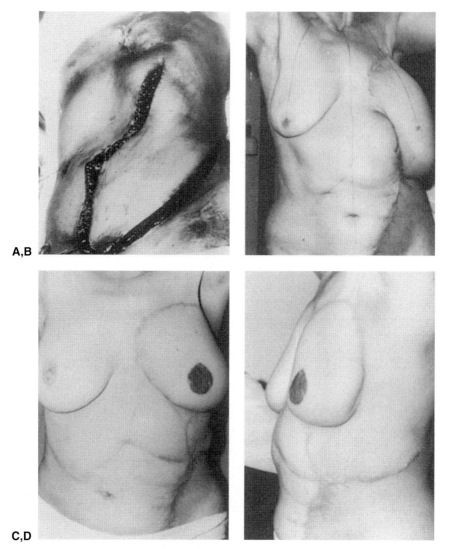

FIG. 2. A: The lateral abdominal skin flap during the first stage. The radical mastectomy included a wide skin excision and had been skin-grafted. **B:** Just before the second stage, preoperative markings should be done on the future submammary fold and the nipple height with the patient standing to compare them to the normal breast. **C,D:** Eight months postoperatively. Apart from the hypertrophic scarring, an adequate mammary volume has been obtained.

wedge, suturing the remaining edges together, and folding that under the rest of the flap (Figs. 1E to G and 2).

CLINICAL RESULTS

There have been few complications. Of nine patients, only one had a partial necrosis that was covered with a skin graft and later revised. Subsequent fat hardening was found in three patients. The patient must be reassured that it softens after several months. A biopsy is helpful to rule out a recurrence. Infection on the undersurface of this partially open flap was seen in three patients, was treated, and had no major consequences or loss of tissue.

SUMMARY

The lateral abdominal skin flap is a reliable flap that can be used without implant in two stages for breast reconstruction.

References

1. Drever JM. Total breast reconstruction with either of two abdominal flaps. *Plast Reconstr Surg* 1977;59:185.
2. Drever JM. Total breast reconstruction. *Ann Plast Surg* 1981;7:54.
3. Daniel RK, Cunningham DM, Taylor GI. The deltopectoral flap: an anatomic and hemodynamic approach. *Plast Reconstr Surg* 1975;55:275.
4. Webster JP. Thoracoepigastric tubed pedicles. *Surg Clin North Am* 1937; 17:145.

CHAPTER 352 ■ MIDABDOMINAL SKIN FLAP

J. M. DREVER

This skin flap is particularly useful for breast reconstruction when there is a considerable redundancy of tissue around the midabdominal area (1–4). It must be noted that a considerable amount of skin and subcutaneous fat can be transferred with this type of reconstruction, and therefore, the use of implants can be avoided. The obvious scarring is a disadvantage (5).

ANATOMY

This is a random or cutaneous flap (6) that receives its vascular supply through perforators that arise from the superior epigastric vessels that pierce the rectus abdominis muscle and fascia to supply an area of skin around the xiphoid. Some supply comes laterally from the terminal branches of the intercostal vascular bundles. The rest of the flap is vascularized from the dermal and subdermal plexus.

FLAP DESIGN AND DIMENSIONS

This is a spear-shaped flap based superiorly just at the costal margin. Here it is about 15 to 20 cm in width, depending on the patient's girth. It tapers down into the pubis, giving it some 25 to 30 cm of total length.

OPERATIVE TECHNIQUE

First Stage

The flap is lifted from the rectus abdominis fascia and delayed for 10 days to the height of the umbilicus, which is transected and everted. When it survives, it can serve as a nipple. Following this period, the lower end of the flap is deepithelialized and tapered to what will form the upper extremity of the new breast. This area is tucked under an undermined upper edge of the thoracic incision. It is a horseshoe design, and its trapdoor is used to line part of the undersurface of the rotated abdominal flap. This arc of rotation is about 130 degrees (Fig. 1B and C).

Closure of the abdominal defect has the effect of a vertical abdominal lipectomy, and a new umbilicus can be made by a defatted 2-cm Z-plasty at the level, suturing the dermis to the fascia.

Second Stage

The pedicle is divided 30 to 40 days later. The lower end is defatted slightly and sutured to the horizontal portion of the T incision. The upper part is marked across what will be the submammary fold, and that portion which is distal to this line is deepithelialized. The previous trapdoor is excised and discarded. The cone shape of the breast is obtained by excising a central wedge, suturing the remaining edges together, and folding that under the rest of the flap (Figs. 1D–F and 2).

CLINICAL RESULTS

Flap necrosis occurred, to some extent, in 5 of my 13 patients. In 1 patient, practically the entire flap was lost. The other 4 patients developed varying degrees of necrosis at the edge. These patients were managed by resection of the necrotic area, upward advancement, and reinsertion of the remainder of the flap. Necrosis of subcutaneous fat alone occurred in two other patients, manifesting as a hardening of the distal part of the flap. This softened after several months.

One patient had a *Pseudomonas* chondritis, managed by high doses of carbenicillin. It took several months to clear. There were two other cases of superficial infection of the raw undersurface of these open flaps, but fortunately, no consequences occurred. There were no function deficits arising after the completed reconstruction.

SUMMARY

The midabdominal skin flap can be used without implants as a two-stage procedure for breast reconstruction.

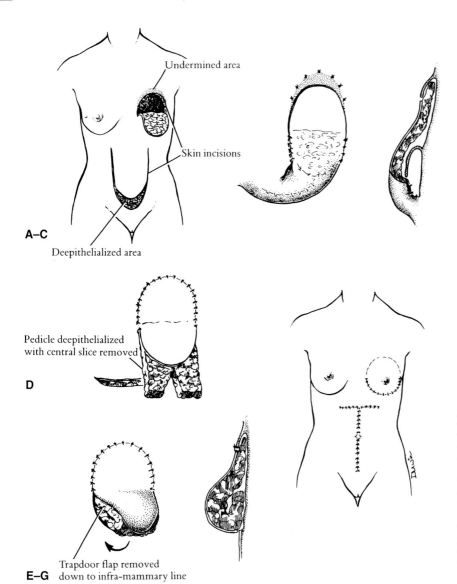

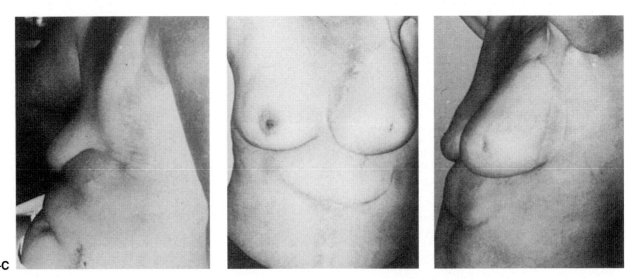

FIG. 1. A: Note the preparation of the breast area, with an inferiorly hinged trapdoor flap and the undermining above it. The midabdominal skin flap end is deepithelialized. **B:** The flap is hinged at the xiphoid, twisted about 130 degrees, and inset. **C:** Cross section shows the undersurface lining provided by the trapdoor flap. **D:** The pedicle is sectioned and deepithelialized from the submammary fold, and a central wedge is removed. **E:** The trapdoor flap is removed, and the deepithelialized pedicle is tucked under the rest of the flap. **F:** Cross section of same. **G:** Finished reconstruction; the umbilicus can be reformed by a 2-cm Z-plasty.

FIG. 2. A: Preoperative view. The flap was delayed for 10 days. **B,C:** Two years postoperatively, the umbilicus (nipple) reinverted and the pigment partially reabsorbed in the areola that had been tattooed. The breast mound is soft and natural looking.

References

1. Drever JM. Total breast reconstruction with either of two abdominal flaps. *Plast Reconstr Surg* 1977;59:185.
2. Gillies H, Millard DR Jr, eds. *The principles and art of plastic surgery.* Boston: Little, Brown, 1957.
3. Fernandes J. Mammary reconstruction. *Bol Trab Acad Argent Cir (Buenos Aires)* 1968;52:86.
4. Fernandes J. Mammary reconstruction immediately following a mastectomy. *Bol Trab Acad Argent Cir (Buenos Aires)* 1969;53:352.
5. Drever JM. Total breast reconstruction. *Ann Plast Surg* 1981;7:B54.
6. Daniel RK, Cunningham DM, Taylor GI. The deltopectoral flap: an anatomic and hemodynamic approach. *Plast Reconstr Surg* 1975;55:275.

Online Chapter

CHAPTER 353. Contralateral Breast Flap *D. R. Marshall*
www.encyclopediaofflaps.com

CHAPTER 354 ■ DEEPITHELIALIZED FLAP FROM ARM TO CHEST

J. R. LEWIS, JR.*

EDITORIAL COMMENT

The turnover flap is most attractive to fill the subclavicular hollow. However, the vascularity is not totally reliable.

Since there is a defect in the upper chest following resection of the pectoralis major muscle, it occurred to me a number of years ago that corrections of chronic lymphedema of the arm and of the defect of the upper chest might be combined by the use of a deepithelialized fat flap from the upper arm onto the chest. It was further felt that this might give some chance of reestablishing lymphatics across the axilla onto the chest, further improving the residual lymphedema. Whether or not this theoretic consideration is actually borne out by the results remains to be proven.

INDICATIONS

The deepithelialized flap from the arm to the chest is used to fill out the infraclavicular hollow after mastectomy. The flap is created during resection of some of the excess fibrofatty tissue of the lymphedematous arm. This procedure has been used, along with breast reconstruction and as an isolated procedure, in an attempt to reestablish lymphatic return and to improve lymphedema.

ANATOMY

The circulation to the flap is derived from branches of the brachial artery, and the return circulation is by accompanying small veins, including branches of the basilic vein. Lymphatics that accompany these vessels and the normal lymphatics in the subcutaneous fat are included with the flap.

FLAP DESIGN AND DIMENSIONS

A length-to-width ratio of 2.5:1 is probably reasonable with a flap of this type. The flap is outlined by parallel incisions along the posteromedial aspect of the upper arm, extending onto the forearm when the lymphedema is more extensive (Fig. 1).

OPERATIVE TECHNIQUE

The incision is carried through the fat and to the fascia, being very careful to avoid injury to the deeper structures, including major arteries, veins, and nerves. The flap is essentially a subcutaneous tissue flap, including at first the skin which is deepithelialized. Ideally, the dermis is left in place on the flap.

The flap is then turned upward, based in the upper arm opposite the axilla. Obviously, the whole length of the flap will not survive on its own circulation, and the flap is resected at the desired point. The residual flap is turned onto the chest into a subcutaneous pocket, which is dissected through a short incision in the axilla or by the planned resection of a chest scar.

---

* Deceased.

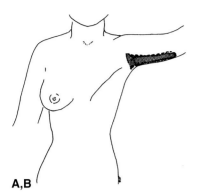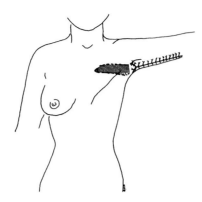

A,B

FIG. 1. **A:** Arm flap outlined on the posteromedial aspect of the upper arm. This flap may extend down into the forearm when the lymphedema is more marked, and the distal portion is usually discarded in such cases. The residual flap is then turned over onto the chest across the axilla. **B:** Following shift of the arm flap onto the upper chest and axilla. The purpose is to give further bulk to the upper chest in breast reconstructions and to help improve the lymphedema of the arm by resecting some of the excess lymphedematous fat. This is also done to improve the transfer of lymphatics across the scar tissue of the anterior axilla.

It is important that the base of the flap not be angled or flexed sharply, so as to ensure circulation into the tissue. Leaving the dermis intact probably salvages some of the more superficial vessels, but the dermis is thin in this area.

The base of the flap at the axilla is generally denuded in order to close the skin. If there is some uncertainty about the circulation, the skin may be left intact at the base, to be corrected later when the flap has healed satisfactorily. This is a variation from the usual technique and is a combination of skin-fat pedicle and deepithelialized fat flap.

Fixation sutures are pulled through at the farthest point medially and at other points along the flap course, and a light tie-on bandage is applied. A small drain is left if desired, and the arm is wrapped snugly, but not tightly, with an elastic bandage from the fingers upward.

CLINICAL RESULTS

The results of this procedure in a small series seem to have been worth the effort (Fig. 2). If the flap is left long, the distal portion of the flap probably "takes" more as a free-fat graft, and there is usually a certain amount of fat necrosis and/or fibrosis, while the proximal portion of the flap apparently survives as a flap. The firmness in the distal portion of the flap in the more medial upper chest gradually resolves, leaving increased fullness in the area of the deficiency of the pectoralis major muscle.

In my series, there have been no complications, except for the obvious "take" in the distal portion of the pedicle as a free graft rather than as a well-vascularized flap. Generally, the results are good. There have been no complications in the arm

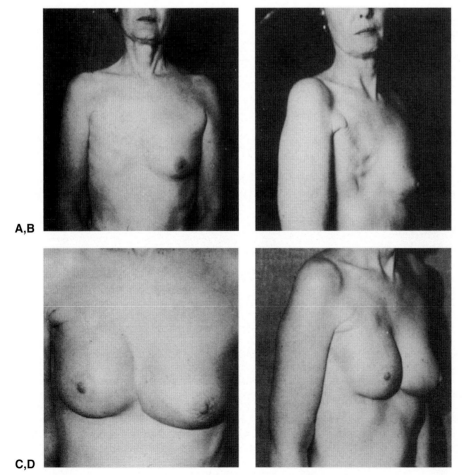

A,B

C,D

FIG. 2. **A,B:** Preoperative appearance of the patient following radical mastectomy. Note that there is lymphedema of the right arm and upper portion of the forearm. Also, there is a hollow in the upper chest. Most of the pectoralis muscles have been resected along with the breast. **C,D:** Following reconstruction of the right breast by an advancement flap from the abdomen, securing the flap onto the chest wall at the proposed inframammary crease. The defect in the upper chest has been corrected by the arm flap turned onto the chest from the right upper arm. This has reduced the bulk of the arm for correction of the lymphedema of the upper arm and forearm and a transfer of tissue containing lymphatics across the axilla onto the chest. The distal part of this flap more medially on the chest probably has taken as a free-fat graft rather than as a flap surviving on its own circulation. The patient has been followed for 4 years.

itself, because of great care to avoid damage to important structures deep to the resected fat and careful postoperative care with dependent drainage of the arm.

SUMMARY

While resecting excess lymphedematous tissue in the post-mastectomy arm, a deepithelialized flap can be created. The flap can be used to help fill out the infraclavicular hollow

resulting from loss of the pectoralis muscle. It is also hoped that the flap will help to improve the transfer of lymphatics across the scar tissue of the anterior axilla in an attempt to reduce the lymphedema.

Reference

Lewis JR Jr. Reconstruction of the breasts. In: Lewis JR, Jr, ed. *The art of aesthetic plastic surgery.* Boston: Little, Brown, 1989;941.

 CHAPTER 355. Tubed Abdominal Skin Flap *J.C. Kelleher and R. V. Janevicius*
www.encyclopediaofflaps.com

CHAPTER 356 ■ OMENTAL FLAP

R. T. ROUTLEDGE AND S. K. DAS

> ### EDITORIAL COMMENT
>
> The omentum obviously can be used for breast reconstruction if so desired, since the anatomic length of the omentum will easily reach to the breast area. The editors are perplexed at the use of omentum over a breast implant, since there are no known advantages to the resurfacing of an implant with omental fat.

After years of intense activity, interest in methods of breast reconstruction following ablative surgery continues to grow, and certainly the last word on the subject has not yet been written. Merely covering the defect of a mastectomy wound with omentum is discussed in Chapter 387. The use of omentum for reconstruction after mastectomy is described here (1–5).

INDICATIONS

The omentum is ideally suited for breast reconstruction because of its shape and unique blood supply. Since it is highly vascular, omentum will protect the overlying skin flap following subcutaneous mastectomy, a flap that is often riddled with the multiple scars of previous biopsies and thereby jeopardized. The omentum also will protect the underlying prosthesis that is most commonly used to replace volume loss following mastectomy and thus reduce the incidence of extrusion. In a

high percentage of patients, the volume of breast tissue removed is so large that no implant made could properly fill the skin envelope. To place too small an implant and hope that the skin envelope will shrink to accommodate it is a certain recipe for aesthetic disaster.

Another use of omentum in breast reconstruction is to replace volume, exploiting the special property of omentum to accept split-thickness skin grafts; the omentum is brought out to the chest, shaped like a breast, and a skin graft is applied.

Indications for the use of the procedure include (1) immediate one-stage breast reconstruction following subcutaneous mastectomy, either unilateral or bilateral, with or without a silicone implant, depending on the size of the breast, and (2) late or delayed breast reconstruction (1) following simple or radical mastectomy when there are no other suitable alternatives, e.g., in patients in whom extensive burns have destroyed local skin or there has been extensive radionecrosis and/or radiodermatitis.

ANATOMY

The arrangement of the two main vessels of the omentum, right and left gastroepiploic vessels, allows the division of the omentum in half on each of these pedicles for bilateral targets (Fig. 1). As far as volume is concerned, however, total omentum may be adequate for reconstruction of only one breast. Since the silicone gel prosthesis is so easily available, the volume problem can be obviated by its use. Omentum, then, will function primarily as a vascular protective apron, but in some cases it will replace volume as well.

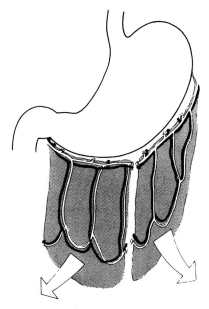

FIG. 1. Construction of two omental flaps, each based on one of the gastroepiploic pedicles. (From Barron, Saad, ref. 7, with permission.)

FLAP DESIGN AND DIMENSIONS

The average size of the omentum in a female is 33 cm in length and 32.5 cm in width. This allows a sheet of omentum at least 16 × 16 cm for each breast cover. Even when a minimum amount of omentum is available, it is still at least 19 × 20.4 cm, thus allowing enough to cover both breasts (6–8).

It is possible to predict the length and width of the omentum from the woman's height and weight before laparotomy (4); the only practical difficulty is if the patient has undergone previous laparotomy and has acquired adhesions of the omentum. Even so, with careful dissection, all the adhesions can be freed.

OPERATIVE TECHNIQUE

The subcutaneous mastectomy is performed through an infero-lateral approach (Fig. 2), separating a thin layer of skin and fat from the surface of the breast up to the level of the clavicle and paying particular attention to the axillary extension laterally and the thinned inner breast quadrants medially. The gland is then elevated from the pectoral fascia and removed, and hemostasis is secured.

Through a midline upper abdominal incision, the omentum is brought out, and its area and vascular pattern are noted (Fig. 2). Previous abdominal disease may have produced multiple adhesions, which have to be painstakingly divided before delivery of sufficient bulk can be effected. The omentum is then freed from the transverse colon along the avascular plane, so that the middle colic vessels will not be damaged (8).

Then the omentum is freed from the greater curvature of the stomach, basing the pedicle on the right gastroepiploic vessels if the omentum is being used for reconstructing only one breast. If both breasts are to be reconstructed, the omentogastrolysis is started in the middle of the greater curvature of the stomach and progresses on either side of the midline, thereby maintaining both right and left gastroepiploic pedicles (8). The plane of dissection runs close to the greater curve of the stomach, making sure that the gastroepiploic arch is preserved with the omentum.

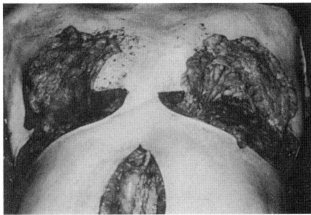

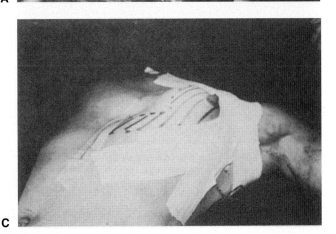

FIG. 2. A: Omentum being inspected after delivery through laparotomy wound, following omentocololysis, and before planning the two breast flaps. **B:** Creation of two omental flaps following division through the middle of the omentum for bilateral breast reconstruction. Each flap is tunneled subcutaneously to the chest and inspected for viability before placing it over the implants. Lower incision is for laparotomy, and upper incisions are for subcutaneous mastectomy. Margins of the omentum are secured peripherally under the skin flap with bolster sutures for permanent fixation. **C:** Elastoplast® dressing to hold omentum and implant in place.

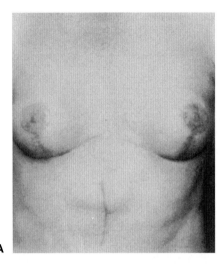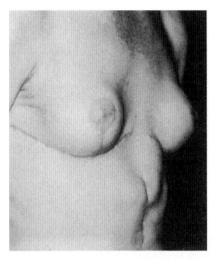

A   B

FIG. 3. Breasts 6 years following breast reconstruction with omentum. In this patient, the size of the skin flaps was reduced following the pattern of a Strombeck reduction mammaplasty.

There should now be sufficient length for the omentum to reach easily from the abdominal incision into the breast pocket by means of a subcutaneous tunnel. Within the breast pocket, the omentum is spread out into a fan to line the skin envelope. The pedicle must be checked to ensure that no torsion exists.

The omental fan can be tacked peripherally by catgut sutures to the deep surface of the skin or secured by peripherally placed sutures brought up through the skin and lightly tied over bolsters. A suitably sized silicone gel prosthesis is inserted deep to the omental layer, and the breast wound is closed in layers, picking up the lower omental edge with subcutaneous sutures. Suction drainage is instituted (Fig. 2C).

The abdominal wound is closed in layers, leaving a small dehiscence superiorly where the omental pedicle runs through. A light dressing is secured with Elastoplast® (Fig. 2C). A bra dressing must be avoided, for fear of compression of the omental pedicle as it runs up over the costal margin.

In big-breasted females, the subcutaneous mastectomy is performed through incisions based on a standard Strombeck pattern for breast reduction (Fig. 3). At first, we kept the nipple-areola complex intact on the dermal pedicles, but although viability appeared secure on the table, subsequent nipple necrosis was the rule. This is hardly surprising when one considers that the nipple-areola complex depends for its vascular supply on two long, attenuated, excessively thin dermal pedicles which themselves are attached to skin flaps of considerably diminished viability. In later cases, we removed the nipple-areola complex, thinned it, and applied it as a free graft to a prepared disk on the reconstructed breast.

CLINICAL RESULTS

There have been very few criticisms about the use of omentum for breast reconstruction. In all, we have treated 26 patients in this manner, 22 unilateral and 4 bilateral, with maximum follow-up of 9 years. Complications have been encouragingly few.

Of the abdominal complications, only one patient developed an abdominal hernia and one patient had a prolonged ileus. Five patients, however, complained of prolonged abdominal discomfort. Of the breast complications, 12 had a minimal skin loss that healed spontaneously. There were 5 implant displacements and 1 extrusion. Four patients developed a hematoma, and 1 patient developed an infection.

There has been only one serious and irreversible set of complications in the series, and this involved one patient

treated by bilateral subcutaneous mastectomy and immediate repair. She was anticoagulated postoperatively for a pulmonary embolus and subsequently developed repeated hematomas. These eventually became infected, despite aspiration, necessitating removal of the implant.

Significant displacement of the prosthesis postoperatively occurred most often in early patients in the series, in whom we erred in reconstructing with implants much too small for the overcapacious breast pocket. Despite carefully applied support, there was significant lateral displacement of the implants. Today we would not hesitate to reduce the size of the skin envelope before implanting.

We are aware of potential dangers and would now advise our patients to undergo, after 3 months, a minor secondary procedure in which the omental pedicle is divided and returned to the abdomen with full closure of the abdominal wall. There have been no long-term disasters resulting from the loss of the "abdominal policeman," even in those few patients in whom, for lack of material, most of the omentum has been transferred out of the abdomen.

SUMMARY

Omentum has proven ideal for breast reconstruction, providing a protective cover both for the skin flaps and for the implant, as well as actually providing some volume.

References

1. Arnold PG, Hartrampf CR, Jurkiewicz MJ. One-stage reconstruction of the breast using the transposed greater omentum. *Plast Reconstr Surg* 1976; 57:520.
2. Woods JE, Irons GB, Mason JK. Use of muscle, musculocutaneous and omental flaps to reconstruct difficult defects. *Plast Reconstr Surg* 1977; 59:191.
3. McColl I. Reconstruction of the breast with omentum after subcutaneous mastectomy. *Lancet* 1(Jan-Jun): 134, 1979.
4. Fissete J. Le lambeau épipldïque darts la reconstruction mammaire. *Acta Chir Belg* 1980;2:115.
5. Depoorter M. Reconstructive procedures after breast cancer surgery. *Acta Chir Belg* 1980;2:119.
6. Das SK. The size of the human omentum and methods of lengthening it for transplantation. *Br J Plast Surg* 1976;29:170.
7. Das SK. In: Barron JN, Saad MN, eds. *Operative plastic and reconstructive surgery.* Edinburgh: Churchill-Livingstone, 1980. Chap. 5;137–147.
8. Das SK. Assessment of the size of the human omentum. *Acta Anat* 1981; 110:108.

CHAPTER 357 ■ LATISSIMUS DORSI MUSCULOCUTANEOUS FLAP

J. M. GRIFFIN

EDITORIAL COMMENT

It was the latissimus dorsi myocutaneous flap that opened up the whole field of breast reconstruction. As initially introduced, it required the use of a prosthesis. Further modifications, such as described in the following chapters, may make it possible to reconstruct the breast without a prosthesis. This flap remains a most reliable one; it can be used with the muscle alone, or with an overlying skin island.

The latissimus dorsi musculocutaneous flap is a remarkably versatile, large, robust flap of many uses. The concept and development of this flap have revolutionized the approach to breast reconstruction (1–20). Although the rectus abdominis flap has reduced its popularity, the latissimus flap can still be quite useful for breast and chest-wall reconstruction.

INDICATIONS

There are several problems to consider when reconstructing a breast after mastectomy: (1) resurfacing of the chest wall with healthy tissue, (2) reconstruction of the breast mound itself, (3) restoration of the infraclavicular defect in the event of ablation or denervation of the pectoralis muscle, (4) reconstruction of the axillary tail of the breast, and (5) reconstruction of the nipple. All these reconstructive steps are performed with the purpose of restoration of normal breast symmetry. The latissimus dorsi flap can be used with considerable success in approaching all the preceding problems except for restoration of the infraclavicular defect.

ANATOMY

The latissimus dorsi muscle, as the name implies, "broadest of the back," has six origins: (1) the lower six thoracic spines and supraspinous ligaments, (2) the posterior layer of lumbar fascia, (3) the tendinous attachments to the iliac crest, (4) strips of muscle interdigitating with the external oblique muscle, (5) muscular slips from the lower four ribs, and (6) muscular slips from the scapula. The anterior and upper borders of the muscle are essentially free. The muscle is deep to the trapezius. The upper edge of the latissimus dorsi forms a "vest pocket" for the inferior angle of the scapula by running horizontally across the angle, from which it receives additional fibers. The insertion of the latissimus dorsi is in a broad ribbon-like tendon about 10 cm long, which inserts into the floor of the bicipital groove of the humerus behind the tendon of the long head of the biceps. The latissimus tendon curves around the lower border of the teres major muscle and forms, therefore, the posterior fold of the axilla, along with the subscapularis muscle.

The blood supply of the latissimus dorsi comes from a terminal branch of the subscapular artery, itself a branch of the third portion of the axillary artery (Fig. 1). The subscapular artery runs about 5 cm before dividing into the scapular circumflex and thoracodorsal arteries (21–23). The thoracodorsal artery is about 2 to 4 mm in diameter, and it courses along the posterior portion of the axilla for about 8 to 14 cm before it actually enters the latissimus dorsi itself. The thoracodorsal artery gives off one or two branches to the serratus anterior muscle and one branch to the skin. The thoracodorsal artery is accompanied by the thoracodorsal nerve and one or two thoracodorsal veins. The neurovascular supply to the latissimus dorsi muscle can be identified at the midpoint between the scapula and the abducted humerus about 0.5 inch from the free border of the muscle. Once the branches of the thoracodorsal artery

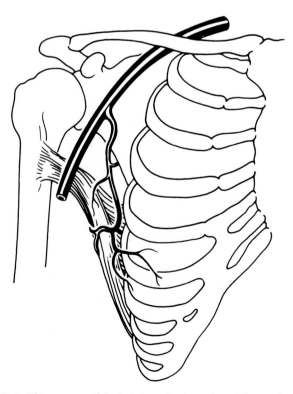

FIG. 1. The anatomy of the latissimus dorsi muscle and thoracodorsal pedicle.

penetrate the muscle, they divide and run parallel to the muscle fibers and, through perforating vessels, supply the entire skin overlying these vessels. The tendon of insertion of the latissimus dorsi can be divided close to the humerus without injury to the bundle. The combined lengths of the subscapular and thoracodorsal arteries, once their branches are divided, provide a very long, resilient pedicle.

A vigorous blood supply to the muscle is also available at its origin (24,25). Perforating vessels from the intercostal and lumbar arteries supply the muscle and overlying skin. These perforators enter the origin of the muscle just lateral to the thoracolumbar fascia, about 8 cm from the midline, at the level of the seventh, ninth, and eleventh vertebral spines. These perforating vessels, usually 1 to 1.5 mm in diameter, supply the so-called reversed latissimus flap.

The flap anatomy also allows the flap to be split and divided into two separate paddles if necessary (26).

FLAP DESIGN AND DIMENSIONS

Generally, when the flap is based at its insertion, the thoracodorsal vessels are not specifically identified and the pivot point is at the level of the midposterior axillary wall (27). When used as an island flap based on the subscapular and thoracodorsal vessels, the pivot point is 1.5 to 2 cm inferior to the pectoral humeral junction. Provided these vessels to the island flap are not rotated 360 degrees, the resulting flap is extremely mobile and can cover from the top of the head to the elbow region. The pivot point of the reversed flap is at the level of T7, T9, or T11, about 4 to 8 cm from the midline, on one or more of the posterior perforating vessels.

A difference in bulk between the latissimus on the operated side and that on the unoperated side may be an indication that the muscle has been denervated.

A skin paddle as large as 12 × 20 cm can be taken along with the muscle with the possibility of direct closure of the donor site. Of course, a skin paddle as large as the muscle itself and extending as far as 5 cm anteriorly and inferiorly to the muscle can be harvested without delay. If a larger skin portion is needed, appropriate surgical delays will be necessary.

When drawing out the skin paddle, one must remember that the further the paddle is from the axillary pivot point, the more difficult the dissection of the entire muscle will be, since considerable subcutaneous tunneling and retraction will be necessary.

With the patient standing or sitting, draw the outline of the latissimus dorsi on the patient using a cloth pattern. Using the pattern or measuring tape, determine the extent of the flap area needed and the mobility required. Determine the inframammary crease on the operated side and shade 3 to 4 cm in area below this crease for dissection and insetting of the muscle portion of the flap. The resulting breast reconstruction would prove to be too high if dissection were terminated at the inframammary crease itself.

Unless surgical considerations necessitate excision of the opposite breast, try to match the reconstruction with the existing breast. Avoid, if possible, the necessity for changing the contour of the existing breast. To this end, it is necessary to provide a reconstructed ptotic, normal-appearing breast. This goal requires that the skin portion of the latissimus flap be placed low and transversely on the reconstructed breast, preferably at the level of the inframammary crease. The shape of the skin paddle should not necessarily be elliptical, but rather should be in the shape of an L or J. This shape will provide a generous amount of tissue inferiorly and can extend up toward the axilla to simulate an axillary tail. One should take care that the skin portion of the flap be inserted low. This will avoid exposure of the flap skin, which is of a different color

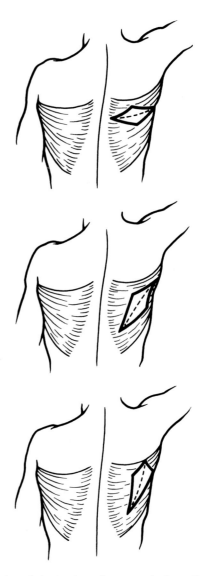

FIG. 2. Various design options diagrammatically outlined over the latissimus muscle.

and texture than breast skin, when the patient is wearing low-cut clothes. If tissue is needed higher on the reconstructed breast to fill out the infraclavicular defect, one should deep-ithelialize the skin portion of the flap and insert it beneath the existing chest skin.

If possible, the design of the skin paddle on the latissimus dorsi flap should be such that the resulting scar on the back is generally in a transverse or oblique position and can be covered by a brassiere (Fig. 2). To achieve this end, it is helpful to make preliminary drawings of the flap with the patient wearing her brassiere. The position of the resulting donor-site scar can be localized in relationship to this garment.

OPERATIVE TECHNIQUE

The easiest position on the operating table for raising the flap is the lateral position with the appropriate shoulder abducted and flexed to 90 degrees. The position may have to be changed after dissection of the flap to facilitate transfer of the flap, breast reconstruction, and possible surgery on the opposite breast. The position provides, however, the best exposure for dissection of the flap.

The incision should be straight down to the underlying muscle and should not undermine the skin flap. The skin inferior and superior to the skin paddle over the muscle must be freed by sharp or cautery dissection. Blunt dissection is extremely difficult in this plane. The muscle can then be defined and dissected sharply from either its anterior or superior free borders. Deep to the muscle anteriorly and perpendicular to the fibers of the latissimus dorsi are the fibers of the serratus anterior insertion. These fibers can be elevated easily with the latissimus dorsi and should be separated under direct vision using sharp dissection. If one starts dissection from the superior free border, blunt dissection usually is effective in elevating only the latissimus and not the surrounding muscles. If the serratus is inadvertently raised with the latissimus, it should be dissected from the latissimus sharply and returned to its proper place on the chest wall. Occasionally, particularly if the dissection is started inferiorly, posteriorly, or anteriorly, the overlying trapezius muscle can be raised with the flap and hinder anterior transposition of the flap.

If, while separating the latissimus muscle posteriorly, perforating vessels are encountered, the perforators should be divided and tied on both the flap and donor sides. One should realize that there are two sets of perforating vessels along the paravertebral area; these produce a considerable amount of bleeding if they are disturbed. For purposes of reconstruction, one needs muscle much more than fascia, and therefore, one should try to move only a small amount of fascia beyond the end of muscle from the paravertebral area. If one dissects only a short way into the paravertebral area and does not dissect as low as the iliac crest, one will avoid many large bleeders. Bleeding also may occur where the rib origin of latissimus dorsi interdigitates with the external oblique muscle. This dissection must be sharp, and appropriate hemostasis is necessary.

Once the edges of the latissimus dorsi are dissected free and the muscle and skin are elevated toward the insertion, the muscle becomes much more mobile. There is no need for direct visual exposure of the thoracodorsal vessels if the flap is elevated only to about midaxillary level. If the flap is elevated beyond this point or used as an island flap, the neurovascular bundle should be visualized. It can be seen entering the muscle about 10 cm from its insertion, or at about the midpoint of the axilla with the arm abducted 90 degrees. The thoracodorsal artery can be further freed just proximal to its entrance to the latissimus dorsi by dividing the branch of the thoracodorsal artery to serratus anterior and by dividing the occasional cutaneous branch of the thoracodorsal artery to the lateral chest wall. The proximal pedicle of the vessel is easily seen and dissected from the areolar tissue adjacent to the muscle itself. Once the vascular pedicle is visualized and protected, the insertion of the muscle can be encircled with the finger. With direct visualization of the vascular pedicle, the insertion can then be divided and transposed and the muscle can be used as an island flap. This greatly increases the flap's range and mobility.

The anterior pocket is dissected with the patient in the same position. Care is taken to dissect 3 to 4 cm inferior to the inframammary crease. Exposure is carried to the sternum medially and well up under the pectoralis remnant superiorly if the muscle is still intact. Dissection should not be carried too far laterally, since the breast reconstruction may be asymmetrical and the donor-site pocket may inadvertently be entered (28).

Once the anterior pocket is prepared, a tunnel is created from the posterior dissection high in the axilla and the flap is passed to the anterior wound. One should take care to avoid twisting the flap, particularly if it is an island flap. Kinking of the island pedicle by the branch of the thoracodorsal artery to the serratus anterior muscle should be avoided by division and ligation of this branch. The tunnel should be large enough to avoid compression of the flap but small enough to avoid lateral and posterior displacement of the prosthesis.

Once the flap is raised and transferred to the recipient site, the donor site can then be closed. The donor site can be closed primarily in the great majority of musculocutaneous flap reconstructions. If the skin paddle is very large, a skin graft may be necessary. Suction drainage should be used in the donor site and should be left in several days.

At this stage, the patient may be turned to the supine position for the breast reconstruction and for surgery on the opposite breast if needed.

Anteriorly, several sutures may be necessary to snug up the exit from the flap tunnel in the axilla. The muscle is then sutured to the sternum medially, to the pectoralis muscle remnants superiorly, and to the chest wall 3 to 4 cm inferior to the inframammary crease. If not enough muscle is available to stretch inferiorly, then the muscle should be sutured to the skin above the crease. Restricting the size of the pocket inferiorly should be avoided. The implant is then inserted under the pectoralis and latissimus muscles. No attempt is made to place the implant beneath the serratus anterior muscle.

At this point, one can attempt to reconstruct the infraclavicular defect. This is a problem that has not been solved satisfactorily. The latissimus dorsi muscle can be attached to the clavicle, but it is relatively thin and would have to be detached from its insertion. Even when the insertion of muscle is attached and folded over twice, it does not provide enough bulk for satisfactory correction of this defect.

Custom silicone implants have been tried to reconstruct the infraclavicular defect, but the implants often form capsular contractures with the edges of the implant palpable and visible.

A dermal graft from excess skin from the island over the latissimus dorsi muscle can be used. The graft can be folded upon itself like a sandwich, to receive blood supply from two directions. The lower abdomen has not been a satisfactory donor site for this sort of graft because of the relatively thin dermis and thick subdermal fat layer.

The axillary tail of the breast can be reconstructed by deepithelializing a portion of the skin paddle and extending it into the axilla or the latissimus muscle can be divided from its insertion (Fig. 3). One must take care to avoid the neurovascular bundle to the latissimus dorsi. The tendon of insertion can be attached to the pectoralis muscle and provide a satisfactory reconstruction.

Nipple reconstruction is usually deferred until maturation of the reconstruction; this subsequent surgery can be performed on an outpatient basis.

CLINICAL RESULTS

Seromas or hematomas can form either at the donor or recipient site. If these occur once the drains have been removed, incisions can be made in the most dependent portions of the wounds. Multiple needle aspirations can be performed, but these may be less effective.

Because of the strong, vigorous blood supply to the flap, flap necrosis is rare, even with ablation of the thoracodorsal artery in previous surgery. Necrosis has been reported when there has been undue tension or torsion on the flap pedicle.

Transient brachial palsy, particularly posterior cord or radial nerve palsy, can be encountered with improper positioning. Vigorous dissection near the takeoff of the subscapular artery from the axillary artery also can produce transient palsy, since this dissection is adjacent to the brachial plexus itself. Unless direct surgical damage has been inflicted on the brachial plexus, the palsy is reversible within several weeks.

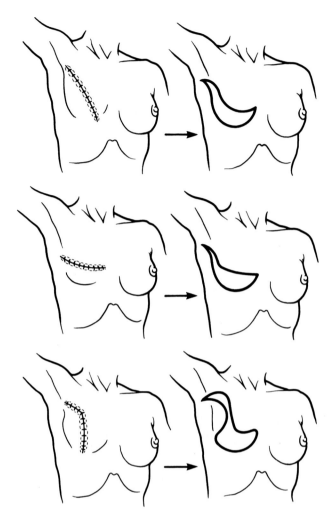

FIG. 3. The latissimus dorsi musculocutaneous unit can be designed and inset in various ways depending on the extent and nature of the recipient defect.

Inadvertent elevation of the serratus or trapezius muscles along with the latissimus muscle will produce limited flap mobility and may restrict shoulder motion.

Vigorously active patients may experience some weakness of the shoulder in lifting themselves from a chair or on parallel bars or may experience weakness in competitive swimming. Crutch walking is not usually affected. The latissimus dorsi may be required by patients with polio who need the muscle to elevate the ipsilateral pelvis in walking.

Results from breast reconstruction using the latissimus dorsi flap have been quite satisfactory. The use of a J-shaped flap, rather than the elliptical flap, and the low placement of this flap on the reconstructed breast have made a significant improvement in the quality of breast reconstructions. Flap viability has been quite predictable, although there have been some flap losses reported, associated with a combination of excessive flap tension and a previously ablated thoracodorsal vessel.

SUMMARY

The latissimus dorsi musculocutaneous flap, combined with an implant, can provide the excess skin and bulk needed for breast reconstruction after mastectomy.

References

1. Schneider WJ, Hill HL Jr, Brown RG. Latissimus dorsi myocutaneous flap for breast reconstruction. *Br J Plast Surg* 1977;30:277.
2. Bostwick J, Vasconez LO, Jurkiewicz MJ. Breast reconstruction after a radical mastectomy. *Plast Reconstr Surg* 1978;61:682.
3. Bailey BN. Latissimus dorsi flap—a practical approach. *Ann Acad Med* 1979;8:445.
4. Bostwick J, Nahai F, Wallace JG, Vasconez LO. Sixty latissimus dorsi flaps. *Plast Reconstr Surg* 1979;63:31.
5. Horton CE, Rosato FA, McCraw JB, Dowden RV. Immediate reconstruction following mastectomy for cancer. *Clin Plast Surg* 1979;6:37.
6. McCraw JB, Bostwick J, Horton CE. Methods of soft tissue coverage for the mastectomy defect. *Clin Plast Surg* 1979;6:57.
7. Olivari N. The latissimus dorsi flap, experience with 51 operations. *Acta Chir Belg* 1980;2:111.
8. Depoorter M. Reconstructive procedures after breast cancer surgery. *Acta Chir Belg* 1980;2:119.
9. Bostwick J. Reconstruction of the breast. *Acta Chir Belg* 1980;2:125.
10. McCraw JB, Maxwell GP, Horton CE. Reconstruction of the breast following mastectomy. *Acta Chir Belg* 1980;2:131.
11. Lejour M, Eder H, De Mey A, Mattheiem W. Breast reconstruction at the Tumor Center of the University of Brussels. *Acta Chir Belg* 1980;2:135.
12. Mendelson BC. The latissimus dorsi flap for breast reconstruction. *Aust NZ J Surg* 1980;50:200.
13. Bostwick J, Jurkiewicz MJ. Recent advances in breast reconstruction: transposition of the latissimus dorsi muscle singly or with the overlying skin. *Am Surg* 1980;46:537.
14. Maxwell GP. Iginio Tansini and the origin of the latissimus dorsi musculocutaneous flap. *Plast Reconstr Surg* 1980;65:686.
15. Bostwick J, Scheflan M, Nahai F, Jurkiewicz MJ. The "reverse" latissimus dorsi muscle and musculocutaneous flap: anatomic and clinical considerations. *Plast Reconstr Surg* 1980;65:395.
16. Bishop JB, Fisher J, Bostwick J. The burned female breast. *Ann Plast Surg* 1980;4:25.
17. Fodor PB, Khoury F. Latissimus dorsi muscle flap in reconstruction of congenitally absent breast and pectoralis muscle. *Ann Plast Surg* 1980;4:422.
18. Pendergrast WJ, Bostwick J, Jurkiewicz MJ. The subcutaneous mastectomy cripple: surgical rehabilitation with the latissimus dorsi flap. *Plast Reconstr Surg* 1980;66:554.
19. Bostwick J, Scheflan M. The latissimus dorsi musculocutaneous flap: a one-stage breast reconstruction. *Clin Plast Surg* 1980;7:71.
20. Vasconez LO, Johnson-Giebink R, Hall EJ. Breast reconstruction. *Clin Plast Surg* 1980;7:79.
21. McCraw JB, Dibbell DG. Experimental definition of independent myocutaneous vascular territories. *Plast Reconstr Surg* 1977;60:212.
22. Rubinstein ZJ, Shafir R, Tsur H. The value of angiography prior to use of the latissimus dorsi myocutaneous flap. *Plast Reconstr Surg* 1979;63:374.
23. Bartlett SP, May JW Jr, Yaremchuk MJ. The latissimus dorsi muscle: a fresh cadaver study of the primary neurovascular pedicle. *Plast Reconstr Surg* 1981;67:631.
24. Levine RA, DeFelice CA. Possible explanation of successful latissimus dorsi flap without the thoracodorsal artery. *Plast Reconstr Surg* 1980;65:532.
25. Maxwell GP, McGibbon BM, Hoopes JE. Vascular considerations in the use of a latissimus dorsi myocutaneous flap after a mastectomy with an axillary dissection. *Plast Reconstr Surg* 1979;64:771.
26. Tobin GR, Schustennan M, Peterson GH, et al. The intramuscular neurovascular anatomy of the latissimus dorsi muscle: the basis for splitting the flap. *Plast Reconstr Surg* 1981;67:637.
27. Dinner MI, Peters CR. The arc of the latissimus dorsi myocutaneous flap. *Ann Plast Surg* 1979;3:425.
28. Vasconez LO. Colloquium: total breast reconstruction. *Ann Plast Surg* 1981;7:62.

CHAPTER 358 ■ EXTENDED COMPOSITE LATISSIMUS DORSI MUSCULOCUTANEOUS FLAP

D. R. MARSHALL

The early results of breast reconstruction with a latissimus dorsi musculocutaneous flap combined with a prosthesis are good (1), but there is a significant complication rate in the long term, capsule formation is common, and outright rejection happens not infrequently (2).

The extended composite latissimus dorsi musculocutaneous flap is most suitable in a woman with a breast of average size. It relies on use of the whole latissimus dorsi muscle to carry a skin paddle for reconstruction of the mastectomy loss and also to carry a deepithelialized portion of skin and dermis to provide the volume usually provided by a prosthesis.

INDICATIONS

The skin and fat of the lower abdomen are excellent donors for a soft-tissue reconstruction (3), but there are many problems in the transfer of this tissue to the breast. The direct flap transfer (4) is too cumbersome, and the external oblique musculocutaneous flap (see Chapter 361) is useful in the patient who is not particularly overweight, but the blood supply is somewhat unpredictable and a delay procedure may be required for the safe transfer of the soft tissue.

The rectus abdominis flap is not without donor-site problems (3), and the risk of thromboembolic complications is significant. It is much simpler to use the highly vascular latissimus dorsi flap to provide the normal muscle and skin required in a postmastectomy reconstruction, and it is possible to carry enough soft tissue with it to provide for the required augmentation.

ANATOMY

See Chapter 357.

FLAP DESIGN AND DIMENSIONS

Various methods have been described for locating the skin incision and for taking the underlying muscle when performing a latissimus dorsi flap (5). Whether a small or large portion of the muscle remains is unimportant, since it is completely denervated and, subsequent to the operation, gradually atrophies. There is thus no reason why one should not transfer the whole of the latissimus dorsi muscle and in doing so carry with it into the breast a much larger volume of skin and subcutaneous tissue than was previously possible. The muscle extends from the angle of the scapula to the

iliac crest, and there is considerably more subcutaneous tissue situated over the lower than the upper part of the muscle.

The whole of the latissimus dorsi muscle and adherent subcutaneous tissue from the loin, equal to the volume of the prosthesis usually employed in breast reconstruction, may be safely raised on the subscapular vascular pedicle and used to achieve a one-stage breast reconstruction without need for a prosthesis.

A large sickle of skin and fat is outlined on the back, lower down than usual. The sickle is planned to be let into the submammary groove and is outlined to lie basically in the skin fold below the scapula, since more tissue can be taken in this plane and the wound can be closed without tension (Fig. 1C).

The large dart of skin marked out beneath the sickle extends down over the lower portion of the latissimus dorsi muscle as far as the iliac crest to provide a T-shaped flap of skin and subcutaneous tissue.

OPERATIVE TECHNIQUE

The operation is carried out in a patient with a breast of moderate size (Fig. 1) and with the patient on her side. The epithelium is removed from the vertical portion of the T of skin and fat (Fig. 2), and then the flap is elevated in the usual way. The muscle is dissected off the underlying serratus anterior and from the overlying skin and fat up to the axilla, but it is not necessary to dissect beyond the branches of the subcapsular vessels to the serratus anterior muscle.

The lower portion of the muscle is dissected off the thoracic and lumbar spines and from the posterior portion of the iliac crest and out laterally to its free border. The muscle is dissected upward off the rib cage where it interdigitates with the external oblique muscle, and the large flap of subcutaneous tissue is left attached to the muscle throughout (Fig. 2B). There is no problem with viability, and at the completion of the dissection, the flap is seen bleeding freely.

It is fortunate that the subcutaneous tissue situated in the loin corresponds in most women to the size of the breast. In a relatively thin woman, there is a small but adequate amount of soft tissue in the loin for breast reconstruction, while in a woman with a larger breast, there is a large amount of subcutaneous tissue in this region both overlying the latissimus dorsi muscle and lying beneath it in the groove adjacent to the erector spinae muscles.

Direct closure of the defect is achieved by mobilizing the skin across the midline and dissecting it off the spines of the lumbar vertebrae. The flap is transferred around anteriorly

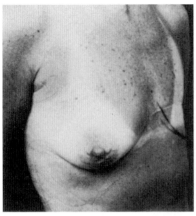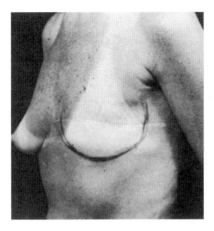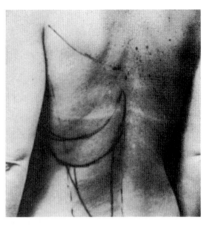

A–C

FIG. 1. A: This patient had a Patey mastectomy for carcinoma of the breast 2 years prior to reconstruction. She has a normal right breast of average size. B: The planned incision is shown, since placing the flap in the submammary groove generally produces a better breast contour. C: The limits of the latissimus dorsi muscle are shown, and the large sickle of skin and fat to replace the skin defect is shown running in the crease line, well below the angle of the scapula. The large dart of skin to be deepithelialized runs inferiorly to this, down to and over the iliac crest.

and is let into the incision in the submammary groove. The skin and subcutaneous tissue are lifted off the chest wall to accommodate the new breast. Any remnant of pectoral muscle is left attached to the skin flap, since problems of viability are more likely to be encountered here than with the composite latissimus dorsi flap.

The sickle-shaped flap of skin is inserted into the defect created in the submammary groove and deepithelialized skin and subcutaneous tissue, and the lower portion of muscle is turned beneath the skin flap and is sutured to the muscle higher up to provide adequate bulk in the upper portion of the reconstructed breast. Only a few sutures are necessary, and the breast tissue is allowed to fall into the somewhat dependent shape of the normal breast. The wounds are closed with drainage.

CLINICAL RESULTS

Complications are extremely rare. Postoperative hematoma and wound infection can be prevented by meticulous tech-

nique. The vascularity of the flap is excellent both for skin replacement and for dermis-fat volume replacement. The usual problems of a deepithelialized dermis as a volume replacement occasionally occur, viz., epithelial cyst formation, but this is very uncommon.

The procedure is well tolerated by the patient, and postoperative recovery is much faster than for a rectus abdominis or external oblique musculocutaneous flap reconstruction. An occasional seroma may develop beneath the skin flaps of the back, but this responds quickly to aspiration. The donor scar, while obvious, is in an area where it is out of sight and it is quite well accepted (Fig. 3).

SUMMARY

A modification of the standard latissimus dorsi musculocutaneous flap makes it a far more acceptable procedure for breast reconstruction. A large paddle of deepithelialized skin and subcutaneous tissue is added so that a prosthesis is not necessary.

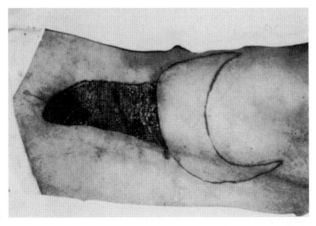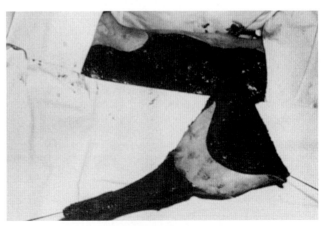

A   B

FIG. 2. A: The sickle-shaped flap and its dermis/subcutaneous extension all overlying the latissimus dorsi muscle and the area that is deepithelialized are shown. B: The whole of the latissimus dorsi muscle is elevated and extends to the limits of the deepithelialized flap.

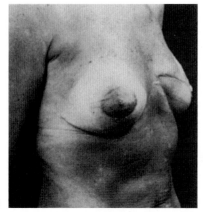
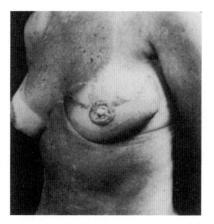
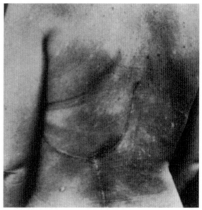

A–C

FIG. 3. A, B: The result 3 months later, with the breast of similar volume to the normal side. A nipple reconstruction has been carried out using a composite graft, and symmetrical breasts of normal consistency are the result. No prosthesis has been used. **C:** Note that the donor-site incisions have been closed primarily. The donor scar can be seen, and although extensive, it is in a position where it is not normally seen by the patient. It is well accepted.

References

1. Bostwick J, Vasconez LO, Jurkiewicz, MJ. Breast reconstruction after radical mastectomy. *Plast Reconstr Surg* 1978;61:682.
2. Marshall DR, Mutimer KA. Complications of breast reconstruction. Presented at the 56th General Surgery Meeting of the Royal Academy, Hong Kong, 1983.
3. Dinner MI, Labandter HP, Dowden RV. The role of the rectus abdominis myocutaneous flap in breast reconstruction. *Plast Reconstr Surg* 1982; 69:209.
4. Marshall DR, Anstee EJ, Stapleton MJ. Postmastectomy breast reconstruction using a direct flap from an abdominal lipectomy. *Br J Plast Surg* 1981;34:280.
5. Wolf LE, Biggs TM. Aesthetic refinements in the use of the latissimus dorsi flap in breast reconstruction. *Plast Reconstr Surg* 1982;69:788.

CHAPTER 359 ■ AUTOGENOUS LATISSIMUS FLAP FOR BREAST RECONSTRUCTION

J. B. MCGRAW, C. A. RHEE, AND B. STRAUCH

EDITORIAL COMMENT

This is an excellent technique for breast reconstruction in which a prosthesis is not used. It does not replace the TRAM or the free TRAM; however, in female patients with very large, thick septocutaneous layers, the latissimus with expanded subcutaneous tissue can be utilized for breast reconstruction without a prosthesis. Howerer, the concavity that is created at the donor site is noticeable, and the opposite side may have to be suctioned for equalization.

The autogenous latissimus flap for breast reconstruction differs from the original design, in that it incorporates full-thickness fat overlying the entire latissimus dorsi muscle, in addition to the myocutaneous paddle of skin, full-thickness fat, and muscle.

INDICATIONS

The standard latissimus flap for breast reconstruction necessitates the additional use of an implant to provide volume and shape. A high incidence of capsular contracture has been described with the use of this technique. The autogenous latissimus flap can be used in partial reconstruction of the breast for contour deformities following partial mastectomy and quadrantectomy. It has also been useful for reconstruction of Poland's chest deformity and post-radiation-induced skin damage.

The method is a reasonable alternative when TRAM reconstruction cannot be performed, due to previous abdominal lipectomy or procedures in which the blood supply to the rectus abdominis muscle or the muscle itself have been disrupted. In addition, the autogenous latissimus flap can be used as a backup following TRAM reconstruction, to restore contour deficiencies following partial flap failure.

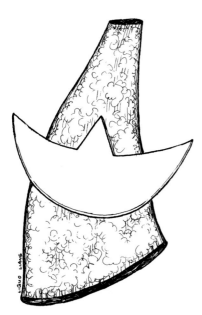

FIG. 1. Fleur-de-lis design. Initially used, but since abandoned because of unfavorable donor-site scar.

The advantages of this flap include the use of autogenous tissue replacement of breast volume, thus offering excellent restoration of the anterior axillary fold and infraclavicular breast, providing all the tissue required for shaping the breast without the use of an implant (in most cases), as well as a good donor-site scar. In all but very thin patients, a breast implant is not needed to restore volume. The procedure is a reasonable alternative to the pedicled TRAM flap in patients who have more than 2 cm of back fat by pinch test (1–3).

The procedure cannot be performed in patients who have had a previous thoracotomy in which the latissimus muscle or blood supply has been disrupted. Prolonged postoperative seroma formation at the donor site can be a problem.

ANATOMY

The latissimus dorsi muscle is a large, flat, triangular muscle, which extends over the lumbar region and the lower part of the thorax. The muscle is supplied by the thoracodorsal artery and intercostal perforators, and it originates from the posterior aspect of the iliac crest, lumbar fascia, spines of the lower six thoracic vertebrae, and from the lower three ribs. Its tendinous portion inserts onto the bicipital groove of the humerus. Its actions are to extend, adduct, and medially rotate the arm.

FLAP DESIGN AND DIMENSIONS

Previously, a three-cornered skin paddle fleur-de-lis skin design (4) was initially used, but has since been abandoned due to its unfavorable donor-site scar (Fig. 1). A crescent-shaped skin paddle is now used. The skin paddle is oriented horizontally over the fat roll of the back (Fig. 2). This places the closure parallel to the lines of skin tension and allows for a favorable scar when closed primarily. The bulk of the flap is provided by the fat carried on the entire surface of the latissimus muscle, including the two adjacent areas: scapular fat overlying the trapezius, and the fat above the iliac crest. The length of the flap varies with the girth of the patient, and the width of the flap is designed in relation to what can be easily closed.

OPERATIVE TECHNIQUE

The skin paddle is incised full thickness through the fat of the back down to the latissimus muscle. The entire muscle is elevated with the overlying full-thickness layer of fat, including the scapular fat overlying the trapezius and the fat above the iliac crest (Fig. 3).

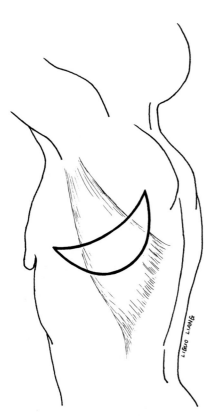

FIG. 2. Crescent-shaped skin paddle oriented horizontally over fat roll of back.

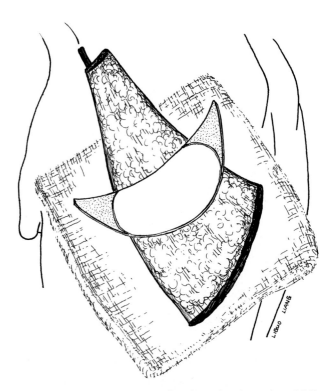

FIG. 3. Latissimus myocutaneous flap elevated with muscle and full-thickness fat from the scapular region and iliac crest.

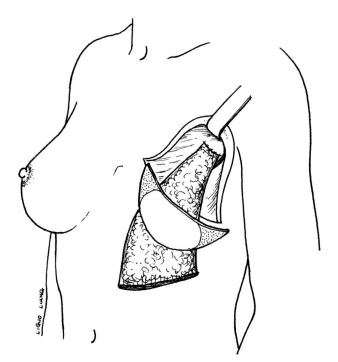

FIG. 4. Flap transposed anteriorly onto chest wall.

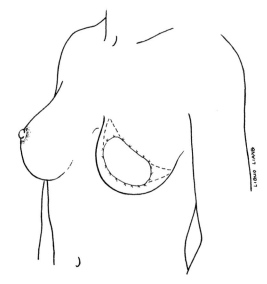

FIG. 6. Final result. Flap inset and lateral limbs deepithelialized and buried.

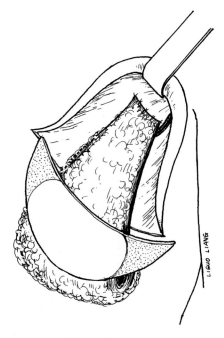

FIG. 5. Lower portion of muscle folded inward to provide breast projection. Inframammary fold to be created by tacking inferior border of fold to chest wall.

The thoracodorsal vessels are dissected completely free in the axilla, to avoid kinking of the pedicle. The muscle, when transposed, reaches beyond the margin of the rib cage anteriorly and has the necessary mobility for folding the muscle on itself (Fig. 4).

Insetting begins by attaching the extensive fat surrounding the latissimus tendon to the tendon of the pectoralis major muscle, to recreate the anterior axillary fold. The insetting is continued by attaching the anterior border of the latissimus muscle to the infraclavicular portion of the pectoralis muscle near the clavicle. Medially, the edge of the muscle forms the cleavage through an inset near the midline on the sternum. The distal margin of the muscle is folded beneath the skin paddle to provide projection, and tacked to the chest wall to recreate the inframammary fold (Fig. 5).

The skin paddle is shaped into a U, deepithelialized, and buried, if there is adequate skin cover (Fig. 6). If there is deficient breast skin, the skin paddle is used to replace the lower breast skin that normally lies between the nipple and inframammary fold.

Prior to closure, the skin of the back is evaluated with 1000 mg fluorescein. Any areas of inadequate vascularity are discarded. Suction drains are placed, and removed when the output is less than 30 cc per day. The back is supported with elastic tape dressing, to provide compression and to allow the skin flap to adhere to the chest wall.

SUMMARY

The autogenous latissimus flap is an improvement of the standard latissimus flap. This technique allows for complete reconstruction of breast volume and, in most cases, obviates the need for implant placement. It offers a feasible alternative to TRAM reconstruction, with acceptable results and minimal donor-site morbidity.

References

1. McCraw JB, Papp C, Edwards A, McMellin A. The autogenous latissimus breast reconstruction. *Clin Plast Surg* 1994;21:279.
2. Papp C, Zanon E, McCraw J. Breast volume replacement using the deepithelialized latissimus dorsi myocutaneous flap. *Eur J Plast Surg* 1988;11:120.
3. Schneider W, Hill L, Brown R. Latissimus dorsi myocutaneous flap for breast reconstruction. *Br J Plast Surg* 1977;30:2277.
4. McCraw JB, Papp C. The fleur-de-lis autogenous latissimuss dorsi myocutaneous flap breast reconstruction. Presented at the Annual Meeting of the American Association of Plastic Surgeons, Scottsdale, AZ, May 1989.

CHAPTER 360 ■ INTERCOSTAL ARTERY PERFORATOR (ICAP) FLAP FOR BREAST RECONSTRUCTION IN POST–BARIATRIC WEIGHT LOSS PATIENTS

S. KWEI, L. J. BORUD, AND B. T. LEE

EDITORIAL COMMENT

This chapter shows how anatomical concepts can be applied to reconstructive efforts in treating an increasing bariatric patient population.

Perforator flaps based on the intercostal vessels along the anterior axillary line were first described for free-tissue transfer to resurface neck burn wounds. The intercostal artery perforator (ICAP) flap has also been reported as a pedicled perforator flap for the reconstruction of partial mastectomy lateral defects. More recently, the ICAP flap has been described for autologous breast augmentation after massive weight loss in bariatric patients.

INDICATIONS

Patients with excessive lateral upper truncal tissue are candidates for the ICAP flap. The flap uses redundant skin and subcutaneous tissue based on the intercostal artery perforators. This extra tissue may be used as a free flap or redistributed regionally to augment the breast or to add volume to a lateral breast defect. Common current applications for the pedicled ICAP flap include (a) reconstruction of lateral and inferior oncologic breast defects (1,2); (b) autologous breast augmentation in bariatric patients after massive weight loss (1–3); (c) contralateral symmetry augmentation reconstruction in unilateral breast cancer patients; and (d) autologous augmentation of a previously reconstructed breast.

ANATOMY

Intercostal flaps were first described in 1978 (1) for torso reconstruction and were designed based on branches originating from the aorta between the T7 and T11 interspaces. These vessels were found to terminate anteriorly, adjacent to branches from the superior and inferior epigastric vessels. The use of the latissimus dorsi myocutaneous flap for breast reconstruction (1) characterized the potential of the thoracodorsal pedicle, and perforator flaps from this system were later introduced in 1995 (1). The distinction between the thoracodorsal artery perforator (TDAP) and intercostal artery perforator (ICAP) flaps was subsequently described for reconstruction of breast defects (2). The intercostal flap described herein originates from the internal mammary vessels, with perforators that penetrate the serratus anterior muscle at the level of the anterior axillary line. This system is adjacent, yet distinct, from the thoracodorsal system.

The blood supply to the lateral chest wall is supplied by the thoracodorsal perforators, the lateral thoracic vessels, and the intercostal artery perforators. The thoracodorsal perforators can be found at the anterior edge of the latissimus muscle, and there can be one or two perforating vessels. The lateral thoracic vessels are located anterior to the latissimus and are more superior on the chest. The intercostal artery perforators are located 2.5 to 5 cm anterior to the latissimus muscle. They emanate from the fifth interspace, and occasionally the fourth interspace, at the anterior axillary line. These vessels penetrate the slips of the serratus and are typically 1.5 mm in size but can be significantly larger in a patient with massive weight loss (4–8).

FLAP DESIGN AND DIMENSIONS

The ICAP flap is based on the fourth or fifth intercostal artery perforators (or both) that are located along the anterior axillary line. With a Doppler probe, the intercostal cutaneous perforators are identified to plan the base of the flap, measuring 6 to 8 cm, depending on the number of perforators incorporated into the flap. The length of the flap extends posteriorly and follows the curvature of the ribs, up to 15 to 20 cm in length. The inferior border of the flap is located just below the inframammary fold and the fifth interspace. Posteriorly, the flap can be angled superiorly, according to the amount of excessive truncal tissue. When used in conjunction with a Wise-pattern mastopexy, the flap is designed as a lateral extension of the inferior pedicle (Fig. 1). Once elevated, the flap can then be rotated 90 degrees to fill the lateral aspect of the breast, or turned over to fill the inferior border.

OPERATIVE TECHNIQUE

Elevation of the ICAP flap begins at its distal apex from posterior to anterior. Patients with massive weight loss may need to be placed in the prone position to gain access to the posterior truncal tissue. Otherwise, some lateral rotation is required for access to the apex of the flap posteriorly. Dissection is carried out through the skin and subcutaneous tissue, with inclusion of the muscle fascia in the flap.

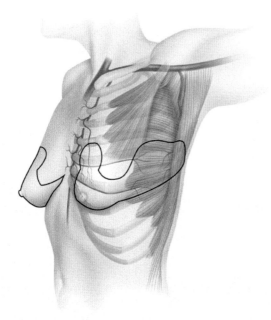

FIG. 1. Schematic illustration of the intercostal artery perforator (ICAP) flap.

If more volume is necessary, the periphery of the flap can be beveled outward. The muscle fascia is then raised from posterior to anterior, and small perforating branches from the thoracodorsal axis are encountered first, lateral to the major intercostal perforators. These thoracodorsal perforators are sacrificed lateral to the serratus muscle. The lateral thoracic vessels can be seen at the superior aspect of the dissection and are divided, as well. On identification of the serratus anterior muscle, great care is taken to identify the intercostal perforators that traverse through the muscle slips. The largest perforator is usually at the fifth interspace, but another perforator can be found at the fourth interspace. A Doppler probe may be used intraoperatively to ensure incorporation of the intercostal perforators in the flap. It is not necessary to isolate the perforators through the interspace.

The flap-donor site is closed in a layered fashion. Depending on the size of the donor-site defect, a drain may be placed. Once the donor site is closed, the patient is returned to the supine position for breast shaping. The flap is then deepithelialized, and the distal perfusion of the flap can be assessed. In mastopexy and autologous augmentation, such as in the patient with massive weight loss, the flap is designed in conjunction with a Wise-pattern mastopexy inferior pedicle. The ICAP flap is rotated superiorly up to the breast and anchored to the chest wall and inferior pedicle, to provide definition to the lateral border of the breast. It has also been described in conjunction with a superior-pedicle mastopexy.

When used to reconstruct a partial mastectomy defect, the flap can be rotated 90 degrees to fill laterally, or turned over to fill inferiorly. It can be designed for replacement of the skin envelope or augmentation of a contour deformity. The flap can also be used for augmentation of a previously reconstructed breast. For this purpose, dissection is carried out under the previous reconstruction, and the flap is tacked into this pocket.

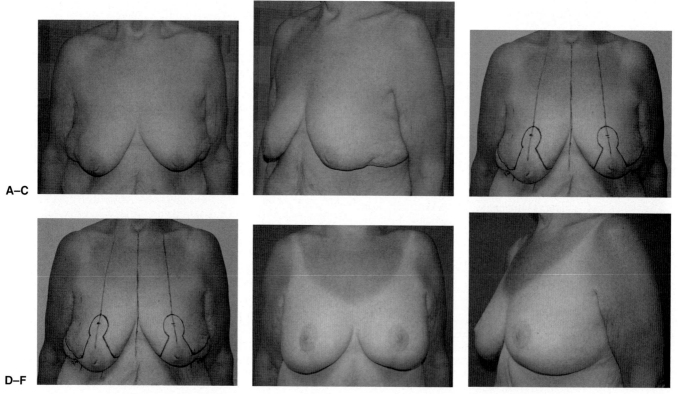

A–C

D–F

FIG. 2. A,B: The intercostal artery perforator flap for autologous augmentation after massive weight loss. C,D: Preoperative markings. Note that the inferior border of the flap extends below the inframammary fold laterally. E,F: One-year postoperative result. Note the improvement in the lateral breast contour.

CLINICAL RESULTS

Successful pedicled ICAP flap reconstruction has been achieved in patients for partial mastectomy defects, for autologous augmentation in patients with massive weight loss (9) (Fig. 2), and for restoration of breast symmetry in a previously reconstructed or contralateral breast. Early reports have noted seroma occurrence, as well as fat necrosis, with a large flap and a long distal component. These early findings have been minimized, as the perforator anatomy is better understood, ensuring more robust survival of the ICAP flap.

SUMMARY

The use of lateral truncal tissue based on the intercostal artery perforators provides an appealing source for extra volume. The ICAP flap can be useful for augmentation or reconstruction of lateral and inferior defects of the breast. Careful identification of the perforating vessels ensures robust, long-term survival of the flap, with minimal fat necrosis.

References

1. Badran HA, Youssef MK, Shaker AA. Management of facial contour deformities with deepithelialized lateral intercostal free flap. *Ann Plast Surg* 1997;37:94.
2. Hamdi M, Van Landuyt K, Monstrey S, Blondeel P. Pedicled perforator flaps in breast reconstruction: a new concept. *Br J Plast Surg* 2004;57:531.
3. Levine JL, Soueid NE, Allen RJ. Algorithm for autologous breast reconstruction for partial mastectomy defects. *Plast Reconstr Surg* 2005;116:762.
4. Hamdi M, Van Landuyt K, de Frene B, et al. The versatility of the intercostal artery perforator (ICAP). *J Plast Reconstruct Aesth Surg* 2006;59:644.
5. Rubin P, Agha-Mohammadi S, O'Toole JP, et al. Breast reshaping after massive weight loss. In: Aly A, ed. *Body contouring after massive weight loss.* St. Louis: Quality Medical Publishing, 2006.
6. Daniel R, Kerrigan CL, Gard DA. The great potential of the intercostal flap for torso reconstruction. *Plast Reconstr Surg* 1978;61:652.
7. Schneider WJ, Hill HL Jr, Brown RG. Latissimus dorsi myocutaneous flap for breast reconstruction. *Br J Plast Surg* 1977;30:277.
8. Angrigiani C, Grilli D, Siebert J. Latissimus dorsi musculocutaneous flap without muscle. *Plast Reconstr Surg* 1995;96:1608.
9. Kwei S, Borud LJ, Lee BT. Mastopexy with autologous augmentation after massive weight loss: the intercostal artery perforator (ICAP) flap. *Ann Plast Surg* 2006;57:361.

 CHAPTER 361. External Oblique Musculocutaneous Abdominal Flap *D. R. Marshall*
www.encyclopediaofflaps.com

CHAPTER 362 ■ RECTUS ABDOMINIS MUSCULOCUTANEOUS FLAP

M. I. DINNER, H. LABANDTER, AND R. V. DOWDEN

EDITORIAL COMMENT

Although supplanted by the TRAM flap, the vertically oriented rectus abdominus myocutaneous flap still has its place in reconstruction of the breast.

The rectus abdominis musculocutaneous flap provides a suitable alternative to the latissimus dorsi flap for breast mound reconstruction under specific circumstances.

INDICATIONS

Patients who require a flap and in whom the latissimus dorsi musculocutaneous flap is not available include the following:

(1) those with a previous thoracotomy transecting the latissimus muscle, those with congenital absence or severe atrophy of the muscle, those in whom the muscle was used previously as a free flap, or those in whom a previous latissimus muscle flap failed; (2) those with a modified radical mastectomy in whom the inferior half of the pectoralis major muscle has been resected or denervated, resulting in atrophy of that muscle; (3) those in whom the pectoralis major muscle is completely intact but inadequate skin is available to allow for adequate mound formation; and (4) those who strongly prefer a donor-site scar on the anterior abdominal wall instead of the back (1–3).

ANATOMY

The rectus abdominis is a long, broad strap muscle, broader above and extending the full length of the anterior abdominal wall [4]. It arises from the fifth, sixth, and seventh costal

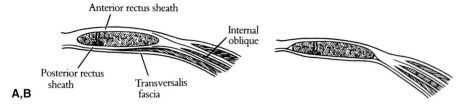

FIG. 1. A: Rectus sheath above linea arcuata. B: Rectus sheath below linea arcuata.

cartilages above and inserts into the crest of the pubis below. It is separated from its fellow by the linea alba in the midline. Three tendinous intersections interrupt the muscle fibers; these are at the level of the umbilicus below, at the free end of the xyphoid process above, and midway between these two.

The rectus abdominis muscle is enclosed in the rectus sheath, which is formed by the splitting of the aponeurosis of the internal oblique muscle. The sheath consists of an anterior and posterior lamina. The anterior lamina is reinforced by the aponeurosis of the external oblique muscle, and the posterior lamina is reinforced by the aponeurosis of the transversus abdominis muscle (Fig. 1). This fascial arrangement exists from the costal margin above to a variable level below, usually midway between the umbilicus and the symphysis pubis. At this level, the posterior sheath ends in a curved margin called the arcuate line (Fig. 1B). This is particularly important in the restoration of abdominal wall integrity after raising the rectus abdominis muscle or musculocutaneous flap.

This muscle has a dual dominant blood supply (Fig. 2). The upper vessel is the superior epigastric artery, one of the two terminal branches of the internal mammary artery. This descends in the space between the costal and xyphoid origins of the diaphragm and enters the rectus sheath at the upper medial extreme of the sheath and continues along the posterior surface of the muscle.

The lower vessel is the inferior epigastric artery that arises from the external iliac artery above the level of the inguinal ligament. It traverses upward and medially on the extraperitoneal tissues, where it perforates the transversalis fascia to pass anterior to the arcuate line and continues between the posterior rectus sheath and the rectus muscle. Within the muscle, these vessels divide into multiple terminal branches that communicate at the level of the umbilicus (Fig. 2A). Both being dominant vessels, either may be ligated and the muscle will survive.

The perforators to the skin overlying the rectus abdominis muscle are of the indirect type and traverse the rectus abdominis muscle to supply the overlying skin (5). These tend to lie along the medial third of the rectus abdominis muscle (see Fig. 1). They are predominantly above the level of the arcuate line, and more than one perforator below the arcuate line is rare.

FLAP DESIGN AND DIMENSIONS

The rectus abdominis musculocutaneous (RAM) flap may be either horizontal or vertical. The vertical flap may be inferiorly based or superiorly based.

Vertical Superiorly Based RAM Flap

The size will depend on the reconstructive requirements, but the skin may include the full length of the anterior abdominal wall, about 30 cm long in the average adult. The width may vary from 10 to 15 cm, still allowing for primary closure of the anterior abdominal wall. The axis of rotation point of the superior rectus abdominis musculocutaneous flap will be the point of entry of the superior epigastric artery into the rectus abdominis muscle at the subcostal margin. However, this point may be extended superiorly by dissection of the superior epigastric vessel proximally to various levels of the internal mammary artery. The arc of rotation is 0 to 180 degrees in either clockwise or counterclockwise direction. The reach of

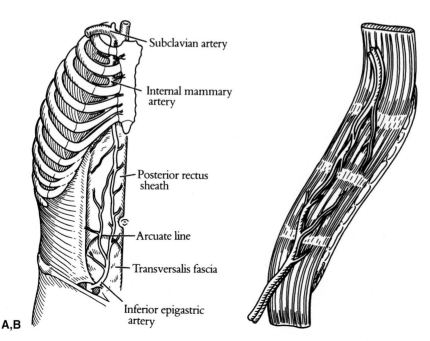

FIG. 2. A,B: Dual dominant blood supply, superior and inferior epigastric vessels.

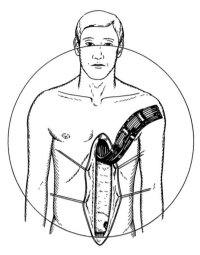

FIG. 3. Arc of rotation of the superior RAM flap.

the flap includes the presternal and premanubrial areas, the lateral chest wall, and the lateral abdominal wall (Fig. 3).

Design begins by delineation of the rectus abdominis muscle by marking the midline and the lateral margin of the muscle about four to five fingerbreadths lateral to the midline. Next, the ellipse of the skin flap required is designed (Fig. 4A).

Inferior Vertical RAM Flap

The inferior axis will be the point of origin of the inferior epigastric vessel from the external iliac artery at the level of the inguinal ligament. The arc of rotation will again be 0 to 180 degrees in either a clockwise or counterclockwise direction. Sites of reach include the lower anterior abdominal wall, the inguinal areas, the iliac areas, and the perineum (6,7).

Extended Vertical and Horizontal RAM Flap

The RAM flap may be extended with an ipsilateral, contralateral, or combination extension in the form of random-pattern flap extension (Fig. 6).

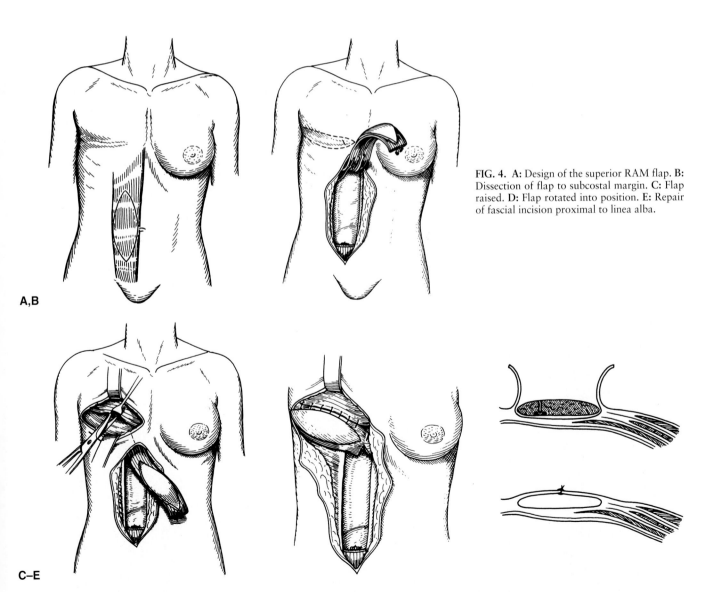

FIG. 4. A: Design of the superior RAM flap. **B:** Dissection of flap to subcostal margin. **C:** Flap raised. **D:** Flap rotated into position. **E:** Repair of fascial incision proximal to linea alba.

A,B

C–E

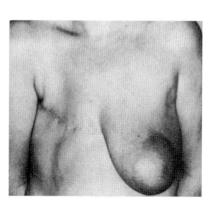
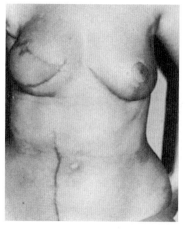
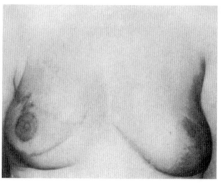

A–C

FIG. 5. **A:** Preoperative view, modified radical mastectomy. **B:** Postoperative view, RAM flap for mound reconstruction, abdominal scar. **C:** Postoperative view.

OPERATIVE TECHNIQUE

Vertical Superiorly Based RAM Flap

The skin is incised through subcutaneous tissue to expose the anterior rectus sheath (3). Sutures are inserted between the dermis and the anterior rectus sheath to prevent a shearing strain on the indirect perforator system. The anterior sheath is incised around the margins of the skin element, and superiorly, the anterior rectus sheath may be incised in the midline, opening the sheath like the pages of a book (Fig. 4E).

The muscle is easily dissected from the subjacent posterior rectus sheath by sharp and blunt dissections. The muscle is raised to the subcostal margin (Fig. 4B). It is not necessary to expose the superior epigastric vessel that enters the muscle medially at the subcostal margin. The superior insertion of the rectus abdominis muscle may be detached from the fifth, sixth, and seventh costal cartilages to facilitate rotation of the

musculocutaneous island element. The distal end of the muscle is raised from the subjacent transversalis fascia, and the inferior epigastric vessels are located, transected, and ligated. The lower aspect of the rectus abdominis muscle is transected with cutting cautery about two to three finger-breadths proximal to the pubic crest (Fig. 4B). The flap is then rotated into the required position (Fig. 4C and D).

Above the level of the arcuate line, the anterior rectus sheath is repaired by direct approximation with nonabsorbable sutures (Fig. 4E). Below the arcuate line, repair of the fascia is vital to prevent a postoperative hernia and may be performed, in most cases, by advancement of the medial free edge of the aponeurosis of the external oblique to the linea alba medially. This creates considerable tension that is released by a relaxing incision in the fascia of the external oblique far laterally. If the defect is too large, a free fascial graft of external oblique fascia harvested from the contralateral side is sutured into position with nonabsorbable sutures under suitable tension. Marlex mesh may be used, but autogenous material is preferable.

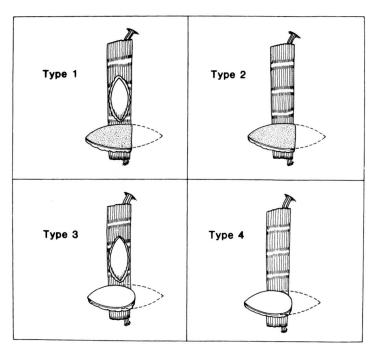

FIG. 6. Variations of horizontal extensions of the RAM flap.

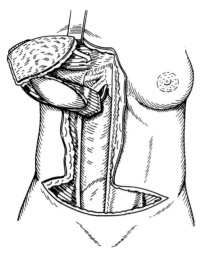
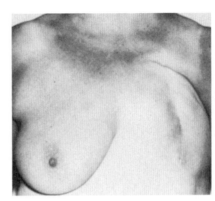
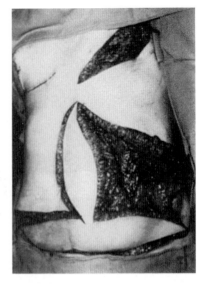

A–C

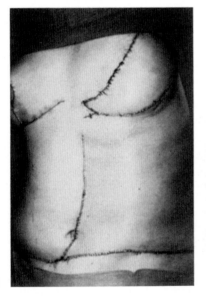
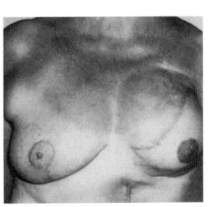

D,E

FIG. 7. **A:** Type I extended horizontal RAM flap for mound reconstruction. **B:** Preoperative view, radical mastectomy. **C:** Intraoperative flap. **D:** Intraoperative view. **E:** Postoperative view at 6 months.

Inferior Vertical RAM Flap

This flap is raised similarly to the superior counterpart. However, in this case, the superior aspect of the rectus abdominis muscle is transected and the superior epigastric artery is ligated. The flap is maintained on the inferior epigastric arteriovenous arcade and rotated into the required position.

Extended Vertical and Horizontal RAM Flap

Extending the RAM flap with ipsilateral, contralateral, or combination extension in the form of random-pattern flap extension allows for safe, reliable transverse of the abdominal panniculus to the anterior chest wall for reconstruction of the breast mound by vascularized autogenous abdominal skin and subcutaneous tissue (Fig. 7).

CLINICAL RESULTS

The rectus abdominis musculocutaneous flap is extremely reliable, and complications are invariably technical in nature. Loss of the flap will be related to violation of the dominant vessels or shearing stresses with injury to the indirect perforator system.

Donor-site functional deficit is minimal (Fig. 5). In the immediate postoperative period, difficulty in sitting from a recumbent position is experienced. However, after a period of 6 weeks, the function is adequately compensated for by action of the external oblique muscles.

Hernia is related to technically inadequate repair of the fascial integrity of the anterior abdominal wall below the arcuate line. Meticulous surgical repair will preclude this complication.

SUMMARY

The vertical or horizontal rectus abdominis musculocutaneous flap can be reliably used to reconstruct the breast.

References

1. Drever JM. The epigastric island flap. *Plast Reconstr Surg* 1977;59:343.
2. Robbins TH. Rectus abdominis myocutaneous flap for breast reconstruction. *Aust NZ J Surg* 1979;49:527.

3. Dinner MI, Labandter HP, Dowden RV. Role of the rectus abdominis myocutaneous flap in breast reconstruction. *Plast Reconstr Surg* 1982; 69:209.

4. Last RJ. The abdomen: the anterior abdominal wall. In: *Anatomy, regional and applied*, 4th ed. London: J&A Churchill, 1966;382–385.

5. McCraw JB, Dibbell DG, Carraway JH. Clinical definition of independent myocutaneous vascular territories. *Plast Reconstr Surg* 1977;60:341.

6. Mathes SJ, Bostwick J, III. A rectus abdominis myocutaneous flap to reconstruct abdominal wall defects. *Br J Plast Surg* 1977;30:282.

7. Bostwick J, III, Hill HL, Nahai F. Repairs in the lower abdomen, groin, or perineum with myocutaneous or omental flaps. *Plast Reconstr Surg* 1979;63:186.

CHAPTER 363 ■ TRANSVERSE ABDOMINAL ISLAND FLAP

C. R. HARTRAMPF, JR. AND L. F. ELLIOTT

EDITORIAL COMMENT

Unquestionably, the introduction of this flap, a most innovative and creative one, changed the field of breast reconstruction, particularly since one could reconstruct a breast of variable size, with the provision of excellent shape and symmetry with the contralateral breast and without the use of an implant. The flap is most reliable when it is pedicled, if one delimits to the ipsilateral half. As extension beyond the midline occurs, the incidence of partial necrosis increases.

In a single operation, the transverse abdominal island flap can produce a completely autogenous breast of practically any size. The donor defect after closure results in an acceptable transverse abdominal scar.

INDICATIONS

The transverse abdominal island flap was devised in response to a perceived need to reconstruct breasts after mastectomy for carcinoma with entirely autogenous tissue (1). Other uses for the flap are replacement of breast tissue after simple and subcutaneous mastectomy and correction of congenital chest-wall defects such as Poland's syndrome.

Since its introduction for breast reconstruction, this flap has been used for additional reconstructive problems. These include sternal wound infection after coronary artery bypass, chest-wall ulcers after irradiation, and the persistent thoracic cavity defect after closure of bronchopleural fistula. The flap also can be based inferiorly for use in pelvic and perineal defects as well as superior thigh and groin defects.

Using microsurgical technique, the transverse abdominal island flap can be transferred to distant sites to provide generous amounts of well-vascularized skin and fat to resolve unsightly contour deformities or to close the problem wound that requires free-flap coverage. The donor site for this free flap is excellent, and the potential size is enormous.

The only absolute contraindication to the use of the transverse abdominal island flap is previous extensive abdominal wall dissection such as abdominoplasty that has disturbed the musculocutaneous perforators essential for the survival of the overlying fat and skin. Abdominal scars limit the availability of flap tissue, since tissue distant to the scarring is unreliable. However, scarring, such as the right subcostal incision, is not necessarily a contraindication to the transverse abdominal island flap based on the right rectus muscle, since it could be transferred as a free-tissue transfer based on the right inferior epigastric pedicle.

Relative contraindications to this procedure include obesity, history of smoking, and the presence of chronic illness or malnourishment.

ANATOMY

The blood supply to the transverse abdominal island flap is through large perforator vessels from the superior and inferior epigastric system coursing through the rectus muscles (Fig. 1). The superior and inferior epigastric vessels are branches of the internal thoracic and external iliac arteries, respectively. The communication between the two vessels is usually an arborized plexus in the rectus muscle at the level of the umbilicus. The larger inferior epigastric artery and vein enter the rectus laterally, near the arcuate line. Below the arcuate line there is a paucity of perforators, while above it, generally in the periumbilical region, there are many perforators. Pressure gradients may not allow flow between the superior and inferior systems in the normal state. However, when one system is ligated proximally, it is perfused by the other. This accounts for the extensive flow throughout this large flap after the superior epigastric vessels are isolated and the inferior epigastric artery and vein are ligated.

The rectus muscle itself is divided by three or four transverse tendinous intersections spaced evenly throughout its length. These intersections segment the muscle into individual sections so that if the muscle is transected, it will not com-

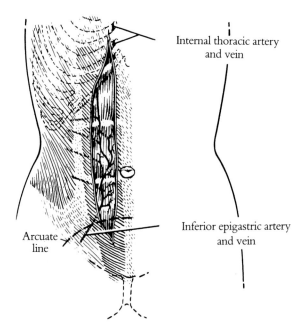

FIG. 1. Diagrammatic representation of the epigastric arcade composed of the superior and deep inferior epigastric vessels as well as the segmentally oriented intercostal vessels.

(Labels on figure: Internal thoracic artery and vein; Inferior epigastric artery and vein; Arcuate line)

pletely contract but will maintain its length as long as muscle is attached to a tendinous intersection.

The nerve supply to the rectus muscle and the abdominal wall enters laterally and is from the lower six or seven thoracic nerves as well as the iliohypogastric and ilioinguinal nerves. These are severed in elevating the island flap; thus this flap is not innervated.

FLAP DESIGN AND DIMENSIONS

Lines of proposed incisions should be drawn on the patient prior to the operation, with the patient preferably in the standing position (Fig. 2). Measurements of the desired breast should be guided either by the contralateral breast, if it is suit-

able to the patient, or by a planned size previously agreed upon. An estimation of skin needed from the abdomen should be based on the pathology report regarding the previously resected mastectomy skin. The dimensions of the needed tissue should then be transferred to the patient's abdomen with the patient in a standing position. In using the flap for problems other than breast reconstruction, the defect should again be measured carefully and transferred exactly to the abdomen, since any excess tissue will prove bulky in the final result.

Planning of the abdominal incision is based on a number of factors: (1) the amount of skin and soft tissue determined by the measurements previously made, (2) the surgeon's judgment with regard to the mass needed to produce the desired breast versus the mass of fat available for transfer, and (3) the presence and location of abdominal scars. For example, a lower midline scar precludes taking the contralateral wing of tissue on one muscle. However, the flap can be developed on both rectus muscles if both sides of the flap are needed for bulk (2).

The horizontal length of the flap is governed by the vertical dimension. However, with the vertical dimension of 14 to 18 cm, the length from the umbilicus in each direction can be 20 to 25 cm to the tip of the flap in each flank. It is safe to retain this prolonged length on the contralateral side without delay in the superiorly located flap. The viable length of the contralateral wing of the lower flap without delay is uncertain at present but probably is not past the lateral border of the rectus sheath on the contralateral side. Observation after fluorescein injection and gross examination of bleeding surfaces can aid in deciding how much of the flap is viable, particularly on the contralateral side.

We prefer to use the rectus muscle that is contralateral to the chest defect. This allows a less twisted route of the pedicle from the costal margin to the chest wall (3). The axis of rotation is near the xiphoid. This generally allows a pedicle length that is more than adequate for the infraclavicular hollow as well as the anterior axillary fold. However, for even more distant filling, resection of the lower costal cartilages can be employed so as to provide for a longer vascular leash.

OPERATIVE TECHNIQUE

The degree to which the transverse island can be inferiorly placed depends on a number of factors and is planned

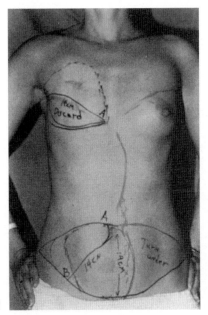

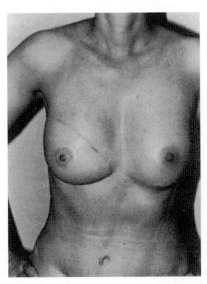

A,B

FIG. 2. A: Preoperative photograph of the planning for reconstruction of the right breast. The takeoff of the breast is determined from the normal contralateral one and is depicted by the dotted line. The flap will be deepithelialized to provide fill in the infraclavicular area. Point A corresponds to the medial aspect of the inframammary fold, and as the flap is rotated, it will correspond to the area of the umbilicus. Point B is similarly marked. The area marked "turn under" is usually deepithelialized and corresponds to the lower and lateral portion of the breast. It will serve to provide bulk and projection to the reconstructed breast. B: Postoperative result demonstrating the reconstructed breast as well as the abdominal wall closure at 1 year.

preoperatively. Factors such as a history of smoking, lower abdominal scarring, and the need for extensive lateral survival of the flap would encourage the operating surgeon to move the abdominal ellipse more cephalad on the abdominal wall.

The abdominal incision is beveled away from the flap to gain additional adipose tissue and needed perforators, particularly at the superior aspect of the flap near the midline over the rectus muscle, which will become the pedicle. The lateral wings are elevated off the external oblique fascia medially to the lateral aspect of the rectus sheath and to the midline on the opposite side if a single-pedicled unilateral reconstruction is planned.

The rectus sheath is then opened at the level of the arcuate line approximately 1 cm medial to the lateral border of the rectus or where the first large perforators are noted. The inferior epigastric vessels are located by splitting the muscle at this location and are ligated and divided. A generous section of rectus muscle is divided at this point, leaving approximately one-fourth of the muscle in situ, both medially and laterally.

The flap is retracted carefully as the muscle is dissected up from the posterior sheath, gradually taking more and more muscle medially, up to the next tendinous intersection. Above this point, all the muscle medially is taken with the flap. A cuff of anterior rectus sheath is left both medially and laterally for closure. As the dissection proceeds superiorly, the pedicle can be avoided by determining the precise location of the arterial channel or channels using the intraoperative Doppler device.

The umbilicus is isolated and left with the abdominal wall for later relocation, as with an abdominoplasty. There are a number of perforators in this area, and therefore, dissection of the periumbilical area should be kept to a minimum.

Once the flap is elevated to the costal margin, the anterior rectus sheath is opened medially, near the midline, up over the costal margin to the fifth rib. The rectus muscle insertion into the lower costal segments can then be divided, with the superior epigastric vessels in view, so as to create a true island flap (Fig. 3A).

The old mastectomy scar is excised, and an adequate pocket is formed. A tunnel is made from the breast pocket over the rectus origin to the abdominal dissection plane and is widened to allow flap passage (Fig. 3B). The flap is delivered through the tunnel and into the pocket (Fig. 3C). One must avoid shearing and tearing of the delicate tissue planes during this passage. An examination of the pedicle for unnecessary kinking, twisting, or pressure is necessary at this point.

Tailoring of the flap is performed to fill the deficient areas appropriately. This is the most demanding and time-consuming aspect of the operation (4) (Fig. 3D).

The flap can be placed with either wing up in the axilla, but it is usually best oriented with the wing contralateral to the blood supply up toward the axilla to enhance venous drainage. The dermis can be either deepithelialized or excised. The flap should be sparingly sutured around the upper circumference of the pocket from the anterior axillary fold and humerus across the infraclavicular space. The flap may be folded on itself or debulked, depending on the exigencies of the situation.

Chest skin below the mastectomy scar may be discarded to a new inframammary line to relieve pressure on the pedicle, to enhance the cosmetic appearance of the new breast, and to preserve superior skin, so that the upper scar will be well below the blouse line (see Fig. 2A).

When only a single rectus muscle is used for the pedicle, the abdominal wall defect can usually be closed directly using the cuff, or sheath, carefully spared on the initial dissection (5). Lateral and medial muscle portions left below the umbilicus assist in closure as well. The periumbilical portion provides the most resistance to direct closure.

Bilateral rectus pedicles leave larger fascial defects. However, in many patients, these defects also can be closed directly (Fig. 4). It is a good idea to attempt closure as far as it is possible in all patients in order to more accurately restore preoperative abdominal anatomy. However, if the surgeon is

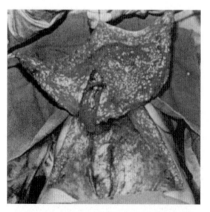
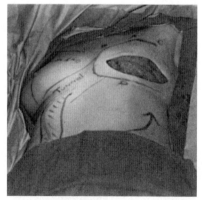

A,B

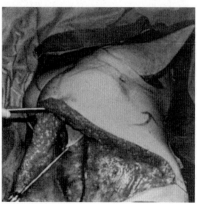
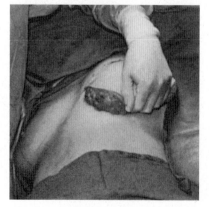

C,D

FIG. 3. A: Intraoperative photograph showing the large flap with the relatively small amount of rectus muscle that has been included. (Note that the rectus muscle is transected at the level of the semicircular line and segments of muscles are left in place medially and laterally in the abdominal wall.) B: Mastectomy defect and tunnel planning. Note that the tunnel extends to the contralateral side and spares disruption of the inframammary line. C: The flap, passed under the tunnel, can be rotated either way, although most often the contralateral tip that is to be discarded extends toward the axilla (see text). D: Shaping of the flap by turning under a wing for projection.

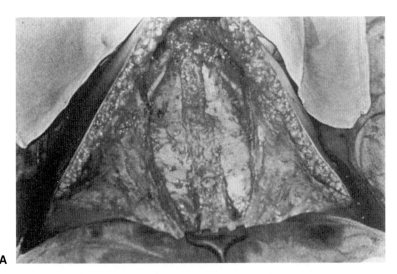
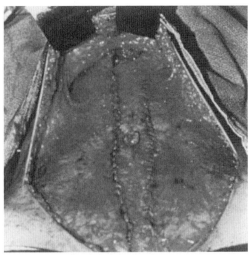

FIG. 4. **A:** Abdominal wall defect after harvest of bilateral rectus pedicles. **B:** Direct primary closure of bilateral defect using overlapping no. 1 nylon without mesh support.

uncertain of the stability of this closure, mesh can be added for security.

Closed suction drains are left subcutaneously in both the chest and abdominal planes of dissection. We also drain the tunnel region where the pedicle passes through to the chest.

In patients with abdominal scarring possibly disruptive to the blood supply in the lower abdominal ellipse, one should consider moving the ellipse higher up on the abdomen. Also, for those requiring quite large flaps or those for whom the location of the scar is of less concern, the higher ellipse may be preferred. The midabdominal transverse scar is acceptable and may be safer in some patients (6,7).

CLINICAL RESULTS

The unilateral mastectomy defect is the most common indication for this flap's use. However, the bilateral deformity is also

suited to this flap technique (Fig. 5). The flap can be used either immediately at the time of mastectomy in selected patients or delayed after healing of the mastectomy site.

The most common causes of immediate postoperative problems are hematoma and kinking of the pedicle. At reexploration, kinking can be managed by rotating the flap in the opposite direction, changing the angle of the pedicle, or, if all else fails, returning the flap to the abdomen.

We routinely use nifedipine, oxygen, and steroids on an empirical basis for assistance in flap survival.

Complications thus far encountered include partial loss of the flap, hematoma, seroma, inequality of size of the breasts, abdominal weakness, and firmness in the breasts. Ventral hernias have been avoided by careful attention to sound two-layer closures of the abdominal wall. If the defect is securely closed, the function deficit is minimal, since the oblique muscles and remaining rectus muscles are adequate for flexing the torso.

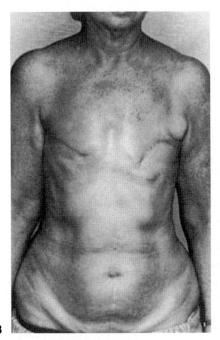
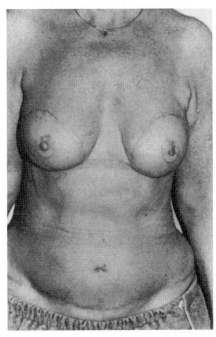

FIG. 5. **A:** Patient who had undergone a bilateral mastectomy and also had a lower midline vertical scar. **B:** Postoperative result following reconstruction of both breasts simultaneously, with bilateral transverse island abdominal flaps, at 1 year.

SUMMARY

The transverse abdominal island flap has provided a dramatic alternative to existing techniques for breast reconstruction as well as other difficult reconstructive problems on the chest wall, pelvis, and distant sites. The benefits of avoiding implant material for breast reconstruction as well as the frequently generous, well-vascularized supply of fat and skin make this flap an attractive answer to a myriad of difficult reconstructive problems.

References

1. Hartrampf CR, Sheflan M, Black PW. Breast reconstruction with the transverse abdominal island flap. *Plast Reconstr Surg* 1982;69:216.
2. Ishii CH Jr, Bostwick J, III, Rain TJ, et al. Double-pedicle transverse rectus abdominis myocutaneous flap for unilateral breast and chest-wall reconstruction. *Plast Reconstr Surg* 1986;76:901.
3. Vasconez LO, Psillakis J, Johnson-Giebink R. Breast reconstruction with contralateral rectus abdominis myocutaneous flap. *Plast Reconstr Surg* 1983;71:668.
4. Elliott LF, Hartrampf CR Jr. Tailoring of the new breast using the transverse abdominal island flap. *Plast Reconstr Surg* 1983;72:887.
5. Hartrampf CR Jr, Bennett KG. Abdominal wall competence in transverse abdominal island flap operations. *Ann Plast Surg* 1984;12:139.
6. Hartrampf CR Jr, Bennett KG. Autogenous tissue reconstruction in the mastectomy patient: a critical review of 300 patients. *Ann Surg* 1987;205:508.
7. Hartrampf CR Jr. Breast reconstruction with the transverse abdominal island flap. *Perspectives Plast Surg* 1987;1:123.

CHAPTER 364 ■ TRANSVERSE RECTUS ABDOMINIS MUSCULOCUTANEOUS FLAP FROM THE SCARRED ABDOMEN

J. M. DREVER

EDITORIAL COMMENT

Dr. Drever supplies proven and reliable methods for transferring the TRAM flap, even in patients who have very scarred abdomens. Readers are encouraged to study this chapter for the safe performance of what otherwise would be a difficult procedure.

The transverse rectus abdominis musculocutaneous flap gives most satisfying results in breast reconstruction. It not only has enabled us to create a breast with autogenous tissues that remain soft and supple and identical to the opposite, but it also improves the looks of the abdomen. It is a torsoplasty in the real sense of the word (1–7).

INDICATIONS

Transverse rectus abdominis musculocutaneous (TRAM) flaps are not the answer for every patient who needs a breast reconstruction. They are for the woman who is physically fit and who would benefit from an abdominal lipectomy. A lean young woman of childbearing age would do better with the expander-implant reconstruction.

It is most important that the patient be free of any disease that might contribute to postoperative complications. Since we are dealing with an elective flap transfer, the patient must have a good pulmonary-cardiovascular status. I do not operate on patients with a previous history of vascular problems, such as hypertension, peripheral vascular disease, strokes, myocardial infarcts, chronic smoking, or any pulmonary insufficiency that might have reduced their vital capacity.

It is a good idea to prepare the patient for this operation by asking her to walk 2 to 3 miles per day or to do the equivalent exercise of her choice. If the patient is obese, make her lose weight through exercise and have her lower her pulse rate. Also, the patient should be psychologically prepared, meaning she should be keen and enthusiastic and well informed of how the operation is done and the possible complications. I show patients preoperative and postoperative photographs and get them in touch with other patients who have had TRAM flap reconstructions done. This communication with someone who has had a first-hand experience is very reassuring. Patients arrive at their surgery with a very positive attitude.

ANATOMY

The rectus abdominis muscle pedicle can feed a random flap of the anterior abdominal skin practically in any direction or shape (see Chap. 362), provided there are enough perforators on the deep epigastric vascular system to the skin. Therefore, it is very important to conserve undisturbed the vascular integrity of this pedicle. This means that our dissections should be carried through natural planes, avoiding even coming near these feeding vessels and maintaining as many musculocutaneous perforators as possible in the base of our flap.

The rectus abdominis muscle pedicle should be a 4- to 5-cm-wide musculofascial strip removed from the most *medial* side of the rectus abdominis muscle with the entire rectus fascia attached to it completely. The muscle and fascia are sectioned transversely at the lower end of the skin flap. In this way, one can preserve the maximum number of perforators available to the skin flap. This muscle-fascia pedicle carries the circulation of two territories: the superior epigastric and the deep inferior epigastric arteries. These traverse the undersurface of the pedicle from the medial side above to the lateral side below. They are both relatively medium sized arteries (with venae comitantes) until they divide and lose themselves as thin arterioles within the substance of the rectus muscle. This occurs at the height of the *middle* transverse septa area, where one has to be most careful with handling of the muscle pedicle by always keeping it protected by the overlying fascia.

FLAP DESIGN AND DIMENSIONS

The best indication for a TRAM flap for breast reconstruction is the middle-aged woman who is healthy and would benefit from an abdominal lipectomy. These patients have an average age of 51 years. Often they have had previous abdominal operations that have transected the right superior epigastric artery. Subcostal scars or other scars can decrease both the pliability and/or the viability of some parts of the flap. Therefore, when I choose the design of the flap, I have to reach a basic compromise between the best possible lipectomy with the most viable flap design. Naturally, the best lipectomy is the one that leaves the shortest and lowest abdominal scar, and the most viable flap design is the midabdominal. Also, whenever possible, I try to use the contralateral muscle pedicle. With these parameters in mind, I will analyze the different choices of flaps in patients with scarred abdominal walls.

Vertical Midline Supraumbilical and the Paramedian Supraumbilical Scar

My first choice in these patients is the lower abdominal transverse rectus abdominis musculocutaneous flap coupled with a vertical excision of the scar above the flap (Fig. 1). The vertical component of this scar is closed with Z-plasties. This technique gives a good lipectomy, and it is an easier operation because when I remove the vertical preexisting scar, it gives me

a direct approach to the muscle pedicle right up to the xiphoid. In patients with a vertical paramedian scar, the contralateral muscle pedicle should be used. A scarred muscle almost invariably has an impaired circulation and should never be used as a pedicle.

Vertical Midline Infraumbilical Scar

This is a very frequently found scar in this age group. It puts out of bounds the contralateral side of a lower abdominal flap, but the choices are as follows:

1. Using the ipsilateral side of a lower abdominal transverse flap (Fig. 2). This is a good choice if there is enough abdominal wall volume to reconstruct the missing breast. In these patients, I leave this scar in the flap and suture it to the inframammary fold, because this scar is often contracted and helps give a round fullness in the lower quadrants of the breast.
2. Using a midabdominal flap when a larger breast is to be reconstructed, necessitating the use of both sides of the flap (Fig. 3). This is a well-vascularized flap, and both sides will survive even if there is still some remaining scar below the umbilicus. Closure of the abdominal wall is done by creating Z-plasties in the remaining scar in the suprapubic area.

Infraumbilical Paramedian Scar

When presented with this scar, one has to gauge if there is enough volume in the lower abdomen to use a LATRAM flap (Fig. 4). Naturally, I always use the side opposite to this scar as the muscle carrier. When this scar is located on the same side as the mastectomy, as it is brought up to the chest, it should be placed in the desired position and observed. Usually not more than one or two fingerbreadths distal to the scar acquire a somewhat pale, cyanotic tinge. All this part should be discarded.

When this scar is on the opposite side of the mastectomy, one is forced to use an ipsilateral muscle carrier. In these patients, I leave the scar on the flap and suture it to the inframammary fold, which contributes to a nice round fullness in the lower quadrants.

If a larger mound is desired, such as that provided by an unscarred flap, then I use the midabdominal flap and close the abdomen by creating Z-plasties in the paramedian scar.

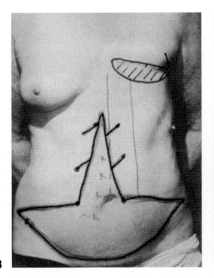
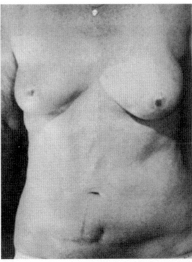

A,B

FIG. 1. **A:** Patients who have vertical, median, or paramedian supraumbilical scars. Use the opposite muscle pedicle, excise the scar in an inverted V-shaped fashion, and use the lower abdominal transverse flap. **B:** The reconstructed breast. The vertical component of the abdominal incision has been closed with Z-plasties.

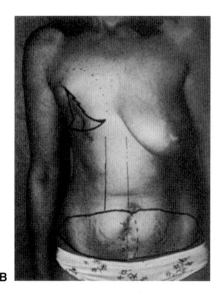
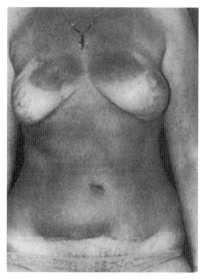

A,B

FIG. 2. A: In patients with a vertical midline infraumbilical scar, I use the ipsilateral side of the lower abdominal transverse flap if there is enough volume there to reconstruct the missing breast. Vertical mastectomy scars are excised in an inverted-T fashion, making an incision on the proposed inframammary fold and undermining the area cephalad to it. B: Appearance 6 years postoperatively. Notice how the nipple in the reconstructed breast tends to descend and in the reduced breast with inferior pedicle technique tends to ascend.

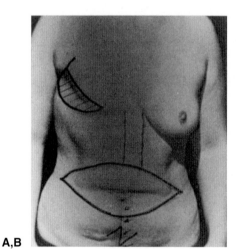
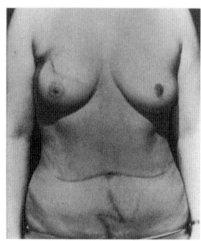

A,B

FIG. 3. A: When there is a vertical midline infraumbilical scar but both sides of the flap are needed for a reconstruction, use a midabdominal flap. Closure of the abdominal skin is done by creating Z-plasties in the remaining scar in the suprapubic area. B: Appearance 2 years postoperatively with some hypertrophic scarring that will settle down with time.

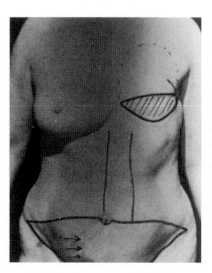
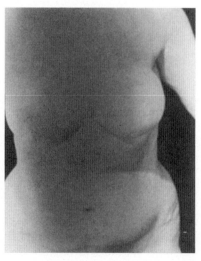

A,B

FIG. 4. A: An infraumbilical paramedian scar. Since there is enough volume to make a breast, I use a LATRAM flap. Always use the opposite side of this scar as the muscle carrier. Suturing the scar to the inframammary fold helps give a nice roundness in the lower quadrants of the breast. B: Appearance 5 years postoperatively. Notice how a nice, well-balanced ptosis is achieved.

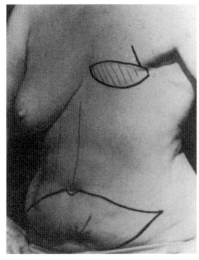
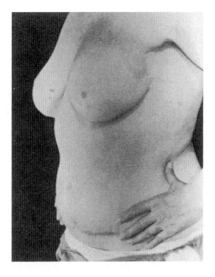

A,B

FIG. 5. **A:** In patients with Pfannenstiel scars, before using the LATRAM flap, find out if the previous surgeon has undermined the area of the perforators. **B:** Appearance 6 years postoperatively after doing all the balancing procedures, such as suction lipectomy, nipple-areola reconstruction, and opposite breast reduction.

Pfannenstiel Scar

The flap of choice here is obviously the lower abdominal transverse, but it is necessary to find out what type of operation was done through the Pfannenstiel incision because, occasionally, some surgeons, after doing the transverse skin incision, undermine the anterior rectus sheath off the subcutaneous tissue and therefore sever important perforators that feed a LATRAM flap (Fig. 5). This may lead to surprising and abundant fat necrosis.

McBurney Scar

This is a frequently found scar that presents no major problems. If it is foreseen that this scar might be included in the new breast area, it is better to use the opposite muscle carrier.

Kocher Scar

This right subcostal scar is the LATRAM flap's worst enemy. The left rectus muscle must be used as the carrier. The breast flap will be viable, but there is a very high chance of necrosis developing in the periumbilical area. The best choice of flap is

the midabdominal flap with the upper incision following the subcostal scar or very near to it (Figs. 6 and 7).

Another possibility when confronted with Kocher scars is to use the left vertical flap. It is very useful when a somewhat conical and ptotic breast is desired.

Patients with Multiple Scar

These situations can pose a real challenge to one's imagination. Every patient is different, and one has to plan for the maximum viability of the flap, coupled with cosmetic improvement to the abdomen and breast. In general, patients in late middle age do not like large breasts; they prefer a better-balanced figure. In fact, one of the most common complaints is their difficulty in finding proper clothing. Also, in the surgeon's favor is the fact that since they already have several scars, they do not mind too much about the location of the next one. This, in fact, allows the surgeon to place the lipectomy excision in practically any direction. Therefore, all redundant abdominal fat and skin should be removed either through vertical and/or horizontal excisions. Always use the muscle pedicle that is not scarred. Finally, consider that two pedicles have a better viability than one, but be well aware that with the use of a double pedicle, the patient must be

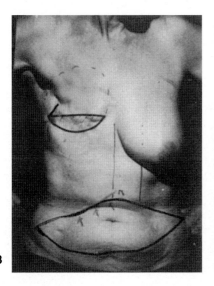
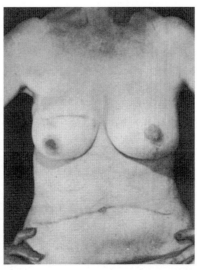

A,B

FIG. 6. **A:** The Kocher or subcostal scar. Use the midabdominal flap, making your superior incision following the subcostal scar. Always use the contralateral muscle carrier. **B:** Appearance 1 year postoperatively.

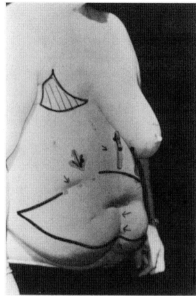
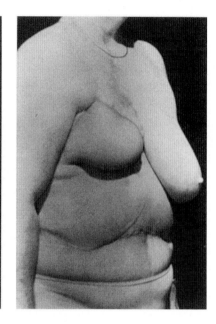

A,B

FIG. 7. **A:** The obese patient with a Kocher and an infraumbilical scar. Use the safest flap, which is the midabdominal, and make the breast only with the tissue overlying the muscle pedicle. **B:** A recent postoperative result. The patient still needs contralateral reduction.

warned that she will have noticeable difficulty for many months moving from a lying-down to a sitting-up position. This weakness diminishes with lots of exercise in patients who are really determined, because the action of the rectus is taken over by the combined efforts of the superior fibers of the external oblique and the psoas muscles.

The Obese Patient

The obese patient is not a good surgical candidate because the thick fatty layer is associated with decreased vascularity coupled with an increased friability of the flap (see Fig. 7). Also, obese patients usually have a poor cardiovascular-pulmonary status which contributes to increased postoperative complications. Nevertheless, you sometimes find an obese person who has great determination and a relatively good cardiovascular status in spite of being overweight.

Before operating on the obese patient, I do a simple cardiovascular fitness test. If the patient passes this, I choose the safest flap, which is the *midabdominal* flap, and I make the breast with only the ipsilateral side of skin and fat and discard the great majority of the contralateral side.

Obese patients will usually indicate that they want small breasts and as much as possible removed from the abdomen. This allows one to make a round mound using only the skin and fat directly over the musculocutaneous perforators (zone 1). Since this fatty subcutaneous layer is so thick, I keep the undermining of the abdominal wall to a minimum. Once the flap is in the breast area, there is usually no need to deepithelialize skin because the thick panniculus itself makes the mound. Therefore, suturing can be done edge to edge and still result in an adequate looking mound. It is important to place these patients on perioperative wide-spectrum antibiotics.

OPERATIVE TECHNIQUE

Raising the Flap

The operation is performed simultaneously by two teams. The mastectomy scar is excised, and a pocket cephalad to this scar is undermined over the pectoralis major fascia. The abdominal island is incised, and the fat is beveled in all areas except over the pubis to bring with the flap as much fat as possible. Then the abdominal wall is undermined until both anterior rectus sheaths are exposed to a height transversely across the base of the xyphoid. Then both surgeons, helping each other, fashion a tunnel right over the anterior rectus sheath from the medial half of the inframammary fold down to the undermined area in the abdomen. A closed fist should pass easily through this tunnel.

Then two vertical lines are marked over the chosen muscle pedicle, one on the lateral edge of the linea alba from the base of the xyphoid down to the umbilicus (or to the upper end of the flap). Another line is then marked parallel to this first one and 4 to 5 cm away, starting at the same horizontal height as the previous, which means 4 or 5 cm above the costal margin, and extending down to the upper end of the flap.

The contralateral side of the skin island flap is then undermined off the anterior rectus sheath and the external oblique aponeurosis up to the midline. All the perforators are clipped; cautery is not used on the flap itself.

The ipsilateral tail side of the island flap is then elevated. This should be done carefully right over the shiny fascia. I stop when I am at the same line of the previously marked lateral incision on the rectus sheath.

The anterior rectus fascia is then incised on the previously marked lateral line that should extend up to the costal margin and down to the lower end of the flap. As the rectus fascia is incised, above the umbilical transverse septa the rectus muscle is seen, but below this septa there is another fascia that must be incised. It corresponds to the internal oblique. It is incised at the same level.

When the umbilical part of the rectus muscle is exposed, it is split along its fibers or slid along its lateral border, and here, floating in the preperitoneal fat, the inferior epigastric artery with its venae comitantes can be seen. They are clipped and divided at this level. The rectus muscle is split, continuing upward toward the umbilical transverse septa and right underneath it. The neurovascular bundle is identified, clipped, and divided.

Many times, above the umbilical transverse septa, the muscle fibers run slightly obliquely to the fascial incision. They should be divided at the same level. On its undersurface, two more lateral neurovascular bundles are identified and divided. Once the middle transverse septa is reached, the splitting of the muscle is continued at the same level as the fascial incision.

Two more neurovascular bundles are then seen lying right on the shiny transversus fascia. These are clipped and divided. The muscle is split upward, and the upper transverse septum, which is located just at the level of the costal margin, is divided. The muscle fiber splitting is continued to where the previous fascial incision ends.

Access to the undersurface of the muscle from the lateral side is now available. It is retracted medially by simple blunt dissection, *taking care to preserve the already clipped neurovascular bundles attached to the undersurface of the muscle.* This will indicate that the dissection is in the correct plane. The dissection is continued as far as it will go medially until the linea alba is reached. Control of the lower limits of the musculofascial pedicle is obtained at this stage by placing fingers in this space. The lower end of the rectus abdominis muscle and the anterior rectus fascia are divided transversely across just at the lower limits of the skin flap.

The next step consists of separating the muscle and fascia from the linea alba. This is best done by retracting the flap and the undersurface of the muscle toward the contralateral side. The anterior rectus sheath is then cut from its undersurface right at its medial junction with the linea alba. As this is being done, one or two veins above the semicircular line of Douglas that perforate the posterior rectus sheath near the midline around the umbilical area are encountered. These are the capitus meducae veins. They should be clipped and divided. The anterior rectus fascia around the umbilical stalk is divided.

Then the medial edge of the fascia is divided from the linea alba above the umbilicus. For this, heavy Mayo scissors are used to cut the anterior rectus sheath right at the junction with the linea alba by placing one tip of the scissors next to the muscle and feeling with it where the medial junction lies.

At this stage, all three edges of the musculofascial pedicle are divided. The next step consists of lifting it from the posterior rectus sheath. This can be done by careful blunt dissection, leaving all the areolar tissue attached to the undersurface of the muscle. The posterior rectus sheath (transversus tendon or fascia transversalis) above the semicircular line of Douglas should appear shiny and devoid of any areolar fatty tissue. When the costal margin is reached, the seventh intercostal neurovascular bundle is identified right under its edge. Ideally, a selective neurotomy of the nerve should be performed, leaving the artery and veins undisturbed. This is possible when doing a lower abdominal flap, but when taking a midabdominal flap, the whole neurovascular pedicle has to be sacrificed in order to avoid tenting from this pedicle. It is not convenient to look for, or dissect, the area of the superior epigastric (internal mammary) pedicle. This might create regrettable vasospasm. *The fascia or muscle should never be divided transversely above the costal margin.*

The flap is transferred by passing first the contralateral point facing cephalad. The skin surface is moistened thoroughly and pushed into the prepared mastectomy area. If it will not pass easily, the tunnel must be enlarged.

Closing the Donor Area

Since a 4- to 5-cm-wide muscle-anterior rectus fascia strip has been removed from the base of the xiphoid down to the lower end of the skin flap, the incised edges should be returned to the preoperative position. Closing a 4- to 5-cmwide aponeurotic gap directly will result in a very tight closure that will change the tone of the oblique muscles, increase the possibility of dehiscence, create considerable postoperative pain, and shift the umbilicus to one side. Only patients with marked fascial laxity can be closed primarily.

Mersilene mesh is preferable because it is strong, pliable, and does not shred. Prolene is too wiry, and Marlex is too hard and can be felt through the skin. The Mersilene comes in sheets that measure 20 × 20 cm. They can be doubled, resulting in a long rectangle (20 × 10 cm).

Below the umbilical transverse septa, it is important to notice that the internal oblique and the transversus abdominis aponeurosis tendons have a tendency to retract deep to the external oblique. They should be drawn back and sutured to the edge of the mesh and thus incorporated into the repair. I believe that a running stitch distributes the forces better than multiple separate stitches because it acts essentially as a complex pulley system. When doing this closure with mesh, the patient should be in a straight supine position and flexed only when the skin is about to be sutured.

The umbilicoplasty is done with a V incision of the abdominal skin in order to avoid a circular contracture. A marked cosmetic benefit can be obtained by removing the fat from the undersurface of this V incision in a radius of about 5 to 7 cm in a tapered fashion.

In patients in whom the two rectus abdominis muscle pedicles have been used, closure is done following the same principles. The area of the fascia, including the linea alba, is replaced with one piece of double Mersilene mesh. The umbilicus is retrieved through a hole in the mesh.

Making the Breast Mound

The first step is to excise the old mastectomy scar, coupled with an incision along the future inframammary fold. If this scar is transverse or slightly diagonal, it is excised together with the skin between it and the inframammary fold, taking into account that the inframammary fold will drop 2 to 3 cm when doing the abdominal closure (see Figs. 1A, 3A, 4A, and 5A). If the mastectomy scar is vertical, it is excised and coupled with an incision on the future inframammary fold, which means that the skin that is removed will have an inverted-T shape (see Fig. 2A).

The pocket cephalad to this scar excision is created in an area symmetrical to that occupied by the opposite breast. The undermining is always done in the subcutaneous layer. (See the dotted line on the upper quadrants of part A of all the figures.)

Once the flap is passed into the mastectomy defect, it is rotated in several directions until the ideal position is found, always considering that the side with the muscle pedicle should be facing downward. In general, when using a LATRAM flap, the periumbilical area of the flap is sutured to the most medial extremity of the inframammary fold incision.

The rest of the flap, the ipsilateral end, is tucked under and a curved line is marked exactly where it falls on the inframammary fold. Naturally, all the buried part of skin is deepithelialized, and the inframammary fold is sutured.

Once this has been done, the amount of the contralateral side (which is going to form the upper quadrants) that is going to be discarded must be determined.

The upper edge of the chest skin is somewhat tight on the flap, and this is released by making a dart in the area of the anterior axillary fold (see Fig. 5A). The length of this dart is usually 2.5 to 3 cm. The corresponding skin edge over the flap is then removed from the pocket and deepithelialized. A drain is placed in the operative site.

In cases of bilateral reconstruction, the flap is transferred ipsilaterally, and the inframammary fold is sutured to what used to be the midline in the abdominal area.

Secondary Procedures

As early as 6 weeks after a TRAM flap reconstruction, one can do the ancillary procedures that will enhance the results. These usually consist of a nipple and areola reconstruction, a better definition of the inframammary fold, the opposite breast reduction, and suction lipectomy to the epigastric and donor-scar areas.

Nipple and Areola Reconstruction

Before marking the future nipple placement, consider that the reconstructed breast tends to *descend* about 1 to 2 cm over the course of 1 year, whereas the nipple placement in a reduced breast with the inferior pedicle technique tends to *ascend* 1 to 2 cm over the course of 1 year. In general, I choose a place on the reconstructed breast mound and move the opposite nipple to the symmetrical place marked on the reconstructed one, taking into account the previously mentioned variations.

The technique of choice to make a nipple is to share half the opposite one. Naturally, this can be done only if there is sufficient projection of the donor. If there is not, in order of preference, I use composite grafts of labia minora, local flaps, or earlobe grafts.

The technique of choice to reconstruct the areola is a full-thickness graft of the perimeter of the opposite areola when it is excessively wide. Adequate color matching also can be obtained by full-thickness grafts removed from the inner surface of the upper thighs. A simpler technique that gives adequate results is tattooing. The light brown or tan pigments should be used in Caucasians, and the opposite areola should also be tattooed. This will result in a much better match. Pigment also can be placed directly on the dermis of a split-thickness skin graft, thus obviating the need for a tattoo machine. It also gives a very even result.

Definition of the Inframammary Fold

With a patient in the standing position, I mark on the reconstructed breast a symmetrical line to the opposite inframammary fold. I then do a lipolysis of the deep and superficial fat along the marked line. I then make a 2-cm incision beveled down to the deep dermis but not through it. Then, using a large needle with O Prolene, I take a bite of the deep fascia and suture it to this exposed dermis and then bury the knot. The inframammary fold should be fixed like this at least in two spots, in the middle and medially.

Opposite Breast Reduction

Depending on the size of the opposite breast, I do either a mastopexy, an inferior or central pedicle reduction, or a free nipple graft. Very frequently I choose the free-nipple graft technique because it is the most versatile with regard to the

shape of the breast and placement of the nipple-areola complex. It also removes the central and lower quadrants of the breast tissue with a consequent oncologic and psychologic benefit for the patient.

Suction Lipectomy Touch-ups

Autogenous breast reconstructions can be looked on as a torsoplasty where cosmetic improvements are brought to the breast and the abdominal area. Suction lipectomy is the ideal technique to complement a TRAM flap reconstruction. Suction can be used to soften up areas of fat necrosis in the reconstructed breast and to define the inframammary fold as described. It is used commonly to decrease the bulge created by the twisted muscle pedicle in the epigastrium and to enhance a natural depression in the periumbilical area. Another favorite place for suction is the area just above the transverse abdominal scar and on both flanks.

SUMMARY

TRAM flap breast reconstruction is intended to be a torsoplasty, a combined thoracoabdominoplasty with the inherent benefits to both areas. It is done on the mastectomy patient who is healthy and who would benefit from an abdominal lipectomy. Maximum viability of the flap is obtained by preserving as many of the musculocutaneous perforators as possible under the skin flap and removing the muscle with the fascia attached to it. The operation is performed by a team, thus allowing each surgeon to concentrate in his or her own area of expertise, with a marked reduction in the operating time.

References

1. Drever JM. The epigastric island flap. *Plast Reconstr Surg* 1977;59:343.
2. Mathes SJ, Bostwick J III. A rectus abdominis myocutaneous flap to reconstruct abdominal wall defects. *Br J Plast Surg* 1977;30:282.
3. Hartrampf CR, Sheflan M, Black PW. Breast reconstruction with the transverse abdominal island flap. *Plast Reconstr Surg* 1982;69:216.
4. Elliott LF, Hartrampf CR Jr. Tailoring of the new breast using the transverse abdominal island flap. *Plast Reconstr Surg* 1983;72:887.
5. Vasconez LO, Psillakis J, Johnson-Giebink R. Breast reconstruction with contralateral rectus abdominis myocutaneous flap. *Plast Reconstr Surg* 1983;71:668.
6. Ishii CH Jr, Bostwick J III, Rain TJ, Coleman JJ III, Hester TR. Double-pedicle transverse rectus abdominis myocutaneous flap for unilateral breast and chest-wall reconstruction. *Plast Reconstr Surg* 1986;76:901.
7. Hartrampf CR Jr. Breast reconstruction with the transverse abdominal island flap. *Perspectives Plast Surg* 1987;1:123.

CHAPTER 365 ■ MICROVASCULAR FREE TRANSFER OF A GROIN SKIN FLAP

K. HARII

Advances in musculocutaneous flaps over the past several years have brought about easy and reliable procedures for reconstruction of breast defects. However, such secondary problems as scars and disfigurement of donor sites after removal of both muscle and skin may occur. For these reasons, the free groin flap becomes a good candidate for reconstruction of the female breast and chest wall, even though the operative procedure is more complex than for musculocutaneous flaps (1–3).

OPERATIVE TECHNIQUE

The most important key to satisfactory results is selection of the recipient vessels (4), because it is usually difficult to expose suitable vessels in the axillary region after a radical mastectomy. Also, vessels may be heavily irradiated and degenerative. Interpositional vein grafts from the axillary artery with end-to-side anastomoses have been used (1) to create a new recipient artery that can form a bridge between the axillary artery and the superficial circumflex iliac artery of the groin flap placed in the breast defect. However, this procedure appears to be hazardous and risky.

In patients in whom recipient vessels are not available in the axillary region, I recommend use of the gastroepiploic vessels. Through an upper median laparotomy, the gastroepiploic vessels are dissected from their attachment to the stomach as a long vascular cord and are transposed to the recipient chest wall through the abdominal wall. A new vascular stump is thus created at an adequate site in the recipient bed (Fig. 1).

Taking the complex vascular anatomy into consideration, a free groin flap of required size is elevated (see Chap. 133). If the patient requires reconstruction of the breast mound after radical mastectomy, as much as possible of the fatty tissue in the groin should be included in the flap to augment the chest wall. Planning usually includes placing a silicone implant of suitable size beneath the flap in a second stage procedure to obtain breast mound symmetry (Fig. 2).

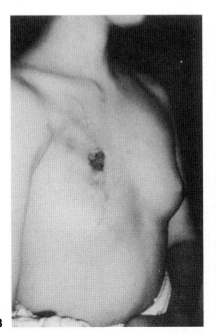
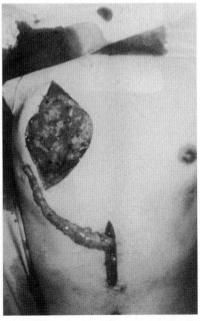

FIG. 1. A 32-year-old woman with breast loss and unstable scars following radical surgery for carcinoma. There was no evidence of recurrence. **A:** Preoperative view. **B:** Defect after debridement and transposed gastroepiploic vessels. The diameters of the artery and vein at the distal stump of the vascular stalk were 1.8 and 2.0 mm, respectively. *(Continued)*

A,B

1053

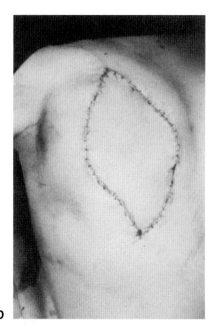
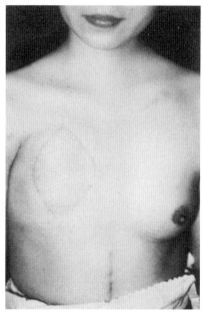

C,D

FIG. 1. *Continued.* **C:** A groin flap 10 × 14 cm was elevated, along with excess fatty tissue, and transferred with vascular anastomoses between the superficial epigastric artery and the cutaneous vein. **D:** Appearance 6 months postoperatively. (From Harii et al., ref. 2, with permission.)

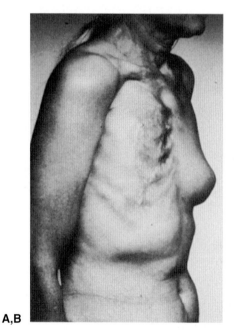
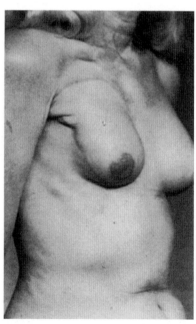

A,B

FIG. 2. **A:** Result following radical mastectomy. Note that the defect was extensively covered with a split-thickness skin graft. **B:** Postoperative result. The recipient vasculature was the axillary artery and venae comitantes. Note the correction of the infraclavicular hollow. The implant and nipple-areola reconstruction are each completed in separate stages. (From Serafin et al., ref. 5, with permission.)

SUMMARY

A free groin flap is an alternative to other methods of breast reconstruction.

References

1. Serafin D, Given, KS. Reconstruction of the thorax and breast following radical mastectomy. In: Serafin D, Buncke HJ, eds. *Microsurgical composite tissue transplantation.* St. Louis: Mosby, 1979;541.

2. Harii K, Ohmori S, Torii S, et al. Free groin skin flaps. *Br J Plast Surg* 1975;28:225.
3. Harii K. Free-Flap Surgery. In: Jackson IT, ed. *Recent advances in plastic surgery.* Edinburgh: Churchill Livingstone, 1981;67.
4. Harii K, Ohmori S. Use of the gastroepiploic vessels as recipient or donor vessels in the free transfer of composite flaps by microvascular anastomoses. *Plast Reconstr Surg* 1973;52:541.
5. Serafin D, Georgiade NG, Given KS. Transfer of free flaps to provide well-vascularized, thick cover for breast reconstructions after radical mastectomy. *Plast Reconstr Surg* 1978;62:527.

CHAPTER 366 ■ MICROVASCULAR FREE SUPERFICIAL INFERIOR EPIGASTRIC ARTERY (SIEA) FLAP

R. J. ALLEN AND MARY E. LESTER

Breast reconstructive surgeons have long recognized the advantages of the lower abdomen as a donor site. In 1982, Dr. Hartrampf (1) introduced the transverse rectus abdominis myocutaneous (TRAM) flap. More recently, the use of the lower abdominal tissues sparing the rectus muscle has reduced donor-site morbidity while providing adequate amounts of tissue for breast reconstruction. A flap based on the superficial inferior epigastric artery (SIEA) harvests tissue superficial to the rectus sheath and provides a direct cutaneous blood supply, allowing more versatility in surgical planning and application.

INDICATIONS

The SIEA flap was first described by Wood (2) as a pedicled flap for burn contracture of the hand in 1863. It was mentioned for use in the lower extremity as a free flap or in the thigh as an island flap (3). As limb reconstruction frequently demands a large, thin, pliable flap, the SIEA flap provides a large area of skin with variable subcutaneous thickness, depending on the body habitus of the patient. The large surface area is useful in covering head and neck defects. Koshima (4)described a deepithelialized SIEA flap to correct facial contour in hemifacial atrophy and other defects. The SIEA flap has been used to reconstruct the trunk, as a pedicled flap to correct contralateral abdominal wall defects, pelvic floor defects, and pressure sores (3). It is ideal for use in breast reconstruction, including partial breast reconstruction (5).

ANATOMY

The superficial inferior epigastric artery is a direct cutaneous artery that supplies the skin of the lower abdominal wall. The SIEA networks with other vessels supplying the abdominal wall, including the superficial and deep circumflex iliac arteries, superior and inferior deep epigastric arteries, and external oblique perforators. Taylor (6) believes that it is this network of choke vessels that allows the entire lower abdomen to be supported by a unilateral deep inferior epigastric artery or SIEA.

Taylor also found the SIEA present in 65% of 46 cadaver dissections. Allen and Heitland's study of 100 cadaver dissections (7) found a 72% presence of the SIEA. In 58% of cadavers, the SIEA was present bilaterally. The average pedicle diameter at the inguinal ligament was 1.6 mm (range, 0.75 to 3.5 mm), and at the origin was 2.9 mm (range, 2.0 to 4.0 mm). Pedicle length can vary between 7 and 11 cm.

The pedicle most commonly shares an origin with the superficial circumflex iliac artery, present in 79% of cadaver dissections, but can also have a separate origin from the femoral artery. In either case, the origin is 2 cm caudal to the inguinal ligament. The artery courses superficially and cephalad through the femoral sheath and pierces the cribriform fascia (8). It then travels just superficial to Scarpa's fascia toward the inguinal ligament. It crosses the inguinal ligament lateral to the midpoint between the pubic tubercle and anterior superior iliac spine (ASIS). It then continues just superficial to Scarpa's fascia as it travels cephalad. The course of the SIEA then varies, as it can travel toward the umbilicus or laterally toward the ASIS.

The superficial inferior epigastric vein (SIEV) supplies venous drainage of the abdomen along with the venae comitantes of the SIEA. The SIEV lies more superficial than the SIEA, often just underneath the skin. It is also found medial to the midpoint between the ASIS and pubic tubercle. Its origin is the saphenous bulb. The comitant vein is more commonly used for anastomosis.

Problems can be encountered when the pedicle diameter is inadequate for flap harvest. The pedicle diameter at the trunk is unknown until the end of the dissection, when the presence or absence of a common trunk is seen. However, the lower abdominal tissue can also be harvested with the deep inferior epigastric artery or the contralateral SIEA. An SIEA of 1 mm or greater at the level of the inguinal ligament is adequate for flap viability (9). Another difficulty can be previous abdominal surgery, including liposuction. We have not offered DIEP or SIEA flaps to patients with previous liposuction. Patients with lower-midline scars are precluded from carrying the entire abdomen with one pedicle; however, most are able to have a DIEP or SIEA if the vessel has not been transected. Preoperative bedside Doppler examination can aid in identifying the presence of the SIEA but is unreliable in assessing its size.

FLAP DESIGN AND DIMENSIONS

The most common flap design is horizontal because the parous patient frequently has an excess of lower abdominal skin and fat. The flap design is drawn on the standing patient from the ASIS to above the umbilicus to the contralateral ASIS. The second portion of the ellipse is drawn from the ASIS to just above the pubic hairline to the ASIS, similar to a

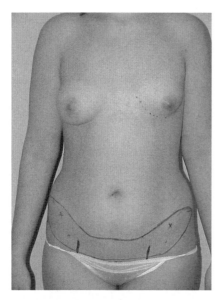

FIG. 1. Modified horizontal flap design with smaller flap design. Superficial inferior epigastric artery (SIEA) marked in red. Patient had a congenital breast deformity and underwent an augmentation with an SIEA flap. She did not need umbilical transposition.

standard abdominoplasty incision. However, if less tissue is needed, the cephalad mark can be drawn below the umbilicus, avoiding umbilical transposition (Fig. 1).

The flap design is drawn on the patient 1 day before surgery. The patient is then placed supine for Doppler examination. The SIEA, SIEV, and deep inferior epigastric perforators are marked. Vertical and oblique patterns have also been described but are typically used with the pedicled technique. These designs are based on the path of the superior inferior epigastric artery determined by Doppler examination.

OPERATIVE TECHNIQUE

The procedure is performed with a two-team approach. If the reconstruction is performed immediately, flap harvest can begin simultaneous with the mastectomy. The second team prepares the skin envelope and the internal mammary recipient vessels. The skin envelope is inspected at the inframammary fold and lateral aspect of the breast. If necessary, these can be recreated with tacking sutures. The internal mammary vessels are exposed by separating the pectoralis major muscle along its fibers above the third rib. The internal mammary perforators are examined and, if of sufficient size, they are then used for recipient vessels. If the internal mammary perforators are inadequate, then the second interspace is explored.

The medial border of the pectoralis major is incised from the sternum, and the second interspace is entered. The intercostal muscles are removed from the second interspace while the dissection remains superficial to the fat pad overlying the internal mammary artery and vein. The artery and vein are then exposed after intercostal muscle removal. Rib cartilage can be removed for a narrow interspace or access to a branching internal mammary vein.

Flap harvest is begun by incising the lower portion of the flap design. The SIEV is preserved because it is frequently used to aid in drainage of venous congestion that occurs in either SIEA or DIEP flaps. The SIEV is usually very superficial and can be seen underneath the skin. Under loupe magnification, the SIEV is dissected to the level of the inguinal ligament. The

SIEA, which lies lateral to the SIEV, is frequently deep within the superficial layer of subcutaneous tissue just superficial to the Scarpa fascia. It is dissected to the level of the inguinal ligament. It takes a sharp turn deep into the subcutaneous tissue around the inguinal ligament as it travels toward its origin. Typically, the superficial circumflex artery joins the SIEA before its origin at the common femoral artery. If the SIEA is inadequate, then the contralateral SIEA or deep inferior epigastric artery is explored.

Further flap design depends on the type of reconstruction (i.e., unilateral or bilateral). If bilateral reconstruction is performed, the flap can be divided in the midline from the contralateral side. Flap harvest is then performed in a similar fashion. If unilateral reconstruction is performed, the flap is elevated from the anterior rectus sheath, and the superior flap design is incised. The flap is weighed to compare with the mastectomy specimen weight and to aid in size approximation.

The extent to which the SIEA flap can cross the midline depends on the course of the SIEA within the abdominal tissue. The network of vessels supplying the abdominal wall (10) can allow the flap to survive past the midline. Traditionally, zones I, II, and III, as described by Rickard (11) and Holm and colleagues (12), survive, and zone IV is in question. However, Ulusal (9) reports good survival rates of zone IV with 92.3% of the abdomen used for SIEA donor vessels. Most authors agree that a previous midline incision precludes extending the SIEA flap across the midline; however, low transverse incisions usually do not interfere with the blood supply of the SIEA or DIEP.

Routinely, the contralateral side is used for flap inset. The flap is rotated 180 degrees clockwise so that the caudal edge of the flap with donor vessels is cephalad. This edge (caudal edge of the flap) is temporarily secured to the breast skin during the anastomoses (Fig. 2). The venous and arterial anastomoses are performed under the operating room microscope. The venous anastomosis is frequently performed with the aid of the Synovis Microvascular Anastomotic Coupler System (Synovis Life Technologies, Minneapolis, MN). The flap is turned 90 degrees counterclockwise for inset, so that the caudal edge of the flap is now medial, and the lateral edge of the flap points toward the axillary tail of the breast.

Skin paddles are used for flap monitoring, if a skin Doppler signal can be identified. Ancillary staff are trained to check Doppler signals, color, turgor, capillary refill, and temperature. If a skin signal cannot be found, an implantable Doppler probe is placed. The breast skin incisions are closed with subcuticular sutures and Dermabond glue; no dressings cover the breast. Breasts are drained with closed suction drainage distant from anastomosis. Surgical bras are placed on patients with pendulous breasts to prevent separation of pedicle from recipient vessels. The abdominal donor site is closed in standard abdominoplasty fashion over suction drainage.

Other options for flap harvest include the bilateral inferior epigastric artery flap (BIEF) or thinning of the flap. The BIEF is a large flap and involves dissection of the SIEA, superficial circumflex iliac artery, and deep inferior epigastric artery (13). The SIEA flap can be thinned relatively safely by relying on its anatomy. The SIEA is superficial to the Scarpa fascia, and therefore, the subcutaneous tissue deep to the Scarpa fascia can be removed.

CLINICAL RESULTS

Microsurgical free flaps are associated with a learning curve that is dependent on surgeon expertise. The SIEA can be challenging, but the dissection of a direct cutaneous artery is less demanding than that of a perforator flap. As SIEA flap applications have increased, the reliability and predictability have

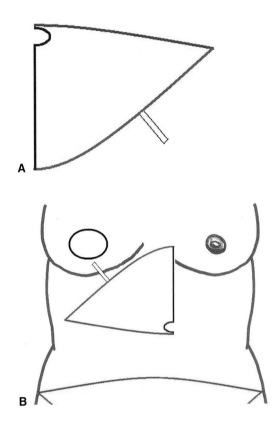

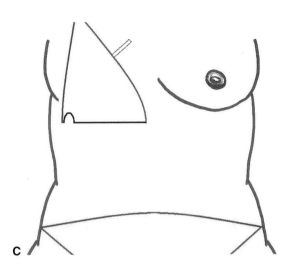

FIG. 2. A: Left hemiabdomen. Flap is weighed and then used to reconstruct the patient's right breast. B: The left hemiabdomen is rotated 180 degrees and secured to the patient with sutures for microvascular anastomosis. C: The left hemiabdomen is rotated 90 degrees counterclockwise for inset. The caudal edge of the flap is now medial, and the lateral corner of the flap points toward the axillary tail of the breast.

also improved. The first reports of the SIEA as a free flap are case reports from the 1970s. One of the earlier series by Hester (3) demonstrated 16 SIEA free-flap attempts with two failures (12.5%). One flap was lost, and one did not have suitable vessels. More recent series show failure rates between 0 and 8.3% (14,15).

Our experience includes 233 flaps for breast reconstruction and augmentation since 1997 with one total flap loss (0.43% flap-loss rate). The age range for patients is 15 to 70 years. Indications include augmentation for symmetry with cancer reconstruction and for congenital breast deformities. Breast-reconstruction cases include immediate and delayed breast reconstruction with 121 and 78 flaps, respectively (Fig. 3). Reconstruction after previous failed implant attempts has

been performed with the SIEA in 34 cases. Bilateral SIEA flap procedures have been performed in 35 patients.

SUMMARY

The SIEA free flap is an ideal flap for breast reconstruction. It allows harvest of a large amount of skin and fat from the lower abdomen while minimizing donor-site morbidity and eliminating the risk of hernia. Its location also allows alternative procedures, such as the DIEP, if the pedicle is inadequate. It has a fairly consistent pedicle that is present in 76% of groins. Its direct cutaneous supply allows a versatile and thin flap that can be applied to many soft-tissue defects.

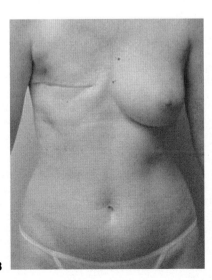
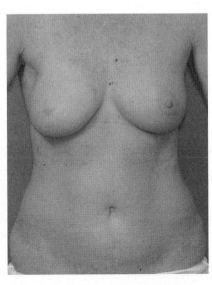

A,B

FIG. 3. A: Preoperative photograph of 51-year-old patient undergoing delayed reconstruction for breast cancer. B: Postoperative photograph of same patient after delayed reconstruction with SIEA.

References

1. Hartrampf CR, Scheflan M, Black W. Breast reconstruction with a transverse abdominal island flap. *Plast Reconstr Surg* 1982;69:216.
2. Wood J. Extreme deformity of the neck and forearm. *Med Chair Trans* 1863;46:161.
3. Hester TR, Nahai F, Beegle PE, Bostwick J. Blood supply of the abdomen revisited, with emphasis on the superficial inferior epigastric artery. *Plast Reconstr Surg* 19847;4:657.
4. Koshima I. Short pedicle superficial inferior epigastric artery adiposal flap: new anatomical findings and the use of this flap for reconstruction of facial contour. *Plast Reconstr Surg* 2005;116:1091.
5. Rizzuto RP, Allen RJ. Reconstruction of a partial mastectomy defect with the superficial inferior epigastric artery (SIEA) flap. *J Reconstr Microsurg* 2004;20:441.
6. Taylor GI, Daniel RK. The anatomy of several free flap donor sites. *Plast Reconstr Surg* 1975;56:243.
7. Allen R, Heitland A. The superficial inferior epigastric artery flap for breast reconstruction. *Semin Plast Surg* 2002;16:35.
8. Ninkovic M. Superficial inferior epigastric artery perforator flap. In: Blondeel PN, Morris SF, Hallock GG, Neligan PC, eds. *Perforator flaps: anatomy, technique and clinical applications.* St. Louis: Quality Medical Publishing, 2006;405–419.
9. Ulusal BG, Cheng MH, Wei FC, et al. Breast reconstruction using the entire transverse abdominal adipocutaneous flap based on unilateral superficial or deep inferior epigastric vessels. *Plast Reconstr Surg* 2006;117:1395.
10. Taylor GI. Discussion: Blood supply of the abdomen revisited, with emphasis on the superficial inferior epigastric artery. *Plast Reconstr Surg* 1984;74:667.
11. Rickard R. TRAM and DIEP flap zones. *Br J Plast Surg* 2001;54:272.
12. Holm C, Mayr M, Hofter E, et al. Perfusion zones of the DIEP flap revisited: a clinical study. *Plast Reconstr Surg* 2006;117:37.
13. Buncke H. Bilateral inferior epigastric artery flap (BIEF). In: *Microsurgery: transplantation-replantation. An atlas text.* Philadelphia: Lea & Febiger, 1991;167–186.
14. Stern HS, Nahai F. The versatile superficial inferior epigastric artery free flap. *Br J Plast Surg* 1992;45:270.
15. Chevary PM. Breast reconstruction with superficial inferior epigastric artery flaps: a prospective comparison with TRAM and DIEP flaps. *Plast Reconstr Surg* 2004;114:1077.

CHAPTER 367 ■ MICROSURGICAL FREE TRANSFER OF A LATISSIMUS DORSI MUSCULOCUTANEOUS FLAP

D. SERAFIN AND D. J. GOODKIND

EDITORIAL COMMENT

Although generally supplanted by the free Transverses Rectus Abdominal Flap (TRAM), this flap still has a place in some selected patients for breast reconstruction.

Breast reconstruction following mastectomy has become a major concern of the plastic surgeon during the past two decades. In recent years, women have been reluctant to accept the mutilating consequence of an ablative mastectomy. As new methods have become available, patients have sought consultation for reconstruction in increasing numbers (1).

INDICATIONS

A radical mastectomy with ligation of the neurovascular pedicle does not preclude the safe transfer of an ipsilateral latissimus dorsi musculocutaneous flap (2,3). Viability of the muscle is ensured, provided a vascular pedicle from the serratus anterior muscle is included with the transferred latissimus dorsi muscle. The muscle is usually atrophic, however, and is less suitable for reconstruction of large defects. The quantitative deficiency that exists following radical mastectomy is accentuated by postoperative irradiation. In these patients, one can sometimes detect upper extremity edema with limitation of abduction and external rotation, radiation osteitis, osteoradionecrosis, and brachial plexus neuropathy (4). Thus the combination of both qualitative and quantitative deficiencies of the anterior thoracic wall would render such a defect not amenable to reconstruction with the ipsilateral latissimus dorsi musculocutaneous flap.

Recently, the rectus abdominis musculocutaneous flap has been popularized for breast reconstruction (5,6). This flap has proven its reliability and is a viable alternative to the latissimus dorsi musculocutaneous flap. In past publications, it was felt that approximately 9 percent of patients requiring reconstruction would benefit most from the microvascular method (7). It would appear that there are fewer indications for the microvascular method following the recent introduction of the rectus abdominis musculocutaneous flap.

The rectus abdominis musculocutaneous flap has an unacceptable flap morbidity rate under certain circumstances: (1) in extremely obese patients, and (2) in patients with midtransverse or lateral oblique abdominal incisional scars (i.e., the longitudinal blood supply of either the ipsilateral or the contralateral rectus abdominis muscle is interrupted).

Finally, with severe qualitative and quantitative deficiency of the anterior thoracic wall, muscle or musculocutaneous flap reconstruction might be indicated to restore an adequate blood supply to this relatively avascular area. Thus patients with skin breakdown, osteoradionecrosis, or brachial plexus neuropathy are best treated with microsurgical muscle transplantation. The rectus abdominis musculocutaneous flap would not be suitable for reconstruction in these patients primarily because of the extensive undermining that is a necessary part of the dissection and the relatively scarce blood supply in the transferred cutaneous paddle.

Another reason to select the microsurgical method is the previous failure of a conventional musculocutaneous flap. In spite of meticulous preoperative preparation, flap morbidity and failure occur with a predictable rate. Salvage of the reconstructive effort can be accomplished with the microsurgical method.

ANATOMY

The latissimus dorsi is a broad, flat muscle that originates from the lower six thoracic vertebrae, the posterior layer of the lumbar fascia, and the medial aspect of the iliac crest. From this extensive origin, the fibers course superolaterally toward the axilla, inserting into the intertubercular groove of the humerus.

The dominant blood supply to the latissimus dorsi muscle is the thoracodorsal artery, a branch of the subscapular artery (Fig. 1). The subscapular artery arises from the second portion of the axillary artery. At its origin, it is approximately 4 to 5 mm in external diameter. At approximately 2 to 3 cm from its origin, the subscapular artery divides into the circumflex

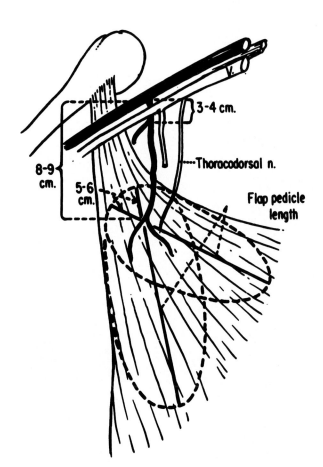

FIG. 1. Illustration depicting the vascular anatomy of the latissimus dorsi muscle or musculocutaneous flap. Note that the effective pedicle length is 8 to 9 cm.

scapular artery, which courses through the triangular space posteriorly, and the thoracodorsal artery, which continues inferiorly and laterally to supply the latissimus dorsi and serratus anterior muscles.

Average diameters of the thoracodorsal artery and vein are approximately 2.7 to 3.4 mm, respectively, at their origin and approximately 1.6 mm as they enter the muscle. The length of the vascular pedicle is approximately 9 cm. In 86 percent of dissected muscles, the artery was found to branch immediately upon entering the muscle body (8). A lateral or longitudinal branch was found to course toward the iliac crest approximately 2.1 cm from the lateral muscle edge. An upper transverse or horizontal branch was noted to course medially 3.5 cm from the upper edge of the muscle. In approximately 14 percent of dissected specimens, no transverse branch could be identified.

The nerve to the latissimus dorsi muscle, the thoracodorsal nerve, arises from the posterior cord of the brachial plexus and can usually be identified approximately 3 cm medial to the subscapular artery in the axillary dissection (8–10).

FLAP DESIGN AND DIMENSIONS

Preoperative markings are always performed with the patient upright and awake. The contracting, viable latissimus dorsi muscle should be identified by palpation and inspection. The proper size of the cutaneous paddle is outlined according to the requirements of the recipient defect. If a cutaneous paddle greater than 9 to 10 cm in width is required, then the donor site cannot be closed primarily. Since postoperative donor-site morbidity is much greater following split-thickness skin grafting, every effort is made to close the donor site primarily.

OPERATIVE TECHNIQUE

The cutaneous paddle and associated muscle on its vascular pedicle can always be isolated through the posterior thoracic incision. The most posterior extent of the donor site is then closed, and the patient is then rotated to a more supine position.

Recipient vasculature can usually be identified in one of three locations: (1) the axilla, (2) the costochondral junction, and (3) the neck. Patients who have satisfactory abduction of the ipsilateral extremity and minimal edema are candidates for axillary exploration of the recipient vasculature (Fig. 2). The latissimus dorsi musculocutaneous flap has a lengthy pedicle, as outlined previously. This facilitates end-to-side anastomoses to the axillary artery and/or vein. Frequently, an axillary vena comitans accompanies the axillary artery and can be isolated. An end-to-end anastomosis is then performed between the thoracodorsal vein and the vena comitans. A frequent finding during axillary exploration is that the thoracodorsal artery was previously ligated, but that the circumflex scapular artery is patent. This permits an end-to-end anastomosis between the thoracodorsal artery of the flap and the recipient circumflex scapular or subscapular artery.

Every attempt is made to identify and isolate the donor nerve to the latissimus dorsi muscle. A neural coaptation is then performed between the transplanted donor tissue and the thoracodorsal nerve following neuroma excision.

Occasionally, recipient vasculature can be isolated at the costochondral junction. A portion of the rib cartilage is excised, exposing the internal mammary artery. Frequently, two veins accompany the artery. This may present some difficulty when the venous anastomosis is performed. The thoracodorsal vein is usually not duplicated and is of large external diameter.

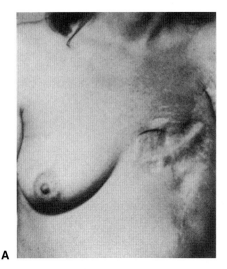

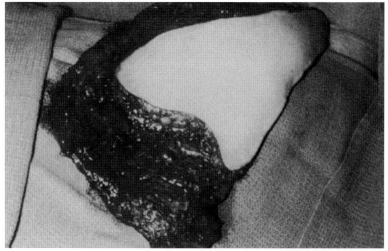

A

B

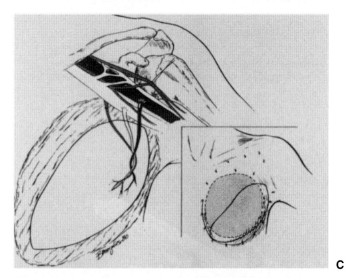

C

FIG. 2. **A:** Preoperative photograph of a patient who had undergone a previous left radical mastectomy with subsequent wound breakdown and healing by secondary intention. The patient also received postoperative irradiation. The latissimus dorsi muscle could not be palpated, indicating injury to the thoracodorsal nerve at the time of mastectomy. **B:** Intraoperative photograph demonstrating the cutaneous paddle attached to the underlying latissimus muscle prior to transplantation. **C:** Illustration depicting transfer of the latissimus dorsi musculocutaneous flap. Note end-to-side anastomosis of the thoracodorsal artery to the axillary artery and end-to-side anastomosis of the axillary vein to the thoracodorsal vein. The neuroma of the thoracodorsal nerve was excised and an anastomosis performed. (*Insert*) Completed reconstruction with silicone prosthesis placed beneath the latissimus muscle. **D,E:** Late postoperative result.

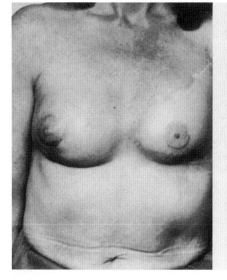

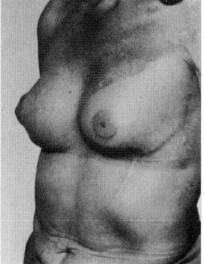

D,E

Patients with radiation changes should have the initial exploration for isolation of the recipient vasculature in the neck. This can be accomplished through a transverse incision exposing branches of the external carotid artery and superficial facial veins. An end-to-end anastomosis is performed to the thoracordorsal artery and vein of the flap. The lengthy vascular pedicle is sufficient to permit placement of the composite tissue on the thorax, obviating the use of an interpositional vein graft.

CLINICAL RESULTS

Using the microsurgical method of reconstruction, the latissimus dorsi musculocutaneous flap has been transplanted in 15 patients without any flap morbidity or failure. This method is both useful and reliable when performed on a certain subgroup of patients requiring reconstruction of the breast and thorax.

SUMMARY

The primary indication for reconstruction of the breast and thorax using the microsurgical method is the failure to employ the ipsilateral island latissimus dorsi musculocutaneous flap and/or either rectus abdominis musculocutaneous flap.

Patients with an extensive qualitative and quantitative deficiency of cutaneous cover associated with sequelae secondary to irradiation are best treated with the microsurgical method.

References

1. Clifford E, Clifford M, Georgiade N. Breast reconstruction following mastectomy: I. Social characteristics of patients seeking the procedure. *Ann Plast Surg* 1980;5:341.
2. Bostwick J, Vasconez LO, Jurkiewicz MD. Breast reconstruction after radical mastectomy. *Plast Reconstr Surg* 1978;61:682.
3. Muhlbauer W, Olbrisch R. The latissimus dorsi myocutaneous flap for breast reconstruction. *Chir Plast* 1977;4:27.
4. Serafin D, Deland M, Lesesne C, et al. Reconstruction with vascularized composite tissue in patients with excessive injury following surgery and irradiation. *Ann Plast Surg* 1982;8:35.
5. Hartrampf CR Jr, Scheflan M, Buck PW. Breast reconstruction with a transverse abdominal island flap. *Plast Reconstr Surg* 1982;69:216.
6. Marino H Jr, Dogliciti P. Mammary reconstruction with bipedicle abdominal flap. *Plast Reconstr Surg* 1981;68:933.
7. Serafin D, Voci VE, Georgiade NG. Microsurgical composite tissue transplantation: indications and technical considerations in breast reconstruction following mastectomy. *Plast Reconstr Surg* 1982;70:24.
8. Tobin GR, Schusterman BA, Peterson GH, et al. The intramuscular neurovascular anatomy of the latissimus dorsi muscle: the basis for splitting the flap. *Plast Reconstr Surg* 1981;67:637.
9. Bartlett SP, May JW Jr, Yaremchuk MJ. The latissimus dorsi muscle: a fresh cadaver study of the primary neurovascular pedicle. *Plast Reconstr Surg* 1981;67:631.
10. Maxwell GP, Manson PN, Hoopes JE. Experience with 13 latissimus dorsi myocutaneous free flaps. *Plast Reconstr Surg* 1979;64:1.

CHAPTER 368 ■ MICROVASCULAR FREE TRANSFER OF A GLUTEAL MUSCULOCUTANEOUS FLAP

T. FUJINO

The gluteus maximus musculocutaneous flap has been proven worthwhile as an alternative technique in breast reconstruction (1–3).

INDICATIONS

Primary indications for the use of this procedure are (1) congenital unilateral absence of the breast, (2) primary reconstruction of the breast after standard radical mastectomy, and (3) secondary reconstruction of the breast after standard radical mastectomy.

ANATOMY

The major gluteal muscle, the largest and most superficial muscle in the region, is a broad and thick quadrilateral mass forming the prominence of the buttock. It arises from the posterior gluteal line of the ilium and the rough area of bone, including the crest immediately above and behind it, from the aponeurosis of the erector spinae, from the dorsal surface of the lower part of the sacrum and the side of the coccyx, from the sacrotuberous ligament, and from the gluteus aponeurosis fascia covering the gluteus medius.

The fibers descend obliquely and laterally. The upper and larger part of the muscle, together with the superficial fibers of the lower part, ends in a thick, tendinous lamina that passes lateral to the greater trochanter and is attached to the iliotibial tract of the fascia lata. The deeper fibers of the lower part of the muscle are attached to the gluteal tuberosity between the vastus lateralis and adductor magnus. Its superficial surface is related to a thin fascia that separates it from subcutaneous tissue, its deeper surface to the ilium, sacrum, coccyx, and sacrotuberous ligament, part of the gluteus medius, piriformis, gemelli, obturator internus, greater trochanter, and the attachments of biceps femoris, semitendinosus, semimembranosus, and adductor magnus.

The superficial division of the superior gluteal artery reaches the deep surface of the muscle between the piriformis and gluteus medius. Then it creeps along the deep surface of the major gluteal muscle and perforates through the muscle, distributing the perforating branches to the subcutaneous adipose tissue and skin.

The major gluteal muscle is innervated by the inferior gluteal nerves L5 and S1 and S2.

FLAP DESIGN AND DIMENSIONS

The upper third of the major gluteal muscle, attached with the subcutaneous adipose tissue and skin, is used as a free musculocutaneous flap. The skin flap is designed within the skin territory of the superior gluteal artery, and its long axis runs from the upper sacrum to the greater trochanteric region (Fig. 1). It measures 15 cm in length, 10 cm in width, and 10 cm in thickness.

The donor flap is outlined in an elliptical fashion from the upper sacrum to the greater trochanteric region. The amount of skin is equal to the proposed skin defect for a standard radical mastectomy. The adipose tissue taken is greater than that of the overlying skin and enough to fill up the subcutaneous tissue defect following the radical mastectomy (Fig. 2).

OPERATIVE TECHNIQUE

Dissection is started from the upper edges of the ellipse, going to, beyond, and returning to the upper edge of the major

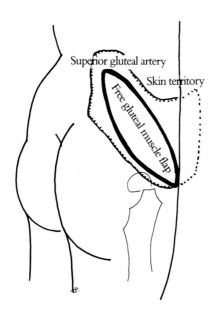

FIG. 1. Free flap designed within the skin territory of the superior gluteal artery.

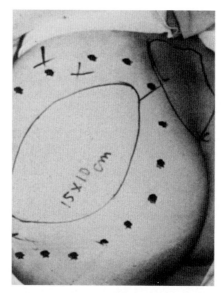

FIG. 2. Free musculocutaneous gluteal flap. Preoperative design on hip. Skin incision corresponds to the size of the skin incision for a standard radical mastectomy. Dotted line is an extension of the adipose tissue resection to fill the subcutaneous tissue defect after surgery.

gluteal muscle. Then blunt dissection is carried out between the major and middle gluteal muscles from the sacral region toward the greater trochanteric region and then split off the upper third of the major gluteal muscle toward the sacrum. The superior gluteal artery and vein are exposed between the middle gluteal muscle and piriformis muscles near the sacrum. The superior gluteal vessels are prepared, and the major gluteal muscle proximal to them is then severed (Fig. 3).

Congenital Unilateral Absence of the Breast

Preoperative angiography is performed in order to determine the size and location of the recipient vessels. Usually, the thoracoacromial vessels are chosen. The thoracoacromial vessels are dissected out through a lateral thoracic incision. The entire anterior chest is undermined by a combination of sharp and blunt dissection techniques. Complete hemostasis is secured prior to microvascular anastomosis (Fig. 4A).

Primary Reconstruction of the Breast After Standard Radical Mastectomy

Because of the complete removal of a lesion, the recipient vessels for microvascular anastomosis are often short. Therefore, an adequate length of donor vessels is sought. The proximal portion of the major gluteal muscle, which includes the perforating branches of the superior gluteal vessels, is trimmed off, and thus several centimeters of vascular length are gained.

Secondary Reconstruction of the Breast After Standard Radical Mastectomy

Detection of recipient vessels is the same as described for primary reconstruction of the breast after standard radical mastectomy. If they are not found, a greater omental pedicle flap is transferred to the region through a celiotomy for microvascular anastomosis.

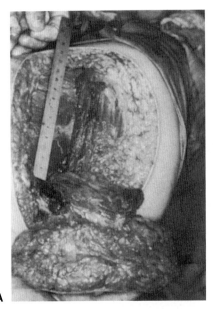 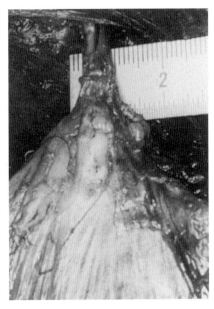

A   **B**

FIG. 3. **A:** Dissection of free flap. The superior gluteal vessels course through the proximal portion of the free flap under the major gluteal muscle. Then, at the middle portion, they penetrate through the muscle layer, becoming the perforator vasculature to supply the overlying skin and adipose tissue. **B:** The superior gluteal artery (2 mm) and vein (3 mm) are ready for severance, just between the middle gluteal and piriform muscles, in order to make the free flap.

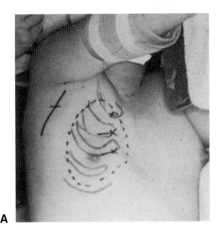 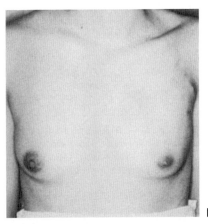

A   **B**

FIG. 4. **A:** First successful transfer of free musculo(sub)cutaneous gluteal flap. A 22-year-old patient with a congenital absence of the right breast and pectoral muscles. **B:** Appearance 4 years after surgery. (From Fujino et al., ref. 1, with permission.)

CLINICAL RESULTS

The success rate of this flap for reconstruction of congenital unilateral absence of the breast is 100 percent (2 of 2); for primary reconstruction, 100 percent (2 of 2); and for secondary reconstruction, 100 percent (1 of 1). There have been no functional deficits.

SUMMARY

The gluteal musculocutaneous flap can be used as a free flap for breast reconstruction.

References

1. Fujino T, Harashina T, Aoyagi FL. Reconstruction for aplasia of the breast and pectoral region by microvascular transfer of a free flap from the buttock. *Plast Reconstr Surg* 1975;56:178.
2. Fujino T, Harashina T, Enomoto K. Primary breast reconstruction after a standard radical mastectomy by a free-flap transfer. *Plast Reconstr Surg* 1976;58:371.
3. Fujino T, Abe O, Enomoto K. Primary reconstruction of the breast by free myocutaneous gluteal flap. *Int Adv Surg Oncol* 1981;4:127.

CHAPTER 369 ■ MICROVASCULAR FREE TRANSFER OF A GLUTEAL MUSCULOCUTANEOUS FLAP

W. W. SHAW AND R. W. LIEBLING

Any breast reconstruction is directed toward restoring natural contour, creating a mound with infraclavicular and axillary fullness, and reanimating the new tissue with more normal temperature, softness, mobility, sensibility, and symmetry to the contralateral breast. Moreover, functional and aesthetic morbidity at the donor site should be kept to a minimum. The buttock region is an abundant source of skin and soft-tissue bulk. In 1975, the use of a gluteus maximus musculocutaneous free flap to correct a case of congenital aplasia of the breast and pectoral region was reported (1). This concept was subsequently expanded for breast reconstruction primarily following radical mastectomy. Recent clinical experience with the gluteus maximus musculocutaneous free flap has generated further enthusiasm for the use of this method (2,3).

INDICATIONS

The advantages of a free composite-tissue flap of sufficient volume, such as the gluteus maximus musculocutaneous free flap, are quite obvious in breast reconstruction. Limited dissection in the axilla minimizes the possibility of aggravating any lymphedema. A free flap does not borrow any functional tissue from the adjacent area, but rather adds substantial tissue to the area from a distance. The gluteal free flap allows much greater freedom in flap design compared to regional pedicled flaps and enables the surgeon to perform immediate living sculpturing until a gratifying result is obtained. The independent arterial supply of the free flap allows the patient to undergo radiation as well as further revision and tailoring. Breasts reconstructed with free musculocutaneous gluteal flaps have proved to be warmer than those reconstructed by free groin flaps with underlying silicone prostheses. In addition, there has been a considerable return of sensation, even without sensory neurorrhaphy. A sense of permanence is enhanced, eliminating some of the disadvantages of silicone implants.

Since the muscle mass taken along with the skin flap is smaller, flap shrinkage becomes minimal, thus making estimation of breast volume easier. The breast mound achieved is soft to palpation and does not change in shape or size after the first few weeks. The skin surface of the reconstructed breast is soft and smooth, unlike the thicker, coarser, and frequently actinic-damaged skin from the back. In the supine position or with motion, the reconstructed breast has a soft, natural bounce approaching that of a normal breast, and it is distinctly superior to most breasts reconstructed with implants.

ANATOMY

The gluteus maximus is a broad, fan-shaped type III muscle that is a strong extensor and lateral thigh rotator. The superior half of the muscle may be used without significant functional loss in the ambulatory patient. It originates on the gluteal line of the ilium and sacrum and inserts on the greater tuberosity of the femur and the iliotibial tract. It is innervated by the inferior gluteal nerve on its deep surface. The superior and inferior gluteal arteries, both separate branches of the hypogastric artery, supply the upper and lower halves of the muscle, respectively. The muscle may be divided into superior and inferior halves based on these two pedicles, and there is ample collateralization between these two systems. The superior gluteal artery courses posteriorly above the piriform muscle. It then gives off a branch to the superior portion of the gluteus maximus muscle. The artery then courses laterally to supply the gluteus medius and minimus muscles. The inferior gluteal artery enters the gluteal region through the sciatic foramen in close proximity to the sciatic nerve. It supplies the inferior portion of the gluteus maximus muscle.

FLAP DESIGN AND DIMENSIONS

The flap is designed after establishing the extent of the gluteus maximus muscle and locating the origin of the superior gluteal artery. The cutaneous portion of the flap may be placed anywhere on the muscle and may even extend beyond it. Skin territories ranging from 8 to 13 cm in width and from 20 to 30 cm in length have been used.

OPERATIVE TECHNIQUE

The patient is marked in an erect position, so that the inframammary crease can be determined. An ipsilateral gluteal flap is used. Once the flap is harvested, the donor site is quickly closed, so that the patient can be brought into a more or less supine position for the microvascular anastomoses on the chest. After completion of the anastomoses, considerable time is spent in the trimming and setting in of the flap to achieve an optimal aesthetic result.

The initial incision starts along the superior and lateral borders, exposing the lateral fibers of the gluteus maximus muscle. After dividing the lateral upper third of the gluteus maximus about 4 cm posterior to the trochanter, the undersurface of the muscle is elevated. By following the branches of the superior gluteal artery and vein, the origin of the vessels can be identified. The skin and muscle incisions are then completed circumferentially. The final stage of dissection involves tedious detachment of the sacral origin of the gluteal muscle and isolation of the vascular pedicle. The superior gluteal artery and vein are usually 2 mm or larger, but very fragile. Dissection must be performed delicately, and small branches should be taken with bipolar forceps at a distance from the main branch or ligated. A vascular pedicle of 2 to 3 cm is dissected free. The donor vessels may be elongated by trimming the proximal portion of the muscle and subcutaneous fat without violating the perforating vasculature within these layers. The donor site is closed after slightly undermining the skin edges just above the fascia over the remaining gluteus to allow for more natural redraping.

A curved incision is used on the chest, with its lowest portion nearly to the inframammary line. In the case of a transverse mastectomy incision, this is simply ignored, and the "hockey stick" incision comes all the way down to the inframammary crease and curves medially. Medial and lateral skin flaps are then raised. If the internal mammary artery is chosen as the recipient vessel, the fifth rib costal cartilage is identified and resected within the perichondrium. The perichondrium and deep fascia are then incised longitudinally, starting inferiorly. The internal mammary vessels are located approximately 1 cm lateral to the edge of the sternum. These vessels are then dissected free from the surrounding bed, and small vascular branches are cauterized by bipolar forceps or tied.

If the recipient vein is too small, a vein graft is harvested from the leg and anastomosis to the axillary vein is performed first. If the patient does not want incisions on the leg and there is no evidence of edema on the arm, then the cephalic vein can be harvested through two small incisions and brought medially into the wound, draining into the thoracoacromial access.

Other recipient vessels, such as the thoracoacromial artery, transverse cervical artery, and branches of the axillary and external carotid arteries (depending on flap geometry and previous zones of irradiation and fibrosis), may be employed with or without vein grafts, accordingly. Drainage may be facilitated through the axillary, thoracoacromial, facial, and external or internal jugular venae comitantes.

It is crucial to stabilize the gluteal flap temporarily in its approximate position low at the fascial level just above the muscle in order to adjust pedicle length correctly. The gluteal flap is placed on its side on the chest, with the skin facing interiorly and the muscle superomedially. The distal (lateral) part of the skin flap is then brought into the axilla to fill out the infraclavicular hollow. If the curved skin incision is designed properly, the bending of the gluteal free flap automatically creates a nice central projection. The medial chest flap is then draped over the side of the gluteal free flap anteriorly. After placing some holding sutures, the gluteal flap can then be trimmed, deepithelialized, and shifted around until the overall contour is pleasing. A suction drain is placed underneath the flap laterally, and the skin is closed (Fig. 1).

The patient is allowed to lie on the buttocks immediately. On or about the third day, ambulation is permitted. About the fifth day, sitting in a chair with full bending of the hip is allowed. Within a week, the patient is generally walking comfortably, and she is discharged between the seventh and tenth postoperative days.

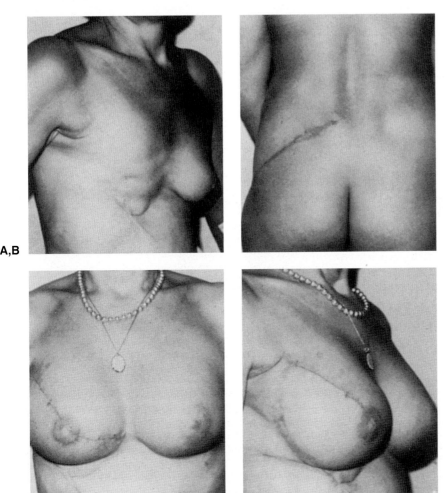

A,B

C,D

FIG. 1. A: Preoperative appearance after a modified radical mastectomy. B: Donor-site scar. C,D: Postoperative appearance. (From Shaw, ref. 2, with permission.)

CLINICAL RESULTS

Up to 13 cm in skin width has been taken from the buttock with fairly tensionless primary closure. The linear superior gluteal scar is well hidden in bathing suits or shorts. No functional muscle weakness has been noted, since only a small portion of the upper part of the gluteus muscle is taken with the skin flap. On late follow-up examination, patients are able to walk up and down stairs, alternately stand on one leg, and jump rope. There is minimal change in the appearance of the gluteal fold. An unexpected bonus of this particular donor site is that the superior gluteal area is not only difficult for the patient to see herself, but is also an area rarely in the conscious minds of most people. Patients have voiced surprising pride and confidence in feeling that the reconstructed breasts are part of their own bodies.

A disadvantage of microvascular transfer is the increasing complexity requiring specialized equipment and experience. A second concern is that of long operating time. For free flaps, the only added time is that of microvascular anastomosis of the artery and vein, adding approximately 1 to 2 hours to the procedure. A fair amount of time is spent in trimming, insetting, and contouring the flap to achieve the optimal aesthetic result. A final disadvantage of free-flap reconstruction is possible failure of the anastomoses, resulting in total loss. However, the current success rate of microvascular free flaps in experienced hands is about 95 percent, including all types of reconstructions, often in extremely difficult circumstances.

SUMMARY

The gluteus maximus musculocutaneous free flap is used increasingly for breast reconstruction. The extra operative time is not excessive, and the results in both recipient and donor sites are superior to many of the other available methods.

References

1. Fujino T, Harashina T, Aoyagi FL. Reconstruction for aplasia of the breast and pectoral region by microvascular transfer of a free flap from the buttock. *Plast Reconstr Surg* 1975;56:178.
2. Shaw WW. Breast reconstruction by superior gluteal microvascular free flaps without silicone implants. *Plast Reconstr Surg* 1983;72:490.
3. Shaw WW. Microvascular free flap breast reconstruction. *Clin Plast Surg* 1984;11:333.

CHAPTER 370 ■ MICROVASCULAR FREE TRAM FLAP

A.-M. FELLER, E. BIEMER, AND H.-U. STEINAU

> **EDITORIAL COMMENT**
>
> Although technically more involved, the advantages of the free TRAM flap include a decreased incidence of fat necrosis, as well as better vascularity beyond the hemilateral flap. See also Chapter 372.

Compared to other free-flap procedures for breast reconstruction following radical or modified radical mastectomy, the free TRAM flap has achieved wide recognition. It provides greater possibilities for breast contouring and a reliable vascular pedicle.

INDICATIONS

The free TRAM flap was used and reported in two cases of breast reconstruction in 1979 (1), but it did not achieve extensive use or a significant literature until the years following the report of Hartrampf et al. in 1982 (2).

Indications for the flap are similar to those for other flaps used in breast reconstruction. In patients with large, ptotic breasts, the flap is the procedure of choice, since the entire transverse flap can be used to achieve the desired breast volume. Special indications include radiotherapy with destruction of skin and soft tissue not only over a mastectomy defect, but also over the sternal area, with an expected hypoplastic vascular system in the internal mammary and superior epigastric vessels.

The free TRAM flap cannot be used in patients with a lower transverse laparotomy with presumably ligated inferior epigastric vessels. In addition, in extremely obese patients or chronic heavy smokers, the procedure is quite risky and is not recommended.

ANATOMY

The rectus muscle is covered by the anterior rectus sheath along its entire length; the posterior rectus sheath ends at the arcuate line. Below this level, the muscle directly overlies a thin layer of transversalis fascia. The blood supply to the rectus abdominis muscle is derived from the superior and inferior epigastric vessels, and because of their longer length and greater diameter, these vessels are useful for free-tissue transfer (3).

The free TRAM flap is supplied by one of the deep inferior epigastric vessels, with diameter of the artery between 2 and 4 mm and that of the vein about 3 mm. Dissection of the

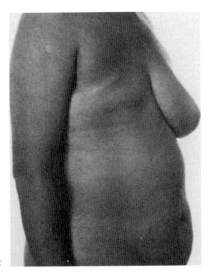
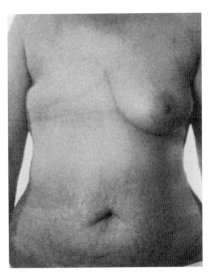
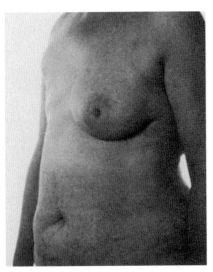

A–C

FIG. 1. A–C: A 50-year-old woman with modified radical mastectomy on the right side.

inferior epigastric pedicle to the level of the external iliac vessels provides a vascular pedicle of about 10 to 12 cm.

Generally, the inferior epigastric artery divides into two large branches below the level of the umbilicus. It passes upward into the muscle to communicate with the superior epigastric system above the level of the umbilicus. The densest network of larger perforators is located over the middle and medial thirds of the muscle in the paraumbilical region.

To ensure a sufficient blood supply to the free TRAM flap, it is necessary to dissect the rectus muscle from the arcuate line upward to the umbilical level. Following such dissection, the largest perforators can be included to guarantee adequate perfusion of the subdermal plexus lateral to the rectus sheath, as well as to the contralateral side.

FLAP DESIGN AND DIMENSIONS

The flap is designed in a horizontal, elliptical manner, as is the pedicled TRAM flap; in both cases, the umbilicus must be included in the ellipse. Flap width from the umbilicus to the pubic area depends on the volume of the contralateral breast.

The lateral flap tips are always situated over the iliac crests, allowing easier closure of the abdominal defect. This also ensures better contouring of the abdominal wall, similar to a regular abdominoplasty.

OPERATIVE TECHNIQUE

The free flap is raised in a manner similar to the pedicled TRAM flap (3–6); flap dimensions must be outlined in a standing patient. The patient is then placed in a supine position, with a slightly elevated shoulder on the mastectomy side. Both arms are abducted.

With two teams working, the scar on the chest wall is excised for histologic examination. The mastectomy defect is undermined and prepared, and the flap is incised on its inferior rim (Figs. 1 and 2). One team explores the axillary region and prepares the recipient vessels, while the other team dissects the inferior epigastric pedicle. In the axilla, we prefer the lateral thoracic artery and vein; however, if they are not available, the circumflex scapular or thoracodorsal vessels represent reliable alternatives.

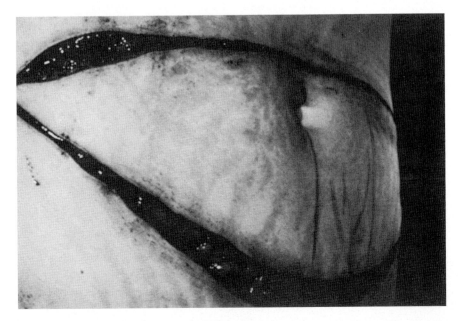

FIG. 2. The free TRAM flap incised including the umbilical region. The inferior epigastric pedicle will be harvested from the left side.

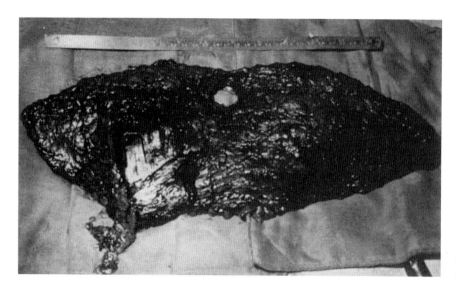

FIG. 3. The free TRAM flap turned over, ready for transfer to the right thoracic wall. Note the small amount of rectus muscle and the fairly long pedicle.

The contralateral rectus abdominis muscle is always taken with the inferior pedicle. The muscle is divided just above the umbilical level, and the complete free TRAM flap is tethered into the mastectomy defect for microsurgical revascularization (Fig. 3). Whenever possible, end-to-end anastomoses are used, but the pedicle is usually long enough to reach even the axillary artery and vein for end-to-side anastomoses.

Once the microsurgical procedures are completed, the patient is raised to a sitting position of about 45 degrees, and the abdominal wound is closed. Final orientation and tailoring of the flap are carried out in this position, allowing the flap to be situated with the desired contour matching that of the contralateral side.

As in all free-tissue transfers, the patient is closely observed postoperatively for adequate flap circulation. To prevent compromised blood flow in the axilla, special attention is paid to the arm on the repaired side, which should be slightly abducted (Fig. 4).

CLINICAL RESULTS

Between 1987 and 1988, 12 mastectomy reconstructions with free TRAM flaps have been carried out by us; none of these flaps failed. None of the patients developed a hernia, probably because of less muscle loss with this procedure than with the pedicled TRAM flap. A well-contoured, ptotic breast was achieved in only 50 percent of patients, requiring reduction of the contralateral breast. Adjustment of the contralateral breast, with nipple-areola reconstruction, is performed 6 months after breast reconstruction.

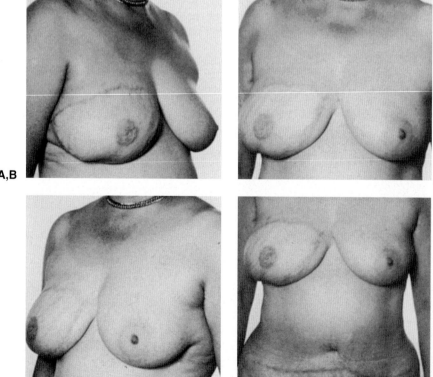

A,B

C,D

FIG. 4. A,B: Postoperative result 6 months after breast reconstruction and 2 months after reconstruction of the nipple-areola complex without necessity of breast reconstruction of the contralateral side. **C,D:** The patient 6 months after breast reconstruction with acceptable scar of the donor area.

Advantages of the free TRAM flap include (1) availability of large vessels for microsurgical anastomoses, (2) a long vascular pedicle (about 10 to 12 cm), (3) ease in raising the flap, (4) better and more vigorous skin circulation than with the pedicled TRAM flap, (5) greater freedom in reconstruction, since the entire transverse flap can be used to achieve the desired breast volume, and (6) avoidance of considerable weakening of the abdominal wall, since the muscle is taken only between the arcuate line and the umbilical level.

In the hands of surgeons well experienced in microsurgery, the microvascular anastomoses involved in the procedure present no great difficulties, and with two surgical teams working simultaneously, operative time is not an issue.

SUMMARY

Even with the requirement of microsurgical technique, the advantages of the free TRAM flap are clear. Compared with other free-flap procedures for breast reconstruction, this flap provides greater freedom in breast contouring and a reliable vascular pedicle.

References

1. Holmström H. The free abdominoplasty flap and its use in breast reconstruction. *Scand J Plast Reconstr Surg* 1979;13:423.
2. Hartrampf CR, Scheflan M, Black PW. Breast reconstruction with a transverse abdominal island flap. *Plast Reconstr Surg* 1982;69:216.
3. Boyd BJ, Taylor GI, Corlett R. The vascular territories of the superior epigastric and the deep inferior epigastric systems. *Plast Reconstr Surg* 1984;73:1.
4. Bunkis J, Walton RL, Mathes SJ. The rectus abdominis free flap for lower extremity reconstruction. *Ann Plast Surg* 1983;11:373.
5. Friedman JR, Argenta LC, Anderson RA. Deep inferior epigastric free flap for breast reconstruction after radical mastectomy. *Plast Reconstr Surg* 1985;76:455.
6. Arnez ZM, Smith RW, Eder E, et al. Breast reconstruction by the free lower transverse rectus abdominis musculocutaneous flap. *Br J Plast Surg* 1988; 41:500.

CHAPTER 371 ■ MICROVASCULAR FREE DEEP INFERIOR EPIGASTRIC PERFORATOR (DIEP) FLAP

C. HEITMANN AND R. J. ALLEN

EDITORIAL COMMENT

This is a major advance in the armamentarium of the plastic surgeon doing breast reconstruction. Nevertheless, pedicle and prosthetic reconstruction still plays an important role in the care of the post-mastectomy patient.

The deep inferior epigastric perforator (DIEP) flap arose as a refinement of the conventional transverse rectus abdominis myocutaneous (TRAM) flap. The DIEP flap can carry the same tissue as the TRAM flap, without the sacrifice of the rectus muscle or fascia, thereby minimizing donor-site morbidity, including bulge, hernia, weakness, and length of recovery time (1,2). The DIEP flap is commonly used for breast restoration to provide a soft, naturally shaped, long-lasting result.

INDICATIONS

An excellent source of soft tissue for free-flap reconstructions is the lower abdomen in women. Generally speaking, women who would benefit from an abdominoplasty are possible candidates for a DIEP flap and, in fact, most women who have had or will have mastectomies for breast cancer are candidates for the DIEP flap. In cases of breast reconstruction, we prefer to have patients complete any radiation therapy, and a delay of 6 months, prior to free-flap procedures. Although perforator flaps usually tolerate radiation well, superior long-term results are typically obtained in reconstructions performed after, rather than before, chest-wall irradiation [3].

Abdominal scarring is probably the most important risk factor for raising DIEP flaps, and can cause major problems during the dissection of perforators and epigastric vessels. Intramuscular scarring is not always diagnosed accurately with preoperative ultrasound, and can spread farther than suspected from the placing and length of a previous incision. Smoking is considered a relative contraindication to raising a DIEP flap (4). Smokers who request elective, delayed reconstructions are required to stop smoking at least 3 months before becoming candidates for surgery. An absolute contraindication for a DIEP procedure in our practice is a history of previous abdominoplasty or abdominal liposuction.

ANATOMY

The deep inferior epigastric artery arises from the external iliac artery, which is just above the inguinal ligament, and approaches the rectus abdominis muscle from its lateral side. The artery is accompanied by two venae comitantes and forms an excellent pedicle for free tissue transfer.

The anatomy of the deep inferior epigastric artery system is quite variable. The average pedicle length is 10.3 cm, and the average vessel diameter is 3.6 mm. Generally, the artery divides into two branches, with a dominant lateral branch (54%). However, if the deep inferior epigastric artery does not divide, the vessel has a central course (28%), with multiple small branches to the rectus abdominis muscle and centrally located perforators. If the medial branch of the artery is dominant (18%), flow appears to be significantly lower than in a central system or in patients with a dominant lateral branch.

Previous studies of abdominal-wall vasculature anatomy have noted that one or two perforators per pedicle can be reliably observed to be greater than 1 mm (5). In addition, all major perforators can usually be found within 8 cm of the umbilicus. The closer a perforator is to the midline, the better the blood supply to zone IV (the area most distant from the vascular pedicle) will be (6). However, the lateral perforators are often dominant and easier to dissect, because they run more perpendicularly through the muscle. The sensory nerve that runs with these perforating vessels is also often much larger. The medial perforators provide better perfusion for the DIEP flap, but they have a longer intramuscular course and require more elaborate dissection, with extensive longitudinal splitting of the muscle. Preference is also given to perforators that pass through the rectus abdominis muscle at the level of the tendinous intersections (7). At this point, the perforators are frequently large and have few muscular side branches. The distance from the subcutaneous fat to the deep inferior epigastric vessels is also shorter, simplifying this most delicate part of the dissection.

FLAP DESIGN AND DIMENSIONS

The patient is usually seen in the office on the day prior to surgery for preoperative markings and Doppler studies. She should assume a standing position, and an elliptical skin island is drawn on the abdomen. The borders of a DIEP flap are generally located at the level of the suprapubic crease, the umbilicus, and both anterior superior iliac spines. A DIEP flap generally measures 12 cm in height and extends 20 to 24 cm from the midline. However, the tension at the donor site following closure should be estimated, as this ultimately limits the size of the flap that can be harvested. The side of the abdomen contralateral to the side to be reconstructed is preferred, as this provides for easier insetting at the time of surgery. With the patient in the supine position, a Doppler probe is used to identify the main perforators of the deep inferior epigastric artery. This road map of the largest perforators helps the surgeon make decisions intraoperatively. The superficial inferior epigastric artery and vein are likewise found with the Doppler and marked. The procedure is performed under general anesthesia, with the patient in the supine position and the arms positioned beside the trunk. Preoperatively, placement of intravenous lines, an indwelling urinary catheter, and deep vein thrombosis prophylaxis with low-dose heparin and sequential pressure hose are recommended

OPERATIVE TECHNIQUE

A two-team approach is used, with simultaneous raising of the flap and preparation of the recipient vessels. For breast reconstruction, the internal mammary artery (IMA) and vein (IMV) are the recipient vessels of choice and are used in more than 90% of our cases. The central position of the IMA and IMV in the chest wall makes medial placement of the flap easier on insetting. The vessels are dissected between the second and third rib spaces. A distance of 2 to 3 cm in width is sufficient to enable anastomosis. If the rib space is less than 3 cm in width, removal of a portion of the lower rib is performed.

The thoracodorsal vessels are used alternatively when the internal mammary vessels prevent proper flap insetting and geometry, such as in cases of partial breast reconstruction. While making the inferior skin incision, care is taken to preserve the superficial epigastric vein.

If venous drainage of the flap is insufficient or thrombosis of the perforator veins occurs after the anastomosis, the superficial epigastric vein can be used as an additional venous conduit (8). The vein is dissected over a length of 4 to 5 cm and ligated with clips to make them easily retrievable later, if needed. If the inferior epigastric vessels are found to be sufficient in size and quality, they are followed down to their origin from the common femoral artery, and a superficial inferior epigastric artery (SIEA) perforator flap procedure can be performed.

For the DIEP flap, the abdominal incisions are continued down to the fascia. Beveling is avoided unless extra volume is required, as this may later lead to a depressed scar in the abdomen. However, the flap may be beveled laterally to include more fat and reduce residual dog ears. Dissection of the vascular pedicle of a DIEP flap can be divided into three different technical stages: suprafascial, intramuscular, and submuscular. The most demanding stage is the intramuscular dissection of the vascular pedicle.

At first, the abdominal skin island is carefully elevated from lateral to medial until the lateral row of perforators is encountered. If a large perforator is found, the flap may be based on this vessel. Additional perforators in the same row may also be dissected and included with the flap for extra perfusion. If no large perforator is found, the medial row is approached in a similar fashion. If no dominant single perforator is found, two or even three smaller perforators in the same medial or lateral row may be taken to carry the flap. In cases in which more than one large perforator is present, the perforator with a more central location to the proposed flap is used. In our experience, approximately 25% of DIEP flaps are based on one perforator, 50% on two, and 25% on three or more perforators. We prefer a flap to be based on a single large perforator. The abdominal muscles must be relaxed at all times and the perforating vessels kept moist with normal saline.

Complete dissection of a perforator helps prevent vessel damage when raising the flap from the contralateral side. In the case of a unilateral DIEP flap reconstruction, if the medial and lateral row perforators on the initially approached side of the abdomen are found to be less than optimal, the perforators on the opposite side of the abdomen are investigated, as the contralateral side often yields a perforator of better quality. Once the appropriate perforators are chosen, the anterior rectus fascia is incised with a pair of microscissors, following the direction of the rectus abdominis muscle fibers at the rim of the tiny gap in the fascia through which the perforating vessel passes. If more than one perforator is dissected, the different gaps can be connected. The division of the fascia is continued superiorly for a distance of 2 to 4 cm, and inferiorly to the lateral border of the rectus abdominis muscle.

It is advisable to fully complete the dissection of the DIEP flap on one side before progressing to the other. This precaution provides a lifeboat in the form of a contralateral DIEP flap, to be used if the perforator is inadvertently damaged. As dissection progresses, the DIEP flap should be secured to the abdominal wall or carefully held by an assistant. The rectus abdominis muscle is spread apart in the direction of the fibers, and care is taken to identify and preserve any intercostal nerves. Dissection continues through the muscle down to the deep inferior epigastric vessels. By so doing, the perforator is liberated from the muscle by blunt dissection, staying close to the vessel at all times, as it remains covered by a thin layer of loose connective tissue.

As a general rule, if resistance to dissection is encountered, a side branch or a nerve is identified. Using bipolar coagulation diathermy and small hemoclips, one continues to ligate all side branches until the inferior epigastric artery is reached on the posterior surface of the rectus abdominis muscle. If two perforators have been selected that run in adjacent perimysial planes, the muscle fibers between have to be cut. In a submuscular dissection, the lateral border of the rectus abdominis muscle is raised to open the plane posterior to the muscle.

The main pedicle of the deep inferior epigastric vessels is exposed and the side branches of the main stem are ligated. The length of the pedicle can be tailored to meet the needs of different recipient sites, or the demands of the shape of the flap. If one is certain that the blood flow through the deep inferior epigastric vessels is sufficient, the remainder of the flap can be raised. The umbilicus is released, and the entire skin flap is raised. The artery and the veins of the pedicle are then clipped and the pedicle slid out underneath any crossing intercostal nerves. Sometimes, it is necessary to divide a crossing motor intercostal nerve to release the vascular pedicle. In these cases, the nerve is repaired with two interrupted 8-0 nylon sutures prior to closure of the abdominal fascia. The flap is then weighted and transferred to the recipient site. Great care is taken to lay the donor pedicle to the recipient vessels without any twists or kinks. Although the overall incidence of vascular complication is low, experience has shown that many cases of venous compromise can be traced to a twisted pedicle. Temporary stay sutures are placed in the flap with the orientation of 180 degrees with the umbilicus inferiorly. This allows for the thicker part of the flap to lie medially on the chest wall. The operating microscope is brought into position.

For the venous anastomosis, we use an anastomotic coupling device. The coupling device makes the anastomosis easier and more rapid, and has the additional benefit of stenting the vein open after the vessels are joined. The arterial anastomosis is typically performed manually with interrupted sutures. After the anastomosis is complete, the flap is checked for bleeding and capillary refill.

Insetting and closure are performed over a suction drain, and great care is taken at all times to monitor the integrity of the pedicle during the insetting of the flap. If a contralateral flap is used, the flap is turned between approximately 90 and 120 degrees so that the medial portion of the abdominal flap becomes the base of the reconstructed breast. Excess skin is deepithelialized superiorly and inferiorly, and the flap inset with a visible skin paddle left in place.

The external Doppler probe is used to identify the locations on the flap with good arterial and venous signals, and these locations are marked for postoperative monitoring in the postanesthesia care unit (PACU) and on the floor with a handheld Doppler probe. For monitoring, it is also possible to use an implantable Doppler probe. This is especially helpful in cases in which a smaller skin paddle is left, or no dominant point can be found on the exposed skin portion of an otherwise healthy flap. Also, in nipple-sparing mastectomies in which no skin island is left, the implantable probe is used. Care must be taken with the placement of these probes. A Doppler sleeve placed too loosely around the vessel may result in loss of signal, despite the presence of good blood flow, whereas a tight sleeve or wire connection may kink or otherwise compromise the vessel's patency.

The abdominal fascia is closed and securely tied with a running size 1 absorbable suture. Mesh or other synthetic materials are not used in abdominal-wall closures. The edges of the umbilicus are tacked down to the fascia with a 2-0 Vicryl suture. The upper abdominal flap is undermined to the level of the xiphoid and costal margin. The patient is then flexed and the wound closed in layers over two closed suction drains. As in an abdominoplasty, the umbilicus is brought out through the abdominal flap and secured in place.

CLINICAL RESULTS

On the basis of our retrospective review and our 10-year experience, we have adopted this method as our standard of care for breast reconstruction (Fig. 1). We have established smoking and postmastectomy radiation therapy as primary risk factors. We now require our patients to refrain from cigarette smoking for 4 weeks, and we delay reconstruction for all patients potentially receiving postmastectomy radiation therapy. Complications are infrequent. In the published series of more than 750 DIEP flap reconstructions (4), 6% of patients were returned to the operating room for flap-related problems. Partial flap loss occurred in 2.5% and total flap loss in less than 1%. Problems

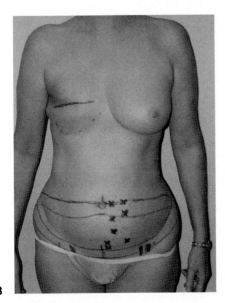
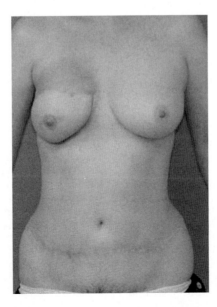

A,B

FIG. 1. **A:** Preoperative view of a patient marked for the deep inferior epigastric perforator (DIEP) flap. **B:** Result 1 year after the DIEP flap procedure and nipple-areola reconstruction.

with the vein or venous anastomosis were almost four times more likely than problems with the arterial anastomosis. Fat necrosis appeared in 12% of flaps. Seroma formation at the abdominal donor site was approximately 3.5%, and abdominal hernia occurred in 0.7 % of cases.

SUMMARY

After more than a decade of experience with the DIEP flap, it has become the preferred choice for breast reconstruction. Better cosmesis can be achieved with skin and soft tissue, and there is no sacrifice of the abdominal musculature, which has led to a marked decrease in the hernia rate. With an average unilateral reconstruction time of 4.66 hours and a bilateral reconstruction time of 7.3 hours, the operative time is not increased, in comparison with the free TRAM flap. Also in comparison with the free TRAM flap, the DIEP flap provides a significantly longer pedicle, which allows tension-free anastomoses. This permits more freedom of design, which results in a centrally located breast mound, especially with anastomoses to the internal mammary system. As microsurgical experience increases, we think that the benefit of this flap will outweigh its risks, and the time spent learning microsurgical techniques will be rewarded with a first-line option for breast reconstruction, affording better patient satisfaction, decreased donor-site morbidity, and shorter hospital stays.

References

1. Allen RJ, Treece P. Deep inferior epigastric perforator flap for breast reconstruction. *Ann Plast Surg* 1994;32:32.
2. Futter CM, Webster MH, Hagen, et al: A retrospective comparison of abdominis muscle strength following breast reconstruction with a free TRAM or DIEP flap. *Br J Plast Surg* 2000;53:578.
3. Rogers NE, Allen RJ. Radiation effects on breast reconstruction: a review. *Semin Plast Surg* 2002;1:19.
4. Gill P, Hunt J, Guerra A, et al: A 10 year retrospective review of 758 DIEP flaps for breast reconstruction. *Plast Reconstr Surg* 2004;113:1153.
5. Heitmann C, Felmerer G, Durmus C, et al: Anatomical feature of perforator blood vessels in the deep inferior epigastric flap. *Br J Plast Surg* 2000;53:205.
6. Blondeel PN, Morris SF, Hallock GG, Neligan PC: *Perforator flaps: anatomy, technique, and clinical application.* St. Louis: Quality Medical Publishing, 2006.
7. Vandevoort M, Vranckx JJ, Fabre B, et al: Perforator topography of the deep inferior epigastric perforator flap in 100 cases of breast reconstruction. *Plast Reconstr Surg* 2002;109:1912.
8. Blondeel PN, Arnstein M, Verstraete K, et al. Venous congestion and blood flow in free transverse rectus abdominis myocutaneous and deep inferior epigastric perforator flaps. *Plast Reconstr Surg* 2000;106:1295.

CHAPTER 372 ■ IMMEDIATE MICROVASCULAR FREE TRAM FLAP

J. C. GROTTING

As experience has been gained in autologous breast reconstruction using the TRAM flap (1–4), its suitability for immediate reconstruction has been increasingly recognized. All the advantages of this donor site for delayed reconstruction are equally applicable in the immediate situation. At present, this flap remains the most versatile flap for matching the opposite breast in a single procedure without implants.

INDICATIONS

Transferring the TRAM flap as a microsurgical procedure based on the deep inferior epigastric artery and vein offers several additional advantages (5). First, the greater blood flow through the larger-caliber artery virtually always irrigates a larger territory of the flap, thereby making more tissue reliably available for the reconstruction. Second, only a small rectangle of the rectus abdominis muscle need be included in the flap, just enough to surround the medial and lateral row of perforating vessels from the deep inferior epigastric pedicle (6–8).

The free TRAM flap is particularly advantageous in immediate breast reconstruction where the subscapular axis is readily available following axillary dissection. By using these vessels as recipient vessels, considerable options are available for folding or molding the flap. In fact, there is less restriction to placing the flap tissue to create a symmetrical breast. The skin and tissue volume of the mastectomy specimen can very accurately be replaced.

FLAP DESIGN AND DIMENSIONS

It is unnecessary to take any muscle below the point where the pedicle meets the muscle (Fig. 1B). This allows a strip of medial and lateral rectus abdominis muscle to be left from the semicircular line to the umbilicus. Above the umbilicus, the entire rectus muscle is left intact and not dissected from its bed. Small twigs of intercostal motor nerves to the rectus muscle are not divided along the semilunar line, thereby leaving intact functional rectus muscle laterally.

Because the upper portion of the rectus muscle does not need to be dissected for this flap transfer, the superior abdominal flap is undermined only as much as necessary to close the donor defect without tension. No tunneling is required

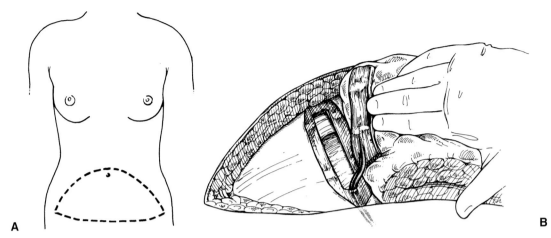

FIG. 1. **A:** The design of the TRAM flap. **B:** It is unnecessary to take any muscle below the point where the pedicle meets muscle.

between the abdominal donor site and the mastectomy wound. This markedly reduces the excess bleeding that can occur during this portion of the conventional TRAM operation. The epigastric bulge produced by the tunneled rectus muscle that is often persistent after the conventional TRAM flap is also eliminated. The medial portion of the inframammary fold can be left intact. Therefore, symmetry is improved.

Immediate breast reconstruction using the free TRAM flap is performed using two surgical teams with separate operative instrument sets. Planning should include a discussion of incisions to spare as much skin of the breast as possible. Usually an incision encompassing the nipple-areola complex and the previous biopsy site, if present, is a sufficient amount of skin to be taken. An oblique extension into the axilla will allow adequate exposure for the axillary dissection.

The TRAM flap is designed on the lower abdominal wall exactly the same as one designs the conventional flap. I prefer to design the flap as if doing a standard abdominoplasty, seeking to keep the scar as low and transverse as possible (Fig. 1A). The contralateral rectus abdominis muscle is routinely used. This allows the small segment of rectus muscle to be placed at the point of maximum projection of the newly formed breast and still leaves a dependable amount of flap available for filling the infraclavicular hollow and to provide fullness inferiorly and inferolaterally. If chest-wall skin must be replaced high in the infraclavicular area, the ipsilateral rectus muscle might be a better choice.

OPERATIVE TECHNIQUE

The umbilicus is incised circumferentially down to the rectus fascia. The superior incision is made by beveling superiorly between the semilunar lines to include a few extra rectus perforators. The ipsilateral side of the flap is raised at the level of the deep fascia beyond the midline by approximately 1 to 2 cm. Elevation stops when the medial row of perforators of the contralateral rectus muscle is reached. The contralateral side of the flap is then raised until the lateral row of rectus perforators is visualized. Inferiorly, the flap is raised to the level of the semicircular line, which is commonly marked by a large rectus perforator. At this point, the anterior rectus sheath is incised, forming a rectangle that encompasses the medial, lateral, and inferiormost rectus perforators. The lateral edge of the rectus muscle is then separated just enough to identify the entry point of the deep inferior epigastric artery (Fig. 2). When this point has been identified, the rectus muscle is split within its fibers just lateral to this entry point, thereby preserving the

lateral row of perforators with the flap. The rectus abdominis muscle can then be divided just inferior to the point where the deep inferior epigastric pedicle meets the muscle. The muscle separation is then continued medially, again including the medial row of perforators, but preserving an intact medial strip of muscle.

Through this window in the muscle deep retractors are placed, and using loupe magnification, the deep inferior epigastric artery and veins (there are usually two) are dissected to their origin through the lateral pelvic wall. Usually, only two or three small branches are encountered during this dissection, and these are easily controlled using small vessel clips.

Before the superior rectus abdominis muscle is cut, the recipient vessels must be explored to determine their adequacy for microvascular anastomoses. Usually, the times required to raise the flap and complete the mastectomy are similar. Therefore, the subscapular axis can be examined following completion of the mastectomy to identify satisfactory recipient vessels. I prefer to use the thoracodorsal artery and vein proximal to the serratus branch for end-to-end anastomoses. I believe that this provides the safest inflow with good size match of vessel caliber and more flexibility to place the flap in the proper position. Also, axial flow to the latissimus dorsi muscle is maintained by retrograde flow through the serratus branch if this muscle were ever required for secondary coverage.

After adequate inflow has been established, the central remaining portion of the rectus abdominis muscle is divided

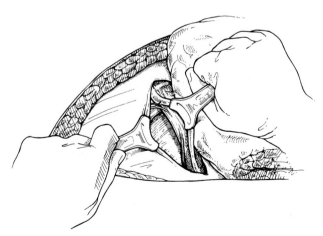

FIG. 2. The lateral edge of the rectus muscle is separated just enough to identify the entry point of the deep inferior epigastric artery.

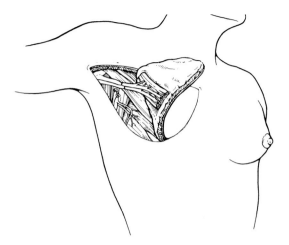

FIG. 3. The flap is anastomosed to the thoracodorsal artery and vein proximal to the serratus branch if possible.

superiorly so that the entire flap is allowed to perfuse only on the deep inferior epigastric artery and accompanying veins. Up to this point, the flap could still be transferred as a conventional TRAM flap. With warming of the flap, its circulation improves, and after 10 to 15 minutes, it can be safely transferred.

The deep inferior epigastric pedicle is then divided at its origin through the lateral pelvic wall. The flap is transferred to the mastectomy site. It can be positioned either on the upper arm, allowing the vessels to fall into the axillary wound, or alternatively, it can be temporarily positioned in the mastectomy wound and the vessels brought into the axillary defect. It may help to tilt the patient toward the contralateral side to improve the visibility into the axilla. Also, I prefer to have the anesthesiologist monitor the patient from the foot of the table using long ventilation tubes. This allows positioning of the microscope and the assistant at the patient's head.

End-to-end microvascular anastomoses are then performed and the flap is allowed to perfuse (Fig. 3). A drain is placed in

the axilla, and the latissimus dorsi muscle is sutured to the serratus in order to partially close the axilla. The axillary skin flap then also can be sutured to close the axilla and help recreate the lateral and inferolateral aspects of the breast. The small segment of rectus muscle is sutured to the pectoralis major muscle at the point where maximum projection of the breast is desired. Care is taken to observe the vessels during this closure to make sure they are under no tension. The flap can then be rotated and folded to replace the tissues removed with the mastectomy specimen. If abundant breast skin is available, most of the flap can be deepithelialized, and only a small monitoring disk of skin can be left at the anticipated position of the nipple-areola complex. Many times the entire flap could be safely used, since zone 4 frequently receives adequate perfusion. However, in my experience, it has never been necessary to use the entire flap to have enough tissue for symmetry with the opposite side.

If a large skin excision is necessary for an adequate mastectomy, it is helpful to make a template of the shape of the skin excision prior to incising the mastectomy flaps. This template can then be used as a guide to reapproximation of the mastectomy flaps over the deepithelialized TRAM flap. A second drain is usually left beneath the flap.

If a reduction or mastopexy is desirable on the opposite side, I prefer to do this prior to molding the TRAM flap. It is best to have a second team perform the opposite breast correction while the mastectomy is being done or while the TRAM flap is being raised. I have found that it is easier to match the corrected opposite breast with the TRAM flap rather than vice versa in a second operation.

The closure of the abdominal wall is straightforward. The anterior rectus sheath and medial and lateral strips of rectus muscle are easily reapproximated. The umbilicus may be pulled over during this closure but can usually be easily recentralized by imbricating the fascia on the opposite side. The entire reconstruction is improved if formal abdominoplasty techniques are used for the abdominal wall closure. This may include correction of a rectus diastasis superiorly and improvement of the waistline using bilateral external oblique

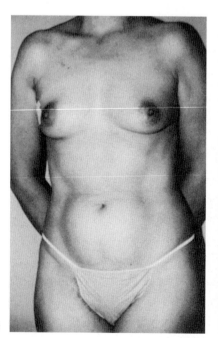
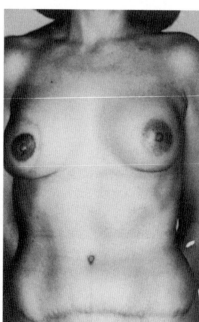
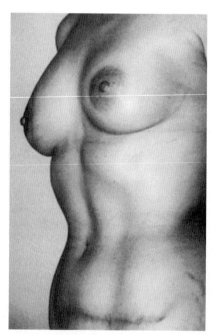

A–C

FIG. 4. A: A 35-year-old woman with biopsy-proven carcinoma of the right breast. Subsequent to this picture, she underwent a modified radical mastectomy and immediate reconstruction with a left free TRAM flap. B,C: Postoperative result 6 months after the initial procedure and 3 months after nipple-areolar reconstruction.

advancement flaps. The superior abdominal skin and subcutaneous tissue are undermined as much as necessary to allow closure of the flap donor site without tension. The umbilicus is sutured to the deep fascia and brought through in an appropriate position. The area around the neoumbilicus is defatted to recreate the periumbilical depression. Two large suction drains are placed on each side and the wound is then closed.

Molding of the breast is best accomplished with the patient in the sitting position so that symmetry can be examined. More time spent molding the breast in the initial operation reduces the likelihood of secondary corrective revisions (Fig. 4). Nipple-areola reconstruction is always performed 3 months later unless chemotherapy has been initiated. In this situation, nipple-areola reconstruction is usually delayed until completion of chemotherapy.

The patient is transferred directly to a hospital bed with the head elevated 20 to 30 degrees and the knees elevated slightly as well. The patient is asked to maintain her arm on the side of the reconstruction between 45 and 90 degrees to avoid compression or stretching of the microvascular anastomoses. This is continued for approximately 10 days. No dextran or other anticoagulants are used with the exception of a single aspirin tablet daily starting in the postoperative period.

SUMMARY

The free TRAM flap can be molded and adapted to the mastectomy defect to create a soft, well-designed breast.

References

1. Hartrampf CR, Scheflan M, Black PW. Breast reconstruction with a transverse abdominal island flap. *Plast Reconstr Surg* 1982;69:216.
2. Drever JM. The epigastric island flap. *Plast Reconstr Surg* 1977;59:343.
3. Robbins TH. Rectus abdominis myocutaneous flap for breast reconstruction. *Aust NZ J Surg* 1979;49:527.
4. Marino H, Dogliotti P. Mammary reconstruction with bipedicled abdominal flap. *Plast Reconstr Surg* 1981;68:933.
5. Shaw WW. Microvascular free-flap breast reconstruction. *Clin Plast Surg* 1984;11:333.
6. Boyd JB, Taylor GI, Corlett R. The vascular territories of the superior epigastric and the deep inferior epigastric systems. *Plast Reconstr Surg* 1984;73:1.
7. Carramenha e Costa MA, Carriquiry C, Vasconez LO, et al. An anatomic study of the venous drainage of the transverse rectus abdominis musculocutaneous flap. *Plast Reconstr Surg* 1987;79:208.
8. Brown RG, Vasconez LO, Jurkiewicz MJ. Transverse abdominal flaps and the deep epigastric arcade. *Plast Reconstr Surg* 1975;55:416.

CHAPTER 373 ■ RUBENS FLAP FOR BREAST RECONSTRUCTION

P. M. GARDNER AND J. C. GROTTING

The Rubens flap is particularly useful for patients who require breast reconstruction when a TRAM flap is not available, either because of a failed attempt or because of previous abdominoplasty.

INDICATIONS

This flap is a soft-tissue free flap found in the peri-iliac area. Described by Hartrampf in 1994 (1), it is useful for breast reconstruction in women who desire autogenous reconstruction, but who do not have sufficient tissue in the more conventional donor sites.

ANATOMY

The blood supply to the flap arises from the musculocutaneous perforators of the deep circumflex iliac artery (DCIA). This artery averages 2 mm in diameter. It originates from the lateral aspect of the external iliac artery just above the inguinal ligament and almost directly opposite the deep inferior epigastric artery. It has a straight course laterally along the posterior margin of the inguinal ligament toward the anterior superior iliac spine (ASIS). Here, it lies between the transversalis fascia and the transversus abdominis muscle.

An ascending branch is found just proximal to the ASIS, which penetrates the internal oblique muscle. Just beyond this branch, the DCIA pierces the transversalis fascia and travels laterally along the inner lip of the iliac crest. At this point, it lies in a fibrous tunnel formed by the fusion of the iliacus muscle and transversalis fascia (2).

The dominant perforator to the Rubens flap arises along the inner lip of the iliac crest 2.5 to 4.0 cm lateral to the ASIS.

A second smaller perforator is usually found 5.5 to 6.0 cm from the ASIS. They travel within millimeters of the bone but do not pass through. The perforators traverse the adjacent abdominal muscle to supply the skin and fat of the flap (1).

FLAP DESIGN AND DIMENSIONS

The flap is taken from the skin and fat overlying the iliac crest. The skin island is designed as an ellipse extending from the ASIS to the posterior axillary line. It parallels the iliac crest superiorly. The inferior extent is determined by the amount of tissue that can be taken with primary closure of the donor site (Fig. 1).

The skin island can be safely designed as a 6- × 12-cm ellipse. A flap up to 9 × 20 cm has been reported (1), and injection studies on cadavers demonstrate an area of 15 × 30 cm supplied by the DCIA (2). The weight of the flap depends on the patient's habitus; weights from 520 to 640 g have been reported (1).

OPERATIVE TECHNIQUE

The patient is placed supine with a bean bag beneath the buttock to elevate the pelvis toward the opposite side. The flap is outlined over the iliac crest with an incision extending anteriorly over the inguinal canal (Figs. 1 and 2). Dissection of the pedicle begins over the inguinal canal with an incision down to and through the external oblique aponeurosis. The round ligament is retracted medially and the pedicle (DCIA) is identified. It is dissected laterally to the ASIS.

Care is taken to avoid the lateral cutaneous femoral nerve, which courses downward medial to the ASIS. The skin island incisions are then made. The upper half is dissected off the external oblique to within 5 to 6 cm of the iliac crest. At this

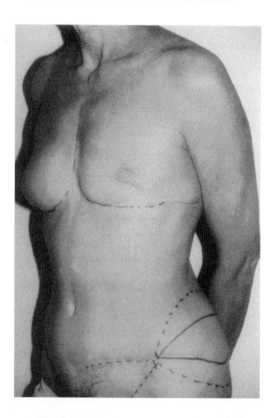

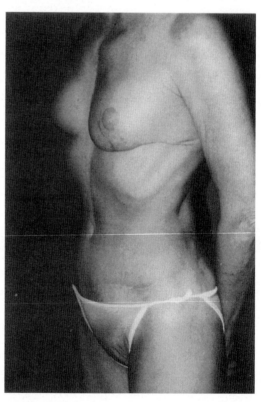

FIGS. 2. AND 3. Pre- and postoperative views demonstrate Rubens fat pad and cosmetically acceptable contour of donor site. The dotted lines show the extent of beveling outward from the incisions (solid lines).

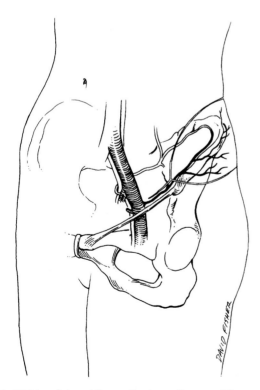

FIG. 1. DCIA pedicle and flap outlined over iliac crest. The two dominant perforators are found after the ascending branch. The anterior incision is made over the inguinal canal. Five centimeters above the iliac crest, the dissection goes through the muscles, which are included as a cuff.

point, the external oblique, internal oblique, and transversus abdominis muscles are incised and taken as a cuff with the flap. The inferior incision is then made and the flap is elevated off the tensor fascia lata and gluteus medius to the lower border of the iliac crest.

Here, the dissection is continued over the lip of the iliac crest directly on top of the periosteum, preserving the musculocutaneous perforators which run within millimeters of the crest. The muscles and pedicle are dissected off the inner surface of the iliac crest, taking a cuff of muscle approximately 10×3 cm. Laterally, beyond the iliac crest, the dissection proceeds above the muscles, but below the fascia, to the posterior axillary line (3). The flap is then transferred to the defect. Microsurgical anastomosis is usually done to the thoracodorsal or internal mammary vessels.

Careful closure of the donor defect is critical to avoid abdominal-wall herniation. Closure is in layers. First, the transversalis fascia is approximated to the iliacus muscle and fascia. Next, drill holes are made in the iliac crest, through which a large suture approximates the transversus and internal oblique muscles to the iliac crest. Finally, the external oblique is closed over the crest to the tensor fascia lata and gluteal fascia. The inguinal incision is closed by approximating the external oblique (1,4).

CLINICAL RESULTS

The Rubens flap is an excellent secondary flap for autogenous breast reconstruction. After abdominoplasty or failed TRAM flap, patients usually have a generous amount of tissue in the peri-iliac area. When harvested, the scar becomes an extension of the abdominoplasty incision. The change in contour of the waist is usually deemed favorable (Fig. 3).

There are several drawbacks to using the Rubens flap. Technically, it is more difficult than the TRAM flap. In comparison to other alternative flaps for breast reconstruction, it is easier than the gluteal flap, and probably equal in difficulty to the lateral thigh flap. The donor site can be more painful in the immediate postoperative period, secondary to drilling the iliac crest during closure (5). Additionally, in order to gain symmetry, the opposite peri-iliac fat pad requires resection. Finally, shaping the flap is considered a bit more difficult.

SUMMARY

The options for autogenous breast reconstruction following abdominoplasty or failed TRAM flap are few. The Rubens flap provides an adequate amount of tissue with a cosmetically acceptable donor site. Although technically more difficult to harvest and shape, it is an excellent choice for the microvascular surgeon.

References

1. Hartrampf CR, Noel TR, Dragan E, et al. Rubens fat pad for breast reconstruction: a peri-iliac soft-tissue free flap. *Plast Reconstr Surg* 1994;93:402.
2. Taylor GI, Townsend P, Corlett R. Superiority of the deep circumflex iliac vessels as the supply for free groin flaps: experimental work. *Plast Reconstr Surg* 1979;64:595.
3. Mathes SJ, Nahai F. Deep circumflex iliac artery (DCIA composite) flap: vascular anatomy. In: *Reconstructive surgery: principles, anatomy, and technique*, Vol. 2. New York: Churchill Livingstone, 1994;967.
4. Taylor GI, Townsend P, Corlett R. Superiority of the deep circumflex iliac vessels as the supply for free groin flaps: clinical work. *Plast Reconstr Surg* 1979;64:745.
5. Elliott LF. Options for donor sites for autogenous tissue breast reconstruction. *Clin Plast Surg* 1994;21:177.

CHAPTER 374 ■ MICROVASCULAR FREE SUPERIOR AND INFERIOR GLUTEAL ARTERY PERFORATOR (SGAP/IGAP) FLAPS FOR BREAST RECONSTRUCTION

M. M. LOTEMPIO AND R. J. ALLEN

EDITORIAL COMMENT

Although free gluteal artery perforator flaps may not be the first choice for many surgeons in breast reconstruction, it is important to have these options available.

Perforator flaps have raised the standard in breast reconstruction. By replacing like with like, permanent natural results with minimal donor-site deformities can be achieved. Being able to choose from many donor-site options makes virtually all patients candidates for this method of autogenous reconstruction. The superior or inferior gluteal artery perforator flap (SGAP, IGAP) was first introduced by our group in 1993.

The advantages of the gluteal flap include preservation of the gluteus maximus muscle and elongation of the pedicle. As with other perforator flaps, donor-site morbidity is minimal, and no sacrifice of muscle is required.

INDICATIONS

For more than a decade, perforator flaps have allowed the transfer of the patient's own skin and fat in a reliable manner, with minimal donor-site morbidity (1). They are evidence of the most recent development in the evolution of flaps for breast reconstruction. Pedicled, axial-pattern flaps, which could reliably transfer greater amounts of tissue, soon substituted for flaps that relied on a random-pattern blood supply. The concept of free-tissue transfer allowed an infinite range of possibilities to match donor and recipient sites appropriately (2).

Women who have undergone mastectomies and wish to have reconstructions with autologous tissue are candidates for SGAP or IGAP flaps. Those in whom the abdomen cannot be used as a donor site, either because of previous abdominoplasty or liposuction, or who have more tissue in the buttock area than in the abdomen, are the best candidates. The buttock has a high fat-to-skin ratio, whereas the abdomen has a high skin-to-fat ratio. Patients who require mostly fat and little skin may be candidates for SGAP/IGAP flaps. A significant amount of tissue may be harvested, and, in our experience, the average final inset weights of our GAP flaps were slightly greater than weights of the mastectomy specimens removed.

Absolute contraindications specific to SGAP/IGAP flap breast reconstruction in our practice include previous liposuction at the donor site and active smoking within 1 month before surgery. Liposuction of the upper buttock is rare, so does not often affect harvesting of the SGAP, but liposuction of the saddlebag area can affect IGAP-flap viability.

ANATOMY

The superior gluteal artery is a continuation of the posterior division of the internal iliac artery. It is a short artery that runs dorsally between the lumbosacral trunk and the first sacral nerve. It emanates from the pelvis above the upper border of the piriformis muscle, where it soon divides into both superficial and deep branches. The deep branch travels between the iliac bone and gluteus medius muscle. The superficial branch continues to give off contributions to the upper portion of the gluteus muscle and overlying fat and skin. Anatomic location is planned when the femur is slightly flexed and rotated inward; a line is drawn from the posterior superior iliac spine to the posterior superior angle of the greater trochanter. The point of entrance of the superior gluteal artery from the upper part of the greater sciatic foramen corresponds to the junction of the upper and middle thirds of this line. Perforating vessels are found off the superior branch of the superior gluteal artery (3,4) (Fig. 1).

The inferior gluteal artery is a terminal branch of the anterior division of the internal iliac artery and exits the pelvis through the greater sciatic foramen (5). Landmarks can also be used to identify the location of the emergence of the inferior gluteal artery outside the pelvis. A line is drawn from the posterior superior iliac spine to the outer part of the ischial tuberosity; the junction of its lower with its middle third marks the point of emergence of the inferior gluteal and its surrounding vessels from the lower part of the greater sciatic foramen (Fig. 1). The artery accompanies the greater sciatic nerve, internal pudendal vessels, and the posterior femoral cutaneous nerve. In this sub-fascial recess, the inferior gluteal vein will receive tributaries from other pelvic veins.

The inferior gluteal vasculature continues toward the surface by perforating the sacral fascia. It exits the pelvis caudal to the piriformis muscle. Once under the inferior portion of the gluteus maximus, perforating vessels are seen branching out through the substance of the muscle to feed the overlying skin and fat. The course of the inferior gluteal artery perforating vessels is more oblique through the substance of the gluteus maximus muscle than the course of the superior gluteal artery perforators, which tend to travel more directly to the superficial tissue up through the muscle. Thus the length of the inferior gluteal artery perforator and the resultant pedicle length for the overlying IGAP flap at 7 to 10 cm is greater than that found with an SGAP flap (5 to 7 cm). Because the skin island is placed inferior to the origin of the inferior gluteal vessels, a longer pedicle is also ensured.

The direction of the perforating vessels can be superior, lateral, or inferior. Perforating vessels that nourish the medial and inferior portions of the buttock have relatively short intramuscular lengths, between 4 and 5 cm, depending on the

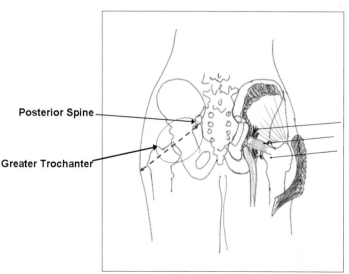

Posterior Spine

Greater Trochanter

SGA
Pyriformis
IGA

Superior Gluteal Artery Flap

FIG. 1. The anatomy of the gluteal region. The superior gluteal artery emerges superiorly, and the inferior gluteal artery emerges inferiorly from the pyriformis muscle. The perforators are identified one-third of the distance from a line drawn from the posterior iliac spine to the greater trochanter.

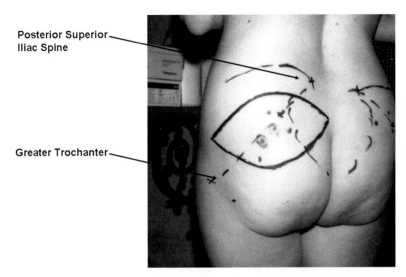

Markings for SGAP

FIG. 2. Skin markings are drawn and perforators are located with a Doppler.

thickness of the muscle. Perforators that nourish the lateral portions of the overlying skin paddle are observed traveling through the muscle substance in an oblique manner 4 to 6 cm before turning upward toward the skin surface. By traveling through the muscle for relatively long distances, these vessels are much longer than their medially based counterparts. The perforating vessels can be separated from the underlying gluteus maximus muscle and fascia and traced down to the parent vessel, forming the basis for the IGAP flap. Between two and four perforating vessels originating from the inferior gluteal artery will be located in the lower half of the gluteus maximus (6).

After giving off perforators in the buttocks, the inferior gluteal artery then descends into the thigh, accompanied by the posterior femoral cutaneous nerve, and follows a long course, eventually surfacing to supply the skin of the posterior thigh (7). The branches of the inferior gluteal nerve (L5, S1–2) supply the skin of the inferior buttock. A neurosensory flap can be elevated if these nerves are preserved in the dissection of the flap (8,9).

The superior gluteal nerve arises from the dorsal divisions of the fourth and fifth lumbar and first sacral nerves. It exits the pelvis through the greater sciatic foramen above the piriformis muscle, accompanied by the superior gluteal vessels, and divides into both superior and inferior branches. The superior and inferior branches of the nerves travel with their corresponding arterial branches to end in the gluteus medius, gluteus minimus, and tensor fasciae latae, respectively.

The inferior gluteal nerve arises from the dorsal divisions of the fifth lumbar and first and second sacral nerves. It exits the pelvis through the greater sciatic foramen, below the piriformis muscle, and divides into branches that enter the deep surface of the gluteus maximus. The posterior femoral cutaneous nerve innervates the skin of the perineum and posterior surface of the thigh and leg. It arises partly from the dorsal divisions of the first and second, and from the ventral divisions of the second and third sacral nerves, and issues from the pelvis through the greater sciatic foramen below the piriformis muscle, along with the inferior gluteal artery. It then descends beneath the gluteus maximus, the fascia lata, and travels over the long head of the biceps femoris to the posterior knee. Finally, it pierces the deep fascia and accompanies the lesser saphenous vein to the middle of the posterior leg. Some terminal branches communicate with the sural nerve. All its branches are cutaneous and distributed to the gluteal region, the perineum, and the posterior thigh and leg.

FLAP DESIGN AND DIMENSIONS

The patient usually is seen in our office 1 day before surgery. The surgical plan is again reviewed with the patient, and any remaining questions answered. The chest is marked in a sitting position. The midline and the inframammary crease on both sides are marked. For patients undergoing immediate breast reconstruction, suggested skin markings are drawn on the breast, which include marks around the nipple–areolar complex and previous biopsy site. In patients who are undergoing a nipple-sparing mastectomy, an inframammary, anterior axillary, or lateral incision is made.

For unilateral SGAP flap markings, the patient is placed in a lateral decubitus position. The Doppler probe is used to locate perforating vessels from the superior gluteal artery. These are usually located approximately one third of the distance on a line from the posterior superior iliac crest to the greater trochanter. Additional perforators may be found slightly more lateral from above. It should be noted that perforators located laterally will produce longer pedicles. The skin paddle is marked in an oblique pattern, from inferior medial to superior lateral, to include these perforators. On average, the flap height and length is 8 to 10 cm and 20 to 24 cm, respectively, and the skin paddle may be as large as 12 × 30 cm. For bilateral SGAP planning, the patient is marked in the prone position (Fig. 2).

For the IGAP flap, the gluteal fold is noted with the patient in a standing position. The inferior limit of the flap is marked 1 cm inferior and parallel to the gluteal fold. The patient is then placed in the lateral position for unilateral reconstruction and prone for bilateral reconstruction. The Doppler probe is used to find perforating vessels from the inferior gluteal artery. An ellipse is drawn for the skin paddle to include these perforators, which roughly parallels the gluteal fold, with dimensions of approximately 8 × 18 cm. For correction of a "saddlebag" deformity, the skin pattern is shifted laterally (Fig. 3).

OPERATIVE TECHNIQUE

For unilateral procedures, the patient is placed in the lateral decubitus position, and a two-team approach is used. The recipient vessels are prepared, as described earlier, while the SGAP/IGAP flap is harvested. For breast reconstruction,

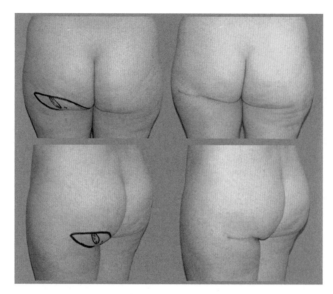

FIG. 3. Pre- and postoperative pictures of the inferior gluteal artery perforator flap.

the internal mammary vessels or internal mammary perforators are preferred, as anastomosis to these vessels allows easier medialization of the flap when it is inset. The IGAP flap often has a long enough pedicle to reach to the thoracodorsal vessels; however, the SGAP may be challenging because of a shorter pedicle. For bilateral simultaneous GAP flap reconstruction, the procedure is started supine. After mastectomy and recipient vessel preparation, the patient is positioned for flap harvest. Then the patient is repositioned supine for anastomosis and insetting.

The skin incisions are made, and Bovie electrocautery is used to divide the flap down to the muscle of the gluteus maximus. Significant beveling is used, as needed, particularly lateral to the muscle superiorly and inferiorly, to harvest enough tissue for width and volume and to create a natural breast shape. The flap is elevated from the muscle in the subfascial plane, and the perforators approached beginning from lateral to medial or medial to lateral. It is preferable to use a single large perforator, if it is present, but several perforators that lie in the same plane and in the direction of the gluteus maximus muscle fibers can be taken together, as well. The muscle is then spread in the direction of the muscle fibers, and the perforating vessels are meticulously dissected free. The dissection continues until both the artery and the vein are of sufficient size to be anastomosed to the recipient vessels in the chest. The artery usually is the limiting factor in this dissection. The arterial perforator is visualized and preserved as it enters the main ascending superior gluteal artery or the descending inferior gluteal artery. The preferable artery and vein diameter for anastomosis is 2.0 to 2.5 mm and 3.0 to 4.0 mm, respectively. When using the IMV perforators as recipient, a shorter pedicle and smaller artery will suffice, thereby simplifying flap harvest.

Harvesting an in-the-crease IGAP allows more beveling superiorly and inferiorly, because soft-tissue deficiency in the crease is normal. Laterally, thicker fat from the trochanteric area can be taken, increasing flap volume and decreasing a saddlebag deformity. When harvesting the IGAP flap, care must be taken to preserve the lighter-colored medial fat pad that overlies the ischium medial to the gluteus maximus muscle. Preservation of this specialized fat pad will prevent possible future donor-site discomfort when sitting.

When the recipient vessels are ready, the gluteal artery and vein are divided, and the flap is harvested and weighed. The skin and fat overlying the gluteus maximus muscle and posterior thigh with the IGAP are elevated superiorly and inferiorly to allow layered approximation of the fat of the donor site and to prevent a contour deformity and give a buttock lift. The donor site is closed in layers over a suction drain with absorbable suture. Adding a permanent removable skin suture increases the strength of the skin closure.

The anastomosis is performed to the recipient vessels under the operating microscope. The flap is inset over a suction drain into the breast pocket, with care taken not to twist or kink the pedicle. To create a spherical flap, the ends of the ellipse are excised. The flap may be inset horizontally, vertically, or obliquely, depending on the situation.

CLINICAL RESULTS

In a review of 377 GAP flaps performed by our unit for breast reconstruction, the incidence of complications was low. The overall take-back rate for vascular complications was 6%. The total flap failure rate was approximately 2%. Donor-site seroma occurred in 15% of patients, and approximately 20% of patients required revision of the donor site (4,5).

SUMMARY

To make these options more available and desirable, there is much room for improvement. The length of the procedure must be decreased, scars must be improved, and complications must be decreased. With improvements in technology and technique, these goals can be realized. The in-the-crease IGAP offers preservation of buttock shape, a scar hidden in a natural crease, and adequate-thickness fat for a youthful, attractive breast. The SGAP flap procedure has little or no postoperative pain and leaves a scar easily concealed with swim wear. The contour can be quite good, without taking a flap too large, and by performing a buttock lift with proper layered closure.

References

1. Allen RJ, Treece P. Deep inferior epigastric perforator flap for breast reconstruction. *Ann Plast Surg* 1994;32:32.
2. Taylor GI, Daniel RK. The anatomy of several free flap donor sites. *Plast Reconstr Surg* 1975;56:243.
3. Guerra A, Metzinger S, Bidros E, et al. Breast reconstruction with gluteal artery perforator (GAP) flaps: a critical analysis of 142 cases. *Ann Plast Surg* 2004;52:118.
4. Strauch B, Yu HL. Gluteal region. In: Strauch B, Yu HL, eds. *Atlas of microvascular surgery: anatomy and operative approaches.* New York: Thieme Medical Publishers, 1993;102–119.
5. Roche NA, Van Landuyt K, Blondeel PN, et al. The use of pedicled perforator flaps for reconstruction of lumbosacral defects. *Ann Plast Surg* 2000;45:7.
6. Granzow JW, Levine JL, Chiu ES, Allen RJ. Breast reconstruction with gluteal artery perforator flaps. *J Plast Reconstr Aesthet Surg* 2006;59:571.
7. Koshima I, Moriguchi T, Soeda S, et al. The gluteal perforator-based flap for repair of sacral pressure sores. *Plast Reconstr Surg* 1993;91:678.
8. Windhofer C, Brenner E, Moriggl B, Papp C. Relationship between the descending branch of the inferior gluteal artery and the posterior femoral cutaneous nerve applicable to flap surgery. *Surg Radiol Anat* 2002;24:253.
9. Blondeel PN. The sensate free superior gluteal artery perforator (S-GAP) flap: a valuable alternative in autologous breast reconstruction. *Br J Plastic Surg* 1999;52:185.

CHAPTER 375. Adipofascial (Anterior Rectus Sheath) Flaps for Breast Reconstruction *S. Sakai, I. Suzuki, and H. Izawa*

www.encyclopediaofflaps.com

CHAPTER 376 ■ NIPPLE RECONSTRUCTION WITH THE MODIFIED DOUBLE-OPPOSING-TAB FLAP

S. S. KROLL

EDITORIAL COMMENT (CHAPTERS 376–378)

The ability to produce a well-projecting nipple reconstruction from locally available tissue brought nipple reconstructions into common usage. No longer need the patient worry about loss of another body part for reconstruction. The following three chapters describe multiple variations.

The modified, double-opposing-tab (MDOT) flap is a method of nipple reconstruction derived from the original double-opposing-tab flap (1,2), using two local flaps containing skin and dermofat. The modifications allow closure of the donor site without a skin graft and increase the blood supply to the flap. The MDOT flap is similar to the S-flap, differing primarily in the shape of the flap tips (3,4).

INDICATIONS

The MDOT technique can be used to reconstruct a nipple on virtually any breast mound, regardless of the original breast reconstruction. It uses two small dermofat flaps to achieve nipple projection, and the only precondition for its use is the presence of enough skin and underlying fat on the breast, to allow elevation of the two flaps.

Most modern methods of nipple reconstruction use similar dermofat flaps to achieve nipple projection. However, unlike most of the other techniques (5,6), the MDOT procedure uses two flaps instead of one, thereby doubling the effective flap-base width and blood supply. This increased supply reduces the risk of flap loss and increases the probability of achieving good projection. The technique also allows for symmetrical closure of the flap donor sites, reducing distortion of the breast mound and eliminating the need for skin grafting. Creation of the areola and pigmentation of the nipple itself are achieved with tattooing (7). The procedure can be easily performed under local anesthesia in the clinic or office.

Contraindications to its use would be the presence of multiple scars cutting across the base of the flaps, or such a severe shortage of breast skin in all directions that using any of it for creation of a nipple would be detrimental to the shape of the breast.

FLAP DESIGN AND DIMENSIONS

The location of the nipple-areolar complex (NAC) is selected, with the patient in the upright position, by carefully noting the position of the NAC on the contralateral breast. The surgeon should attempt to position the NAC, so that it has the same relationships to the inferior, medial, and lateral borders of the breast, as does the NAC on the normal side. This is more difficult, if the reconstructed breast has a different shape from the normal one. Obviously, the surgeon should try to make the reconstructed breast shape as similar as possible to the opposite breast prior to beginning nipple reconstruction.

The flaps are designed, as shown in Figure 1A, with the long axis parallel to any preexisting scar. This will minimize possible interference with the flap blood supply. If no scars are present, the flaps are oriented in whatever direction best improves or maintains breast symmetry. Knowing that the MDOT flaps will tighten breast-mound skin by 1.8 cm at right angles to the long axis of the flaps, the surgeon orients the flaps horizontally to reduce breast ptosis, or vertically to maintain ptosis but slightly narrower breast width. The typical dimensions of the flaps are shown with a width of 1.8 cm; however, flap length or width can be altered slightly, to match an atypical contralateral nipple, if necessary.

OPERATIVE TECHNIQUE

The flaps are elevated with a No. 15 scalpel, and including some subcutaneous fat, so that total flap thickness is about 6 mm (Fig. 1B). The flap base is freed only enough to allow the flaps to be moved into opposition, leaving the blood supply as intact as possible. Buried key sutures (4-0 polyglycolic acid) are placed from the base of one flap to the midpoint of the opposite one (Fig. 1C and D), so that the flaps are brought into opposition like two hands held in prayer.

The donor sites are closed primarily with 4-0 polyglycolic acid buried sutures (in a straight line or by W-plasty, varying with each patient and depending on which closure produces the least distortion). The skin is closed with 5-0 chromic running sutures. The tips of the flaps interdigitate and are closed with 5-0 chromic interrupted sutures (Fig. 1E and F). Bacitracin ointment is then applied to the wound, followed by a gauze dressing to protect the patient's clothing.

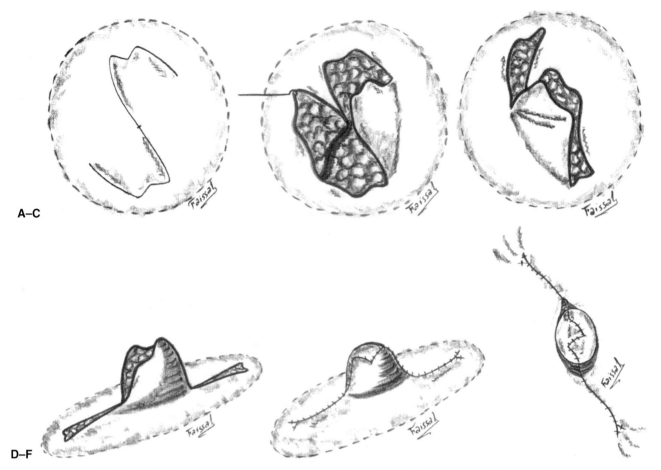

A–C

D–F

FIG. 1. **A:** Plan for nipple-areolar reconstruction with the modified double-opposing-tab flap. Each flap is generally 1.8 cm in width. **B:** Flaps are elevated with skin and subcutaneous tissue. **C,D:** After two key sutures are tied, the opposed flaps support each other. **E,F:** Skin closure with 5-0 chromic sutures.

CLINICAL RESULTS

At the end of nipple reconstruction using this technique, nipple projection is usually 10 to 12 mm. Tattooing can be performed immediately, but we usually prefer to wait 4 weeks for healing to be completed. There is usually some early distortion of the breast-mound shape where the flaps have been harvested. This disappears over the next few weeks, as the weight of the reconstructed breast stretches the skin. Nipple projection varies, gradually decreasing over the next several months. Some nipples will shrink to a projection of only 1 or 2 mm; a few will remain excessively long and need to be trimmed; but most will remain in the 2- to 4-mm range, which is satisfactory to most patients (Fig. 2).

If the correct amount of fat was included in the flaps, the nipple can be perfectly round. If too much was included, closure will be difficult, and the flaps will require thinning intraoperatively. If too little fat was included, the nipples will have an oval shape; this can be corrected in a second stage. It is best to do any necessary revision before tattooing the areola, so that its circular shape is not altered.

Loss of part of one or both flaps will lead to poor nipple projection and is more likely in patients who smoke. The effects of smoking can be mitigated by making the flaps slightly wider than normal, to increase the blood supply. A tight closure at the flap base can also impede blood supply. If this is noted intraoperatively, a suture can be removed and the base left open at one side to reduce skin tension, with revision planned later, as previously described.

Dog-ears at the donor sites and temporary distortion of breast shape are common, but usually disappear spontaneously with stretching of the breast skin, unless the breast is unusually small and tight.

SUMMARY

The MDOT flap can be used on any type of reconstructed breast and allows primary closure of the donor site. It creates a projecting nipple with two local flaps containing skin and dermofat.

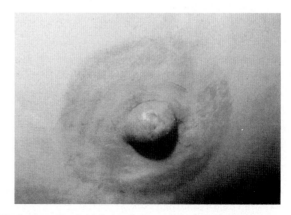

FIG. 2. Completed nipple-areolar complex, after scar maturation and stabilization of projection.

References

1. Kroll SS. Nipple and areolar reconstruction. In: Kroll SS, ed. *Reconstructive plastic surgery for cancer.* Philadelphia: C.V. Mosby, 1996;314–318.
2. Kroll SS, Hamilton S. Nipple reconstruction with the double-opposing-tab flap. *Plast Reconstr Surg* 1989;84:520.
3. Cronin ED, Humphreys DH, Ruiz-Razura A. Nipple reconstruction: the S flap. *Plast Reconstr Surg* 1988;81:793.
4. Weiss J, Herman O, Rosenberg L, Shafir R. The S nipple-areola reconstruction. *Plast Reconstr Surg* 1989;83:904.
5. Little JW. Nipple-areolar reconstruction. *Adv Plast Reconstr Surg* 1987; 3:43.
6. Anton MA, Hartrampf CR Jr. Nipple reconstruction with the star flap. *Plast Surg Forum* 1990;13:100.
7. Spear SL, Convit R, Little JW. Intradermal tattoo as an adjunct to nipple-areolar reconstruction. *Plast Reconstr Surg* 1989;83:907.

CHAPTER 377 ■ PROPELLER FLAP: ONE-STAGE PROCEDURE FOR NIPPLE-AREOLA RECONSTRUCTION

B. TEIMOURIAN, R. B. KARP, AND S. MALEKZADEH

A single-stage technique for long-term nipple projection is described. It uses a local skin flap that provides a good color match and satisfactory projection, compared with the contralateral breast (1).

INDICATIONS

Reconstruction of the nipple and areola continues to be a surgical challenge, despite the many procedures described in the literature over the past 60 years. Free grafts and local skin flaps are the two principal methods currently in use. Free grafts utilize tissue from another site to create a new nipple; donor sites that have been described include the opposite nipple, ear lobe, toe, thumb, labia minora, and mucous membranes (2–7). Local skin flaps have also produced acceptable results (8–13). However, these methods leave a donor-site defect and may require a full-thickness skin graft for closure, thereby creating a second wound. In addition, these reconstructive techniques are multi-staged procedures.

The primary objectives of nipple-areola reconstruction include: (1) optimal position, symmetry, and color match with the contralateral breast; (2) a good color match between the nipple and areola; and (3) adequate nipple projection. Tattooing of the breast-mound skin prior to its elevation in flap reconstruction achieves these requirements and eliminates the need for skin grafts and donor sites (14). Stable nipple projection remains the most difficult aspect of the reconstruction.

The use of the propeller flap is indicated in either immediate single-stage breast reconstruction, or as a second-stage procedure after the breast mound is created. The advantages of the propeller flap, combined with tattooing for nipple-areola reconstruction, include: 1) the fact that this is a simple one-stage procedure; 2) a secondary procedure after creating the nipple-areola complex is eliminated; and 3) a skin graft and second wound are eliminated. This technique can produce a nipple of adequate size, good color match, and satisfactory projection.

OPERATIVE TECHNIQUE

With the patient in a semi-Fowler or sitting position, the location of the new nipple and areola are outlined to match the contralateral side. The proper color dye is selected, and the areola (circle) is tattooed. Tattooing is performed first, thus eliminating the difficulty of coloring the skin after the papule has been raised. In the center of the new areola, we draw a smaller circle, approximating the diameter of the nipple, and two opposing propeller shapes (Fig. 1A). The two limbs of the propeller-shaped flap are raised, leaving the central core undisturbed (9,15). The central core is elevated after sharp dissection, beveling the incision away from the center, and thereby creating a broad pedicle base (Fig. 1B). The flaps are then rotated around the center, creating height for the new nipple (10,12). The donor areas are closed first, and further tattooing is done to correct the distorted circle (areola) (16,17) (Fig. 1C). The elevated new nipple is supported with a Keith needle through the base, and a light dressing is applied.

CLINICAL RESULTS

The propeller flap has been used to reconstruct the nipple-areola complex in over 200 patients during the second stage of breast reconstruction with implant placement. Patients have been followed for up to 6.5 years. There have been no complications of skin-flap necrosis, hematoma, or infection. Compared to the contralateral breast, there is a good color match and satisfactory nipple projection, with minimal changes during the follow-up period (Fig. 2A and B). The amount of nipple created with the propeller flap will vary with the length and width of the flaps and the amount of pull on the central core. Nipple projection is produced by a column of subcutaneous tissue and skin raised above the surface of the breast mound.

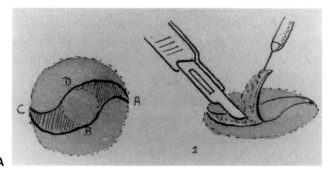

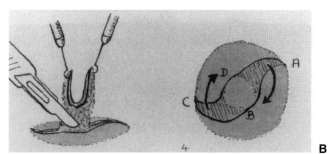

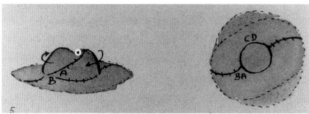

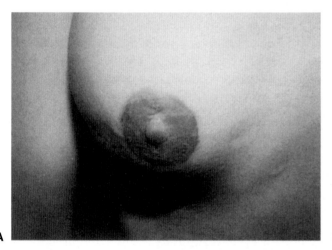

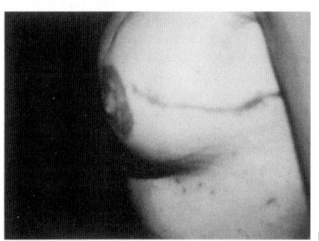

FIG. 1. A–C: Illustrative steps of the one-stage propeller flap procedure. (From Teimourian, Duda, ref. 1, with permission.)

FIG. 2. A,B: Six-and-a-half years after nipple-areola reconstruction.

The skin flaps of the propeller flap are designed so that the skin defect can be closed first, obviating the need for a skin graft or a second wound. Complications associated with skin grafts and secondary procedures are eliminated.

Good color match between nipple and areola and with the opposite breast has been possible with tattooing (3). This has eliminated the need for a second procedure in the reconstruction of the nipple-areola complex with the propeller flap.

SUMMARY

The propeller flap is a new and simple one-stage procedure that provides good color match and satisfactory nipple projection, when compared to the contralateral breast.

References

1. Teimourian B, Duda G. The propeller flap: a one-stage procedure for nipple-areola reconstruction. *Aesthet Plast Surg* 1994;18:81.
2. Millard DR. Nipple and areola reconstruction by skin graft from the normal side. *Plast Reconstr Surg* 1972;50:4.
3. Spear SL, Convit R, Little JW III. Intradermal tattoo as an adjunct to nipple-areola reconstruction. *Plast Reconstr Surg* 1989;83:907.
4. Klatsky SA, Manson PN. Toe pulp free grafts in nipple reconstruction. *Plast Reconstr Surg* 1981;68:245.
5. Weiss J, Herman O, Rosenberg L, Shafir R. The S nipple-areola reconstruction. *Plast Reconstr Surg* 1989;83:904.
6. Adams WM. Labial transplant for correction of loss of the nipple. *Plast Reconstr Surg* 1949;4:295.
7. Gruber RP. Nipple-areola reconstruction: a review of techniques. *Clin Plast Surg* 1979;6:71.
8. Little JW. Nipple-areola reconstruction. *Adv Plast Reconstr Surg* 1986;3:43.
9. Chang WHJ. Nipple reconstruction with a T flap. *Plast Reconstr Surg* 1984;73:140.
10. Cronin ED, Humphreys DH. Nipple reconstruction: the S flap. *Plast Reconstr Surg* 1988;81:783.
11. Little JW III, Munasifi T, McCulloch DT. One-stage reconstruction of a projecting nipple: the quadrapod flap. *Plast Reconstr Surg* 1983;71:126.
12. Cohen IK, Ward JA, Chandrasekar B. The pinwheel flap nipple and barrier areola graft reconstruction. *Plast Reconstr Surg* 1986;77:995.
13. Hartrampf CR Jr, Culbertson JH. A dermal-fat flap for nipple reconstruction. *Plast Reconstr Surg* 1984;73:982.
14. Wong RKM, Banducci DR, Feldman S, et al. Pre-reconstruction tattooing eliminates the need for skin grafting in nipple areolar reconstruction. *Plast Reconstr Surg* 1993;92:547.
15. Brent B, Bostwick J III. Nipple-areola reconstruction with auricular tissues. *Plast Reconstr Surg* 1977;60:353.
16. Dubin DB. A new simplified method for nipple reconstruction. *Plast Surg Forum* 1980;3:32.

CHAPTER 378 ■ NIPPLE RECONSTRUCTION WITH THE SKATE FLAP AND MODIFICATIONS

W. R. STAGGERS, L. O. VASCONEZ, R. J. FIX, AND S. TERKONDA

The skate flap and its modifications, permutations of local flaps fashioned from the reconstructed breast, require ample donor tissue. A satisfactory nipple reconstruction can be simply and reliably achieved, with minimal donor defect, in patients with submuscular implants and with varying methods of autologous reconstruction.

INDICATIONS

Nipple reconstruction should be delayed until the reconstructed breast has been allowed to realize its final position (1,2). Three to 6 months is usually sufficient to allow the breast to settle, probably decreasing the risk of retraction or malposition of the reconstructed nipple, which is a frequent problem. Nipple reconstruction is performed as a second stage and is usually done using local or general anesthesia, the latter if a modification of the reconstructed or normal breast is required to obtain symmetry.

The method of choice should be carefully considered, assuring adequate soft tissue to obtain the desired nipple form. If such tissue is lacking, other methods of reconstruction should be undertaken. Over-correction of flap design will allow for anticipated shrinkage of up to 50 percent (3,4). Patients who smoke, have irradiated donor sites, or have medical issues that affect tissue microcirculation deserve special consideration.

ANATOMY

The skate-flap family consists of a pedicle of epidermis, dermis, and subcutaneous fat centered at the site of the future nipple. The subcutaneous plexus and subdermal plexus provide the major blood supply to the flap (3). Intradermal sources and inosculation provide sustenance to the partial-thickness skin flaps. The thickness of the reconstructed breast mound is directly affected by the method of reconstruction used and affects the abundance of tissue available for use.

FLAP DESIGN AND DIMENSIONS

The location of the nipple is marked preoperatively by visually positioning it in a location agreed upon by the surgeon and patient. This is confirmed by photography that shows even slight abnormalities in position. The location is verified by triangulating landmarks from the opposite nipple in the operating room. A final position is ultimately determined by the surgeon during the procedure.

A circle matching the diameter (D) of the desired nipple and areola is drawn about the nipple mark (Fig. 1). Symmetry may be verified by observing the patient in a sitting position from the foot of the patient's bed. The orientation of the flap is assessed, and scars are positioned to decrease risk to flap vascularity (2,4,5–8). Minimal tension should be transferred to the breast mound. The base of the flap is at 12 o'clock, if no scarring or tension exist. A line is drawn perpendicular to the base of the flap, three nipple diameters in length. The central third of this line will be the future site of the composite flap. The length of the flap is measured as twice the height (H) of the desired nipple (Fig. 1).

A small excess may be added to the flap, to be deepithelialized and incorporated into the nipple. Two lines are drawn parallel to the proposed composite flap, converging distally. A curved line connects the ends of the base line to the apex of the composite flap (3) (Fig. 2A).

Modified Skate Flap

The nipple and areola are marked, as previously described. The flap limbs are drawn as parallel lines from the nipple circle, converging at the areolar margin. These are marked at the 3, 6, and 9 o'clock positions (1,9) (Fig. 3A).

Modified Fish-Tail Flap

This variation is demonstrated in Figure 4A. The angle between the limbs may vary, according to individual circumstances, in an effort to assure flap safety (2).

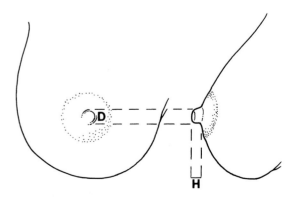

FIG. 1. Normal breast serves as a template for the desired nipple dimensions. Nipple diameter (*D*) and height (*H*) are shown.

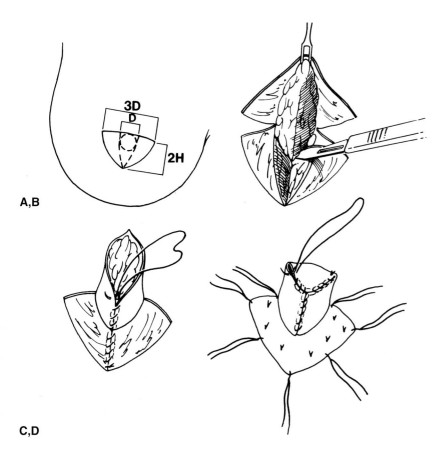

FIG. 2. A: Skate flap is marked for elevation. **B:** The flap is elevated gently, with care taken at the base to avoid vascular compromise. **C:** Donor defects are closed. Deepithelialized skin may be advanced toward the nipple. The skate wings circumscribe the pedicle and are secured. **D:** Tip of the skate flap is deepithelialized and buried within the nipple or trimmed as needed. Closure is complete. Areola grafting is done if necessary.

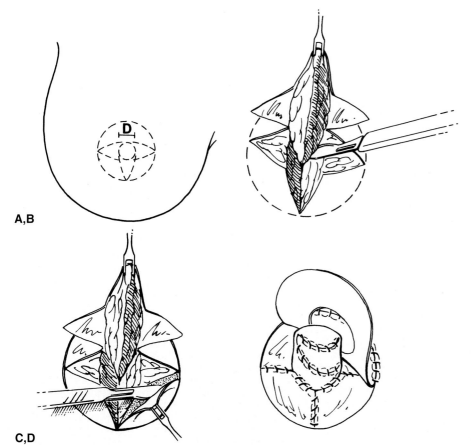

FIG. 3. A: Diagram of modified skate flap on the breast. Flaps extend to the neo-areola margin. **B:** Flap elevation is complete, with care taken near the flap base to avoid vascular compromise. **C:** Neo-areola is deepithelialized and grafted. Donor sites may be closed primarily. **D:** Tip of the dermal-fat flap may be deepithelialized and buried if needed. Closure is complete. Optional areolar grafting is shown.

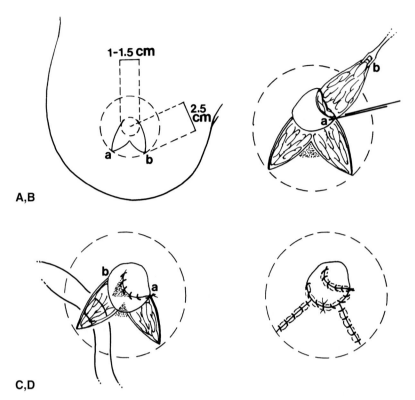

A,B

C,D

FIG. 4. **A:** Diagram of modified fish-tail flap on the breast. The angle between flaps may vary according to local conditions. **B:** Flaps are elevated, with care taken at the flap base to avoid vascular compromise. Flap "a" is rotated into position and secured. **C:** Flap "b" is deepithelialized and passed beneath flap "a." Flap "b" is secured and donor defects are closed. **D:** Completed nipple construct.

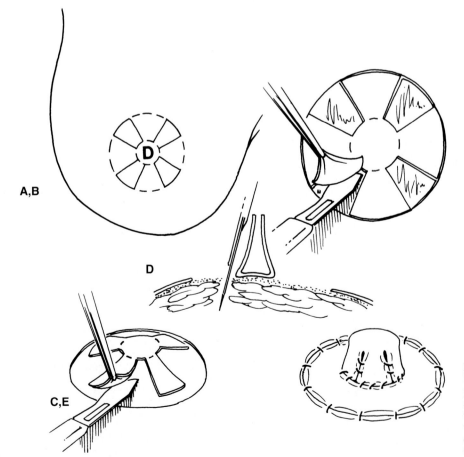

A,B

C,E

FIG. 5. **A:** Quadrapod flap diagrammed on the breast. **B:** Intervening trapezoids are removed as partial-thickness grafts. **C:** Flap limbs are elevated as partial-thickness grafts. Dissection deepens at the nipple disk. **D:** Dissection toward the chest wall is done about the nipple disk as an inverted cone. **E:** Areola grafting is necessary to complete the final construct.

[The **double-opposing-tab flap** variation was designed to help circumvent the problem of surgical scars frequently found crossing the proposed nipple site (10) (see Chapter 376).]

Quadrapod Flap

The nipple location is identified, as previously described. The areola is marked about the nipple point. A concentric circle marking the proposed nipple is drawn within the areola circle. Trapezoid-shaped flaps are marked radiating from the nipple circle to the areola mark (6) (Fig. 5A). Care should be taken to avoid scars that might affect flap vascularity.

Occasionally, there is some concern because of the amount of tissue underlying the breast mound, or when implants are at risk for exposure. The following modifications minimize the extent of subcutaneous intrusion to achieve the desired nipple form (4,7,8).

H Flap

The nipple and areola are marked. Rectangular tabs are drawn on opposing sides of the nipple disk. The width of the rectangle is the desired projection (H) and the length is half the desired nipple circumference (C) (4) (Fig. 6A). The flaps must avoid scarred areas and should rest on healthy donor tissue.

T Flap

The nipple and areola are marked in a satisfactory position. A T-shaped flap is outlined, as indicated (Fig. 7A). Nipple height is determined by varying the length of the transverse limbs of the T. Nipple diameter is determined by the width of the verti-cal limb of the T. The width of the distal transverse limb should be three nipple diameters long; the proximal transverse limb is two nipple diameters in length (7).

Mushroom Flap

The nipple and areola are marked, with the nipple disk as a circle one-quarter the surface area of the neo-areola. The width of the nipple disk may be enlarged, if donor-tissue viability is a concern (8) (Fig. 8A).

OPERATIVE TECHNIQUE

Local anesthetic with vasoconstrictors is infiltrated into the area of the proposed flap. The wings of the skate flap are first developed as a medium-thickness split-thickness graft attached to the composite flap. Dissection ends when the markings outlining the composite flap are reached. The dissection is deepened into the subcutaneous plane, and the composite flap is carefully elevated to its base. If the breast mound is thin, a layer of muscle may be included in the flap (Fig. 2B); however, this is not recommended when using implants because of the risk of implant exposure.

The wound is closed by advancing the skin edges toward the nipple with fine absorbable suture. This may completely close the defect, although the breast must not be deformed in an effort to avoid grafting at the donor site. The subcutaneous defect is closed in a similar manner (Fig. 2C). The wing tips circumscribe the subcutaneous portion of the flap and are approximated at the base with fine suture. The tip is then trimmed and sutured into position. If bulk is required, the tip may be deepithelialized and buried in the nipple (Fig. 2D). The nipple base is stabilized by suturing to the donor-site dermis.

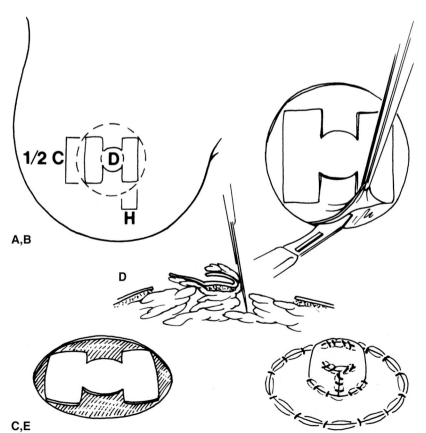

FIG. 6. **A:** H flap diagrammed on the breast. **B:** Areola is deepithelialized to the margin of the H flap. **C:** Deepithelialization of areola completed. **D:** Flap is elevated as a dermal-fat flap. Dermis about the nipple disk is incised to allow complete flap elevation. **E:** Limbs of the H are wrapped about the subcutaneous pedicle and secured. Areola grafting is required to complete the construct.

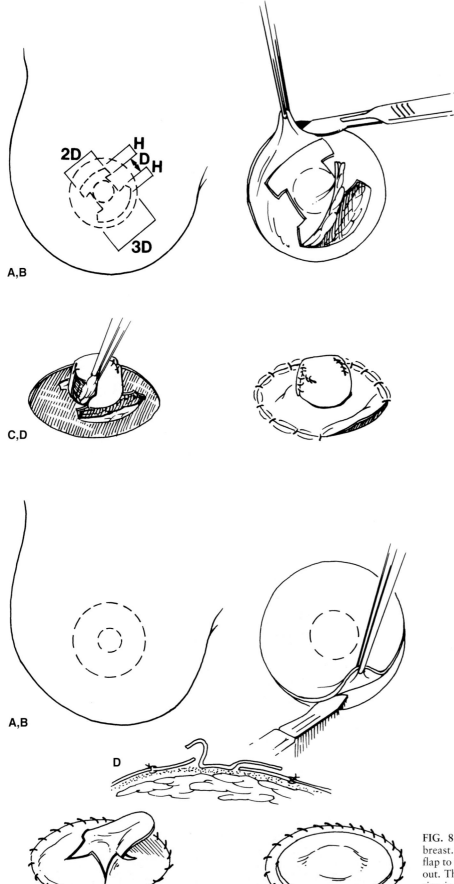

FIG. 7. A: T flap diagrammed on the breast. B: Flap is elevated as a dermal-fat flap, with care taken to avoid vascular compromise near the flap base. The areola is deepithelialized. C: Flap limbs are wrapped about the subcutaneous pedicle and secured. D: Areola grafting completes the construct.

FIG. 8. A: Mushroom flap diagrammed on the breast. B: Flap is elevated as a partial-thickness flap to the nipple disk. C: Areola grafting is carried out. The flap is delivered through a cruciate incision in the areola graft. D: Completed flap shown in cross section. E: Completed mushroom flap ready for dressing.

Full-thickness grafts may be taken for scar revision from the breast or from another suitable donor site. Grafts are applied in the usual manner, and petroleum-jelly-impregnated gauze is applied to the graft. A rigid nipple guard may be fashioned from a 5-cc syringe barrel cut 2 cm in length. The flange is padded with gauze prior to application. Bolster dressings are applied and may be removed in 4 days.

Modified Skate Flap

Full-thickness skin grafts are developed at the 3 and 9 o'clock positions. Elevation stops at the nipple circle. The 6-o'clock flap is raised with a generous subcutaneous fat layer and elevated to the 12-o'clock position (Fig. 3B). The areola is deepithelialized (Fig. 3C). The wing flaps are wrapped about the composite flap and sutured with fine suture, and donor defects are closed with fine absorbable suture. Areola size is verified and trimmed, as needed. The composite flap is trimmed and closed in a similar manner (Fig. 3D). This harvested skin or skin from other suitable donor sites may be used to graft the neo-areola and remaining donor defect.

Modified Fish-Tail Flap

Similar principles for flap elevation have been previously described. Full-thickness flaps are raised with a generous subcutaneous fat pad. Dissection stops at the nipple margin. The dissection is deepened into the subcutaneous fat. The nipple base must not be undermined further. The tip of flap "a" is inset at the base of flap "b" (Fig. 4B). Flap "b" is marked and deepithelialized to allow passage beneath flap "a." Flap "b" is then secured to the base of flap "a" as indicated (Fig. 4C). The donor sites are closed with fine suture (Fig. 4D). Postoperative dressings and wound care have been previously described.

Quadrapod Flap

Intervening trapezoids are deepithelialized (Fig. 5B). The remaining flaps are elevated as medium-thickness split-thickness grafts toward the nipple circle (Fig. 5C). The flaps are widened to include the intervening dermis as the nipple disk is approached. The plane of dissection is now deepened into the subcutaneous tissue and carried as an inverted cone toward the chest wall (Fig. 5D). The nipple should easily elevate to the height of the flap limbs. Dissection may extend to the underlying muscle, if nipple mobility is limited. The areola is then grafted in the usual manner. A cruciate incision is made, and the nipple is delivered from beneath the neo-areola graft (Fig. 5E). Fine suture is used to join the flap limbs at each corner along the length of the nipple. The nipple base is secured to the dermis of the neo-areola using fine suture. Postoperative dressings and wound care have been previously described.

H Flap

The skin between the areola and the flap is deepithelialized (Fig. 6B and C). Rectangular flaps are elevated in the subcutaneous plane to the nipple circle. The remaining dermis about the nipple circle is incised into the subcutaneous fat (Fig. 6D). The nipple disk is now freely mobile; it is elevated, and the tabs of the H are wrapped about the base of the elevated nipple. The flaps are fixed to the opposing flap limbs with fine suture (Fig. 6E). A full-thickness skin graft is obtained, and a small cruciate incision is made, through which the nipple is passed. The graft is sutured into position, and the nipple is

secured to the dermis of the neo-areola with fine suture. Postoperative dressings and wound care have been previously described.

T Flap

The flap is raised as a dermal-fat flap with a generous subcutaneous fat layer. Careful handling is needed to avoid vascular injury. The remainder of the skin between the neo-areola and the flap is deepithelialized (Fig. 7B). The flap limbs are wrapped about the nipple, approximating the subcutaneous layers, and sutured with fine suture (Fig. 7C). The areola is grafted and the nipple secured to the dermis of the neo-areola with fine suture (Fig. 7D). Postoperative dressings and wound care have been previously described.

Mushroom Flap

The areola is incised and elevated as a medium-thickness split-thickness graft to the nipple disk, leaving a thin layer of reticular dermis in the donor bed (Fig. 8B). The neo-areola is then grafted with a full-thickness skin graft and sutured into position. A small cruciate incision is made over the nipple disk. The flap is delivered through the wound (Fig. 8C–E). A dressing is made of petroleum-jelly-impregnated gauze placed between the areola graft and flap. A cover dressing is made with layered gauze, with a central hole created to protect the flap. Soft bulky dressings cover the bolster and remain in place for 6 to 10 days. The undersurface of the mushroom flap requires no dressing, as the areola graft and dressing preclude adherence. Contraction of the elevated flap occurs with time, giving a satisfactory projection.

CLINICAL RESULTS

Nipple projection and size are well-maintained, although shrinkage may occur. This is overcome by slight flap oversizing, but may require secondary amputation if a size discrepancy persists after healing is completed. A generous wedge of subcutaneous tissue should accompany composite flaps to provide adequate blood supply, and careful handling is necessary to protect the delicate vasculature from injury. Tension-free advancement of the donor margins is required to prevent deformation of the breast mound. Prior periareolar mastectomy and reconstruction may negate the need for marking a neo-areola. Meticulous closure of the donor sites will permit tattooing as a next step.

Flattening, malposition, and shrinkage, although improved using current techniques, still continue to occur. Allowing the breast position to stabilize over 3 to 6 months and slight flap oversizing may help to compensate for these sequelae. Flaps with a centrally-attached core are thought to resist radial tension from the breast mound and its deforming forces on the nipple. The generous size of these flaps offers relatively greater vascular reliability. Scars should be carefully avoided, as the local blood supply may be adversely affected. Skin grafts are frequently necessary to cover the denuded neo-areola; these are taken from easily hidden local donor sites.

SUMMARY

The skate flap and its modifications provide reliable methods of producing durable nipples with adequate projection and length. The procedures are simple, reliable, and produce minimal donor defects.

References

1. Kon M. Latissimus dorsi three-flap nipple reconstruction. *Aesthet Plast Surg* 1984;8:243.
2. Grotting JC. Reoperation following free flap breast reconstruction. In: *Reoperative aesthetic and reconstructive plastic surgery.* St. Louis: Quality Medical Publishing, Inc., 1995.
3. Little JW. Nipple-areola reconstruction and correction of inverted nipple. In: Noone RB, ed. *Plastic and reconstructive surgery of the breast.* Philadelphia: BC Decker, 1991;481–490.
4. Hallock GG, Altobelli JA. Cylindrical nipple reconstruction using an H flap. *Ann Plast Surg* 1993;30:23.
5. Georgiade GS, Reifkohl R, Georgiade NG. To share or not to share. *Ann Plast Surg* 1985;14:180.
6. Little JW, Munasifi T, McCulloch D. One-stage reconstruction of a projecting nipple: the quadrapod flap. *Plast Reconstr Surg* 1983;71:126.
7. Chang WH. Nipple reconstruction with a T flap. *Plast Reconstr Surg* 1984;73:140.
8. Smith JW, Nelson R. Construction of the nipple with a mushroom-shaped pedicle. *Plast Reconstr Surg* 1986;78:684.
9. Chang BW, Slezak S, Goldberg NH. Technical modifications for on site nipple areola reconstruction. *Ann Plast Surg* 1992;28:277.
10. Kroll SS, Hamilton S. Nipple reconstruction with the double-opposing tab flap. *Plas. Reconstr Surg* 1989;84:520.

CHAPTER 379 ■ TRANSPOSITION AND ADVANCEMENT SKIN FLAPS

D. P. ARMSTRONG

Resurfacing of axillary defects following excision of burn scars with contracture release or following excision of localized disease can be accomplished by the use of local flaps, with or without the concomitant use of split-thickness skin grafts.

INDICATIONS

Although direct primary closure can be accomplished following excision of localized disease (1,2), well-designed local flaps can provide a means of closure of larger defects by redistributing the local tissues to avoid limitation of motion or distortion of adjacent structures (3–12). When used in combination with skin grafts, random-pattern flaps allow the surgeon to transfer skin and subcutaneous tissue into the axilla in the area of greatest motion while placing the skin graft onto the adjacent chest or arm in an area requiring no splinting and having little or no influence on axillary flexibility.

ANATOMY

The successful use of random-pattern flaps in and around the axilla is made possible by the abundant branches of the axillary artery and their liberal penetration to the dermal-subdermal plexus.

OPERATIVE TECHNIQUE

Burn Scars and Contractures

The patterns of distribution of scars about the axilla are multiple, and the possibilities for flap reconstruction depend on the availability of uninvolved adjacent skin. Local flaps alone (Fig. 1) or in combination with split-thickness skin grafts (Figs. 2 and 3) are helpful in the correction of burn scar contractures.

Four flap patterns for correction of both anterior and posterior axillary contractures are shown in Figures 1 to 3. Figure 1 demonstrates the advancement of a double flap from the axillary skin to relieve a more limited, localized contracture band anteriorly (11). Figs. 2 and 3 demonstrate methods of shifting transposition flaps into areas of greatest motion, the soft flap bases providing the pivot points for motion within or adjacent to the axilla. The medial aspect of the arm is often spared from the burn and provides a generous flap for breaking up a moderate contracture anteriorly or posteriorly,

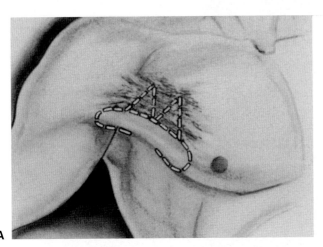
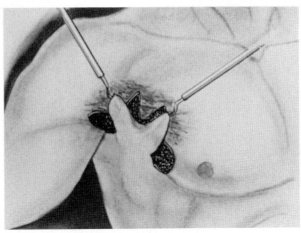

A

B

FIG. 1. Local axillary flap using skin from the axilla to relieve moderate contractures anteriorly or posteriorly. **A:** Design of flaps for elevation. Triangles are areas of scar to be excised. **B:** After excision of scar and mobilization of flaps. (From Converse, ref. 5, with permission.)

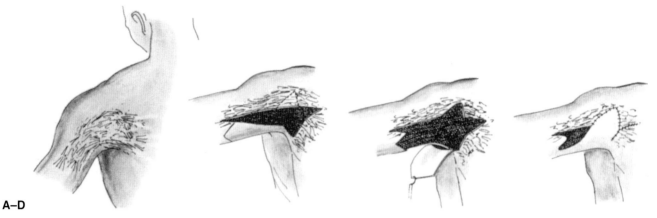

A–D

FIG. 2. **A:** Burn scar contracture involving posterior axillary fold. **B:** Contracture relieved by excision of the thickest band of scar tissue. **C:** Medial arm flap elevated. (May be shifted anteriorly, if appropriate.) **D:** Flap transposed across the posterior axillary fold, leaving a defect on the arm for repair with a split-thickness skin graft. (From Converse, ref. 5, with permission.)

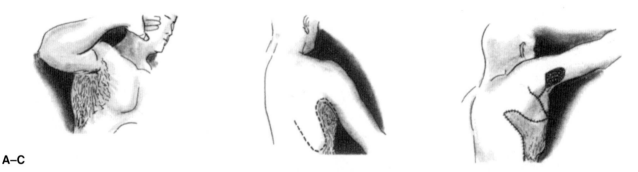

A–C

FIG. 3. **A:** Burn scar of infraaxillary skin extending into axilla. **B:** S-shaped incision elevating superiorly based back flap with release of axillary contracture. (Similar anterior flap could be used if more appropriate to the burn distribution.) **C:** Flap transposed across posterior axillary fold into axilla. Skin graft to arm defect. (From Colson et al., ref. 3, with permission.)

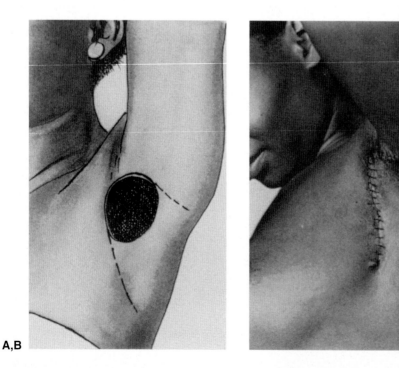

A,B

FIG. 4. **A:** Left axillary hidradenitis defect following excision with outline of posterolaterally based advancement flap. **B:** Result 7 days postoperatively. (From Armstrong et al., ref. 7, with permission.)

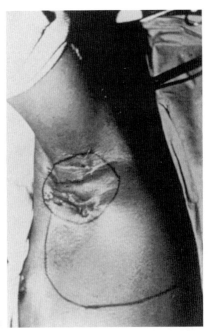
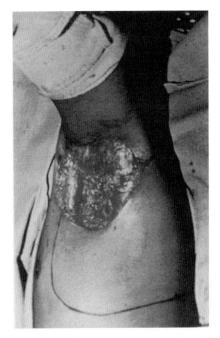
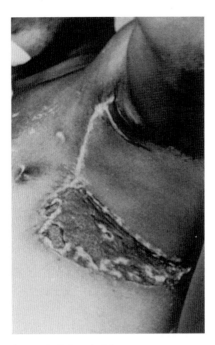

A–C

FIG. 5. A: Left axillary hidradenitis with outline of proposed area of excision and posteriorly based sliding flap. B: Defect following excision. Note enlargement of defect. C: Result 2 weeks postoperatively with a skin graft on the donor site. (From Armstrong et al., ref. 7, with permission.)

leaving a relatively small defect on the arm for resurfacing by means of a split-thickness skin graft (11). A superiorly based flap from the skin of the back just posterior to the posterior axillary fold has been described (Fig. 3) (3). This is rotated anteriorly to interrupt the contracture involving the posterior axillary fold. A similar flap from the anterior chest can be used if burn scars and flap sites favor this approach.

Hidradenitis Suppurativa and Other Localized Disease

Five specific flaps have been found helpful in resurfacing defects following the excision of hidradenitis suppurativa, a disease generally localized to a portion of or all of the hair-bearing skin of the axilla. These principles could be applied in treating other localized tumors. Specific selection of the method of resurfacing

depends on the extent of the disease. Direct primary closure of axillary defects is a well-accepted alternative (1,2).

Fig. 4 illustrates a very conservative advancement flap whose base is very broad in relation to flap length and with the resulting scar positioned to avoid banding with the elevation of the arm (7,9).

Very extensive involvement of the axillary skin may require a larger, posteriorly based sliding flap, as shown in Fig. 5, combined with a split-thickness skin graft in the flap bed. Note that the base of the flap is positioned to avoid limitation of shoulder motion.

The skin and subcutaneous tissue from the anterior and posterior extremes of the wound can be shifted on a subcutaneous pedicle into the central portion of the defect to aid in complete closure (Fig. 6).

Moderate to large axillary defects can be covered by well-designed infraaxillary rotation flaps (Fig. 7) with primary closure of both the defect and the flap bed (4,6,7,9). This flap is

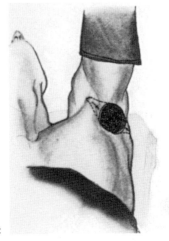
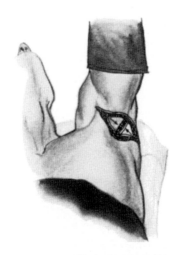
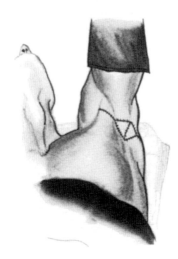

A–C

FIG. 6. A: Defect of left axilla following excision of hidradenitis. B: Triangular flaps from the extremes of the wound are shifted centrally on subcutaneous pedicles. C: Closure. (From Lipshutz, ref. 8, with permission.)

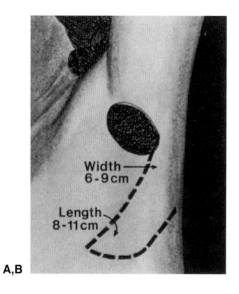
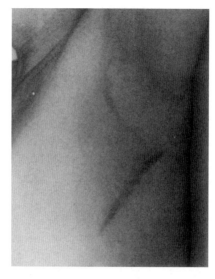

A,B

FIG. 7. A: Drawing of axillary defect from excision of local hidradenitis and projected flap from the infraaxillary area. Note that the inferior outline of the flap terminates at a pivot point slightly anterior to the defect for greatest ease of closure of the flap bed and in order to leave a generous flap base. This flap has an average width of 6 to 9 cm with a length of 8 to 11 cm. B: Postoperative result.

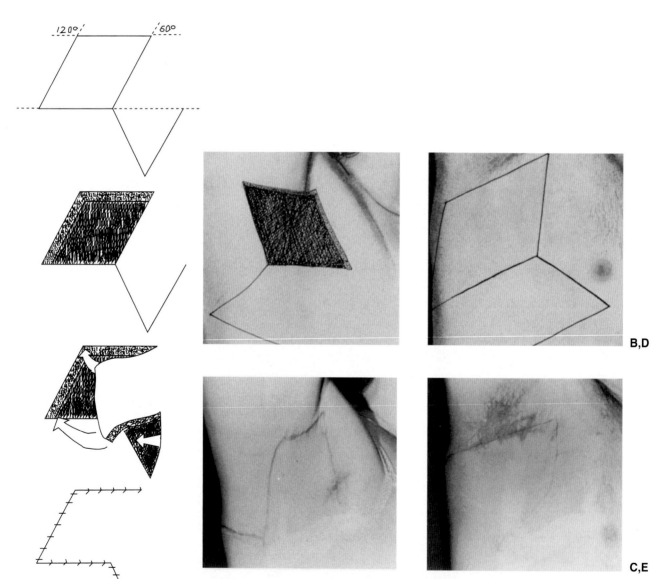

B,D

C,E

A

FIG. 8. A: Limberg flap design. B: Defect after excision in a female patient with an anteriorly based Limberg flap designed. C: Postoperative result. Note scar anteriorly from recent excision of additional focus of disease. D: Male patient with proposed area of excision and posteriorly based Limberg flap. E: Large flap well healed 2½ years postoperatively.

based posteriorly and slightly superiorly and extends toward the submammary fold. The incisions are staggered slightly, as illustrated, to facilitate closure of the flap bed. Final adjustment of the pivot point superiorly can be made after the chest defect is closed and the flap is transferred into its axillary position. Encroachment into the flap base must be avoided to prevent disruption of the blood supply. Hidradenitis tends to occur in slightly obese females who have an abundance of soft tissue in this location. However, a generous flap can be mobilized in the thin male as well. Owing to an abundant dermal-subdermal plexus in this area, an average width of 6 to 9 cm at the flap base and a flap length of 8 to 11 cm have been well tolerated without necrosis.

The Limberg flap is an excellent means of closing axillary defects (10–12). A posteriorly based flap is generally used in the male patient, and an anteriorly based flap is used in the female patient (Fig. 8). This is comparable to the infraaxillary flap described earlier and has the advantage of permitting development of a flap with a width and length up to 12 cm. The flexibility of the adjacent structures permits rotation of this conservative flap into the axillary defect.

Excision of localized hidradenitis disease rarely extends through the axillary fascia, and therefore, the infraaxillary or Limberg-type flap can be elevated in the same plane of dissection. Careful tissue handling, obliteration of the dead space, securing of the flap to the base of the defect with absorbable material, and suction or soft rubber drainage are helpful adjuncts to proper wound healing. Limited shoulder motion during the first postoperative week generally completes the wound care of this versatile flap pattern.

SUMMARY

Several types of transposition and advancement flaps can be used, depending on the extent of the defect, for burn contractures and hidradenitis in the axilla.

References

1. Pollack WJ, Vimelli FR, Ryan RF. Axillary hidradenitis suppurativa. *Plast Reconstr Surg* 1972;49:22.
2. Anderson DK, Perry AW. Axillary hidradenitis. *Arch Surg* 1975;110:69.
3. Colson P, Gangolphe M, Houot R, et al. Correction des retractions par brûlure de l'aisselle: valeur de rotations de lambeau dans les cas de gravité moyenne. *Ann Chir Plast* 1960;5:1.
4. Paletta FX. Hidradenitis suppurativa: pathologic study and use of skin flaps. *Plast Reconstr Surg* 1963;31:307.
5. Converse JM, ed. *Reconstructive plastic surgery,* Vol. 4. Philadelphia: Saunders, 1964;1606–1607.
6. Harrison SH. Axillary hidradenitis. *Br J Plast Surg* 1964;17:95.
7. Armstrong DP, Pickrell KP, Giblin TR, Miller F. Axillary hidradenitis suppurativa. *Plast Reconstr Surg* 1965;36:200.
8. Lipshutz H. Closure of axillary hidradenitis defects with local triangular flaps. *Plast Reconstr Surg* 1974;53:667.
9. Grabb WC, Myers MB, eds. *Skin flaps.* Boston: Little, Brown, 1975;437–446.
10. O'Brien J, Wysocki J, Anastasi G. Limberg flap coverage for axillary defects resulting from excision of hidradenitis suppurativa. *Plast Reconstr Surg* 1976;58:354.
11. Borges A. Choosing the correct Limberg flap. *Plast Reconstr Surg* 1978;62:542.
12. Rossi A, Jeffs J. The rhomboid flap of Limberg: a simple aid to planning. *Ann Plast Surg* 1980;5:494.

CHAPTER 380 ■ FIVE-SKIN FLAP

B. HIRSHOWITZ AND A. KAREV

EDITORIAL COMMENT

These multiple, relatively small flaps are reliable even though most of the designs are made through scar tissue.

The triangular flaps of two Z-plasties and a V-Y advancement flap constitute the five-skin flap. They are best applied for correction of a web contracture, most frequently caused by burns. Generally, the skin on the underside of the web is relatively unscarred and is used for advancement into the scarred area for its release.

INDICATIONS

The sites on the body that lend themselves best to the five-skin flap procedure appear to be thumb webs (see Chap. 315) (1,2), finger webs, and bridle scars of the axilla (3,4). In the latter situation, the apex of the axilla is left intact and in situ, thus avoiding the transfer of unattractive tufts of hair to unusual sites.

FLAP DESIGN AND DIMENSIONS

The design of the five-skin flap as applied to the axilla is shown in Fig. 1A. Flap *CDE* encloses the apex of the axilla and its tip *D* lies at the midpoint of the line *AB* that runs along the ridge of the web. *GA* and *HB* complete the outline of the two Z-plasties; the angles 1 and 2 are about 70 degrees. The incision *DF* opens into a triangular defect, into which *CDE* is advanced.

OPERATIVE TECHNIQUE

In preparing the Z-plasty flaps, the web is incised midway, so that an equal thickness of subcutaneous tissue is retained on both sides of the web.

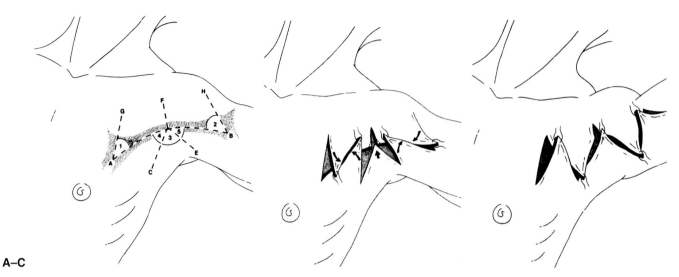

A–C

FIG. 1. **A:** The incisional lines. The procedure consists basically of two Z-plasties with an intervening V-Y advancement. **B:** Flaps raised. **C:** The flaps transposed and advanced.

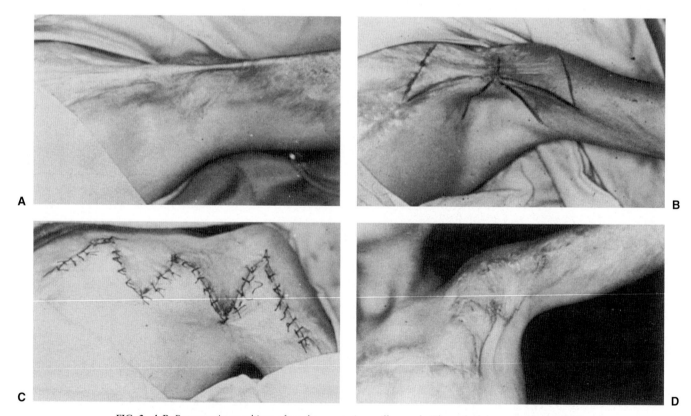

FIG. 2. **A,B:** Preoperative markings of postburn anterior axillary web. The end of the central inverted V can be seen to lie on the undersurface of the web. This will form the flap to be advanced. The inverted V encompasses the apex of the axilla, and accordingly, the hair-bearing skin is left undisturbed. **C:** Immediately postoperatively. **D:** One month postoperatively. A fairly normal contour has been obtained. (From Hirshowitz et al., ref. 4, with permission.)

The part that is advanced and is the only part undermined lies on the underside of the web; thus no change in position of the axillary apex occurs. The length *DF* is adjusted for the best fit. Because the ridge of the web is curved, the angles *ADF* and *BDF* are slightly larger than 90 degrees, and some trimming of excess may be necessary.

SUMMARY

Scar contractures creating a web across the axilla can be released by a procedure that involves the creation of five flaps: two Z-plasties and a V-Y advancement flap.

References

1. Hirshowitz B, Karev A, Rousso M. Combined double Z-plasty and Y-V advancement procedure for the repair of thumb web contractures: five-flap technique. *Hand* 1975;7:291.
2. Rousso M. Brûlures dorsales graves de la main. Reconstruction de la commissure. Technique à cinq lambeaux. Ire partie: La première commissure. *Ann Chir* 1975;29:475.
3. Glicenstein J, Bonnefous G. La plastie en trident. *Ann Chir Plast* 1975; 20:257.
4. Hirshowitz B, Karev A, Levy Y. A five-flap procedure for axillary webs leaving the apex intact. *Br J Plast Surg* 1977;30:48.

CHAPTER 381 ■ PARASCAPULAR FASCIOCUTANEOUS FLAP FOR RELEASE OF AXILLARY BURN CONTRACTURE

G. G. HALLOCK

EDITORIAL COMMENT

It is always preferable to resurface axillary contractures by using a flap. Where burn contractures are concerned, the parascapular area is often uninvolved, and this flap can be used with reconstructive advantages.

The parascapular flap is a true fasciocutaneous flap from the posterolateral chest wall overlying the lateral border of the scapula. In addition to its widespread use as a free flap, its attributes permit a wide range of utility as a local pedicled flap, including coverage of the axilla (1–4).

INDICATIONS

When used as a vascularized flap for axillary reconstruction, the risks of contracture or recurrence, as often follow skin grafting in this region, are avoided (2). Postoperative splints are unnecessary, early mobilization of the shoulder joint is unimpeded, and the period necessary for rehabilitation is diminished. The parascapular flap, as a single-staged alternative, is excellent for resurfacing large defects involving the posterior axillary web, or after the total axillary obliteration that frequently occurs with significant burn injuries (2,3).

ANATOMY

The vascular plexus of the dorsal thoracic fascia has an orientation along the direction of the terminal branches of the cutaneous branch of the circumflex scapular artery (5). This cutaneous branch first courses through the triangular space bounded above by the teres minor, below by the teres major, and laterally by the long head of the triceps muscle, to pierce the deep fascia as a true septocutaneous perforator. Shortly after or sometimes just before this (6), the branch divides into three distinct branches—ascending, horizontal, or transverse, or descending—and each, in turn, ramifies on the surface of the fascia (Fig. 1) (7,8). The descending branch supplying the

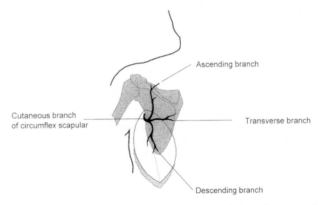

FIG. 1. Schematic diagram of the usual pattern of the trifurcation of the terminal branches of the cutaneous branch of the circumflex scapular artery, after it has passed through the triangular space at the lateral border of the middle third of the scapula. A parascapular flap has been drawn, centered about the descending branch, with its near vertical axis (*dotted line*) paralleling the lateral border of the scapula. (The author thanks Carol Varma, medical illustrator, the Lehigh Valley Hospital, Allentown, PA, for providing the diagram.)

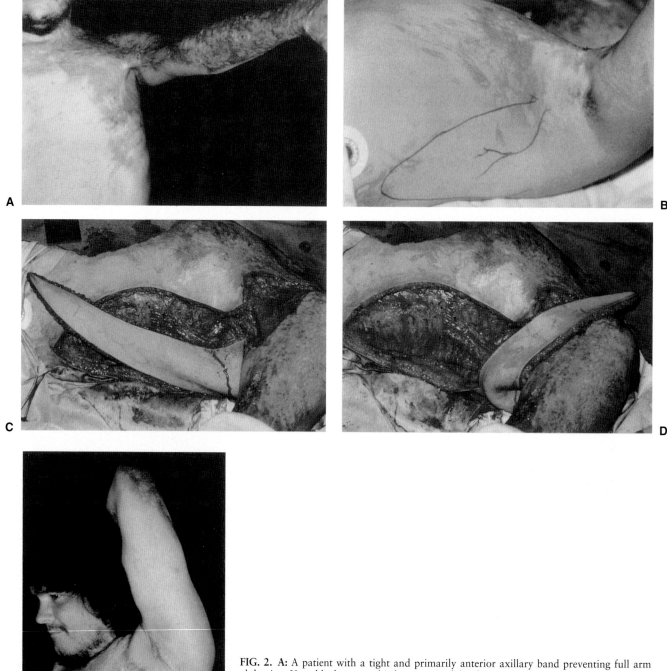

FIG. 2. A: A patient with a tight and primarily anterior axillary band preventing full arm abduction. Unstable, hypertrophic burn scars of the chest and inner arm prevented the selection of alternative local flaps from these regions, after the anticipated contracture release. **B:** Large parascapular flap designed on the posterolateral chest with patient in a lateral decubitus position. **C:** Contracture after release, with a 25-cm × 12-cm parascapular flap elevated in situ, **(D)** then transposed into the large area of axillary-skin deficiency. Flap has a broad skin base that safely obviates the need for actual identification of the vascular pedicle, **(E)** to allow unrestricted arm movement, but resulting in some superior displacement of the cupula. Primary donor-site closure was possible, with the linear scar partially seen laterally. (Fig. 2A and C from Hallock and Okunski, ref. 2, with permission.)

parascapular flap descends toward the tip of the scapula, paralleling its lateral border, and represents the central axis of any such flap.

The descending branch departs occasionally from the circumflex scapular vessels, before reaching the triangular space, and descends beneath to exit below, rather than above, the teres major muscle (5–7). Although the circumflex scapular pedicle is more usually located approximately two-fifths of the distance between the spine of the scapula and the scapular tip (2), this branch can still exit the triangular space anywhere along the middle third of the lateral border of the scapula.

FLAP DESIGN AND DIMENSIONS

The parascapular flap encompasses that portion of the dorsal thoracic fascia nourished by the descending branch of the cutaneous branch of the circumflex scapular artery. Based at the site of this perforator arising from the triangular space, the vertical or slightly oblique design of the flap has a caudal orientation that follows a vascular axis paralleling the lateral border of the scapula.

Using an audible Doppler flowmeter or color duplex imaging, as necessary, the location of the origin of the branch to the parascapular flap can be predetermined (8). The proposed point of rotation or base of the flap corresponds to this site. Flap design is then centered about this vascular axis, which consistently parallels the lateral border of the scapula. Flap width should slightly exceed that of the given defect (Fig. 2). Flaps up to 30 cm long and 15 cm wide, not exceeding a 3:1 ratio, have proven to be successful (2,4). If flap width exceeds about 10 cm (less in more obese patients), primary closure of the donor site will not be possible (3,4).

Using the horizontal (scapular flap) (9) or vertical (ascending scapular flap) (10) branches as alternatives usually requires a conversion to island flaps, which cannot reach the axilla without almost an 180-degree twist about their pedicles, a risk totally avoided by the wide base of a pedicled parascapular flap, where rotation into the axilla follows a shorter, more natural, course (Fig. 2). The pedicled version of the parascapular flap could even reach the side of the face, posterior scalp, shoulder, and upper arm, if desired, with a range similar to the latissimus dorsi muscle (4). A major bonus is that no muscle need ever be expended.

OPERATIVE TECHNIQUE

With the patient in a lateral position, the anterior chest, axilla, and scapular region can all be exposed simultaneously. After assessing the demands of the recipient site, the flap borders are correspondingly outlined (Fig. 2). Dissection should begin inferiorly, to include the latissimus dorsi muscle fascia with the tip of the flap. Retrograde dissection then continues toward the triangular space, being wary of anatomic variations, especially an aberrant descending branch at the inferior border of the teres major muscle (5–7). If present, this muscle may have to be divided, to gain additional length of the vascu-

lar pedicle for unimpeded flap transfer. Otherwise, dissection toward or even along the main vascular pedicle is extended, until insetting can be achieved without tension. Normally, the length of the flap can easily exceed that required, so that actual dissection into the triangular space, discrete vessel identification, and possible vascular injury can be totally avoided (Fig. 2).

CLINICAL RESULTS

Small axillary scars are preferably released with Z-plasties, Y-V plasties, local random flaps, etc. (11). Solitary anterior webs are better treated by an inner-arm (12) or anterior trunk flap; a parascapular flap, if so used, would destroy or displace the hair-bearing cupula. Of course, if the axilla has been totally obliterated or predominantly has a posterior axillary contracture, the parascapular flap would be a primary initial consideration anyway (11). Previous burns or skin grafts of the trunk are not a contraindication to using this flap, as long as excision-to-fascia techniques were not previously utilized (13).

SUMMARY

The large vessel caliber, anatomic consistency, and length of the vascular pedicle permit the design of a large local flap, very convenient for providing vascularized skin coverage for the adjacent axilla.

References

1. Nassif TM, Vidal L, Bovet JL, Baudet J. The parascapular flap: A new cutaneous microsurgical free flap. *Plast Reconstr Surg* 1982;69:591.
2. Hallock GG, Okunski WJ. The parascapular fasciocutaneous flap for release of the axillary burn contracture. *J Burn Care Rehab* 1987;8:387.
3. Yanai A, Nagata S, Hirabayashi S, et al. Inverted-U parascapular flap for the treatment of axillary burn scar contracture. *Plast Reconstr Surg* 1985; 76:126.
4. Kim PS, Lewis VL. Use of a pedicled parascapular flap for anterior shoulder and arm reconstruction. *Plast Reconstr Surg* 1985;76:942.
5. Cormack GC, Lamberty BGH. The anatomical vascular basis of the axillary fasciocutaneous pedicled flap. *Br J Plast Surg* 1983;36:425.
6. Upton J, Albin RE, Mulliken JB, Murray JE. The use of scapular and parascapular flaps for cheek reconstruction. *Plast Reconstr Surg* 1992;90:959.
7. Maruyama Y, Ohsaki M. Anatomical investigations of the cutaneous branches of the circumflex scapular artery and their communications. *Br J Plast Surg* 1993;46:160.
8. Hallock GG. Color duplex imaging for identifying perforators prior to pretransfer expansion of fasciocutaneous free flaps. *Ann Plast Surg* 1994; 32:595.
9. Dimond M, Barwick W. Treatment of axillary burn scar contracture using an arterialized scapular island flap. *Plast Reconstr Surg* 1983;72:388.
10. Maruyama Y. Ascending scapular flap and its use for the treatment of axillary burn scar contracture. *Br J Plast Surg* 1991;44:97.
11. Hallock GG. A systematic approach to flap selection for the axillary burn contracture. *J Burn Care Rehab* 1993;14:343.
12. Budo J, Finucan T, Clarke J. The inner arm fasciocutaneous flap. *Plast Reconstr Surg* 1984;73:629.
13. Hallock GG. The role of local fasciocutaneous flaps in total burn wound management. *Plast Reconstr Surg* 1983;72:388.

CHAPTER 382 ■ TRANSPOSITION AND ADVANCEMENT SKIN FLAPS

J. E. WOODS

Chest-wall reconstruction may be achieved by many means. Following one of the older dicta of reconstructive surgery—to use local tissue when available—leads one seriously to consider use of transposition and advancement flaps as a relatively high priority. Since chest-wall reconstruction is often carried out for radiation necrosis, bringing in tissue with a relatively unaffected blood supply is appropriate (1).

The flaps to be considered here include laterally and medially based flaps, oblique or transverse flaps, and the contralateral breast flap (2). In addition, using a reverse abdominoplasty technique, the abdominal skin may be advanced considerably in conjunction with other techniques or used alone where the defect is only moderate in size (3).

INDICATIONS

Contrary to common opinion, even very sizable defects, including the absence of ribs, with consequent concern for flailing, may be repaired using the flaps to be described. Full-thickness flaps with underlying subcutaneous tissue provide enough substance to minimize flailing without the use of underlying synthetic mesh, except in unusual circumstances. The possibility of subsequent foreign body-reaction and/or extrusion is thus minimized.

Even very large laterally based flaps can be elevated without delay with some back-cutting at the lateral base for greater mobility (see Fig. 1). While the laterally based flap is preferable in most instances, if the area that might serve as its base has been compromised by surgery, radiation, or both, the medially based flap is most useful. Again, surprisingly large defects can be reconstructed. Like the lateral flap, the medially based flap may be elevated without delay, providing it does not extend beyond the anterior axillary line (see Fig. 3). Unlike the laterally based flap, however, the donor defect of

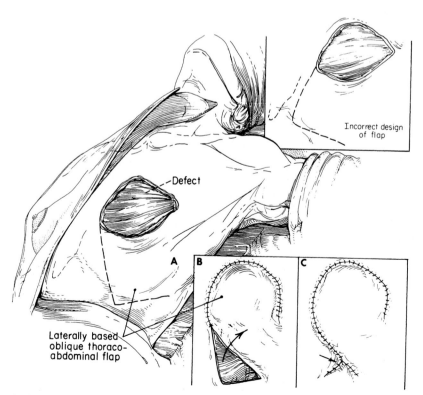

FIG. 1. Design of flap. **A:** Flap is oblique, and medial incision also must be oblique if closure without skin grafting is to be accomplished. Incorrect design is shown in upper right inset. Not only is it impossible to close the donor defect without grafting, but the flap will not reach as high. **B:** Flap rotated into position. To gain more length, some limited back-cutting of the base is permissible. **C:** Closure of the defect is possible by closing the V-shaped defect in part **B** to form a Y or T.

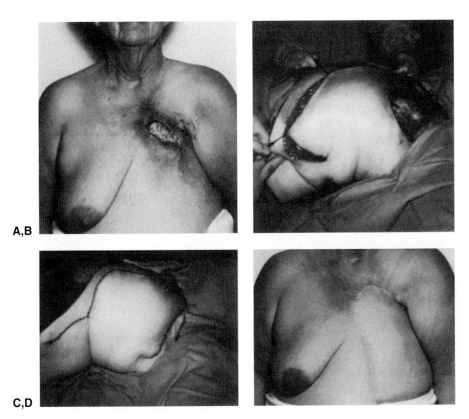

A,B

C,D

FIG. 2. **A:** Radiation necrosis of chest wall following radical mastectomy and radiation therapy. **B:** Defect after excision of affected area showing design of flap. Note oblique medial border (patient's head is to the right). **C:** Reconstruction of defect and closure of donor defect without skin grafting. **D:** Final result.

the medially based flap cannot usually be closed primarily, and a skin graft is frequently required.

The contralateral breast flap may be an alternative when other flaps are not available (see Fig. 5). It is perhaps more readily tolerated in the debilitated patient than the latissimus dorsi muscle or musculocutaneous flap, where the procedure is for palliation and a less extensive and briefer procedure is desirable. However, with all the other options currently available, this flap has not been employed in my practice for several years. In my experience, the contralateral breast flap can be elevated without delay and without subsequent necrosis (see Fig. 6). However, skin grafting to the donor defect is often necessary.

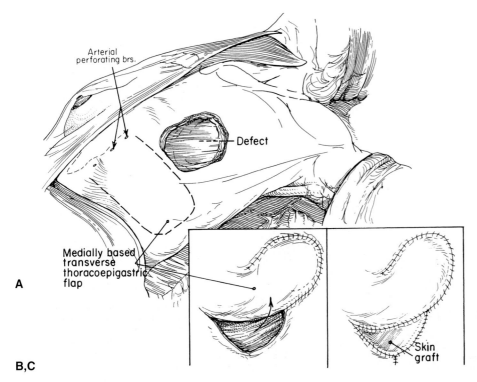

A

B,C

FIG. 3. **A:** Chest-wall defect and design of medially based transverse upper abdominal or thoracoepigastric flap based on medial perforators. **B:** Flap rotated into defect. **C:** Defect closed by advancement of donor defect edges and split-thickness skin grafting.

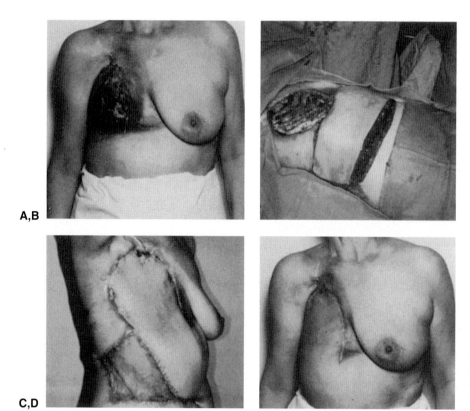

A,B

C,D

FIG. 4. A: Advanced radiation necrosis and recurrent cancer of chest wall. B: Chest-wall defect and flap design. C: Immediate postoperative result showing lateral skin-grafted donor area. D: Late postoperative result.

FLAP DESIGN AND DIMENSIONS

Most commonly, the laterally based flap should be designed as an oblique flap extending downward and medially, so that rotation or transposition occurs at a favorable angle. It is important that the inferomedial border also be oblique (Figs. 1 and 2), so that even with very large flaps, the donor defect can be closed with some mobilization of the skin at the inferior perimeter with a V-Y closure. If the medial border of the flap is not directed obliquely in the inferior and lateral direction, primary closure is impossible and skin grafting becomes necessary, obviating one of the special advantages of this very useful flap. To enlarge or extend this flap, a portion of the external oblique muscle may be included, where appropriate.

The medially based upper abdominal or thoracoepigastric flap differs from the lateral flap in that it is essentially an axial flap based on perforators from the superior epigastric artery by means of the rectus muscle. It is for this reason that the flap is designed in a transverse orientation, taking full advantage of the medial blood supply. The flap is designed with a width to fit the defect and a length to reach it.

OPERATIVE TECHNIQUE

The laterally based flap (Figs. 1 and 2) is incised down to fascia as marked and elevated to the anterior axillary line. As the flap is developed more laterally where large penetrating vessels are seen, these may be spared, although this is essentially a random flap with a favorable base (width) to length ratio. Once elevated, the flap is rotated into the defect with mobilization of the inferior and lateral defect skin, as necessary, and with some back-cutting, if needed.

The medially based flap (Figs. 3 and 4) is elevated with the underlying fat down to fascia from its lateral extreme toward the midline, with the dissection stopping about 2 cm from the

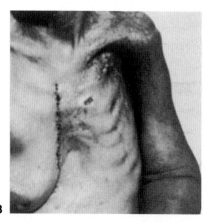

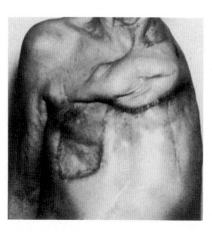

A,B

FIG. 5. A: Advanced radiation necrosis of shoulder and upper chest wall rendering upper extremity painful and useless. B: After shoulder disarticulation and closure of defect with opposite breast. In this case, breast flap was delayed. Nipple-areola complex was removed.

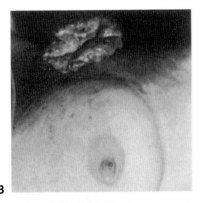
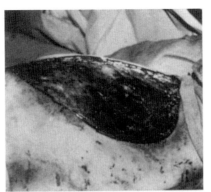

A,B

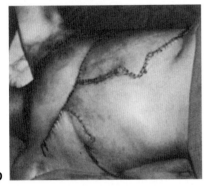
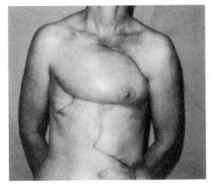

C,D

FIG. 6. **A:** Large local recurrence of breast cancer after mastectomy. **B:** Defect after removal of recurrence. View from left lateral aspect. **C:** Closure of defect with combination of undelayed contralateral breast and laterally based oblique flaps, with closure of all defects without skin grafting. **D:** Final result. This patient was last seen at 3 years without evidence of recurrence.

midline in order to avoid damaging its perforating blood supply. The dissection approaching this area is done very carefully with blunt and scissor-spreading dissection. The flap is rotated into place and sutured appropriately. The skin edges of the donor defect are mobilized, advanced to minimize the open area, and sutured to the underlying fascia. A split-thickness skin graft is used to cover the remaining defect, with bolus dressing for graft immobilization (Fig. 4).

Since the operative technique for the contralateral breast flap is straightforward, no description is given (Figs. 5 and 6) (see Chap. 385).

CLINICAL RESULTS

For the contralateral breast flap, disadvantages include the appearance, the transfer of tissue at risk for cancer, and the unaesthetic donor site. In one instance, after successful use of the breast flap, the nipple-areola complex and underlying remnant of breast tissue were removed at a subsequent time at the patient's request.

SUMMARY

Musculocutaneous flaps with their flexibility and reliability would appear to be a first choice in many cases of definitive chest-wall reconstruction. However, in some patients undergoing palliative resections for recurrent breast cancer, the lesser procedures described herein may be successfully used, even for very large defects. Properly designed and executed primarily for purposes of wound management, the laterally based oblique and medially based transverse thoracoepigastric flaps may be expected to achieve success with minimal significant morbidity.

References

1. Brown JB, Fryer MP, McDowell F. Application of permanent pedicle blood-carrying flaps. *Plast Reconstr Surg* 1951;8:335.
2. Woods JE, Arnold PG, Masson JK, et al. Management of radiation necrosis and advanced cancer of the chest wall in patients with breast malignancy. *Plast Reconstr Surg* 1979;63:235.
3. Lewis JR. Use of a sliding flap from the abdomen to provide cover in breast reconstructions. *Plast Reconstr Surg* 1979;64:491.

CHAPTER 383 ■ CONTRALATERAL TRANSVERSE THORACOABDOMINAL SKIN FLAP

R. L. BAROUDI

A transverse thoracoabdominal skin flap is rotated 90 degrees to cover the defect resulting from radical mastectomy. It avoids the need for skin grafts for closure of the donor area, and the flap can be mobilized and directly rotated without delay. Also, it provides good cover for a future mammaplasty.

INDICATIONS

Use of this flap should be selective, and it should not be used to close all postmastectomy wounds. Patients on whom I have used it were principally those with stage III tumors (79 percent) and those with tumors located in the outer quadrant (35 percent). However, some patients were closed by this procedure even without fitting these qualifications because of the greater ease of repair after wide tumor resection.

ANATOMY

One peculiarity of this flap is that it crosses the midline. The blood circulation within the flap is not clear when examined in the light of current knowledge about the vascularization of skin flaps. However, a careful review of the literature permits some tentative hypotheses without much experimental substantiation (1–4).

The flap does not resemble the axial type of flap but is more like a random flap. The pedicle receives flow from the lateral branches of the segmental arteries at the T6 to T10 level and from the supraumbilical and infraumbilical plexus formed by the perforating musculocutaneous branches that originate in the arcade of the upper and lower deep epigastric arteries (Fig. 1).

Still unclear is the manner in which the lateral branches of the segmental arteries are joined to those on the subaponeurotic plane of the epigastric arcade. The subaponeurotic and subdermal anastomotic network that joins the arcades of the superior and inferior epigastric arteries to the navel must be very important to the circulatory dynamics of the flap (5).

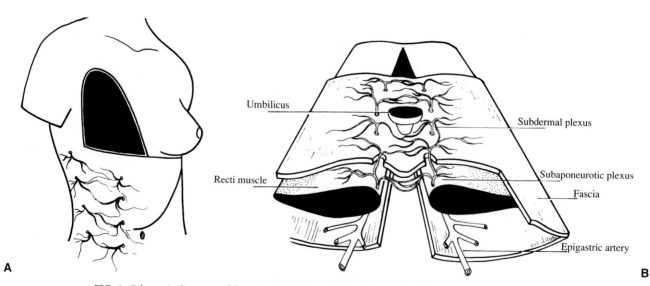

A   Umbilicus   Recti muscle   Subdermal plexus   Subaponeurotic plexus   Fascia   Epigastric artery   B

FIG. 1. Schematic diagrams of flap circulation from the lateral branches of T6 to T10 segmental arteries and from the adjacent plexus and epigastric arteries.

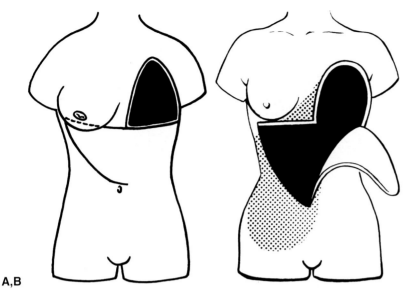

FIG. 2. A: The base of the triangle is along the inframammary sulcus, and the other two convex sides are united at the vertex below the clavicle. The thoracoabdominal skin flap is also triangular in shape. The distal end of the flap is situated at the contralateral hypochondrium. **B:** The dotted area indicates the undermining necessary to close the flap donor site by direct suture.

A,B

My conclusion is that the circulatory system that supplies the flap is based on the direct flow it receives from the segmental branches, from the subdermal and the subaponeurotic infraumbilical plexus at the side of the pedicle, and from the whole subdermal system of the areas adjacent to the pedicle. The subdermal and subaponeurotic plexus, in turn, must be fed by the arcade of the deep epigastric branches of the same side. The superficial and deep anastomoses of the contralateral side also permit the blood flow to cross the midline to serve the biologic requirements of the flap (6).

FLAP DESIGN AND DIMENSIONS

The tumor area and the areola, as well as incision lines, are marked within the oncologic safety margin (Fig. 2). The excision lines resemble a triangle with convex sides. The base of the triangle is along the inframammary sulcus, and the other two convex sides are united at a vertex below the clavicle (the distance varying according to the individual patient). The thoracoabdominal skin flap is outlined, also in a triangular shape (Fig. 2B). The length of the flap may vary from 30 to 40 cm and its base from 20 to 25 cm. Its maximum length-to-width ratio is 2:1, and its size is limited by two transverse parallel lines. One of these lines passes along the inframammary sulcus; the other passes through the navel. The distal end of the flap is situated at the contralateral hypochondrium. The lower edge, which begins very close to the navel, is convex and longer than the upper edge. The flap reaches from one hypochondrium to the other, passing through the epigastric region (Fig. 2B) (7–10).

OPERATIVE TECHNIQUE

Mobilization of the thoracoabdominal flap is shown in Fig. 3. The incisions are perpendicular to the skin plane, and dissection is done at the level of the aponeurosis, from the distal end back to the base of the flap. The dissection and rotation are tested repeatedly and delicately until the flap end reaches the highest part of the surgical wound (Fig. 3D) (9).

To prepare for closure of the donor area, the subcutaneous tissue covering the anterolateral wall of the abdomen is dissected almost to the inguinal fold. The umbilical pedicle is sectioned at its base during this dissection. Suturing of the rotated flap is done in two layers over various drains.

CLINICAL RESULTS

In all patients, the mastectomy was performed according to oncologic safety limits, whatever the location of the tumor in the breast quadrants. The position of the resultant defect on the thorax varied with the location and size of the resection, and thus the width and length of the flap also varied, as it did with patient biotype (longer for tall patients and shorter for short patients). In tall patients with tumors in the upper outer quadrant of the breast, the length of the flap was about 40 cm, and in shorter patients, the length was about 24 to 30 cm.

Thirty-four patients were treated. In 15 patients, seromas occurred. These were drained for 1 or 2 weeks with no residual effect. Postoperative care was routine, and no special surgical treatment was needed.

Some flap necrosis occurred in 10 patients. In 6 of these, the necrosis prolonged healing time. Both superficial and deep necrosis was observed, principally at the free ends of the flaps. In all these patients, there had been more tension in the sutures and more excessive dissection of the flaps. In the six instances of deep necrosis, the maximum extension was 8 cm from the end of the flap and across the entire width. All these patients were reoperated. Necrotic material was excised, and the area was covered with a split-thickness skin graft. Superficial necrosis occurred in 4 patients, slightly affecting the epithelium and the dermis at the flap end. They healed by secondary intention.

Suture dehiscence occurred at the flap end in 11 patients. This varied in length from 2 to 10 cm and occurred where the tension was greater or after early removal of stitches. Seven of these patients were resutured, and four healed by secondary intention. No hematomas were noted in the surgical area. None of these patients developed any major or primary infection.

The site of the tumor and the patient's biotype are of major importance to the results, because they determine the requirements for longer or shorter flaps. Upper outer quadrant tumors in tall patients required greater undermining and longer flaps, and all cases of deep necrosis that occurred were in this group. Four of these patients were tall and two were average in height. The size of the tumor was not a limiting factor in the closure of defects.

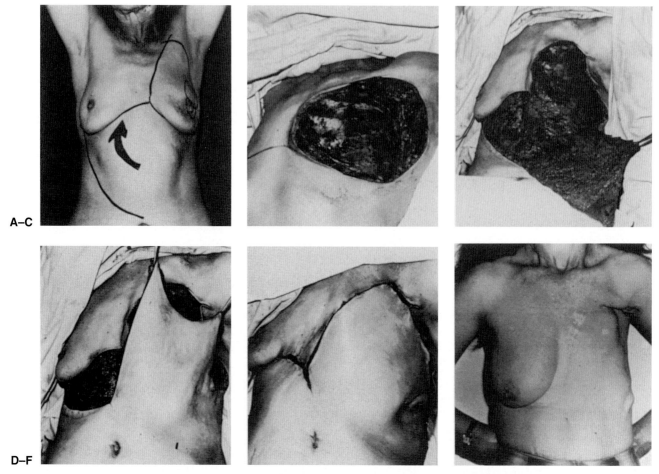

A–C

D–F

FIG. 3. **A:** Triangular area of demarcation surrounding the tumor with oncologic safety margin. **B:** Typical appearance of the wound area immediately after tumor resection of the breast. **C:** The flap elevated. **D:** Cranial traction on the flap. Evaluation of the amount of undermining and umbilical pedicle amputation that must be done at this stage. **E:** Suture of the skin flap is done in two layers. **F:** Postoperative result.

SUMMARY

The transverse thoracoabdominal skin flap can be used for the large chest defects that result after a radical mastectomy, especially when skin also must be excised.

References

1. Bakamjian VY. A two-stage method for pharyngoesophageal reconstruction with a primary pectoral skin flap. *Plast Reconstr Surg* 1965;36:173.
2. Haddad CM. Ensaios sobre a rede arterial da parede anterolateral do abdome (Estudo radiologico). *Rev Assoc Med Bras* 1969;110:225.
3. Smith PJ, Foley B, McGregor LA, Jackson IT. The anatomic basis of the groin flap. *Plast Reconstr Surg* 1972;49:41.
4. Brown RG, Vasconez LO, Jurkiewicz JM. Transverse abdominal flap and the deep epigastric arcade. *Plast Reconstr Surg* 1975;55:416.
5. McGregor IA, Morgan G. Axial and random pattern flaps. *Br J Plast Surg* 1973;26:202.
6. McGregor IA, Jackson IT. The groin flap. *Br J Plast Surg* 1972;2:3.
7. Veronesi U, Lovo GF. Tecnica operatoria dell'exereci di metastasi mammarie interne isolate, in paziente operate di mastectomia radicale. *Tumori* 1963;49:443.
8. Spadafora A. Cierre de brechas producidas por mastectomias amplias. *Prensa Med Argent* 1964;51:552.
9. Baroudi R, Pinotti JA, Keppke EM. Radical mastectomy: new technique for closing wound areas. *Panminerva Med* 1967;9:463.
10. Tai Y, Hasegawa H. A transverse abdominal flap for breast cancer. *Plast Reconstr Surg* 1974;53:52.

CHAPTER 384 ■ BIPEDICLE SKIN FLAPS

L. C. ARGENTA AND E. C. DUUS

Bipedicle flaps of skin and subcutaneous tissue are easily developed on the thorax and are simple solutions to coverage of many superficial defects (1–3). Because of the multiple systems supplying blood to the chest wall, such flaps may be oriented equally well in a vertical or horizontal direction depending on the needs of the patient. When properly designed, bipedicle flaps are robust flaps, allowing mobilization of well-vascularized tissue. However, because of their design, they are limited as to the distance they can be moved.

INDICATIONS

Vertically oriented bipedicle flaps lend themselves extremely well to defects of the sternum. The juxtaposition of two bipedicle flaps, one from each side of the defect, is especially useful for the closure of large defects. Such flaps may be used in combination with underlying synthetic material such as Marlex or homologous muscle flaps. Most defects of the anterior chest wall are best closed with transversely based flaps.

ANATOMY

The blood supply to the skin and subcutaneous tissues of the chest wall is derived from branches of the lateral thoracic, internal mammary, superior epigastric, thoracoachromial, and intercostal arteries (Fig. 1). An understanding of the distribution of these vessels is important so that as many of these vessels as possible may be incorporated into the flap.

The lateral thoracic arteries are tributaries of the second portion of the axillary artery, which descends to the anterior and lateral portions of the chest, turning around the free edge of the pectoralis. Multiple perforators supply the overlying skin. In the female patient, this tends to be a significantly more substantial vessel than in the male patient.

The internal mammary artery gives off the anterior intercostal vessels. The upper six intercostal spaces are supplied by two such anterior intercostal vessels. The perforating branches of these vessels supply the overlying skin, with the second, third, and fourth being dominant.

The superior epigastric artery anastomoses with the internal mammary artery and supplies the area of the rectus sheath and overlying skin. The pectoral branch of the thoracoacromial supplies the pectoral muscles, and its perforators supply the overlying skin. Posterior intercostal arteries send branches to the posterior and lateral chest wall, to the breast, and to the overlying skin and subcutaneous tissue.

FLAP DESIGN AND DIMENSIONS

The anterior and lateral chest walls are usually best covered with a transversely based flap, taking advantage of the transverse orientation of the intercostal vessels. Defects of the midsternum are best covered with vertically oriented bipedicle flaps (Fig. 2).

Obviously, the quality of tissue adjacent to the defect is critical. The inclusion of heavily irradiated, scarred, inflamed, or traumatized tissue with the advancement flap invites failure.

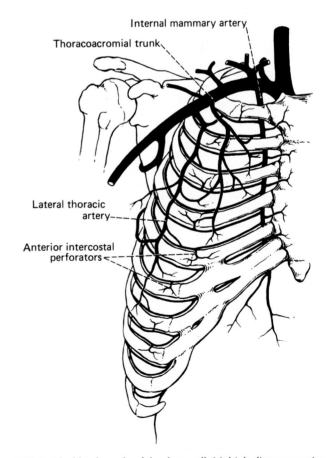

FIG. 1. The blood supply of the chest wall. Multiple discrete arteries and their tributaries supply the thoracic wall. A considerable amount of overlapping of vessels allows safe development of transversely or vertically based flaps on the chest wall.

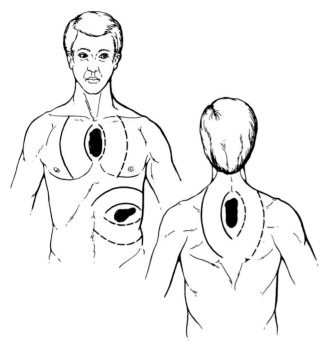

FIG. 2. Most defects of the anterior and posterior chest wall are best closed with transversely based flaps. Defects of the midsternum are expeditiously covered with bilateral flaps on either side of the defect. These are best based in the vertical direction.

The presence of such tissue is best treated with distant vascularized flaps.

The flap should always be at least 25 percent, and preferably 50 percent, larger than the defect. The larger flap allows overlap of the defect so that some contact may be made with adjacent vascularized tissue. Since all bipedicle flaps include some random area, a flap width of at least half the length of the flap is recommended.

OPERATIVE TECHNIQUE

The success and ease of mobilization of this flap largely depend on the initial relaxing incision that is made parallel to the defect. To avoid tension and kinking of the flap, the relaxing incision should be at least twice as long as the defect. Curving the relaxing incision, with the concave side toward the defect, facilitates mobilization of the flap.

Undermining may be done bluntly or sharply at the level of the fascia. While inclusion of the fascia may preserve additional blood supply, it limits mobilization. As many perforating vessels as possible are left intact, as long as the transposition can be accomplished. When the flap is transposed to the defect, extension of the relaxing incision or even judicious backcutting of the flap may be required.

If there is any suspicion of compromise after transposition, fluorescein should be used. If significant areas of the flap fail to fluoresce, the flap should be returned to its donor site for 5 to 7 days as a delay procedure.

After transposition of the bipedicle flap, the donor defect should always be closed with a split-thickness skin graft. At times, undermining of adjacent tissue may give the illusion that the defect may be closed primarily. However, the resultant tension may prove disastrous, with subsequent necrosis or dehiscence of the flap.

SUMMARY

Bipedicle skin flaps, either vertically or transversely oriented, can be used to close chest-wall defects.

References

1. Starzynski T, Snyderman R, Beattie EJ. Problems of major chest-wall reconstruction. *Plast Reconstr Surg* 1969;44:525.
2. Martini N, Starzynski T, Beattie E. Problems in chest-wall resection. *Surg Clin North Am* 1969;49:313.
3. Gingrass R. Flaps for chest wall reconstruction. In: Grabb WC, Myers MB, eds. *Skin flaps.* Boston: Little, Brown, 1975;447–458.

CHAPTER 385 ■ BREAST FLAPS

R. P. GINGRASS

Given the great variety of musculocutaneous, muscle, and skin flaps developed in recent years, the role of the breast flap for chest-wall reconstruction is limited.

INDICATIONS

The breast flap may still have a place in reconstruction of an anterior defect in a woman with radiation necrosis and/or recurrent cancer after mastectomy (1). An appropriate candidate might well be an older woman with a chronic, painful, ulcerating wound who is not concerned about the aesthetic deficiency of the transposed breast (2–4). Another indication might be in a woman who wants a minimum of additional

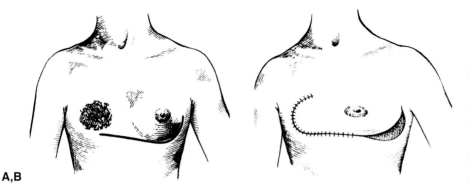

FIG. 1. A: Incision for the breast flap. The superolateral end is determined by rotating the breast into the defect and extending the incision just high enough to allow the flap to cover the defect without tension. **B:** Breast flap rotated into the defect. The shaded area can be closed primarily if this does not cause tension on the flap. If tension results, a split-thickness skin graft is necessary.

scars that cannot be covered easily. These include those which result from flaps taken from the chest, upper abdomen, back, and arm. One additional use of the flap is as a fall-back procedure if an initial flap reconstruction fails, especially if an open chest wound is present.

The breast flap has several advantages over other flap techniques. It is comparatively uncomplicated and can be done expeditiously. The flap usually has a good blood supply that is not jeopardized. Scarring is low on the anterior chest wall, thereby allowing the woman to wear clothes that expose the upper anterior chest, back, and abdomen. The cyclops breast deformity can be decreased by judicious thinning of the transposed breast and by excision of the nippleareola complex, which can be replaced appropriately on the remaining breast mound.

OPERATIVE TECHNIQUE

The incision for the breast flap is usually made in the inframammary crease and is extended as far laterally in the crease as is necessary to allow the flap to rotate into the defect without tension (Fig. 1). The flap is undermined over the pectoralis and serratus fascia, again only as far laterally and superiorly as necessary. If the defect is large and lateral, and/or the donor breast is small, the breast flap may be transposed as well as rotated. This requires a split-thickness skin graft to close the lateral donor site.

A variety of modifications can be used, depending on the size and location of the defect and of the donor breast.

Extended coverage can be obtained by one or several incisions on the deep surface of the breast to allow the skin component to be advanced further laterally. A bibbed flap can be created by an additional skin incision from the crease toward the areola or beyond, with excision of the nipple-areola complex (2,4–6) (Fig. 2).

If the defect is small and medial or the donor breast is large, only the medial portion of the breast may be needed (7) (Fig. 3). If the breast is very large or ptotic, there may be sufficient tissue in the inferior quadrants to use as a medially based pedicle flap (7,8). This creates a long, narrow flap, and a delay procedure may be necessary. In either case, the remaining breast can be rotated into the defect created at the donor site to minimize the deformity and avoid the cyclops problem. A little ingenuity on the part of a thoughtful breast surgeon with experience in reconstruction, reduction mammaplasty, and mastopexy should minimize the donor-site deformity.

For a larger defect, or in a patient with a small breast, additional skin beyond the breast may be needed (Fig. 4). The skin beneath the inframammary crease can be included, either as part of the rotation flap or by creation of a transposition flap (2,9,10) (Fig. 5). The skin beyond the midline may be necessary for an extensive lateral defect (Fig. 6), but a delay procedure may be wise.

SUMMARY

The breast flap may occasionally be the procedure of choice for closing chest-wall defects.

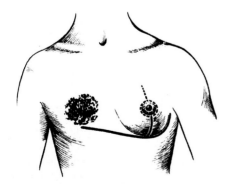

FIG. 2. Breast-splitting incision (*solid line*) creating a bilobed flap. The medial component can thereby be advanced further laterally to the patient's right. For even further advancement, the nipple-areola area can be excised and the incision extended superiorly (*broken line*).

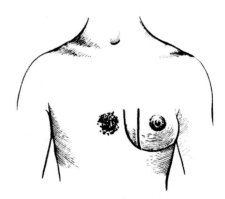

FIG. 3. For a very small medial defect, a transposition flap from the medial portion of the breast may be all that is necessary.

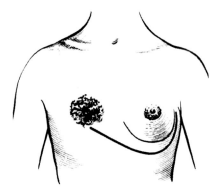

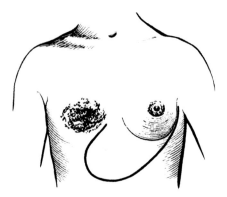

FIG. 4. For a large or lateral defect, or in a patient with a very small breast, the skin beneath the inframammary crease may need to be included with the breast to provide sufficient skin to cover the defect.

FIG. 6. For an extensive lateral defect, the breast flap can be extended across the midline. A delay procedure is strongly recommended.

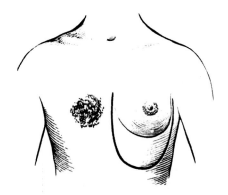

FIG. 5. In selected patients, a transposition flap including the inframammary skin may be more appropriate than the usual rotation flap.

References

1. Gingrass R. Flaps for chest wall reconstruction. In: Grabb WC, Myers MB, eds. *Skin flaps.* Boston: Little, Brown, 1975.
2. Maier HC. Surgical management of large defects of the thoracic wall. *Surgery* 1947;22:169.
3. Pierce GW, Wiper T, Magladry G, et al. Reconstruction of a large defect on the entire thickness of the chest wall. *Am J Surg* 1961;102:720.
4. Rees TD, Converse JM. Surgical reconstruction of defects of the thoracic wall. *Surg Gynecol Obstet* 1965;121:1066.
5. Urban JA. Radical excision of the chest wall for mammary cancer. *Cancer* 1951;4:1263.
6. Whalen WP. Coverage of thoracic wall defects by a split breast flap. *Plast Reconstr Surg* 1953;12:64.
7. Latham WD. Operative treatment for postradiation defects of the chest wall. *Am Surg* 1966;32:700.
8. Pickrell KL, Kelly JW, Mazzoni FA. The surgical treatment of recurrent carcinoma of the breast and chest wall. *Plast Reconstr Surg* 1948;3:156.
9. Davis JS, ed. *Surgery: its principles and practice.* Philadelphia: Blakiston, 1919. Chap. 23.
10. Bennett JE, Carter D. The surgical management of extensive necrosis after Radiation therapy. In: *Transactions of the Third International Congress of Plastic Surgery.* Amsterdam: Excerpta Medica, 1964;113.

CHAPTER 386 ■ DEEPITHELIALIZED TURNOVER DELTOPECTORAL FLAP

A. G. LEONARD

The standard deltopectoral flap (1) can be modified to cover chest-wall defects. The end of the flap is deepithelialized and then turned over like the pages of a book (2,3). In medial defects, the procedure can be completed in one stage; however, in lateral defects, the flap pedicle is returned after 3 weeks.

INDICATIONS

The classic deltopectoral flap can be used in reconstruction of defects of the anterior chest wall (4), although this may give

rise to difficulty with twisting of the pedicle to reach the defect. If the chest-wall excision has been full-thickness, skeletal support may be required, and the dermis of a deepithelialized flap can be used to provide this (5). The flap may be planned simply to turn over into the defect after removal of its epithelium. If the defect is located medially, a one-stage reconstruction can be achieved. However, if the defect is located more laterally, a longer flap is required, and division and return of the pedicle are preferred. Where the former is possible, it has the advantage of retaining the blood supply to the flap in patients in whom the surrounding tissues have been

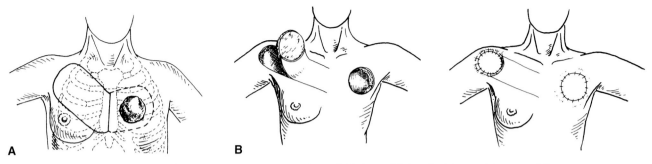

FIG. 1. A: Plan of a one-stage reconstruction of a medially located defect. **B:** A longer deltopectoral flap with a distal deepithelialized paddle for reconstruction of a laterally located defect.

irradiated. If the flap is deepithelialized using the drum dermatome, this allows use of the removed skin to graft the undersurface of the flap, thus reducing the amount of skin to be taken from a distant site.

ANATOMY

See Chapter 124.

FLAP DESIGN AND DIMENSIONS

If the contralateral breast is large and pendulous, the flap should be planned preoperatively with the patient sitting up to avoid inclusion of a large amount of breast tissue in the flap. In any case, the flap should be planned slightly longer than might at first be apparent to allow for some shortening when it is turned over (Figs. 1A and 2).

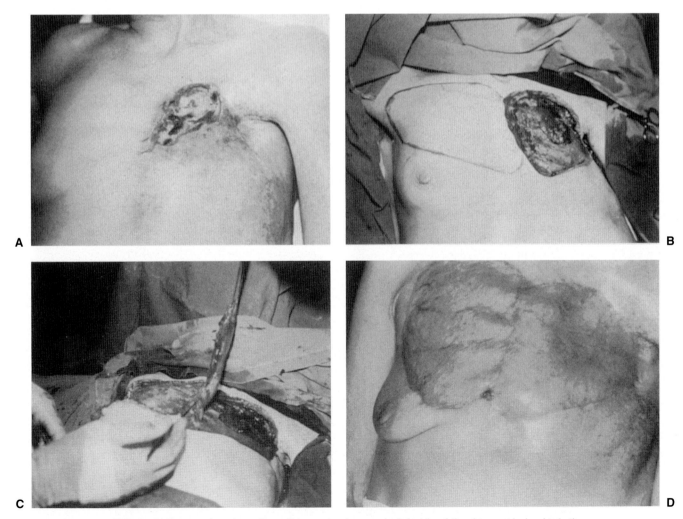

FIG. 2. A: Preoperative view of a radionecrotic ulcer on the left side of the chest, with the third rib exposed in the depth of the wound. **B:** The ulcer has been excised with the full thickness of the chest wall where necessary. The medial margin of the excision extends to the midline, and the deltopectoral flap is outlined on the right side of the chest. **C:** The deepithelialized deltopectoral flap is turned over like a page of a book to lie in the defect. **D:** Postoperative view of the repair.

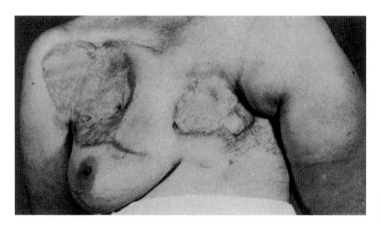

FIG. 3. Postoperative result in a two-stage repair after division and return of the pedicle.

Where the defect is placed so far laterally that extension of its medial margin to the midline would require sacrifice of a large area of normal skin, it is preferable to use a longer flap, with division and return of the pedicle at 3 weeks (Figs. 1B and 3). It also may be preferable to use this technique in a medially located defect in a patient with a very large contralateral breast, in whom the medial part of the flap will be very thick.

OPERATIVE TECHNIQUE

Medially Located Defects

After creation of the defect by excision of radionecrotic ulcer or extirpation of tumor, the medial margin of the defect should be extended at least to the midline or, if there is a great thickness of subcutaneous fat, to the contralateral border of the sternum (Figs. 1A and 2). In the latter case, care should be taken not to damage the perforating branches of the internal mammary artery.

The flap is then raised in the usual way, with dissection carried medially until the perforating branches of the internal mammary artery are seen. It can conveniently be deepithelialized using the drum dermatome. It is then turned over like a page of a book to lie in the defect, where it is sutured in place (6). The previously removed skin is used to graft the exposed undersurface of the flap, and the secondary defect is grafted with split-thickness skin taken from a distant site.

Laterally Located Defects

In this case, only a paddle at the end of the flap, of an area corresponding to the defect, is deepithelialized, planning

on division and return of the pedicle at 3 weeks (Figs. 1B and 3).

CLINICAL RESULTS

Where the defect is medially located, the one-stage technique provides a rapid reconstruction with skeletal support provided by the flap dermis and retention of the vascular axis. Where this is not possible, the two-stage technique provides a satisfactory reconstruction at the expense of longer hospitalization. Paradoxical movement of the reconstructed segment is minimal except on deep inspiration, but this has not reduced exercise tolerance in normal activities.

SUMMARY

The deltopectoral skin flap can be deepithelialized and turned over to cover chest-wall defects in either one or two stages.

References

1. Bakamjian VY. A two-stage method of pharyngeal reconstruction with a primary pectoral skin flap. *Plast Reconstr Surg* 1973, 1965:36.
2. Dinner MI, Anderson R, Kay PP. Repair of defect of anterior chest wall with a turnover dermal-fat deltopectoral flap. *Plast Reconstr Surg* 1978;61:115.
3. Leonard AG. Reconstruction of the chest wall using a deepithelialized "turnover" deltopectoral flap. *Br J Plast Surg* 1980;33:187.
4. Robinson DW. The deltopectoral flap in chest wall reconstruction. *Br J Plast Surg* 1976;29:22.
5. Tamoney HJ, Stent PA. Dermal graft for chest wall repair. *Surg Gynecol Obstet* 1964;118:289.
6. Pakiam AI. The reversed dermis flap. *Br J Plast Surg* 1978;31:131.

CHAPTER 387 ■ OMENTAL FLAP

R. S. STAHL AND M. J. JURKIEWICZ

In no discipline have the recent advances in the knowledge of surgical anatomy and technique enabled more bold and aggressive extirpation of tumor, infection, and radionecrosis than in chest-wall reconstruction. With the use of regional muscle flaps, omental transposition, and free-tissue transfer, most restrictions on chest-wall surgery have been eliminated (1–6). The use of pedicled omentum has proven a reliable method of reconstruction of difficult thoracic defects with highly revascularized tissue and minimal morbidity (7–14).

INDICATIONS

The omentum has many utilitarian virtues: it readily accepts skin grafts, has an extended range, and leaves a minimal donor defect. The omentum typically brings highly vascularized tissue to necrotic, irradiated, malignant, or infected wounds with extreme reliability. Its rich lymphatic supply offers the theoretical advantage of increased resistance to infection and malignancy. Indeed, recurrence of tumor in wounds covered with omentum usually occurs at the margins (13).

Not only does the omentum offer an effective means of reconstruction in curative procedures, but it improves the quality of life in patients with the ulcerated, foul, weeping, miserable wounds of terminal disease. For example, it can be used in reconstruction of excisional defects in many lesions of the chest wall: primary tumors, recurrent breast carcinomas, or progressive radionecrosis. It offers a reliable means of breast reconstruction or infected sternal dehiscence repair when other tissues, such as the latissimus dorsi or pectoralis major, are unavailable or inadequate.

ANATOMY

The greater omentum, having developed from the dorsal mesogastrium, is supplied by the right and left gastroepiploic arteries. These vessels, arising from the gastroduodenal and splenic arteries, respectively, join along the greater curvature of the stomach to form the gastroepiploic arch. This arch typically gives rise to the right, middle, and left omental arteries, as well as multiple short omental vessels. Each of the omental arteries then contributes to another vascular arcade in a more dependent portion of the omentum (15). Knowledge of the five major variants of the vascular arcade (16) allows for preservation and utilization of collateral blood flow in selective division and lengthening for more distant pedicle applications (see Fig. 3).

FLAP DESIGN AND DIMENSIONS

The omentum will reach the nipple in 75 percent of patients, the level of the sternal angle in 40 percent of patients, and the inguinal ligament in 10 percent of patients after lysis of its colonic attachments only (17) (Fig. 1). The omentum has been applied in the treatment of wounds of the back and flank by passing it through retroperitoneal tunnels, further extending its range (18). With attention to the vascular anatomy, the omentum may be divided and lengthened to reach the skull, the midleg, and the midforearm. However, progressive sacrifice of "tip size" corresponds with lengthening, making free microvascular transfer a more practical means of using omentum for distant wounds.

OPERATIVE TECHNIQUE

Prior to operative treatment, the difficult wound should be biopsied for appropriate microbiologic and histopathologic examinations. Such information will, of course, dictate proper antibiotic coverage, as well as appropriate width of resection.

The operative strategy in omental chest-wall reconstruction consists of assessing and mobilizing the omentum prior to manipulating the contaminated thoracic wound or committing to an extensive resection. After a thorough peritoneal exploration by means of a transverse abdominal incision, the first assistant places the omentum on traction, while the surgeon begins lysing its relatively avascular attachments to the colon.

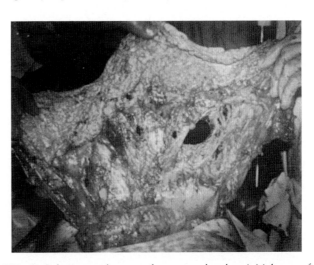

FIG. 1. Colonic attachments of omentum lysed as initial step of omental mobilization.

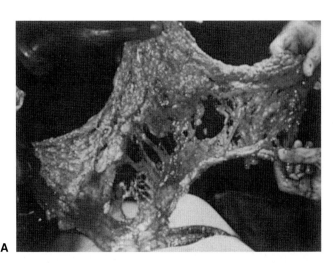

A

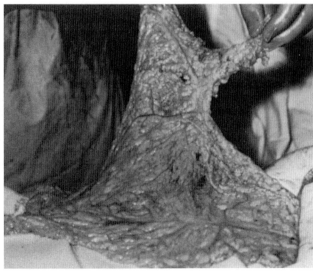

B

FIG. 2. After division of gastric attachments, the omentum may be based on either the right (**A**) or the left (**B**) gastroepiploic vessel, markedly extending omental range.

Since there is usually less fusion of the leaves of the omentum to the tail and body of the pancreas, most surgeons advocate beginning omental mobilization on the left. It is also important to avoid injuring diverticula coli, appendices epiploica, and the transverse mesocolon and middle colic vessels. Immediate ligature of vessels, with avoidance of the use of electrocautery, prevents injuries to these delicate vessels and resultant damage to the gastroepiploic arcade by hematoma formation.

If the range of omental mobilization is not adequate, several steps may be taken to extend this. Division of gastric attachments and one of the gastroepiploic vessels is the simplest and most commonly used method of omental elongation (Fig. 2). Care must be taken not to distort the gastroepiploic vessels during division and ligation of the omental attachments to the stomach. The short vessels between the gastroepiploic system and the stomach may be individually clamped and ligated as far distally as the antrum and duodenum. Furthermore, the right

and left gastroepiploic vessels should be alternately occluded to determine competence of the arch. The right gastroepiploic artery is usually the larger and more pulsatile of the two; consequently, the left gastroepiploic vessel is usually sacrificed. The final option for augmenting omental range consists of selective omental division, described in the discussion of anatomic considerations (Fig. 3).

Having achieved adequate omental length, a generous tunnel is created in the subcutaneous space for passage of the omental flap through the laparotomy incision, through a separate incision in the rectus sheath, or between ribs adjacent to the recipient site. The latter two choices are thought to diminish chances of herniation. Many surgeons place the pedicle through the body wall just to the left of the falciform ligament in an effort to prevent herniation as well. Care should be taken during this transposition of the flap to avoid twisting the pedicle or distorting the duodenum or antrum. The placement of tacking sutures from the omentum to the margins of the exit wound helps to prevent extrusion and excess mobility of the flap.

Once omental range and position are deemed adequate and the omentum is placed in its tunnel readily accessible to its recipient site and covered with a moist pad, the abdominal wound is closed and attention is turned to the chest-wall lesion. A generous resection of all necrotic, infected, irradiated, or malignant tissue is performed. It is especially important to resect involved costal cartilages widely.

Chest-wall rigidity may be restored by suturing one or two layers of Prolene mesh to the inner surface of the rib cage after placement of chest tubes (19). This material seems to tolerate contamination relatively well. For larger full-thickness defects, rib grafts are added to provide bony support, preventing paradoxical motion as well as an unnatural chest-wall contour (Fig. 4).

After the omentum is sutured to the wound margins, covering Prolene, rib grafts, and chest tubes, meshed split-thickness skin is applied directly to the omental surface, allowing for the transudation of fluid that typically occurs postoperatively. The procedure is then concluded with the application of a moist but noncompressive dressing.

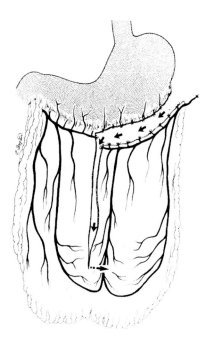

FIG. 3. Knowledge of omental vascular anatomy allows for pedicle lengthening with preservation of blood supply.

CLINICAL RESULTS

Surprisingly few complications arise from use of the omentum for the foregoing purposes, in spite of the need for invasion of

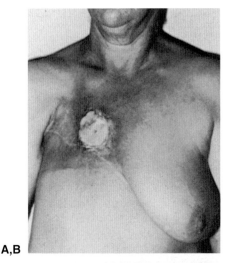
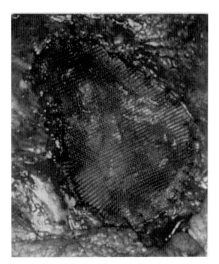

A,B

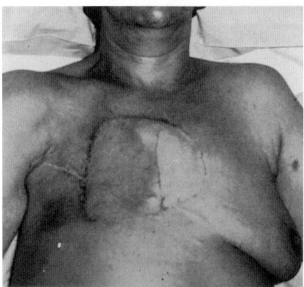

C

FIG. 4. **A:** Ulcerated, irradiated chest-wall recurrence of carcinoma of the breast. **B:** Prolene mesh is sutured to margins of full-thickness chest-wall resection after placement of chest tubes. For larger wounds, rib grafts may be added to restore contour and prevent paradoxical motion. (From Jurkiewicz, Arnold, ref. 11, with permission.) **C:** Healed wound after placement of omentum (plus meshed skin graft) over Prolene mesh.

the peritoneal cavity, the advanced, contaminated wounds for which its application is often reserved, and the debilitated state of many patients in whom it is used.

Most sequelae and complications of use of the omentum are minor and resolve with expectant treatment. These include a brief gastric ileus, partial omental or skin-graft separation or loss, and occasional recurrence of infection. Periodically, elevation of the flap, debridement, and reinsetting may be required, although most of these marginal wounds rapidly granulate and epithelialize.

Possible complications of pedicled omental reconstruction include incisional hernia formation and omental migration of the peritoneal exit site. As with any intraabdominal procedure, a finite risk of adhesive bowel obstruction exists, although this has not seemed a prominent problem. Lysis of omental adhesions has been reported as the cause of cecal volvulus in the mortality of one patient who underwent pedicled omental chest-wall reconstruction (12). However, adherence to the principles outlined earlier should prevent most complications.

SUMMARY

The omentum is especially useful in managing wounds of the chest wall, where dependable, adequate coverage of vital organs and vessels is essential.

References

1. Starzynski TE, Snyderman RK, Beattie EJ. Problems of major chest-wall reconstruction. *Plast Reconstr Surg* 1969;44:5.
2. Martini N, Starzynski TE, Beattie EJ. Problems in chest wall resection. *Surg Clin North Am* 1969;49:313.
3. Woods JE, Arnold PG, Masson JK, et al. Management of radiation necrosis and advanced cancer of the chest wall in patients with breast malignancy. *Plast Reconstr Surg* 1979;63:235.
4. Leonard AG. Reconstruction of the chest wall using a deepithelialized "turn over" deltopectoral flap. *Br J Plast Surg* 1980;33:187.
5. Dingman RO, Argenta LC. Reconstruction of the chest wall. *Ann Thorac Surg* 1981;32:202.
6. Arnold PG. Reconstruction of the sternum and anterior chest wall: aesthetic considerations. *Clin Plast Surg* 1981;8:389.
7. Kiricuta I, Goldstein MB. Das Omentum als Ersatzmaterial der blasenwand bei durchstrahlen verursachten Blasenscheidenfisteln. *Krebsarzt* 1961;16:202.
8. Kiricuta I. L'emploi du grand épiploon dans la chirurgie du sein cancereux. *Presse Med* 1963;71:1.
9. Dupont C, Menard Y. Transpositions of the greater omentum for reconstruction of the chest wall. *Plast Reconstr Surg* 1972;49:263.
10. Arnold PG, Hartrampf CR, Jurkiewicz MJ. One-stage reconstruction of the breast using the transposed greater omentum. *Plast Reconstr Surg* 1976;57:520.
11. Jurkiewicz MJ, Arnold PG. The omentum: an account of its use in the reconstruction of the chest wall. *Ann Surg* 1977;185:548.
12. Hakelius L. Fatal complication after use of the greater omentum for reconstruction of the chest wall. *Plast Reconstr Surg* 1978;62:796.
13. Newing RK, Pribaz JJ, Bennett RC, Buis J. Omental transposition and skin graft in the management of chest-wall recurrence of carcinoma of the breast. *Aust NZ J Surg* 1979;49:546.

14. Arnold PG, Irons GB. The greater omentum: extensions in transposition and free transfer. *Plast Reconstr Surg* 1981;67:169.
15. Powers JC, Fitzgerald JF, McAlvanah MJ. The anatomic basis for the surgical detachment of the greater omentum from the transverse colon. *Surg Gynecol Obstet* 1976;143:105.
16. Alday ES, Goldsmith HG. Surgical technique for omental lengthening based on arterial anatomy. *Surg Gynecol Obstet* 1972;135:103.
17. Das SK. The size of the human omentum and methods of lengthening it for transplantation. *Br J Plast Surg* 1976;29:170.
18. Arnold PG. Chest-wall reconstruction. Presented at the Medical Association of Georgia Conference, Atlanta, Ga., November 21, 1981.
19. Graham J, Usher FC, Perry JL, Barkley HT. Marlex mesh as a prosthesis in the repair of thoracic wall defects. *Ann Surg* 1960;151:469.

CHAPTER 388. Pectoralis Major Muscle and Musculocutaneous Flaps *S. Ariyan*
www.encyclopediaofflaps.com

CHAPTER 389 ■ ROTATION-ADVANCEMENT SPLIT PECTORALIS (RASP) MAJOR MUSCLE TURNOVER FLAP FOR MEDIAN CHEST WOUNDS AND MEDIAN STERNOTOMY DEHISCENCE AND INFECTION

D. A. STAFFENBERG

EDITORIAL COMMENT

Surgeons need several options when considering the extent of the deformity in median sternotomy defects. This and the following chapter show how important it is (a) to have knowledge of what was actually done in previous surgery and (b) to analyze what vessels are still intact and how to plan appropriately.

The rotation-advancement split pectoralis (RASP) turnover flap is a valuable technique to reconstruct median sternotomy infections and wounds with large amounts of dead space.

INDICATIONS

Mediastinitis, sternal dehiscence with or without sternal osteomyelitis, is a known complication of cardiothoracic surgery. The advantages of early diagnosis and reconstruction have been reported (1). If the wound is divided into vertical thirds, difficulty in providing reliable coverage of the lower third of the chest wound has led many surgeons to use rectus abdominis muscle flaps or omental flaps to provide reliable coverage of the wound. This adds the morbidity and pulmonary issues that follow invasion of the abdominal wall.

The split pectoralis major muscle turnover flap, used in conjunction with a contralateral pectoralis major muscle island advancement flap, has been a reliable and safe method to reconstruct these complex wounds completely, while eliminating the need for additional flaps. By splitting the turnover flap along its fibers, we bring its rotation point closer to the problematic lower third. Once this lower turnover flap is brought into position, the middle third is filled with the advancement flap from the contralateral side. This technique has been particularly helpful in cases of cardiac reoperation, in which the incision is extended farther toward the abdomen, to allow the cardiac surgeon safe reentry into the mediastinum. For smaller wounds, a bilateral pectoralis myocutaneous flap closure is usually sufficient (2).

ANATOMY

The pectoralis major muscle is a large fan-shaped muscle on the anterior chest wall. The muscle has its origin from the clavicle and the anterior surface of the sternum, as low as the cartilage of the sixth or seventh rib, and from the anterior leaf of the rectus abdominis and the aponeurosis of the external oblique muscle. From this wide origin, the fibers converge laterally toward their insertion at the crest of the greater tubercle of the humerus.

The vascular pedicles that allow its transfer as a muscle flap define the pectoralis major muscle as a type V muscle (3).

The thoracoacromial pedicle extends medially into the muscle from the acromion. The descending pectoral branch from the thyrocervical trunk emerges from between the clavicle and the second rib in the midclavicular line. From here, it courses inferiorly and laterally on the undersurface of the muscle within the subpectoral fat pad. When the pedicle reaches the line drawn between the xiphoid and the acromion, it turns 90 degrees medially and follows that line (4). Finally, perforators from the internal mammary vessels reach the medial aspect of the pectoralis major muscle by extending into the undersurface of the muscle in the interspaces at the lateral border of the sternum.

OPERATIVE TECHNIQUE

The particular vessels used for coronary revascularization must be ascertained, and the reconstructive plan altered when necessary. Most frequently, the left internal mammary artery (LIMA) has been used, leaving potentially unreliable perforators on the left side. This is the most common scenario, and the following description is consistent with such a case. It should be noted that the plan described could be reversed left to right, in the unlikely event that the right internal mammary artery is used, rather than the left. The technique described can also be used safely if neither internal mammary artery has been dissected.

An advancement flap is designed on the patient's left side (Fig. 1). Dissection is carried laterally on the superficial surface of the pectoralis major muscle to the anterior axillary line, cephalad to within 2 cm of the clavicle and caudal to the anterior rectus sheath. Next, the surgeon's index finger is placed beneath the inferolateral border of the pectoralis major muscle to identify the subpectoral space. The caudal and medial attachments of the muscle are then divided.

Dissection then follows the undersurface of the pectoralis major muscle toward the clavicle. The plane of dissection must be maintained deep to the subpectoralis fat pad to preserve the pedicle, but the pectoralis minor muscle is left undisturbed. To advance this muscle beyond the midline, the lateral aspect is divided from the humeral attachment, with care not to injure the descending pectoral branch as it courses laterally on the undersurface of the pectoralis major muscle before its medial turn at the imaginary line joining the acromion and the xiphoid. A lighted retractor and long tip for the electrocautery

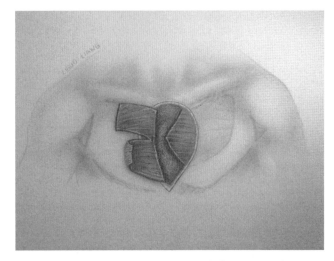

FIG. 2. Split pectoralis major muscle flap is elevated.

is helpful. The clavicular attachment is divided laterally and medially. Because the pedicle is on the deep surface of the muscle, a true island muscle flap can safely be created with care, if required. This island muscle flap will span the chest defect and cover the middle third of the wound.

The right pectoralis major muscle flap is used as a turnover flap. Dissection is carried laterally on the superficial surface of the pectoralis major muscle to the anterior axillary line, cephalad to within 2 cm of the clavicle and caudal to the anterior rectus sheath. The surgeon's index finger is placed beneath the inferolateral border of the pectoralis major muscle to identify the subpectoral space. The lateral aspect of the pectoralis major muscle is divided to provide sufficient length for coverage. Working from lateral to medial, the clavicular attachment is released, including the descending pectoral branch found under the middle third of the clavicle. The turnover flap is elevated (Fig. 2) and held vertically on gentle stretch between two penetrating towel clamps. The muscle is then split along the length of its fibers, resulting in two, now separate, turnover flaps. One perforator for each flap is adequate for viability. The caudal flap is turned over to cover the caudal third of the wound, whereas the cephalad flap is turned over to cover the cephalic third of the wound (Fig. 3).

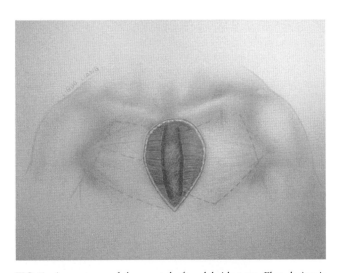

FIG. 1. Appearance of the wound after debridement. Flap design is shown.

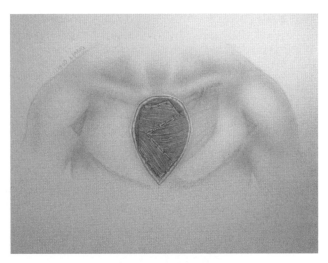

FIG. 3. Split pectoralis major muscle flap is turned over into position, and contralateral advancement is brought into the middle third of the wound.

Suction drains are left laterally in the subcutaneous space, under the flaps in the midline and subcutaneously in the midline. Viability of the muscle flaps is confirmed, and they are gently secured to each other with 3-0 absorbable sutures. Tension is to be avoided. The skin is then closed primarily with 2-0 undyed absorbable sutures. Staples or sutures are used for the final layer.

CLINICAL RESULTS

The rotation-advancement split pectoralis major muscle turnover flap technique has proven to be a safe and reliable method to reconstruct large infected sternal wounds. Although in the past, the inferior third of the wound frequently required additional flaps from the abdomen, this has been addressed by dividing the turnover flap to lower the rotation point. By bringing the rotation point closer to the inferior third defect, reliable coverage has been provided.

SUMMARY

The RASP turnover flap is a valuable technique to reconstruct median sternotomy infections and wounds with large amounts of dead space. It is a recommended method, especially for treating complex median sternotomy wounds with sternal osteomyelitis.

References

1. Jurkiewicz MJ, Bostwick J III, Hester TR, et al. Infected median sternotomy wound: successful treatment by muscle flaps. *Ann Surg* 1980;191:738.
2. Ascherman JA, Hugo NE, Sultan MR, et al. Single-stage treatment of sternal wound complications in heart transplant recipients in whom pectoralis major myocutaneous advancement flaps were used. *J Thorac Cardiovasc Surg* 1995;110:1030.
3. Mathes SJ, Nahai F. Classification of the vascular anatomy of muscles: experimental and clinical correlation. *Plast Reconstr Surg* 1981;67:177.
4. Ariyan S. The pectoralis major myocutaneous flap: a versatile flap for reconstruction in the head and neck. *Plast Reconstr Surg* 1979;63:73.

CHAPTER 390 ■ RECTUS ABDOMINIS MUSCLE FLAPS FOR MEDIAN STERNOTOMY INFECTIONS

M. S. WONG AND T. R. STEVENSON

Several options are available for reconstruction of debrided median sternotomy wounds, including rectus abdominis muscle or musculocutaneous flaps, pectoralis major muscle advancement and turnover flaps, omental flaps, and latissimus dorsi flaps. The caudal aspect of the debrided sternotomy wound is subject to high stresses during respiration and is difficult to fill by using pectoralis major or latissimus dorsi musculocutaneous flaps. The rectus abdominis flap successfully addresses wound-healing concerns in this caudal portion while simultaneously providing closure for the entire wound.

INDICATIONS

Based superiorly, the rectus abdominis muscle flap provides soft-tissue fill and a robust vascular supply, both important in the reconstruction of infected median sternotomy wounds. This flap may be elevated, either as a musculocutaneous or as a muscle flap, depending on soft-tissue requirements of the debrided sternal wound.

ANATOMY

The paired rectus abdominis muscles are long and flat. These muscles originate from the anterior surfaces of the fifth to seventh costal cartilages and the xiphoid process. Each muscle measures 6 to 10 cm in width. The rectus abdominis muscle retains much of this width throughout its course. Narrowing to approximately 5 cm in the lower hypogastric region, the muscle transitions to a tendon, before terminating at its attachment to the pubis between the crest and symphysis. The muscle has a total length of 24 to 30 cm. Medial aponeurotic extensions of other abdominal muscles (the external oblique, internal oblique, and the transversus abdominis) form the rectus sheath that encloses the rectus abdominis muscles. Several intimate attachments or tendinous inscriptions exist between the anterior surface of the rectus abdominis muscle and the overlying anterior rectus sheath, not present on its posterior surface.

A type III muscle, the rectus abdominis has dual blood supplies: the deep superior epigastric artery (DSEA) and the deep inferior epigastric artery (DIEA). These two arterial systems are connected by a series of intervening choke vessels. The superior DSEA pedicle is a terminal extension of the internal mammary artery (IMA), whereas the inferior DIEA pedicle is a branch of the external iliac artery. The DSEA originates beneath the sixth costal cartilage, courses behind the seventh costal cartilage on the transversus abdominis muscle, and enters the rectus sheath. Veins (venae comitantes) are usually paired and accompany the similarly named arteries. Innervation is accomplished by motor branches of the seventh through twelfth intercostal nerves. These paired muscles assist in abdominal flexion. Unilateral use for sternal reconstruction is well tolerated, with little detectable loss of function (1).

FLAP DESIGN AND DIMENSIONS

When used for sternal reconstruction, the pedicle is based on the DSEA, allowing easy rotation into the thoracic defect. If the IMA has been harvested unilaterally (most often on the left) for a cardiac revascularization procedure, the right rectus abdominis muscle may be used for reconstruction. If, however, both IMAs have been transected, the DSEAs can be supplied through a rich collateral circulation from the musculophrenic and lower intercostal arteries (2).

Depending on the skin requirements of the sternal wound, the rectus abdominis muscle may be transposed as either a muscle or a musculocutaneous flap. The cutaneous portion of the flap may be oriented transversely or obliquely, based on underlying musculocutaneous perforators. In general, the vertical design is more useful for sternal wound reconstruction after debridement. When designing a skin island over the rectus abdominis muscle, it is important to remember that the greatest density of skin perforators is in the periumbilical region.

OPERATIVE TECHNIQUE

Muscle Flap

A paramedian skin incision is used to provide adequate exposure of the entire anterior rectus sheath. The sheath is incised 1 cm lateral to the linea alba, revealing the rectus abdominis muscle. The medial leaf of the sheath is dissected off the rectus muscle superiorly and inferiorly, completely exposing the medial border of the rectus abdominis muscle. Similarly, the lateral leaf of the sheath is dissected in a medial-to-lateral direction, exposing the lateral border of the muscle. Care is taken when detaching the anterior rectus sheath from the adherent horizontal inscriptions.

The DIEA and its accompanying veins are isolated, ligated, and divided. These vessels are found entering the posterior portion of the rectus abdominis muscle along its inferolateral

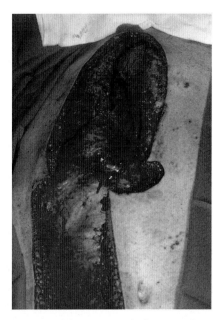

FIG. 2. Right rectus abdominis muscle flap turned over to fill the debrided sternal wound.

aspect, just deep to the thin transversalis fascia. The muscle is divided distally and elevated off the transversalis fascia. Superiorly, the dissection is carried above the arcuate line, ligating and dividing segmental neurovascular structures along the way. As the costal margin is approached, the DSEA pedicle is visualized originating behind the sixth costal cartilage, coursing behind the seventh costal cartilage, lying on the transversus abdominis muscle.

The dissected muscle may be turned over or rotated into the debrided sternal defect. Once freed from its residence within the rectus sheath, the muscle contracts to approximately two thirds to three fourth of its native length (Figs. 1 and 2). If the wound requirements demand more superior fill, the muscle may be stretched by placing segmental tacking stitches to the surrounding tissues of the chest wall. Drains are placed deep and superficial to the muscle flap, and the skin is closed in layers (Fig. 3).

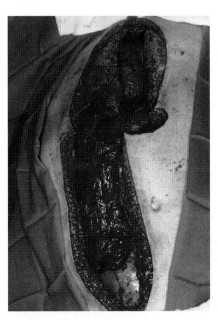

FIG. 1. Contracted right rectus abdominis muscle flap freed from all rectus-sheath attachments.

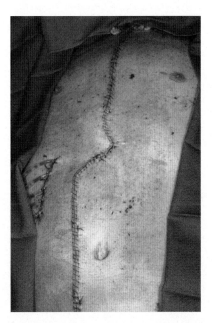

FIG. 3. Primary skin closure over multiple drains.

The anterior rectus sheath is repaired primarily over a closed suction drain, and the skin is repaired in layers over another similar drain. Drains are initially placed on low continuous wall suction, and transitioned to bulb suction after 48 hours. Suction drainage facilitates adherence of tissues and lessens seroma formation.

Musculocutaneous Flap

Dimensions of the skin paddle required for the sternal wound are determined by measuring the skin deficit (Fig. 4). A cutaneous paddle of similar size is drawn over the rectus abdominis muscle, bearing in mind the goal of primary donor-site skin closure. The medial skin-flap margin is incised, exposing the linea alba and anterior rectus sheath. The anterior rectus sheath is incised lateral to the linea alba, abutting the cutaneous paddle, leaving a minimum cuff of 1 cm. If the cutaneous portion of the flap is positioned over the anterior rectus sheath, such that no such cuff is possible, careful elevation of the skin off the anterior rectus sheath is performed, until either the first row of medial perforators is encountered or a cuff of 1 cm is established, whichever is achieved first. This medial rectus sheath incision is carried the full length of the skin paddle. The medial cuff of the anterior rectus sheath is carefully separated from the rectus abdominis muscle, completely freeing its medial border.

The lateral skin incision is made, exposing the abdominal-wall fascia and identifying the lateral edge of the anterior rectus sheath. A minimum lateral cuff of 2 cm is planned. If the skin paddle precludes this cuff, the skin component of the flap may be elevated in a lateral-to-medial direction to the level of the first row of lateral perforators. A vertical incision through the anterior rectus sheath is made, and the lateral cuff of anterior rectus sheath is dissected off of the rectus abdominis muscle, thus exposing the entire length of its lateral border. The deep inferior epigastric vessels and the distal muscle are divided, and the flap is elevated, as described earlier for the muscle flap alone.

The pedicle is identified, and the flap is rotated 180 degrees into position over a drain (Fig. 5). Unlike the muscle flap, the

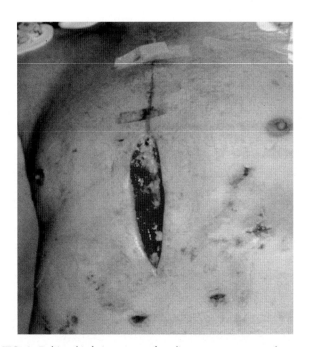

FIG. 4. Dehisced inferior aspect of median sternotomy wound.

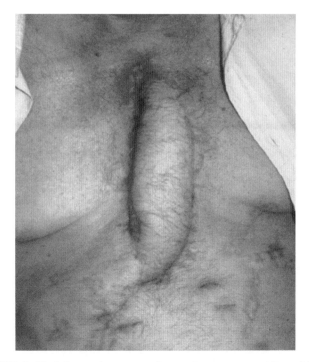

FIG. 5. Healed musculocutaneous flap used to reconstruct this caudal sternal wound.

musculocutaneous flap does not contract as significantly, because of tension in the overlying skin. A layered closure is then performed. The abdominal donor site is similarly closed in layers. The anterior rectus sheath is closed primarily over a drain. Depending on the quality of the fascial closure, consideration should be given to using mesh to supplement the closure (3).

CLINICAL RESULTS

In our reported 10-year clinical experience, 34 patients with infected median sternotomy wounds were treated with aggressive sternal debridement and reconstruction by using a rectus abdominis musculocutaneous flap (4). The 17 male and 17 female patients ranged in age from 13 to 82 years (mean, 55 years) and weighed between 42 and 165 kg (mean, 82 kg). Eighty percent of these patients had three or more medical comorbidities, most commonly diabetes mellitus, hypertension, and atherosclerosis. Twenty-two (65%) patients had coronary artery bypass grafting procedures, with 60% of these using an IMA as a vascularized bypass; 10 (29%) patients had cardiac valve replacements; and 3 (9%) patients had tumor resections requiring median sternotomy.

Flap complications occurred in 10 (29%) patients, including f5 (14%) hematomas and 5 (14%) infections. Six of these patients required a second operative procedure. Eight patients experienced partial distal skin flap loss. All eight of these wounds healed secondarily, after local wound care. Two patients experienced donor-site complications, with one ventral abdominal hernia and one infection. The former patient declined surgical repair, whereas the latter was successfully treated with incision and drainage, followed by a split-thickness skin graft. Four patients died within the first postoperative month; none of the deaths was attributable to the reconstructive procedure. All surviving patients, whether or not they experienced a postoperative complication, achieved complete sternal wound healing, after rectus abdominis musculocutaneous flap reconstruction.

Although our small sample size precluded statistical analysis, several trends were noted. Patients with greater age, weight, number of medical comorbidities, and of female gender, appeared to have more complications, with 45% of morbidly obese patients experiencing postoperative complications, compared with 22% of nonobese patients.

SUMMARY

For reconstruction of median sternotomy wounds, the rectus abdominis muscle (or musculocutaneous) flap is easy to elevate. Further, it offers satisfactory wound coverage in the lower aspect of the sternal wound, an area difficult to address through transposition of the more commonly used pectoralis major muscle flap. Inclusion of an overlying skin paddle has the added advantage of transferring vascularized skin to the sternal wound, decreasing skin tension at the recipient site, and eliminating the need for skin grafting. Disadvantages of

this flap include inconsistent viability of the distal skin island and donor-site morbidity that includes abdominal-wall weakness or hernia formation. We now reserve use of the rectus abdominis musculocutaneous flap for nonobese patients, who have large skin or soft-tissue deficits in the inferior aspect of their sternal wounds.

References

1. Netscher DT, Eladoumikdachi F, HcHugh PM, et al. Sternal wound debridement and muscle flap reconstruction: functional implications. *Ann Plast Surg* 2004;51:115.
2. Netscher DT, Eladoumikdachi F, Goodman CM. Rectus abdominis muscle flaps used successfully for median sternotomy wounds after ipsilateral internal mammary artery ligation. *Ann Plast Surg* 2001;47:223.
3. Kuntscher MV, Mansouri S, Noack N, Harmann B. Versatility of vertical rectus abdominis musculocutaneous flaps. *Microsurgery* 2006;26:363.
4. Oh AK, Lechtman AN, Whetzel TP, Stevenson TR. The infected median sternotomy wound: management with the rectus abdominis musculocutaneous flap. *Ann Plast Surg* 2004;52:367.

CHAPTER 391 ■ SERRATUS ANTERIOR MUSCLE AND MUSCULOCUTANEOUS FLAP

J. C. GROTTING

SEE CHAPTER 151.

Regional use of the serratus muscle is more limited than that of the latissimus muscle because it is only one-fourth the size. The two muscles can be mobilized together for either local use or when a large vascularized free-muscle flap is required.

The serratus anterior muscle also may be used as a transposition flap to close tracheobronchial fistulas by passing the muscle through the chest wall. Since many thoracic surgeons retract and save the serratus anterior muscle during thoracotomy, while dividing the latissimus dorsi, the serratus is usually available for use.

CHAPTER 392 ■ RECTUS ABDOMINIS MUSCLE AND MUSCULOCUTANEOUS FLAP

H. LABANDTER, M. I. DINNER, AND R. V. DOWDEN

The rectus abdominis musculocutaneous or muscle flap provides a suitable alternative for immediate or delayed coverage of sternal or other chest-wall defects (1–3). Most other methods are more complicated and require several procedures or the sacrifice of major areas of surrounding tissue.

INDICATIONS

In patients requiring upper or lower (4) anterior chest-wall reconstruction extending to the posterior axillary line laterally or to the sternal notch superiorly, the rectus abdominis muscle or musculocutaneous flap can be used.

Care must be taken to ascertain that the internal mammary artery on the side of the muscle to be used has not been damaged, particularly in the case of infected sternum after cardiac surgery, where the artery may have been used in bypass. The critical factor remains the removal of all the necrotic, infected costochondral cartilage and ribs. A decision is then made as to whether muscle alone or muscle and skin are required for closure of the defect, and the flap is raised in the standard manner (Fig. 1).

The rectus flap is usually less complicated than other methods, such as the use of omentum (5–7), pectoralis muscle (8–10), latissimus muscle (11,12), or local skin flaps (13–17) and leaves a more acceptable donor-site appearance (Figs. 2 and 3). The patient remains in the supine position, simplifying intraoperative maneuvering.

ANATOMY

See Chapter 362.

FLAP DESIGN AND DIMENSIONS

See Chapter 362.

OPERATIVE TECHNIQUE

See Chapter 362.

CLINICAL RESULTS

The rectus abdominis musculocutaneous flap is extremely reliable, and complications can be avoided by attention to technical detail. Loss of the flap can occur after injury to the indirect perforator system.

Donor-site functional deficit is minimal. In the immediate postoperative period, difficulty is experienced in sitting from a

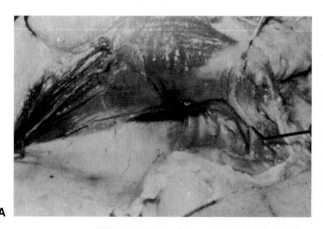
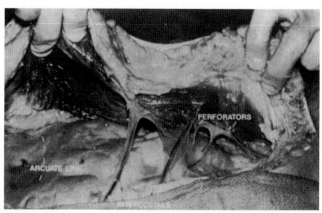

FIG. 1. A: View of the superior pedicle entering and running along the posterior surface of the muscle.
B: The perforators entering medially above the arcuate line.

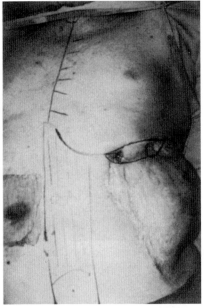 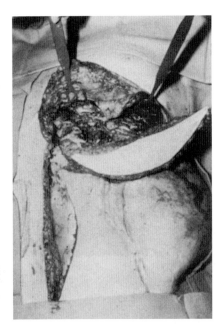 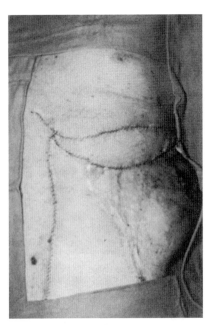

A–C

FIG. 2. A: Lower chest wall with chronic infected costochondritis following x-ray therapy and excisions for recurrent basal carcinoma. **B:** Following extensive debridement, including resection of diaphragm and pleura, the flap has been raised and is to be inserted transversely. **C:** Rectus abdominis musculocutaneous flap in place.

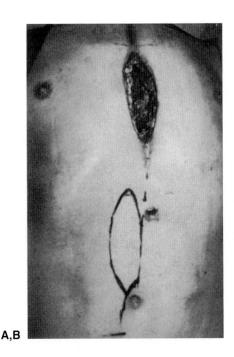 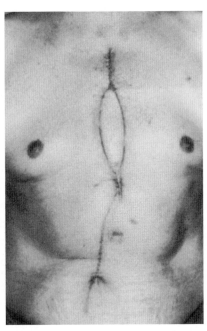

A,B

FIG. 3. A: Infected sternum and costochondral junction following coronary bypass surgery. **B:** Six months after repair with the rectus abdominis musculocutaneous flap.

recumbent position. However, for a period of 6 weeks, the function is adequately compensated for by the external oblique muscles.

The development of a hernia is usually related to breakdown of the fascial repair of the anterior abdominal wall below the arcuate line. Meticulous surgical technique can reduce the incidence of this complication.

SUMMARY

The rectus abdominis muscle and musculocutaneous flaps can be reliably used to close chest-wall defects.

References

1. Drever JM. The epigastric island flap. *Plast Reconstr Surg* 1977;59:343.
2. Neale HW, Kreilein JG, Schreiber JT, Gregory RO. Complete sternectomy for chronic osteomyelitis with reconstruction using a rectus abdominis myocutaneous island flap. *Ann Plast Surg* 1981;6:305.
3. Dinner MI, Labandter HP, Dowden RV. Role of the rectus abdominis myocutaneous flap in breast reconstruction. *Plast Reconstr Surg* 1982; 69:209.
4. Mathes SJ, Bostwick J III. A rectus abdominis myocutaneous flap to reconstruct abdominal wall defects. *Br J Plast Surg* 1977;30:382.
5. Dupont C, Menard Y. Transposition of the greater omentum for reconstruction of the chest wall. *Plast Reconstr Surg* 1972;49:263.
6. Lee AB, Schimert G, Shatkin S. Total excision of the sternum and thoracic pedicle transposition of the greater omentum: useful stratagems in managing

severe mediastinal infection following open heart surgery. *Surgery* 1976;80:433.

7. Jurkiewicz MJ, Arnold PG. The omentum. *Ann Surg* 1977;185:548.
8. Arnold PG, Pairolero PC. Use of pectoralis major muscle flaps to repair defects of anterior chest wall. *Plast Reconstr Surg* 1979;63:205.
9. Jurkiewicz MJ, Bostwick J III, Hester TR, et al. Infected median sternotomy wound. *Ann Surg* 1980;191:738.
10. Arnold PG. Reconstruction of the sternum and anterior chest wall. *Clin Plast Surg* 1981;8:389.
11. McCraw JB, Dibbell DG, Carraway JH. Clinical definition of independent myocutaneous vascular territories. *Plast Reconstr Surg* 1977;60:341.
12. McCraw JB, Penix JO, Baker JW. Repair of major defects of the chest wall and spine with the latissimus dorsi myocutaneous flap. *Plast Reconstr Surg* 1978;62:197.

13. Cervino AL, Bales HW, Emerson GL. Tissue transfers for functional reconstruction in thoracic surgery. *Plast Reconstr Surg* 1974;54:437.
14. Lewin LR, Guthrie RH, Kovachev D. One-stage coverage of the large chest-wall defect with a giant bipedicled flap. *Plast Reconstr Surg* 1975; 56:336.
15. Davis WM, McCraw JB, Carraway JH. Use of a direct, transverse thoracoabdominal flap to close difficult wounds of the thorax and upper extremity. *Plast Reconstr Surg* 1977;60:526.
16. Baroudi R, Pinotti M, Keppke EM. A transverse thoracoabdominal skin flap for closure after radical mastectomy. *Plast Reconstr Surg* 1978; 61:547.
17. Daniel RK, Kerrigan CL, Gard DA. The great potential of the intercostal flap for torso reconstruction. *Plast Reconstr Surg* 1978;61:653.

CHAPTER 393 ■ INTERCOSTAL NEUROVASCULAR MUSCULOCUTANEOUS-RIB FLAP

J. W. LITTLE, III

EDITORIAL COMMENT

The complexity of the dissection has made this flap underutilized; most problems can be solved with microvascular surgery.

The intercostal neurovascular island skin flap has been introduced as a mobile and versatile tissue system for general and sensory reconstruction of the trunk (1–4).

An expanded transpleural technique has been recommended that allows one-stage transfer of the entire upper-quadrant abdominal wall with attached contralateral upper quadrant or ipsilateral lower-quadrant extensions (5,6). This expansion was designed to allow undelayed transfer of large, extended paddles (see Chapter 451).

This expansion is not required for flaps limited to or slightly beyond the costal margin, as is true of rib-containing flaps transferred to thoracic defects. However, while the extrapleural technique suffices, I continue to recommend the transpleural one for greater ease and speed of execution and a greater measure of safety when larger skin islands are elevated on a single intercostal bundle.

INDICATIONS

A skeletal strut across a significant thoracic defect can serve only to reduce paradoxical motion and would therefore appear indicated in those defects, where available. Unfortunately, the most disabling functional defects occur along the anterior thoracic midline after loss of the manubrium, sternum, and costal cartilages and thus remain out of reach of this flap.

Conversely, dorsal defects that are within easy reach rarely demonstrate significant paradoxical impairment because of the limited excursion of the posterior component of the thoracic bellows, the greater stability of its heavier musculature and scapula, and the purely bony nature of its ribs.

Therefore, defects most likely to be helped by this technique are those of the anterolateral thorax (Fig. 1). Here, in truth, the major impact of skeletal support is likely to be aesthetic rather than functional in nature. Isolated lateral thoracic defects with significant functional impairment through paradoxical motion would be of such large size as to effectively exceed the ability of the described flap to achieve meaningful stabilization.

While the extrapleural technique can be used in raising these shorter flaps, there are certain advantages to the transpleural method. The rib segment remains protected on its exposed deep aspect by a layer of parietal pleura, with the soft parts of the paddle covered by fascia. Inclusion of the entire interspace, as well as abdominal wall, both speeds and simplifies dissection and ensures survival of the larger paddles on a single bundle. In the primary repair of full-thickness defects, the thorax is already breached and a chest tube is already a requirement.

Rib also can be transferred to other areas such as the spine, where hard-tissue protection or stabilization may be desired (Fig. 2).

ANATOMY

See Chapter 451.

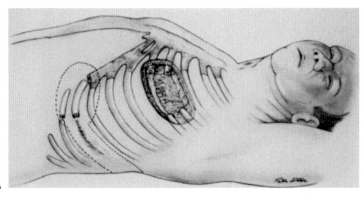
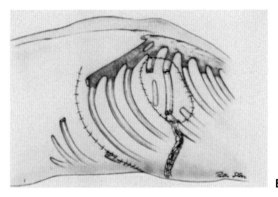

FIG. 1. **A:** Defect involving loss of anterolateral fourth and fifth ribs; T9 pedicle outlined to transfer ninth rib (including small portion of tenth). **B:** Defect stabilized and closed.

FLAP DESIGN AND DIMENSIONS

Rib length within the flap is determined by the requirements of the skeletal defect and limited by the requirements of pedicle length that remains as the difference between total rib length (measured from sacrospinalis to costal margin) and the desired length for transfer. The skin paddle can extend in length across the midline, but rarely exceeds much beyond the costal margin. Paddle width is determined by the requirements of the defect. A typical paddle measures up to 15 × 15 cm. The pivot point of this island flap occurs at the intersection of the selected interspace with the lateral border of the

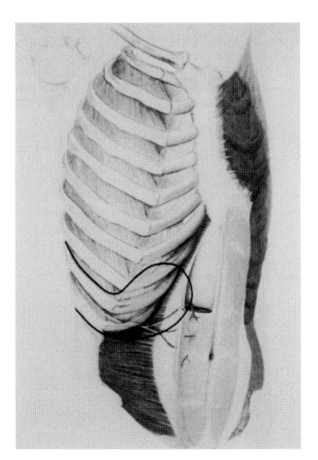

FIG. 2. Planned incision.

sacrospinalis muscle, one handbreadth off the spine. The arc of rotation falls some few centimeters within the free border of the pectoralis major muscle, thus excluding most of the thorax covered by this muscle, as well as the manubrium, sternum, and xyphoid (Fig. 1).

OPERATIVE TECHNIQUE

The terminal portion of the ninth, tenth, or occasionally another rib is selected for transfer to the thoracic defect and is indicated on the chest wall to an appropriate length. The skin paddle is then marked with the rib segment central and with its length and width expanded to meet skin requirements that may be in excess of skeletal ones. The intercostal space of the selected rib becomes the flap pedicle, and the spaces above and below are marked as superior and inferior margins and are blended to the composite paddle (Fig. 3).

The pedicle margins are incised to fascia and carried at this level down to the selected rib above and up to its inferior neighbor below, where they are deepened through muscle and periosteum onto the ribs themselves. The selected rib is removed subperiosteally from the sacrospinalis muscle to the measured point beyond which the rib will be maintained and carried in the paddle.

The thorax is entered through the midportion of the periosteal bed over this extent. The superior border of the lower rib is then freed subperiosteally, and without removing this rib, the superior aspect of its bed is similarly entered behind the rib.

Once the pedicle has been completed by rapid, full-thickness cuts into the thoracic cavity, the composite paddle is dissected. That portion overlying the thorax is incised through skin, fat, and fascia onto muscle and is elevated with the fascia from denuded slips of serratus anterior and external oblique abdominis muscle until reaching the inter-space superior to the selected rib above and the neighboring inferior rib below. That portion extending beyond the costal margin is incised through skin, fat, and abdominal wall muscle onto peritoneum, except for any portion overlying rectus muscle. Because the skin paddle of this shortened, composite flap rarely extends to the midline, it is unnecessary to include rectus muscle within the flap, anterior rectus sheath alone sufficing.

The dissection is carried between transversus abdominis muscle and peritoneum, continuing laterally beneath the costal margin until the diaphragm is reached. The paddle and the pedicle are then joined. Above, the incision through periosteal rib bed is shifted upward to the interspace above

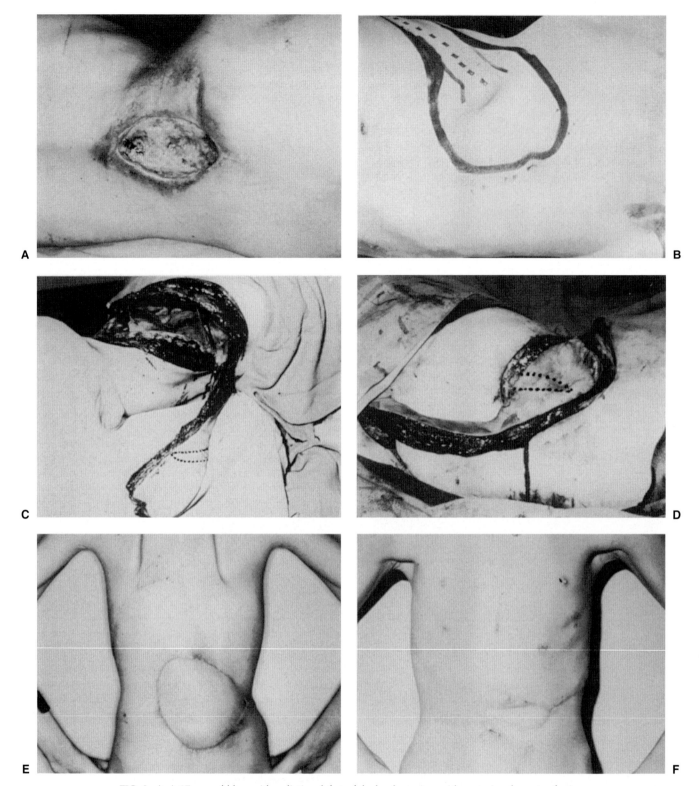

FIG. 3. A: A 17-year-old boy with radiation defect of the lumbar spine, with posterior elements of spine missing and cord unprotected. **B:** T9 pedicle flap will carry portion of tenth rib to spine. **C:** Flap elevated with rib segment indicated; secondary abdominothoracic defect. **D:** Rib segment will be fixed to remaining laminae over cord. **E,F:** Wounds healed at 6 weeks.

and is made full-thickness through that interspace until joined to the abdominal part. Below, the incision continues through the periosteal bed of the lower retained rib until that structure curves upward at the costal margin to cross the intercostal bundle of the selected interspace as it leaves the thorax to enter the abdominal wall.

Here, the lower incision is continued at the same transverse level, cutting across the terminal curved portion of the lower rib and including it within the flap. This situation occurs regularly when the ninth interspace is used, including a portion of chondral tenth rib in the flap. It does not occur when the lower tenth interspace is used. A small portion of diaphragmatic muscle is included as thoracic and abdominal portions are joined, ensuring full inclusion of transversus muscle. The flap can be raised in less than 1 hour.

The thoracic and abdominal defect is closed as described in Chapter 451. As long as the flap has not been expanded, direct closure of the muscle layers in the abdominal wall should suffice.

CLINICAL RESULTS

Rib-containing flaps have been raised to and beyond the midline in six instances without tissue loss (see Chapter 451). There have been no complications following the transfer of such rib-containing flaps. All chest tubes were removed during the first week, following an unremarkable pulmonary course in all patients. Vertical shortening of the hemithorax through rib resection and intercostal closure has produced no postural deformity.

SUMMARY

The intercostal neurovascular island skin flap can be extended to include rib for anterolateral and posterior chest-wall reconstruction. Its application, although limited, is useful when larger flaps (see Chapter 451) including abdominal wall are deemed unnecessary.

References

1. Dibbel DG. Use of a long island flap to bring sensation to the sacral area in young paraplegics: case report. *Plast Reconstr Surg* 1974;54:220.
2. Daniel RK, Terzis JK, Cunningham DM. Sensory skin flaps for coverage of pressure sores in paraplegic patients: a preliminary report. *Plast Reconstr Surg* 1976;58:317.
3. Daniel RK, Kerrigan CL, Gard DA. The great potential of the intercostal flap for torso reconstruction. *Plast Reconstr Surg* 1978;61:653.
4. Kerrigan CL, Daniel RK. The intercostal flap: Anatomical and hemodynamic approach. *Ann Plast Surg* 1979;2:411.
5. Little JW, Fontana DJ, McCulloch DT. The upper quadrant flap. *Plast Reconstr Surg* 1981;68:175.
6. Daniel RK. The upper quadrant flap (Discussion). *Plast Reconstr Surg* 1981;68:183.

ABDOMINAL WALL AND PELVIC-REGION RECONSTRUCTION

CHAPTER 394 ■ LOCAL SKIN FLAPS

W. C. TRIER

The abdominal wall and groin are more commonly thought of as donor sites for skin flaps and skin grafts rather than as recipient sites to which transfer of local flaps is required.

INDICATIONS

Abdominal skin is the most appropriate source of a skin flap to another area of the abdomen if the defect is not too large. Of prime importance is whether or not the deep fasciae of the abdominal wall are intact (1–8).

Suprafascial Skin Defects

Long experience with use of the abdomen as a donor site for skin flaps makes it quite obvious that when suprafascial skin defects cannot be closed by simple undermining of the abdominal skin in the fascial–subcutaneous tissue plane, reconstruction ordinarily should be accomplished using a partial-thickness skin graft.

In the presence of radiation dermatitis or necrosis, however, skin grafts may fail to vascularize or survive. Flaps are then required. Local flaps (which carry their own blood supply) not only survive, but remain viable, since their pedicles do not require division. Furthermore, such flaps may improve blood supply to the recipient site.

Subfascial Skin Defects

Subfascial abdominal skin defects require reconstruction of the supporting deep fasciae of the abdominal wall as well as skin coverage. Such defects result from trauma (commonly shotgun wounds), tumor resection, and radiation necrosis.

Free fascial grafts and synthetic allografts of tantalum, Mersilene®, or Marlex® require cover by well-vascularized skin and subcutaneous tissue (1–10).

ANATOMY

The skin of the ventral surface of the body is loose and quite mobile over both the thorax and the abdomen, but more adherent over the flanks and back and just caudal to the inguinal ligaments.

The more superficial layer of subcutaneous tissue, Camper's fascia, contains adipose tissue of varying thickness. This layer is continuous with subcutaneous fasciae of the thorax, back, and thighs, becoming tougher and more dense over the back. The deeper layer, Scarpa's fascia, is described as membranous in nature, contains little or no adipose tissue, and is composed largely of elastic tissue fibers. Scarpa's fascia forms a continuous layer over the abdomen and is attached to the linea alba in the center of the lower abdomen as well as to the investing fascia of the thigh muscles at a level one or two fingerbreadths below the inguinal ligament (11,12).

Vascular Anatomy

Cutaneous Arteries

Except for the area of the abdomen and groin supplied by branches of the femoral artery, the only large cutaneous arteries of the abdominal wall emerge medial to the semilunar lines of the abdomen (11). This suggests that medially based flaps nourished by these vessels might be similar to such flaps as the deltopectoral flap, based on perforating branches of the internal mammary artery. Flaps based laterally, anterior to the latissimus dorsi muscle, appear to be cutaneous (random pattern) in nature (Figs. 1 and 2).

Musculocutaneous Arteries

Transversely disposed segmental series of perforating musculocutaneous branches of intercostal, subcostal, and lumbar arteries provide blood supply to the subcutaneous tissue and skin across the entire abdominal wall, except for the area of the abdominal skin overlying the rectus muscles medial to the semilunar lines, which receive blood from the musculocutaneous branches of the deep superior and inferior epigastric vessels.

The perforating branches of the intercostal, subcostal, and lumbar arteries arise as two main branches, posterior and lateral. The lateral branches penetrate the oblique abdominal muscles just anterior to the latissimus dorsi muscle and pass obliquely downward to provide blood supply to the anterior abdominal wall. The posterior branches supply the back muscles and skin (12), as do the primary arterial pedicles of such muscles as the latissimus dorsi.

The vertical arterial supply is provided by branches of the superior deep epigastric artery, the continuation of the internal mammary artery, and from the inferior deep epigastric artery, a branch of the external iliac artery. These vessels pass through the rectus muscles and their fasciae to the subcutaneous fasciae and skin. Thus flaps, arterial in type, may be raised transversely based on these perforating vessels, while musculocutaneous flaps can be raised in the vertical direction.

Arterial Flaps

The superficial vertical abdominal and inguinal vascular branches of the femoral artery provide two axial flaps: the hypogastric flap (13), based on the superficial inferior epigastric vessels, and the groin flap (14,15), based on the superficial circumflex iliac vessels (Fig. 2).

FLAP DESIGN AND DIMENSIONS

Transposition or rotation flaps based laterally in the lower thorax, back, or upper or lower abdomen must be considered cutaneous flaps. Local arterial skin flaps, suitable for the reconstruction of suprafascial abdominal defects, include the deltopectoral (16), thoracoepigastric (17), groin (14,15,18), and superficial epigastric flaps (13,19). Scrotal flaps can be useful on occasion (20,21).

The deltopectoral flap may be used to repair upper medial abdominal defects (16) (see Chapter 124). The thoracoepigastric flap (17), felt to be the equivalent of the medially based

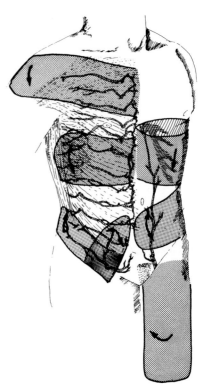

FIG. 2. To the left (right side of torso) are arterial flaps based on cutaneous arteries, deltopectoral, thoracoepigastric, groin, and hypogastric, superimposed over their intrinsic arteries. To the right (left side of torso) are bipedicle advancement flaps (both arterial and cutaneous) and laterally based cutaneous flaps. (Redrawn from Brown et al., ref. 11, with permission.)

deltopectoral flap, is supplied by the perforating vessels of the rectus abdominis muscle. Measuring up to 12 × 30 cm, it extends distally to the anterior axillary line. However, its use is avoided when based below the level of the umbilicus, because of the dominance of the external oblique circulation in that area.

The groin flap (14,15,18), based on the superficial circumflex iliac artery, may be prolonged beyond the anterosuperior iliac spine (see Chapter 300). The hypogastric flap (13,19) may be used untubed as a local arterial flap. Based on the superficial epigastric artery, the flap may measure up to 7 cm in width and 18 cm in length. Adjustment to the point of origin of the medial and lateral incisions bordering the flap permits rotation of the flap medially or laterally.

SUMMARY

The abdomen and groin are traditional donor areas for skin flaps, both cutaneous and arterial. However, local skin flaps infrequently may be required for the reconstruction of these areas.

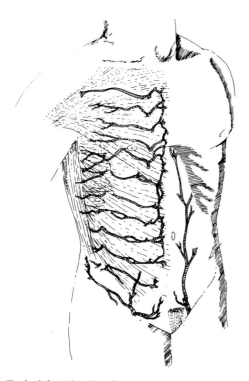

FIG. 1. To the left (right side of torso) are anterior and lateral perforating branches of the cutaneous vascular supply of the anterior abdominal wall. Inferiorly, in the inguinal region, are the cutaneous branches of the femoral, superficial epigastric, superficial circumflex iliac, and superficial external pudendal arteries. To the right (left side of torso) are the superior deep epigastric and inferior deep epigastric arteries. (Redrawn from Brown et al., ref. 11, with permission.)

References

1. Wangensteen OH. Repair of large abdominal defects by pedicled fascial flaps. *Surg Gynecol Obstet* 1946;82:144.
2. McPeak CJ, Miller TR. Abdominal wall replacement. *Surgery* 1960;47:944.
3. Hershey FB, Butcher HR. Repair of defects after partial resection of the abdominal wall. *Am J Surg* 1964;107:586.
4. Medgyesi S. The repair of large incisional hernias with pedicle skin flaps. *Scand J Plast Reconstr Surg* 1972;6:69.
5. Mansberger AR, Kang JS, Beebe HG, Le Flore I. Repair of massive acute abdominal wall defects. *J Trauma* 1973;13:766.

6. Pokorny WJ, Thal AP. A method for primary closure of large contaminated abdominal wall defects. *J Trauma* 1973;13:542.
7. Wilson JSP, Rayner CRW. The repair of large full-thickness postexcisional defects of the abdominal wall. *Br J Plast Surg* 1974;27:117.
8. Earle AS, Blackburn WW. Closure for abdominal hernia with a groin flap lined with a dermal graft. *Plast Reconstr Surg* 1975;56:447.
9. Ye RC, Devine KD, Kirklin, JW. Extensive recurrent desmoid tumor of the abdominal wall: radical excision followed by reconstruction of the abdominal wall with plastic procedure. *Plast Reconstr Surg* 1953; 12:59.
10. Pridgen JE, Tennison CW. Reconstruction of the entire abdominal wall in the presence of postradiation changes. *Am J Surg* 1956;92:54.
11. Brown RG, Vasconez LO, Jurkiewicz MJ. Transverse abdominal flaps and the deep epigastric arcade. *Plast Reconstr Surg* 1975;55:416.
12. Nahai F, Brown RG, Vasconez LO. Blood supply to the abdominal wall as related to planning abdominal incisions. *Am Surg* 1976;42:691.
13. Shaw DT, Payne RL. One-staged tubed abdominal flaps. In: Grabb WC, Myers MB, eds. *Skin flaps.* Boston: Little, Brown, 1975.
14. McGregor IA. The groin flap. In: Grabb WC, Myers MB, eds. *Skin flaps.* Boston: Little, Brown, 1975.
15. McGregor IA, Morgan G. Axial and random pattern flaps. *Br J Plast Surg* 1973;26:202.
16. McGregor IA. Skin flaps. In: McGregor IA, ed. *Fundamental techniques of plastic surgery,* 7th ed. Edinburgh: Churchill Livingstone, 1980.
17. McCraw JB, Dibbell DG, Carraway JH. Clinical definition of independent myocutaneous vascular territories. *Plast Reconstr Surg* 1977;60:341.
18. Bogart JN, Rowe DS, Parsons RW. Immediate abdominal wall reconstruction with bilateral groin flaps after resection of a large desmoid tumor. *Plast Reconstr Surg* 1976;58:716.
19. Aston SJ, Pickrell KL. Reconstructive surgery of the abdominal wall. In: Converse JM, ed. *Reconstructive plastic surgery.* Philadelphia: Saunders, 1977.
20. Arconti JS, Goodwin WE. Use of scrotal skin to cover wound defects in the groin and pubic area. *J Urol* 1956;75:292.
21. Lanier VC, Neale HW. Necrosis of penis with decubitus ulcer: Debridement and closure with scrotal flap. *Plast Reconstr Surg* 1974;54:609.

CHAPTER 395 ■ TRANSPOSITION SKIN FLAP TO THE GROIN

M. B. CONSTANTIAN

A transverse lower abdominal flap can comfortably reach the groin and anterior thigh regions. The flap may be based medially or laterally, depending on the shape and location of the defect.

INDICATIONS

Deep wounds or pressure ulcers of the anterior trochanteric or anterior thigh regions may require a flap for repair.

ANATOMY (1)

Perforating muscular branches of the intercostal, subcostal, lumbar, deep epigastric, and superficial inferior epigastric arteries supply the flap from each end.

FLAP DESIGN AND DIMENSIONS

Based medially, the transverse abdominal flap has an axial blood supply. A surgical delay is not necessary, providing that the perforating branches of the deep epigastric arcade are preserved.

Based laterally, delay is mandatory if the flap is long. The dimensions required of the flap depend, of course, on the size and orientation of the defect but can safely approach 10 × 30 cm if the appropriate precautions regarding delay and tissue handling are observed.

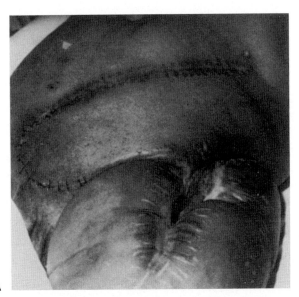

A

FIG. 1. **A:** Deep anterior thigh defect resulting from wound dehiscence after proximal femoral resection. Design of delayed abdominal flap. (*Continued*)

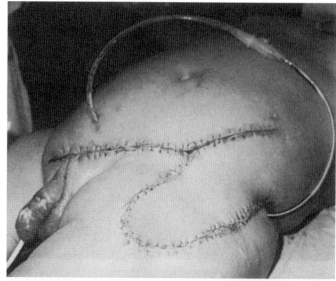

B

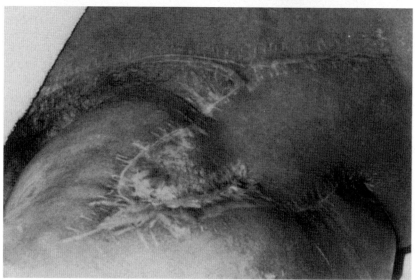

C

FIG. 1. *Continued.* B: Defect excised, and the flap inset. C: Result 7 months postoperatively.

OPERATIVE TECHNIQUE

If a delay is required, it is usually performed in two stages, by first raising the flap as a bipedicle flap and then sectioning the distal end separately 7 to 14 days later (Fig. 1B).

The surgeon should raise the flap at the level of the deep fascia, mobilizing the pedicle only enough for transfer. The donor site can be closed primarily if the noted dimensions have been observed. Adequate suction drainage is advisable, since the area of the dissection is large.

CLINICAL RESULTS

The complications that follow this procedure relate to the flap and the defect. The surgeon can minimize flap loss, seroma, and infection by careful wound preparation and tissue handling, proper drainage, and the use of antibiotics where indicated (2).

Further, the surgeon should be sensitive to the peculiarities of the defect regarding joint involvement, heterotopic calcifications, and abnormalities of any of the local bursae (which occur between the greater trochanter and the gluteus maximus, between the gluteus medius and gluteus minimus muscles, and between the tendons of the gluteus maximus and vastus lateralis muscles).

SUMMARY

A transposition skin flap from the abdomen can be used to cover groin defects.

References

1. Brown RG, Vasconez LO, Jurkiewicz MJ. Transverse abdominal flaps and the deep epigastric arcade. *Plast Reconstr Surg* 1975;55:416.
2. Constantian MB, Jackson HS. In: Constantian MB, ed. *Pressure ulcers: principles and techniques of management.* Boston: Little, Brown, 1980.

CHAPTER 396 ■ GROIN SKIN FLAP FOR COVERAGE OF ABDOMINAL WALL DEFECTS

A. S. EARLE AND C. VLASTOU

The groin flap (1) is used regularly by many reconstructive surgeons, particularly for covering soft-tissue defects of the hand. It is also used as a free flap, perhaps more frequently in the past than at present. The groin flap and related lower abdominal flaps also can be used to resurface abdominal wall defects (1–3).

INDICATIONS

Extended groin flaps will reach any portion of the abdomen and above the ipsilateral rib margin to include the lower anterior chest. The groin flap may be the method of choice for covering radiation and other chronic ulcerations of the abdominal wall.

By including free fascia lata or dermis, the groin flap can be used to repair an associated abdominal wall hernia (2).

ANATOMY

The groin flap is a vascularized axial flap based on the superficial circumflex iliac artery (SCIA) arising from the femoral artery just below the inguinal ligament. The SCIA passes through the deep fascia into the subcutaneous tissues lateral to the fossa ovalis at or close to the lateral border of the sartorius muscle. The artery then passes diagonally upward and laterally parallel to and 2 to 3 cm below the inguinal ligament. This relationship is maintained as far lateral as the ligament attachment at the anterior superior iliac spine (ASIS).

The vessel can be dissected or followed with a Doppler probe in many subjects to the point at which it divides into several branches supplying the skin and subcutaneous tissues. It also anastomoses with branches of the superficial epigastric artery (SEA), with the deep circumflex iliac artery, and with the lateral femoral circumflex arterial system.

The superficial circumflex iliac venous drainage is variable laterally, but a discrete vessel follows the proximal artery. The vein remains in the subcutaneous tissues, however, rather than becoming subfascial and then joins the saphenous vein in the fossa ovalis.

It should be mentioned that the SCIA and the SEA are parallel arterial systems and that one or the other may be dominant and able to replace the other vessel to some extent. The higher SEA may be considerably larger and, at times, is the only one that can be picked up with the Doppler probe. If so, the groin flap may then be designed to make use of the SEA, rather than the SCIA, as the axial vessel of the flap (see Fig. 1).

FLAP DESIGN AND DIMENSIONS

In designing the flap, the inguinal ligament is palpated and marked in its course between the pubic tubercle medially and the ASIS laterally (Fig. 1). The ligament may be found considerably higher than the visible groin crease, particularly in older or obese patients. Whenever possible, the SCIA is identified with the Doppler probe and appropriately marked. (If the SCIA cannot be identified, the SEA may be sought, passing across the inguinal ligament and angling diagonally upward; see Fig. 3).

The flap should then be marked out extending upward and outward, beginning at the projected lateral border of the sartorius and with the upper and lower borders of the flap 5 cm (more or less as needed) above and below the vessel axis. Length can then be determined by planning backward from the defect to be covered. An undelayed flap will survive dependably for at least 5 cm beyond the ASIS and may be used to cover ipsilateral lower abdominal wall defects. A defect of the upper abdomen or lower anterior chest will require the use of an extended, delayed flap. If this further length is required, the flap outline may be carried laterally at least to the lateral margin of the sacrospinalis muscle as a delayed bipedicle flap.

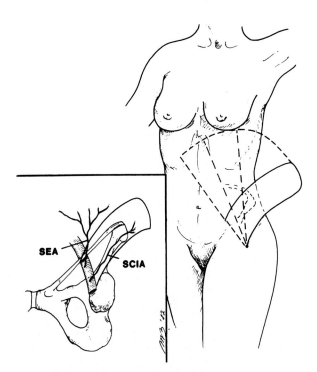

FIG. 1. The extended (delayed) groin flap and the vascular anatomy are outlined. The arc of rotation reaching above the ipsilateral margin of the chest wall is also indicated.

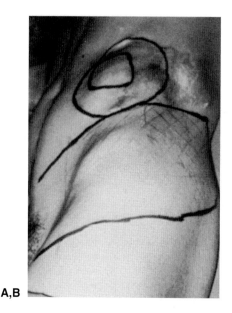
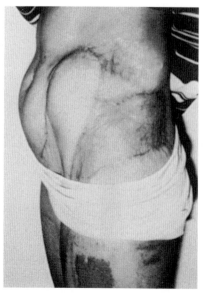

A,B

FIG. 2. **A:** This 41-year-old-woman presented with a painful left upper quadrant hernia, the result of a shotgun wound, repaired with tantalum mesh. The skin over the mesh was paper-thin, with protruding fragmented wire ends. The proposed large groin flap is outlined below. The area occupied by tantalum mesh is the larger area above, with the inner circle representing the herniation. **B:** One year later, the hernia is shown repaired, with dermal graft-lined extended groin flap. The site of the repair bulges less than the remainder of the abdominal wall. (From Earle, Blackburn, ref. 2, with permission.)

OPERATIVE TECHNIQUE

Although the flap is elevated at the level of the deep fascia medially (watch for and avoid injury to the SCIA in approaching the lateral margin of the sartorius during the medial dissection), this plane is lost laterally in the flank, where the subcutaneous tissue should be thinned appropriately. In some patients, direct closure of the donor-site defect is possible, but if the flap is large, the defect will require skin-grafting.

If the groin flap is used for coverage of a hernial defect, support must be provided at the level of the hernial ring. Free fascia lata or dermis are preferred; synthetic mesh is, in our opinion, a poor second choice. We have successfully used dermis to line a groin flap in the repair of an upper quadrant hernia with skin breakdown secondary to fragmentation of tantalum mesh (2) (Fig. 2).

CLINICAL RESULTS

Abdominal defects are, in our experience at least, far less common than those of the chest wall. We have had occasion to use three groin flaps for treatment of sizable abdominal wall defects (one hernia and two radiation reactions). The flaps have proven successful in each patient. In one of our patients, the flap was designed above the inguinal ligament, as described earlier, and carried into the flank based on the SEA vessel, which apparently was a dominant vessel arising from the groin (Fig. 3). We have skin-grafted the donor area in all our patients, but our flaps have necessarily been wide to cover sizable defects. We have experienced no significant complications.

SUMMARY

The groin flap represents a good and safe method for covering defects of the abdominal wall.

References

1. McGregor IA, Jackson IT. The groin flap. *Br J Plast Surg* 1972;25:3.
2. Earle AS, Blackburn WW. Closure of an abdominal hernia with a groin flap lined with a dermal graft. *Plast Reconstr Surg* 1975;56:447.
3. Bogart JN, Rowe DS, Parsons RW. Immediate abdominal wall reconstruction with bilateral groin flaps after resection of a large desmoid tumor. *Plast Reconstr Surg* 1976;58:716.

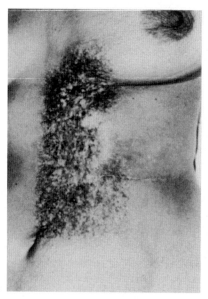
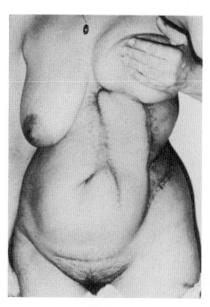

A,B

FIG. 3. **A:** This 57-year-old woman 10 years earlier received orthovoltage radiation for melanoma with subsequent development of severe radiation reaction and early ulceration. Note the extent of the radiation changes reaching from umbilicus to breast. **B:** An extended flap based in this patient on the SEA rather than the SCIA was used for coverage of the defect after excision of the radiated area.

CHAPTER 397 ■ GROIN SKIN FLAP FOR CONTRALATERAL GROIN DEFECTS

I. A. MCGREGOR AND D. S. SOUTAR

The application of groin skin flaps for abdominal wall defects was discussed in Chapter 396. This chapter illustrates how the groin flap can be used to cover defects in the opposite groin.

INDICATIONS

The indications for local transposition of a groin flap are rare, but it is available for this purpose, should the need arise.

FLAP DESIGN AND DIMENSIONS

The flap can be transferred within a range approximating a circle around its base, and this would bring the contralateral groin within its compass (1). With the pivot point of any transfer established, the geometry necessary to calculate the dimensions of the flap appropriate to the transfer are easy to establish (Fig. 1).

For other details of the groin flap, see Chapter 300.

Reference

1. McGregor IA, Jackson, IT. The groin flap. *Br J Plast Surg* 1972;25:3.

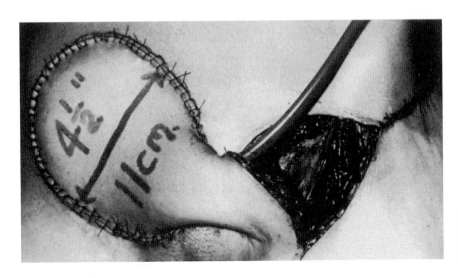

FIG. 1. A groin flap that is 11 cm wide has been used to cover a contralateral groin defect. Note that the donor site is being closed primarily.

CHAPTER 398. Omental Flap for Coverage of Exposed Groin Vessels *R. H Samson*
www.encyclopediaofflaps.com

CHAPTER 399 ■ RECTUS FEMORIS FLAP

W. Y. HOFFMAN AND G. TRENGOVE-JONES

The rectus femoris flap, with its wide arc of rotation, allows reconstruction of the lower abdominal wall, perineum, and trochanteric regions (1–5). It can be used with its overlying cutaneous territory or isolated as a free flap in microvascular transfer (6).

INDICATIONS

The rectus femoris will easily reach the trochanteric, ischial, and perineal regions for closure of pressure sores. In reconstruction of the lower abdominal wall, the rectus femoris is preferred over the tensor fasciae latae, which must pivot further laterally and has a less reliable skin island. Several reports refer to the use of an anterior skin and muscle flap in reconstruction following hemipelvectomy for posterior tumors (4). Obviously, the femoral vessels must be preserved during dissection to guarantee flap survival. The flap also has been used for closure of dead space after a failed total hip arthroplasty (5) and as a free neurovascular flap for replacement of lost forearm muscles (6).

ANATOMY

The rectus femoris is the most anterior muscle of the quadriceps group, originating in two heads from the anterosuperior iliac spine and the upper crest of the acetabulum and inserting conjointly into the patellar tendon with the vastus lateralis, medialis, and intermedius. The muscle fibers attenuate into tendon approximately 6 cm above the upper border of the patella.

The vascular supply is from the descending branch of the lateral circumflex femoral artery (a branch of the profunda femoris) that is 1.5 to 2.0 mm in diameter, accompanied by paired venae comitantes and located approximately 8 cm below the level of the inguinal ligament. It enters the muscle on its deep surface. If the main pedicle is preserved, one or two minor pedicles distal to the main vascular trunk can usually be divided.

A branch of the femoral nerve innervates the muscle and enters the muscle at the same level as the vascular pedicle. The overlying skin is innervated by the intermediate cutaneous nerve of the thigh, a sensory branch of the femoral nerve that can be used to create a neurosensory flap.

Three to four musculocutaneous perforators that arise in the proximal portion of the muscle and, to a lesser extent, in the fasciocutaneous vessels arising in the intermuscular septae vascularize the skin. Thus the lower two-thirds of the muscle can be disassociated from the underlying muscle to increase the surface-covering capacity of this flap.

FLAP DESIGN AND DIMENSIONS

This muscle will support a skin island that can include the anterior third of the thigh. Flaps as large as 15 × 40 cm have been reported, and if the skin island is less than 6 to 7 cm wide, primary closure can be achieved. The skin island is designed directly over the muscle, taking care to include the important proximal musculocutaneous perforators (2,3).

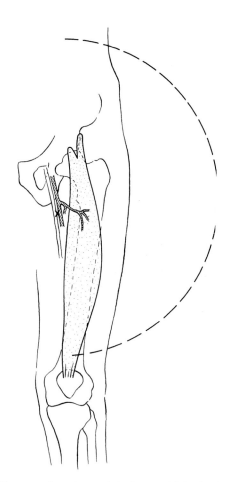

FIG. 1. The rectus femoris muscle is shown with its dominant vascular pedicle, a branch of the profunda femoris. Note that the pivot point is 8 to 10 cm *below* the inguinal ligament, and this limits the superior rotation of the flap.

1140

The muscle pivots about the neurovascular pedicle located some 8 cm from the inguinal ligament (3); this limits the arc of rotation somewhat (Fig. 1). Within easy reach of the rectus femoris are the trochanteric region, the perineum, and the pubic symphysis. However, because of the low pivot point, the umbilicus represents the upper limit of the abdominal wall that can be reconstructed with this flap.

OPERATIVE TECHNIQUE

The skin flap is incised down to the muscular fascia, and the skin edges are sewn to this fascia to prevent shearing of the important musculocutaneous vessels. The muscle or musculocutaneous unit should be elevated from distal to proximal and from lateral to medial until the dominant pedicle is identified. By dividing the muscle at least 6 cm above the patella, the tendinous insertion is preserved. The tendons of the vastus lateralis and medialis are centralized with stout sutures to preserve full knee extension, and the donor defect is closed primarily or, if it is too wide to permit direct closure, with a skin graft.

CLINICAL RESULTS

The rectus femoris flap has been shown to be extremely hardy and reliable in a small clinical series of patients. Skin loss was rare, but a few patients reported some weakness in the terminal extension of their knees. Most others had no discernible deficits, and all patients were ambulatory.

SUMMARY

The rectus femoris flap can be used even in ambulatory patients to reconstruct defects around the lower abdominal wall, perineum, and trochanter.

References

1. McCraw JB, Dibbell JB, Carraway JH. Clinical definitions of myocutaneous vascular territories. *Plast Reconstr Surg* 1977;60:341.
2. Bhagwat BM, Pearl RM, Laub DR. Uses of the rectus femoris myocutaneous flap. *Plast Reconstr Surg* 1978;62:698.
3. Mathes SJ, Nahai F, eds. *Clinical applications for muscle and musculocutaneous flaps.* St. Louis: Mosby, 1982.
4. Sugarbaker PH, Chretien PA. Hemipelvectomy for buttock tumors utilizing an anterior myocutaneous flap of quadriceps femoris muscle. *Ann Surg* 1983;197:106.
5. Arnold PG, Witzke DJ. Management of failed total hip arthroplasty with muscle flaps. *Ann Plast Surg* 1983;11:474.
6. Schenck PR. Rectus femoris muscle and composite skin transplantation by microneurovascular anastomoses for avulsion of forearm muscles: a case report. *J Hand Surg* 1978;3:60.

CHAPTER 400 ■ RECTUS ABDOMINIS FLAP FOR GROIN DEFECTS

J. BUNKIS AND R. L. WALTON

EDITORIAL COMMENT

Extreme care must be taken to avoid an area of potential weakness or frank hernia at the pivot point of the muscle, particularly if that point is below the semicircular line. At times, it may be better to remove the entire muscle as an island and thus obtain a more secure closure of the rectus sheath. Consideration should also be given to a transversely oriented skin paddle.

The rectus abdominis provides ample tissue for closure of groin defects. This arterialized flap can be used either as a muscle or musculocutaneous flap (1–4).

INDICATIONS

The inferiorly based rectus abdominis flap can be used to close any lower abdominal wall or groin defect caused by trauma, radiation injury, or surgical extirpation of tumor or infection. It is particularly useful following injury to the femoral vessels (with injury to the major vascular pedicles of the common thigh muscle flaps) or with exposed vascular prostheses as a result of infection or trauma (see Fig. 5A). The island modification allows the flap to reach defects over the greater trochanter. We also have employed the inferiorly based rectus abdominis musculocutaneous unit as a free flap for more distal lower extremity defects.

ANATOMY

The rectus abdominis muscles are paired anterior paramedian flexors of the vertebral column (particularly the lumbar spine), and they also serve to tense the anterior abdominal wall. Each muscle originates from the lateral head of the pubic crest and the anterior portion of the symphysis pubis (Fig. 1). The muscles each insert as three distinct slips into the costal cartilages of the fifth, sixth, and seventh ribs, deep to the lower origins of the pectoralis major muscles.

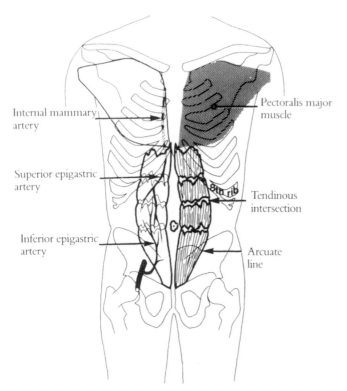

Internal mammary artery

Superior epigastric artery

Inferior epigastric artery

Pectoralis major muscle

8th rib

Tendinous intersection

Arcuate line

FIG. 1. Surgical anatomy of the rectus abdominis muscle. For coverage of groin defects, the flap is based on the ipsilateral inferior epigastric pedicle.

The rectus sheath covers the muscle along its entire length, but at the level of the anterior superior iliac spine, the posterior sheath ends at the arcuate line. Below this point, the muscles lie directly on a thin layer of transversalis fascia overlying the parietal peritoneum. Medially, the muscles are separated by the linea alba.

The width and thickness of the rectus abdominis muscle depend on the patient's physique, but generally each muscle is approximately 8 cm wide and 1 cm thick.

The lateral border of the rectus abdominis curves superiorly from the pubic tubercle through a point midway between the umbilicus and the anterior superior iliac spine and across the inferior costal margin to the fifth rib. The muscle is generally slightly broader at its insertion than at its origin.

The rectus muscle is divided into four segments by three transverse tendinous intersections. The lowest intersection is located at or just below the level of the umbilicus; the other two are equally interspersed superiorly between the umbilicus and the uppermost insertion into the fifth rib. The motor nerve supply to this muscle is segmental through branches of the seventh to the twelfth intercostal nerves, which enter the muscle on its deep surface. These branches are transected during flap elevation, and this will result in subsequent denervation atrophy of the muscle. Sensibility to the cutaneous territory is provided by anterior and lateral cutaneous nerves (T8 to T12), which are also transected during flap elevation, making this an insensate flap.

The rectus abdominis flap can be based on the vascular territory of its superior or inferior vascular pedicle. The superior epigastric artery and vein are continuations of the internal mammary vessels below the costal region. The inferior epigastric artery branches from the anteromedial surface of the external iliac artery, just above the inguinal ligament. Venous drainage from the rectus abdominis superiorly and inferiorly parallels its arterial supply. Inferiorly, two venae comitantes usually accompany the artery and empty into the external iliac vein.

The entire flap can survive on either pedicle, but for coverage of lower abdominal or groin defects, the flap is based on the ipsilateral inferior epigastric pedicle. This pedicle courses across the floor of the inguinal canal and continues in a superomedial direction (beneath the internal oblique muscle) to the lateral border of the rectus abdominis muscle at the level of or slightly below the arcuate line. The vascular pedicle can be seen clearly on the posterior surface of the muscle to the level of the umbilicus. Above this point, the pedicle enters the substance of the muscle and continues upward to anastomose with the superior epigastric vessels.

Our cadaver and clinical dissections have demonstrated considerable anatomic variations in the superior epigastric pedicle at the lower costal margin. At this level, the superior epigastric artery can usually be located within the medial third of the muscle substance. Just below this level, however, the artery may divide into a plexus of tiny arterial branches that converge inferiorly within the muscle to form the inferior epigastric artery. While raising the flap, numerous arterial and venous branches will be encountered piercing the posterior rectus sheath; these may be safely ligated.

The skin overlying the rectus abdominis is well supplied by musculocutaneous perforators. The abundant perforators, plus a reliable random territory laterally, allow transverse extensions of the skin and subcutaneous portions of the flap to be extended to the ipsilateral anterior axillary line without a prior delay procedure. Experience with superiorly based rectus abdominis musculocutaneous flaps in breast reconstruction has demonstrated that the cutaneous extension can be safely carried across the midline to the contralateral midclavicular line (Fig. 2).

FLAP DESIGN AND DIMENSIONS

Key anatomic landmarks are the fifth, sixth, and seventh costal cartilages, subcostal margin, xyphoid process, abdominal

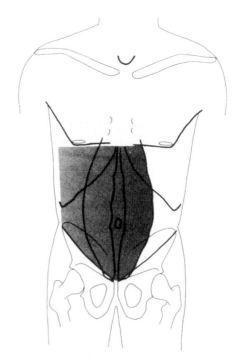

FIG. 2. Skin territory that can safely be taken with the right rectus abdominis muscle without a prior delay procedure. Extensions beyond the borders of the underlying muscle may preclude primary wound closure by approximation.

midline, pubic tubercle, lateral border of the rectus abdominis muscle (halfway between the umbilicus and the anterosuperior iliac spine), inguinal ligament, and course of the inferior epigastric vascular pedicle (Fig. 1).

The design of the flap varies according to the demands for coverage. Flaps can be designed with lengths of up to 30 cm and/or with medial or lateral cutaneous extensions, as mentioned above. The flap can be safely transposed as a peninsular flap or as an island pedicle modification. For coverage of groin defects, it is important to visualize the insertion of the inferior epigastric vascular pedicle at the lateral border of the rectus abdominis before elevation of the muscle. Below the level of the umbilicus, there is a danger of separating the vascular pedicle from the muscle.

As an ipsilateral rectus abdominis flap is rotated toward a groin defect, it passes over the inferior epigastric vessels and their origins from the external iliac artery and vein. With peninsular flap designs, the origin of the rectus abdominis muscle from the symphysis pubis will limit the flap reach. A cone of rotation is inherent in this type of flap and also will limit the reach (Fig. 3). Island pedicle modification and dissection of the inferior epigastric pedicle to the iliac vessels will extend the flap reach an additional 10 cm.

OPERATIVE TECHNIQUE

If a simple muscle flap is chosen, an incision is made along the lateral border of the ipsilateral rectus abdominis. The anterior rectus sheath is opened along its lateral margin, and the inferior epigastric pedicle is identified below the arcuate line. The muscle is then sharply dissected from the pocket of the rectus sheath. Posteriorly, below the arcuate line, the muscle is dissected from the transversus abdominis fascia. Care is exercised to avoid injury to the inferior epigastric pedicle and its attachments to the overlying muscle. After the appropriate flap length

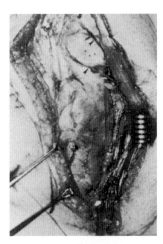

FIG. 4. Raising the flap. Lateral incision has been carried through the anterior rectus sheath and the inferior epigastric pedicle has been identified (*white arrow*). Note continuation of vascular pedicle along undersurface of rectus muscle and anastomoses with terminal branches of intercostal vessels (*black arrows*). Stay sutures secure the skin to the underlying muscle fibers and anterior rectus sheath.

is chosen, the muscle is divided superiorly (usually at one of its tendinous insertions) and transposed to the recipient defect.

Peninsular musculocutaneous versions of this flap incorporate the skin and anterior rectus fascia directly overlying the rectus muscle. A vertical incision is made along the lateral flap margin and extended through the lateral margin of the rectus sheath (Fig. 4). After identification of the inferior epigastric pedicle, the medial incision is performed, and this is extended through the medial edge of the rectus sheath. It is helpful to leave a 1-cm or greater cuff of rectus fascia medially to provide an adequate margin for subsequent fascial closure.

Several sutures are then placed through the skin margins medially and laterally to anchor the cutaneous portion of the flap to the underlying fascia and muscle. The rectus muscle is then dissected from its posterior attachments, as described above. At this point, it may be wise to occlude the superior epigastric pedicle by finger pressure and to observe the flap for capillary refill to ensure adequate inflow from the inferior epigastric system.

The flap is then divided superiorly at the appropriate level and transposed to the recipient defect. To avoid a cone of rotation and gain additional length, the cutaneous portion of the flap can be converted to an island. The rectus muscle also can be divided at its origin on the symphysis pubis to create a true musculocutaneous island pedicle flap. The flap pedicle can be lengthened by incising the internal oblique muscle laterally and dissecting the inferior epigastric vessels to their origin at the external iliac artery and vein.

The cutaneous territory of the rectus abdominis flap can be extended laterally to the anterior axillary line and medially to the contralateral midclavicular line. Elevation of these flaps begins by dissecting the cutaneous paddle above the abdominal fascia to the lateral and/or medial margin of the rectus fascia. The flap is then elevated as described above.

In positioning the flap into the groin defect, care must be taken to avoid twisting or stretching the inferior epigastric vessels. If a skin bridge separates the defect from the flap, the bridge can be divided or a portion of the flap can be deepithelialized, and the flap can be passed through a subcutaneous tunnel into the defect.

In most cases, the external oblique muscle, with its overlying fascia, can be advanced medially and sutured to the medial cuff of rectus fascia and the linea alba. If the donor fascial defect cannot be closed primarily without tension, it is best to employ a free fascial graft or synthetic mesh repair to avoid a hernia.

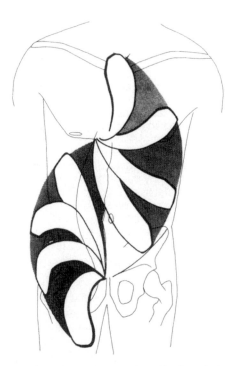

FIG. 3. Arcs of rotation of superiorly and inferiorly based rectus abdominis peninsular flaps. Note possible coverage of groin defects with an ipsilateral inferiorly based rectus flap. Island modification based on the inferior epigastric pedicle will extend the flap reach an additional 10 cm.

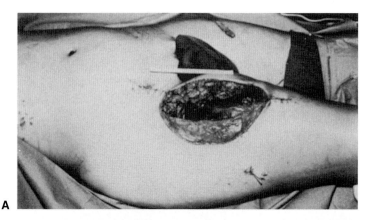

A

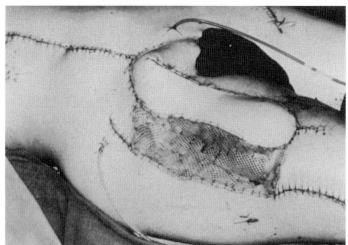

B

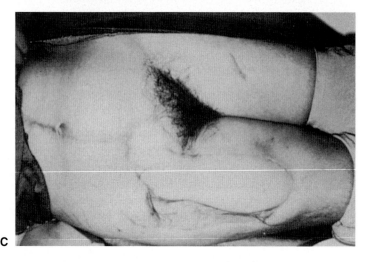

C

FIG. 5. A: Right groin defect in 45-year-old female patient following close-range 12-gauge shotgun injury. The common femoral, superficial femoral, and profunda femoris arteries have been reconstructed with a combination of autogenous and alloplastic vascular grafts. The grafts were partially covered with injured adjacent sartorius and adductor longus muscle fibers. Arteriography following vascular reconstruction demonstrated disruption of major vascular pedicles to lateral thigh muscles. B: An ipsilateral inferiorly based rectus abdominis peninsular flap has been transposed to provide coverage of the exposed vascular prostheses. A meshed skin graft was placed on the muscle lateral to the grafts to complete the reconstruction, and the wounds healed per primum. C: Postoperative result at 7 months.

If the cutaneous paddle does not extend beyond the lateral borders of the muscle, the skin can usually be closed by primary approximation. Use of an extended skin island may require a skin graft to close the secondary cutaneous defect. Generally, transversely oriented cutaneous donor sites are easily closed without complication (Fig. 5).

CLINICAL RESULTS

This is a safe, reliable flap that can be elevated expediently with the patient in a supine position. To date, we have not lost any of our rectus abdominis flaps. One must exercise caution, however, in the face of nearby previous surgical incisions.

Care also must be taken to identify the inferior epigastric vessels along the lateral border of the rectus abdominis and to ensure that the vascular pedicle maintains its attachment to the posterior muscle surface as the flap is elevated.

Attention must be paid to the closure of the donor site, particularly inferiorly, to avoid a hernia. Most unilateral flap defects can be closed without fascial grafts or mesh, but in one patient, following bilateral rectus abdominis musculocutaneous flaps, we employed Marlex® mesh to secure closure of the abdominal wall. If the abdominal wall is closed under some tension, patients will often complain of a temporary tightness.

The rectus abdominis muscle is used to flex the spine and to tighten the abdominal wall, particularly when sitting up from the supine position. We have not noticed a clinically significant functional deficit in any patient following a unilateral procedure. A major disadvantage of this flap is its lack of sensibility.

SUMMARY

The rectus abdominis muscle or musculocutaneous flap is well suited for closing lower abdominal wall or groin defects.

References

1. Drever JM. The epigastric island flap. *Plast Reconstr Surg* 1977;59:343.
2. Mathes SJ, Bostwick J III. A rectus abdominis myocutaneous flap to reconstruct abdominal wall defects. *Br J Plast Surg* 1977;30:282.
3. Mathes SJ, Nahai F, eds. *Clinical atlas of muscle and musculocutaneous flaps.* St. Louis: Mosby, 1979.
4. Nahai F, Bostwick J III, Hester TR. Experiences with the rectus abdominis flap. *Plast Surg Forum* 1980;3:157.

CHAPTER 401 ■ TENSOR FASCIAE LATAE MUSCULOCUTANEOUS FLAP FOR ABDOMINAL-WALL RECONSTRUCTION

G. W. CARLSON

The tensor fasciae latae (TFL) musculocutaneous flap is useful to provide soft-tissue coverage and fascial integrity in abdominal-wall reconstruction. It can definitively repair lower abdominal-wall defects.

INDICATIONS

The TFL musculocutaneous flap is a reliable and versatile method of reconstructing full-thickness defects of the abdominal wall. It is generally used in contaminated operative fields in which nonabsorbable synthetic mesh cannot safely be used. In clean cases, such as those seen after tumor resection, it can provide soft-tissue coverage of synthetic mesh.

ANATOMY

The tensor fasciae latae is a short flap muscle of the lateral thigh, measuring 12 to 15 cm in length. It has a large fascial extension that inserts on the iliotibial band, approximately one-third of the way down the lateral thigh. The origin of the TFL muscle is the anterior iliac spine and the greater trochanter of the femur. The muscle serves as an accessory flexor and medial rotator of the thigh. Occasional knee instability is noted with flap harvest, but suturing the distal cut margin into the fascia of the vastus lateralis muscle may reduce this complication.

The flap is supplied by the transverse branch of the lateral femoral circumflex vessels, which enter the deep surface of the muscle approximately 10 cm below the anterior superior iliac spine. The branch usually arises from the profunda femoral artery, although it may originate from the common femoral artery. The artery divides into several branches before entering the muscle. Inferior branches course superficial to the fascia lata. These vessels send perforating branches to supply the overlying skin.

The skin territory is supplied by two sensory nerves: the lateral cutaneous branch of T12, which innervates the skin overlying the iliac crest, and the lateral cutaneous branches of L2,3, which innervate the skin of the lateral thigh. Both nerves are easily identifiable and may be included in a sensory flap.

FLAP DESIGN AND DIMENSIONS

The skin territory is large, measuring up to 15 × 40 cm. The center of the flap is a line from the greater trochanter to the lateral knee at the margin of the biceps femoris muscle. Anteriorly, the flap may include skin over the rectus femoris muscle. A line drawn from the greater trochanter distally to the head of the fibula marks the posterior margin of the skin territory. The donor site can be closed primarily, if the flap width is less than 10 cm.

The arc of rotation of the pedicled flap will reach the costal margin, if the tensor muscle is completely detached from its origin and raised as an island flap. The problem with using the flap in the upper abdomen is that the distal third of the skin island has a random blood supply and is unreliable. The blood supply to this area is normally via the superior lateral genicular artery branch of the popliteal artery, which is severed during flap elevation. If this portion of the flap is used, a delayed procedure is planned before flap elevation.

OPERATIVE TECHNIQUE

The flap dimensions are diagrammed on the lateral leg, not to extend farther than 5 to 8 cm above the knee. An incision is made through the skin, subcutaneous tissue, and fascia lata at the distal skin border. The fascia is temporally secured to the overlying dermis with sutures. The anterior and posterior skin borders are incised distal-to-proximal through the fascia lata.

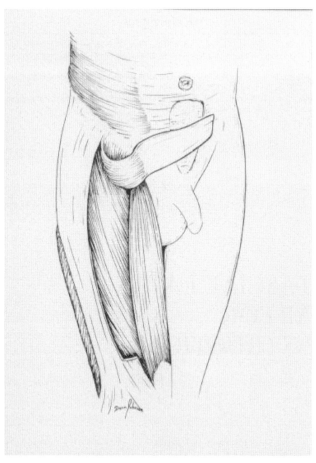

FIG. 1. Schematic of full thickness TFL flap. The distal end will reach across the lower abdomen for fascial closure and closure of skin defect.

The flap is elevated distal-to-proximal in a plane deep to the fascia lata overlying the vastus lateralis (Fig. 1).

The vascular pedicle is visualized on the deep medial aspect of the muscle 8 to 10 cm below the anterior superior iliac spine by medial retraction of the rectus femoris muscle. If an island flap is planned, a superior branch of the lateral femoral circumflex artery must be divided before dividing the muscular insertion on the iliac crest and its attachments to the gluteus minimus muscle. To increase upward mobility, the origin of the rectus femoris can be divided. The donor site is most often closed with a skin graft, which is unaesthetic.

CLINICAL RESULTS

Careful patient selection and planning are necessary to avoid complications. Partial flap necrosis occurred in six of 24 patients, when a TFL flap without vascular delay was used for abdominal-wall reconstruction, in my experience. Fascial herniation is not an uncommon complication, especially when the flap is used to reconstruct the upper abdomen.

SUMMARY

The TFL flap can reliably reconstruct full-thickness lower abdominal-wall defects by providing soft tissue and fascia.

References

1. Nahai F, Hill L, Hester TR. Experiences with the tensor fascia lata flap. *Plast Reconstr Surg* 1979;63:788.
2. Williams JK, Carlson GW, deChalain T, et al. Role of tensor fasciae latae in abdominal wall reconstruction. *Plast Reconstr Surg* 1998;101:713.
3. Gosain AK, Yan JG, Aydin MA, et al. The vascular supply of the extended tensor fasciae latae flap: how far can the skin paddle extend? *Plast Reconstr Surg* 2002;110:1655.

CHAPTER 402 ■ DEEP INFERIOR EPIGASTRIC ARTERY ISLAND RECTUS MUSCULOCUTANEOUS FLAP

G. I. TAYLOR, R. J. CORLETT, AND J. B. BOYD

The rectus abdominis musculocutaneous flap, based on the deep inferior epigastric artery, is an extremely versatile flap for use as either an island or a free flap.

INDICATIONS

The procedure is speedy, simple, and safe. There is a minimal donor-site defect, especially if the anterior rectus sheath is repaired as described. This flap may be used to provide muscle only, as a musculosubcutaneous flap, or as a large skin flap with a variable amount of muscle.

ANATOMY

Contrary to previous views, the major blood supply to the abdomen is from the deep inferior epigastric artery (DIEA)

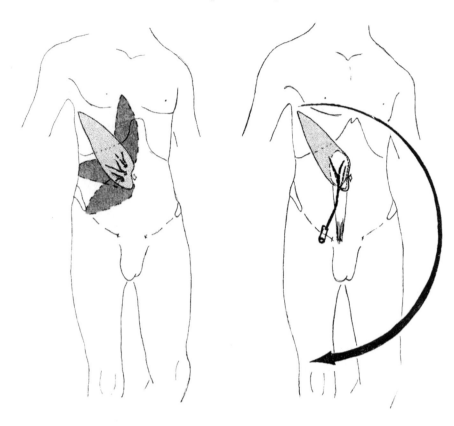

FIG. 1. Left: The various flaps that can be based on the paraumbilical perforators of the DIEA, with the optimal flap radiating toward the inferior angle of the scapula, parallel to the ribs. Right: Arc of rotation of the inferior rectus abdominis thoracoumbilical flap (when dissected to the groin).

(1–3). This artery has an intimate relationship with the rectus abdominis muscle and, in the region of the umbilicus, provides major perforating vessels that pass directly through the muscle to reach the overlying skin. Below this level, the DIEA can be dissected from the muscle to provide a vascular pedicle of 10 to 15 cm in length.

The greatest density of major musculocutaneous perforators emerges from the rectus muscle in the paraumbilical region, especially from its middle and inner thirds. They radiate like the spokes of a wheel to communicate with other vessels supplying the abdominal wall. These vessels are directed predominantly upward and laterally, and as they approach the costal margin, they connect with the lateral intercostal perforators. They connect with the superior epigastric, the lateral intercostals, the deep circumflex iliac artery (DCIA), the superficial circumflex iliac artery (SCIA), and the superficial inferior epigastric artery (SIEA). However, the predominant outflow is directed upward and laterally, parallel to the ribs.

Although the superior epigastric artery (SEA) is currently in vogue for breast reconstruction, in fact, the DIEA supplies a much larger vascular territory, and this is reflected in the relative diameters of these two arteries (DIEA: 3.4 mm; SEA: 1.6 mm). The DIEA flap would appear to be the abdominal equivalent of the versatile latissimus dorsi flap.

FLAP DESIGN AND DIMENSIONS

The deep inferior epigastric flap may be raised in one stage from the groin to the anterior axillary fold. As an island, it will reach the knee on the same side, the distal third of the opposite thigh, the buttocks, or the pelvic floor (Fig. 1). It will more than adequately repair the genitalia in both sexes. Alternatively, it may be used as a free flap, giving it many advantages (Fig. 2). The flap has a long pedicle with large vessels that are ideal for microvascular anastomosis.

A large skin flap can be designed on the perforating vessels, provided that the segment of rectus muscle and its anterior sheath that contain these perforators are preserved. The pedicle

can be dissected to its origin from the external iliac vessels. The flap has a long pedicle with vessels of large diameter (the artery averages 3.4 mm and there are always two venae comitantes that usually exceed 3 mm in diameter). Muscle may be taken alone and skin-grafted at the recipient site. Or the muscle can be combined with a large skin flap. Many designs are available (Fig. 3). The donor defect is minimal, and if care is taken when harvesting the graft, the anterior rectus sheath can be repaired directly in each case.

Because the paraumbilical perforators of the DIEA radiate like the spokes of a wheel, an axial skin flap can be designed in any direction with its base at the umbilicus. However, the longest flap is planned along a line between the umbilicus and the inferior angle of the scapula, because this places the flap along the dominant vascular axis. The width of the flap is determined by a "pinch test," so that the wound can be closed directly.

OPERATIVE TECHNIQUE

The distal end of the flap is elevated first, and the areolar layer on the deep surface of the subcutaneous fat is included. This is an important anastomotic layer between the vascular territories incorporated in this flap. The flap is dissected medially until the lateral border of the rectus sheath is reached. Then it is carefully dissected from the outer third of the sheath to leave a sufficient fringe of this structure to facilitate direct repair of the donor defect. During this part of the dissection, fasciocutaneous perforators that appear from the lateral border of rectus muscle will be divided.

Next, a disk of the rectus muscle and its sheath is isolated to preserve the cutaneous blood supply. The sheath and muscle at the upper border of the flap are divided, and the connections between the superior and inferior epigastric systems are ligated. The sheath is incised medially to leave a 5- to 10-mm fringe to the midline (again, to aid the donor-site repair). The tendinous intersection adjacent to the umbilicus is detached, and the muscle is separated easily from its posterior sheath.

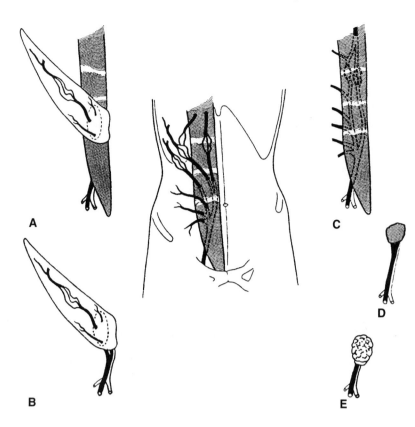

FIG. 2. Diagram of several of the various combinations that we have used for free transfer designed on the DIE system and its paraumbilical perforators. **A,B:** A musculocutaneous flap with varying amounts of muscle. **C,D:** Note the versatility as a muscle flap with the potential for segmental reinnervation. **E:** A musculosubcutaneous flap.

Next, the lateral border of the rectus muscle is defined from its deep surface. The anterior sheath is divided in this region, just lateral to the major skin perforators, leaving an outer fringe of rectus sheath 1 to 2 cm wide. Finally, the lower part of the skin flap is divided and the incision in the anterior rectus sheath is completed, taking care to incise the sheath above the level of the arcuate line.

This isolates the skin flap, which is now attached to the underlying muscle by a disk of the anterior sheath through which emerge the supplying perforators. This disk will be sited approximately over the middle fifth of the length of the rectus muscle.

The pedicle is dissected last. This can be achieved through a paramedian incision, but we usually employ a transverse suprapubic (lipectomy) incision to isolate the pedicle. The anterior abdominal skin is then elevated from the muscle layers to join the upper dissection. A longitudinal incision is made in the anterior rectus sheath and the muscle is dissected from its confines. The DIEA and its paired venae comitantes are found plastered to the undersurface of the muscle.

Near the pelvis, the DIE vessels diverge laterally toward the external iliac vessels. Most of the rectus muscle, except the disk through which the skin perforators course, can be discarded or left in situ. This requires a careful dissection of

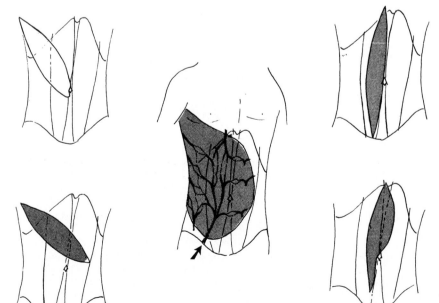

FIG. 3. The clinical cutaneous vascular territory of the DIEA (*center*), which extends by means of captured adjacent arterial territories to the midaxillary line laterally and superiorly to the axilla and crosses the midline to the lateral border of the opposite rectus muscle. Several of the free skin flap designs that we have used successfully within this territory are illustrated, based on the perforators emerging through the anterior rectus sheath.

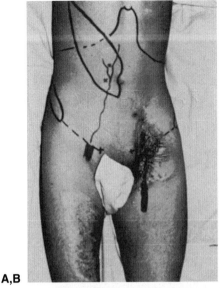
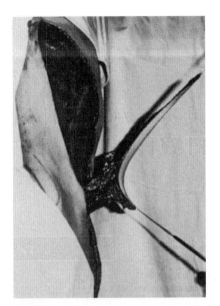

A,B

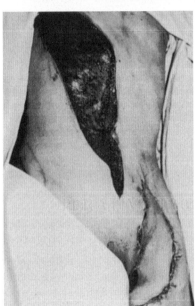
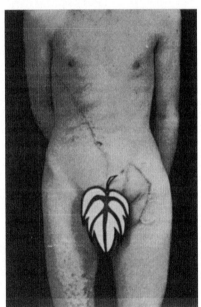

C,D

FIG. 4. **A:** A hypertrophic ulcerated groin scar with the external iliac-femoral artery reconstruction outlined, together with the contralateral flap planned for repair. **B:** A 32 × 11 cm thoracoumbilical flap was designed from the contralateral side. The tip extended to the midaxillary line. The flap was elevated to within 5 cm of the midline, at which stage two large perforators were identified. The skin island was raised with its disk of anterior rectus sheath, and the vascular pedicle was dissected, retaining the rectus muscle and the perivascular connective tissues down to the pubis. The latter was done to provide good cover for the reconstructed femoral artery and to introduce a possible lymphatic bridge that, if successful, would drain the lymphedema to the contralateral normal groin. **C:** The scar was excised and the flap was tunneled to the opposite side, using the rectus muscle to fill the deep cleft in the groin and thigh. The skin flap was sutured in place, and the donor site was closed as a linear scar, with direct repair of the rectus sheath. **D:** The result. Note how the flap has assumed the groin contour. There has been no recurrence of infection, and the swelling of the leg has resolved.

the pedicle, with ligation of multiple branches. Nevertheless, it does provide a large skin flap with a small amount of muscle and a very long pedicle of 10 to 15 cm. Alternatively, the muscle can be retained in the flap and simply filleted from its sheath. This latter method is a very quick and simple dissection.

Closure of the anterior rectus sheath above the arcuate line may be unnecessary. However, as an added precaution to prevent abdominal herniation, we have preserved a cuff of the anterior sheath both medially and laterally that has allowed us to restore its integrity in every case. As another precaution, we suture the anterior and posterior sheaths together at the arcuate line (Fig. 4).

CLINICAL RESULTS

In a series of over 30 patients, the success rate has been 100 percent, with an average operating time of 4¼ hours. Disadvantages are those of a bulky flap in an obese patient

and the possible onset of a late hernia. However, to date, this latter problem has not occurred.

SUMMARY

The deep inferior epigastric artery island flap has an extensive arc of rotation and offers a viable alternative to the reliable latissimus dorsi flap. As a free-muscle or musculocutaneous flap, it has almost limitless possibilities.

References

1. Taylor GI, Corlett RJ, Boyd JB. The extended deep inferior epigastric flap: a clinical technique. *Plast Reconstr Surg* 1983;72:751.
2. Boyd JB, Taylor GI, Corlett RJ. The vascular territories of the superior epigastric and deep inferior epigastric systems. *Plast Reconstr Surg* 1984;73:1.
3. Taylor GI, Corlett RJ, Boyd, JB. The versatile deep inferior epigastric (inferior rectus abdominis) flap. *Br J Plast Surg.* 1984;37:330.

CHAPTER 403 ■ MICROVASCULAR AND PEDICLED ANTEROLATERAL THIGH FLAP FOR ABDOMINAL-WALL RECONSTRUCTION

Y. KIMATA

The anterolateral thigh (ALT) flap has been used to reconstruct various types of defects. The indications and surgical procedures for use of the free or pedicled ALT flap in reconstructing abdominal-wall defects are discussed.

INDICATIONS

Because of its wide vascular tissue territory, the free or pedicled ALT flap is indicated for reconstruction of extremely large, full-thickness defects of the upper and lower abdominal wall (1,2). The cutaneous territory of the ALT flap may extend from a horizontal line at the level of the greater trochanter to a parallel line just above the patella, and includes half the surface of the thigh. The lateral border is the lateral intermuscular septum (3). This vascular territory also includes the iliotibial tract without the tensor fasciae latae muscle. The strong subcutaneous fascia component (iliotibial tract) of this flap can be used to repair defects of the peritoneum and the abdominal wall, and the wide vascularized skin component can be used to repair abdominal skin defects. If the distance or area of an abdominal defect is too great, a pedicled ALT can be converted to a free flap (4).

ANATOMY

The cutaneous perforators of the ALT flap are usually derived from the descending branch of the lateral circumflex femoral artery (Fig. 1). This descending branch runs downward through the intermuscular space between the rectus femoris and vastus lateralis muscles and terminates in the vastus lateralis muscle near the knee joint by branching into several cutaneous perforators at the lateral aspect of the thigh. These cutaneous perforators can be divided into septocutaneous perforators and musculocutaneous perforators that penetrate the vastus lateralis muscle. Musculocutaneous perforators requiring complicated dissection procedures are much more common than are septocutaneous perforators. The perforators are usually near the midpoint of the thigh (5).

The skin of the thigh is supplied by two vascular plexi: the subdermal plexus and the plexus above the deep fascia. These two plexus systems supply blood to large areas of both the skin and the deep fascia.

FLAP DESIGN AND DIMENSIONS

First, the possibility of using a pedicled ALT flap to repair abdominal defects should be assessed in each patient. The pivot point of the pedicled ALT flap is approximately 2 cm

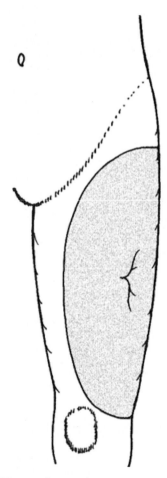

FIG. 1. Diagram showing the territory of the ALT flap.

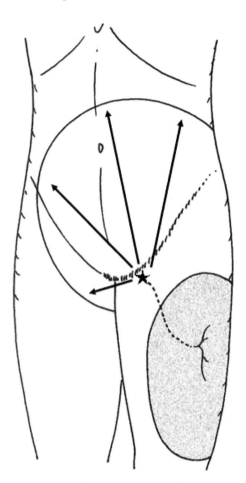

FIG. 2. A pedicled ALT flap raised as an island and its arc are shown. Pivot point of the flap is indicated by an *asterisk*.

below the inguinal ligament on the femoral artery and correlates with the origin of the lateral circumflex femoral artery, which supplies the cutaneous perforators to the ALT flap. Because a perforator of the ALT flap arises near the midpoint of the thigh, the pedicled ALT flap can reach 8 cm above the umbilicus; in contrast, the pedicled tensor fasciae latae flap cannot reach either above the umbilicus or beyond the midline (6). Therefore the pedicled ALT flap can cover the entire groin and the perineum to the anus, reach the contralateral inguinal area, and extend into the contralateral lower abdomen (Fig. 2). One disadvantage of the pedicled ALT flap for reconstruction of abdominal-wall defects is its limited range of orientation on the abdominal wall. Although a vertically oriented pedicled ALT flap allows tension-free placement of the flap pedicle, a horizontally oriented pedicled flap requires a larger skin paddle than does a free flap.

If the distance or area of an abdominal defect is too great, a pedicled ALT can be converted to a free flap. The free ALT flap is indicated for reconstruction of upper-abdominal defects and large horizontal defects.

OPERATIVE TECHNIQUE

Because detailed surgical techniques for the ALT flap have been reported (1,2), some technical aspects of using these flaps for abdominal-wall reconstruction are described. Because the selection of the perforators is related to the length of the pedicle, distal perforators near the midpoint of the thigh are preferred. After the pedicled ALT flap and the fascia lata have been elevated, this island flap and its vascular pedicle are passed under the rectus femoris and sartorius muscles and moved to the abdominal-wall defect. The flap is sutured firmly to the margins of the defect.

When a free ALT flap is used, recipient vessels for microanastomosis must be selected carefully. Because they are easy to dissect and have suitable diameters for microsurgical anastomosis, the inferior epigastric vessels and gastroepiploic vessels are preferred.

After reconstruction with either a pedicled or a free ALT flap, the patient is restricted to bed rest for 5 days and to non–weight-bearing status for 14 days.

CLINICAL RESULTS

In a series of 13 patients, nine pedicled ALT flaps and five free ALT flaps were successfully transferred to repair abdominal-wall defects. However, in two of these patients who underwent resection of the bilateral rectus abdominis muscles, postoperative pseudohernia was recognized. For these patients, dynamic reconstruction of the rectus abdominis muscle may be considered.

SUMMARY

The pedicled or free ALT flap enables satisfactory reconstruction of large abdominal-wall defects.

References

1. Koshima I, Fukuda S, Yamamoto H, et al. Free anterolateral thigh flaps for reconstruction of head and neck defects. *Plast Reconstr Surg* 1993;92:421.
2. Kimata Y, Uchiyama K, Ebihara S, et al. Versatility of the free anterolateral thigh flap for reconstruction of head and neck defects. *Arch Otolaryngol Head Neck Surg* 1997;123:1325.
3. Zhou G, Qiao Q, Chen GY, et al. Clinical experience and surgical anatomy of 32 free anterolateral thigh flap transplantations. *Br J Plast Surg* 1991;44:91.
4. Kimata Y, Uchiyama K, Sekido M, et al. Anterolateral thigh flap for abdominal-wall reconstruction. *Plast Reconstr Surg* 1999;103:1191.
5. Kimata Y, Uchiyama K, Ebihara S, et al. Anatomic variations and technical problems of the anterolateral thigh flap: a report of 74 cases. *Plast Reconstr Surg* 1998;102:1517.
6. Williams JK, Carlson GW, Howell RL, et al. The tensor fasciae latae free flap in abdominal-wall reconstruction. *J Reconstr Microsurg* 2007;13:83.

CHAPTER 404 ■ INTERNAL OBLIQUE MUSCLE FLAP

W. M. SWARTZ AND S. S. RAMASASTRY

The internal oblique muscle, based on the deep circumflex iliac artery, may be used as a pedicle flap for coverage of the groin, pubis, anterior perineum, or greater trochanter (1).

INDICATIONS

Potential uses for this flap include coverage of radiation necrosis ulceration of the pubic area following vulvectomy or primary coverage of defects following treatment of vulvar cancer. The technique is also useful for covering the exposed femoral vessels following arterial surgery. When using this flap for coverage of vascular prostheses in the groin, it is necessary to ensure that the deep circumflex iliac artery is indeed patent. Arteriograms prior to surgery are helpful. The artery can be seen coursing in an oblique direction toward the anterior superior iliac spine. This vessel is not expected to be suitable in patients who have undergone aortoiliac or aortofemoral vascular reconstructions.

ANATOMY

The muscle originates from the lumbosacral fascia, the iliac crest, and the lateral half of the inguinal ligament and inserts into the rectus sheath and the pubis. The muscle lies between the transversus abdominis muscle and the external oblique muscle (Fig. 1). The primary blood supply to this muscle is the deep circumflex iliac artery (DCIA). In approximately 80 percent of patients, a separate blood vessel, the ascending branch of the deep circumflex artery, enters the muscle approximately 1 cm medial to the anterior superior iliac spine. In the remainder of patients, smaller branches from the DCIA supply the muscle along the border of the iliac crest (Fig. 2) (2,3).

FLAP DESIGN AND DIMENSIONS

The maximum size of the muscle flap is approximately 10 × 20 cm when the muscle is detached from its origin along the lumbar-sacral fascia. Its arc of rotation based on the DCIA at its origin from the external iliac artery extends to the greater trochanter, the ipsilateral groin, and the pubis (Fig. 3).

OPERATIVE TECHNIQUE

The internal oblique muscle is exposed through an incision approximately 2 cm above the inguinal ligament, extending beyond the anterior superior iliac spine. The external oblique fascia is incised and the muscle is immediately identified. Dissection of the muscle is made at first superiorly, dividing the muscle along the direction of its fibers. Care must be taken not to penetrate the transversus abdominis muscle, since these fibers interdigitate particularly near the insertion along the rectus border.

Dissection is then continued inferiorly along the rectus sheath, carefully separating the muscle from the underlying transversus abdominis. At this point, the ascending branch is easily identified on the underside of the muscle, originating approximately 1 cm medial to the anterior superior iliac spine in the majority of patients.

If this vessel is not identified, then the entire deep circumflex iliac system along the inner border of the ilium must be kept with the muscle. This is accomplished by identifying the main trunk of the DCIA and then dissecting distally along the inner border of the ilium just beneath the transversalis fascia. Following this, the muscle may be elevated and detached from the inner border of the ilium based on the vascular pedicle alone (Fig. 4).

The pedicle is developed as proximally as necessary to provide adequate rotation of the muscle for coverage of the ipsilateral groin or pubic area. The donor site is closed by suturing the external oblique fascia over a suction drain and closing the wound directly (Fig. 5).

SUMMARY

The internal oblique muscle flap, supplied by the deep circumflex iliac vessels, is an excellent flap for coverage of lower abdominal or groin defects.

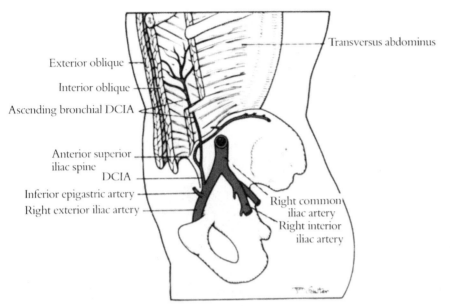

FIG. 1. Internal view of the anatomy of the abdominal wall. The internal oblique muscle lies between the external oblique muscle and transversus abdominis. Its primary blood supply is the deep circumflex iliac artery.

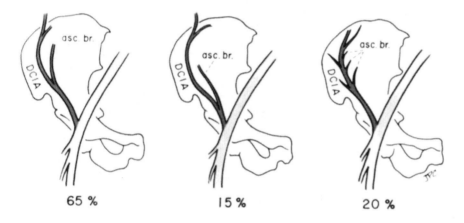

FIG. 2. Anatomic variations in the ascending branch of the DCIA. When this branch is absent, the entire DCIA must be included as the vascular pedicle of the internal oblique muscle.

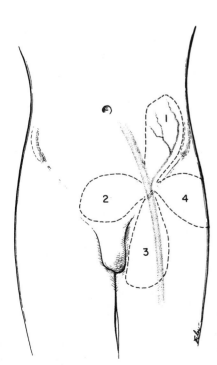

FIG. 3. 1, Arc of rotation of the internal oblique muscle. 2, The muscle will reach the pubis, 3, the ipsilateral groin, and 4, the greater trochanter.

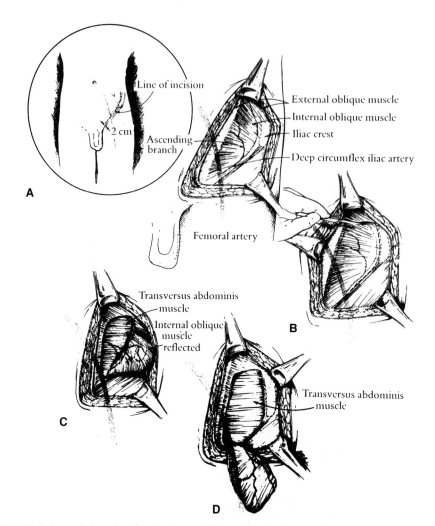

FIG. 4. Technique of dissection for the internal oblique muscle flap. **Inset:** The incision in the groin is made parallel to and slightly above the inguinal ligament, extending laterally beyond the anterior superior iliac spine. **A:** The internal oblique muscle is identified immediately below the external oblique fascia. **B:** Dissection is begun superiorly and medially, taking care not to penetrate the fibers of the transversus abdominis muscle. **C:** The ascending branch is identified on the underside of the muscle prior to dividing the muscle from the iliac crest. **D:** The DCIA is dissected as the pedicle for a rotation flap.

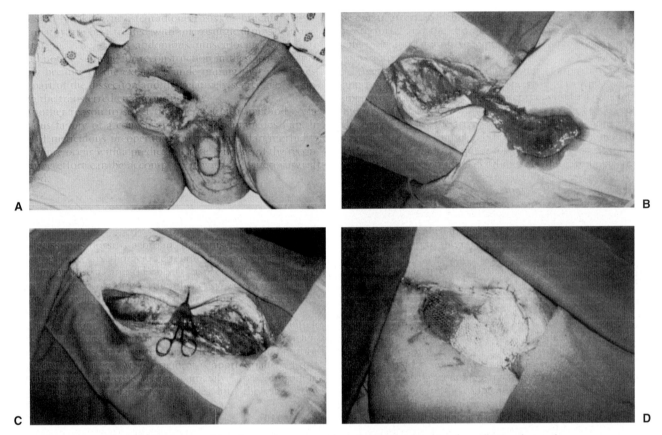

FIG. 5. A: An 86-year-old patient underwent a right radical groin dissection for palliation during the treatment of an extensive penile carcinoma. **B:** Isolation of the internal oblique muscle flap on the DCIA. **C:** Muscle flap rotated as a turnover flap to cover groin vessels. Note vessels on underside of muscle. **D:** Muscle immediately skin-grafted. Six-month follow-up has shown this wound to remain satisfactorily healed without hernia or tumor recurrence.

References

1. Ramasastry S, Tucker J, Swartz W, Hurwitz D. The internal oblique muscle flap: an anatomic and clinical study. *Plast Reconstr Surg* 1984;73:721.

2. Taylor GI, Townsend P, Corlett R. Superiority of the deep circumflex iliac vessels as the supply for free groin flaps: experimental work. *Plast Reconstr Surg* 1979;64:595.

3. Taylor GI, Townsend P, Corlett R. Superiority of the deep circumflex iliac vessels as the supply for free groin flaps: clinical experience. *Plast Reconstr Surg* 1979;64:745.

CHAPTER 405 ■ COMPONENT SEPARATION FOR ABDOMINAL-WALL DEFECTS

V. T. NGUYEN, K. K. AZARI, AND K. C. SHESTAK

EDITORIAL COMMENT

This modification shows how important it is to understand vascular anatomy and apply those principles to extend the value of previously described procedures. Including the abdominal perforators increases the reliability of this reconstructive procedure.

Multiple authors have advocated and published the "components separation" or "separation of parts" procedure for reconstruction of the anterior abdominal wall. Proposed benefits of this procedure focus on its use of innervated, vascularized, autologous tissue for the reconstruction of anterior abdominal-wall defects. Additionally, beyond providing a tensionless closure, the use of these innervated, myofascial flaps helps to recreate the dynamic nature of the native abdominal wall.

INDICATIONS

At our institution, the separation-of-parts procedure, first advocated in 1990 by Ramirez and colleagues (1), has become a mainstay for the closure of complicated or recalcitrant midline and paramedian abdominal-wall defects. For complex reconstructions, patients are addressed by a team approach in conjunction with our general surgery colleagues. Before embarking on the reconstruction, it is critical to assess whether significant portions of the abdominal wall are missing, either from the initial disease process or as a result of prior operative resection. Abdominal computed tomography can greatly assist in the evaluation of the presence or absence of the rectus muscle complex, particularly in cases of massive midline defects, in which the recti can be situated at the lateral extremes of the abdomen. These and other aspects have contributed to a body of literature citing a recurrence rate averaging around 10% to 15% (2–4).

ANATOMY

The anterior abdominal wall consists of paired rectus and oblique muscles that coalesce in the midline, to create a dynamic, myofascial sling that resists internal pressure yet provides a stable platform for core movement and assistance with respiratory excursion. Flexion of the abdominal wall is facilitated mainly by the paired, midline rectus abdominis muscles, with their origin at the pubic symphysis and their insertion at the xyphoid process and the fifth through seventh-costal cartilages.

Lateral support of the abdomen is provided by the trilaminar construct consisting of the external oblique, internal oblique, and transversus abdominis muscles. Bilaterally, these muscles interdigitate toward the midline, to form the anterior and posterior rectus sheaths, with their corresponding insertion medially into the linea alba or white line. Above the umbilicus, the aponeuroses of these muscles divide, with the external oblique providing fibers to the anterior rectus sheath, the transversus abdominis muscle donating its fibers posteriorly, and the internal oblique splitting to contribute fibers to both anterior and posterior sheaths. However, below the umbilicus at the arcuate line, located at the inferior fourth of the rectus sheath, all three aponeuroses run anterior to the rectus muscle, with only the transversus abdominis fascia providing posterior support.

A neurovascular plane exists within the anterolateral abdominal wall, traversing between the internal oblique and transversus abdominis muscles. Coursing within this plane is the innervation to the oblique and rectus muscles, provided by the inferior six thoracic nerves (T7 to T11, and the subcostal nerve T12), and the iliohypogastric and ilioinguinal nerve branches of L1. This anterolateral configuration allows a relatively avascular and nerve-sparing plane to exist between the external and internal oblique muscles on either side of the midline.

OPERATIVE TECHNIQUE

While in the operating room, the general surgeons are allowed first to define the defect, dissecting out the hernia sack and reducing its contents back into the abdominal cavity. Once they are satisfied with their lysis of adhesions and have completed any required intraabdominal procedure, the plastic surgery service assumes control of the patient for definitive closure of the abdomen.

The procedure is begun by elevating adipocutaneous flaps off the underlying abdominal musculature in a lateral direction toward the anterior axillary line (Fig. 1). Next, the linea semilunaris is noted, along with the insertion of the external oblique fascia.

Two to 3 cm lateral to the linea semilunaris, a vertically oriented incision is made through the external oblique fascia and parallel with the linea semilunaris, extending from the inguinal ligament to the level of the costal margin, and often above the costal margin. This superior extension is critical in cases of defects extending up to the xyphoid process, to obtain adequate release of tissue for these superior closures.

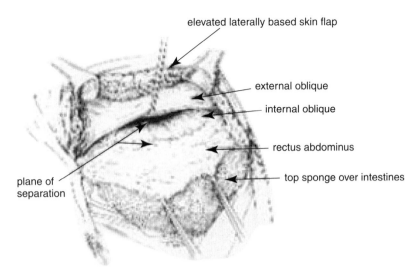

elevated laterally based skin flap

external oblique

internal oblique

rectus abdominus

top sponge over intestines

plane of separation

FIG. 1. Diagrammatic illustration showing elevation of skin flap laterally and development of the plane between the external oblique and internal oblique. This plane was opened all the way to the posterior axillary line.

The incision should be made well lateral to the linea semilunaris, at just medial to the musculofascial junction of the external oblique muscle itself. In a small number of cases, it has been noted that the fascia of the external oblique, internal oblique, transverse abdominis muscles, or a combination of these, coalesce a short distance from the lateral edge of the rectus muscle. In such circumstances, incising directly adjacent to the linea semilunaris risks inadvertent division of the underlying internal oblique and transversalis fascia, and raises the possibility of subsequent spigelian-type hernias.

After division of the external oblique fascia, the deep surface of the external oblique muscle is identified, and the plane between the external oblique muscle and internal oblique muscle is developed (Fig. 2). When making the initial incision in the oblique fascia, the surgeon must be careful not to dissect deep to this layer of external oblique fascia, to avoid injuring the internal oblique fascia or muscle. Generally, the planes are quite distinct.

The dissection proceeds in this relatively avascular intermuscular plane and is continued in a lateral direction beyond the area of skin, undermining to at least the level of the midaxillary line. At this point, the mobility of the innervated rectus abdominis–internal oblique–transversus abdominis muscle complex is determined. If additional mobility of these structures on either side of the midline is desired, then the dissection in the intermuscular plane can be continued to the posterior axillary line. In our experience, each ipsilateral complex can be advanced toward the midline 4 cm in the upper abdomen, 8 cm at the waist, and 3 cm in the lower abdomen (Fig. 3).

In the rare instance that additional advancement is needed, the rectus muscle can be elevated off the posterior rectus sheath in its entirety. Two centimeters of additional advancement can be obtained at each level by using this maneuver. However, the surgeon must leave the anterior rectus fascia intact to allow secure suture placement.

The muscles are joined together in the midline with an interrupted closure, by using strong nonabsorbable suture. During closure of the fascia, peak airway pressures are noted by the anesthesia team. Marked elevations above baseline may indicate some element of respiratory restriction, necessitating prolonged postoperative intubation or paralysis or both. A decision should be made as to whether small increases in peak airway pressures are tolerable to achieve final closure, or if adjunctive maneuvers (e.g., interposition mesh or grafts) are instead necessary. If, after fascial closure, increases in peak airway pressure occur, in addition to alterations in systemic function, such as hypotension or diminished urine output or

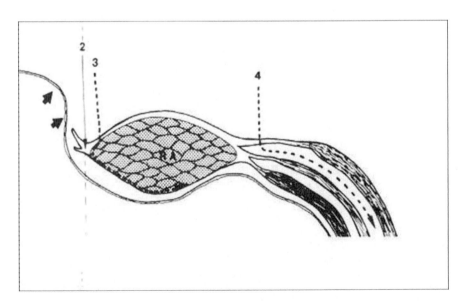

FIG. 2. Plane of dissection (indicated by *dashed line 4*) as it proceeds posteriorly to the posterior axillary line. *Dashed line 3* shows plane of dissection to use the medial aspect of the rectus abdominis muscle, giving an extra 2 cm of tissue at the waist level.

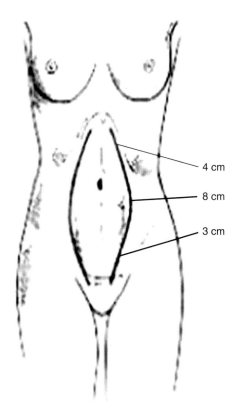

FIG. 3. The distances that the innervated complex of rectus abdominis–internal oblique–transversus abdominis muscles can be moved on one side of the abdomen.

both, one should be cognizant of the possibility of abdominal compartment syndrome. Release of the fascial closure is necessary to restore hemodynamic stability, and fascia or mesh/biologic graft should be used to bridge any remaining defect.

Once the surgeon is convinced of a stable fascial closure and stable patient, the skin flaps are then advanced to the midline and approximated in a layered closure. Three to four suction drains are used routinely, and these are positioned in the plane between the oblique muscles and beneath the skin flaps on each side of the midline and brought out through separate stab incisions in the pubic area, lateral abdomen, or both. An abdominal binder is placed before the patient leaves the operating room.

One obvious drawback of the original procedure is the need for extensive dissection of the skin and subcutaneous layer laterally, to provide adequate exposure for subsequent external oblique division. Such widely undermined cutaneous flaps are subject to ischemia and adipocutaneous flap necrosis, risking exposure of the underlying myofascial closure. To address this issue, other authors developed modified versions of the separation-of-parts technique (5,6). As in the original procedure, they used lateral dissection from the defect edges, to expose the linea semilunaris and to gain access to the external oblique. However, in distinct contrast to the original technique, the periumbilical perforators of the epigastric system are preserved, via subcutaneous dissection performed both superior and inferior to the umbilicus, after which these two areas are connected by a tunnel coursing lateral to the perforators (Fig. 4). This allows access to the external oblique for division, from the inguinal ligament

inferiorly to above the costal margin. We advocate the use of this method in patients who may be at high risk for wound complications, including patients who are significantly obese, patients with previous abdominal incisions off the midline, and diabetic patients.

On some occasions, medialization of the rectus abdominis edge is under undue tension after components separation, or the rectus fascia is deemed to be of poor quality. These clinical situations are thought to be a predisposition to potential reconstructive failure. To achieve the goal of a tension-free and stable closure, augmentation of components separation with biologic mesh substitutes has been advocated (7). With this technique, a biologic mesh substitute is placed as a retrofascial underlay and held with interrupted horizontal mattress sutures. Subsequently, the rectus abdominis fascial edges are reapproximated in a tension-free manner. Next, another layer of biologic mesh can be added above the repair; however, in our significant experience with this components-separation technique modification, only an underlay graft is necessary.

Postoperative Management

Suction drains are maintained until the drainage decreases to less than 30 mL per 24 hours for 2 consecutive days, which is usually at an average of 7 to 14 days. Patients are maintained on nothing-by-mouth status until the resumption of bowel function. Nasogastric tubes are used if extensive intraabdominal dissection is required as part of the procedure.

Although not widely practiced at our institution, consideration should be given to those patients with existing ostomies within the rectus sheath. Division of the external oblique muscle can be achieved via laterally placed incisions, thus leaving the paramedian ostomy undisturbed or allowing placement of new ostomies or both.

Additionally, the literature supports the practice of various techniques to preserve the periumbilical, musculocutaneous perforators, citing a reduced incidence of midline wound complications. We have adopted this practice in many patients.

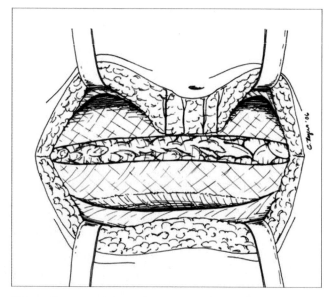

FIG. 4. Illustration showing the technique of periumbilical perforator preservation. Note the dissections superior and inferior to the umbilicus, which meet laterally, above the external oblique fascia.

SUMMARY

Despite some limitations, we believe the components-separation technique to be a powerful method for the closure of extensive or recalcitrant abdominal-wall defects or both. The ideal reconstruction of the abdominal wall should adhere to four requirements: (a) prevent visceral eventration; (b) incorporate the abdominal wall; (c) provide a tensionless repair; and (d) provide dynamic muscle support. These criteria are fulfilled by the components-separation technique through its translocation of vascularized, and innervated, rectus–internal oblique–transversus abdominis muscle complexes. Its use of autologous tissue has obvious benefits, when compared with the use of synthetic mesh, particularly when faced with contaminated or infected wounds. Furthermore, its superiority over other flap methods of reconstruction rests in its preserved innervation and lack of significant donor-site morbidity.

References

1. Ramirez OM, Ruas E, Dellon AL. "Components separation" method for closure of abdominal-wall defects: an anatomic and clinical study. *Plast Reconstr Surg* 1990;86:519.
2. Ewart CJ, Lankford AB, Gamboa MG. Successful closure of abdominal wall hernias using the components separation technique. *Ann Plast Surg* 2003;50:269.
3. Shestak KC, Edington HJ, Johnson JJ. The separation of anatomic components technique for the reconstruction of massive midline abdominal wall defects: anatomy, surgical technique, applications, and limitations revisited. *Plast Reconstr Surg* 2000;105:731.
4. Losanoff JE, Richman BW, Sauter ER, Jones JW. "Component separation" method for abdominal wall reconstruction. *J Am Coll Surg* 2003:196:825.
5. Sukkar SM, Dumanian GA, Szczerba SM, Tellez MG. Challenging abdominal wall defects. *Am J Surg* 2001;181:115.
6. Saulis AS, Dumanian GA. Periumbilical rectus abdominis perforator preservation significantly reduces superficial wound complications in "separation of parts" hernia repairs. *Plast Reconstr Surg* 2002;109:2275.
7. Nguyen V, Shestak KC. Separation of anatomic components method of abdominal wall reconstruction: clinical outcome analysis and an update of surgical modifications using the technique. *Clin Plast Surg* 2006;33:247.

CHAPTER 406 ■ UMBILICAL RECONSTRUCTION USING A CONE-SHAPED FLAP

Y. ITOH

EDITORIAL COMMENT

In diverse cases where loss of the umbilicus has occurred following an operative procedure or sacrifice of the umbilicus, this technique offers an excellent method of reproducing an appropriately-shaped and well-camouflaged neo-umbilicus.

The goals of umbilical reconstruction should be the creation of an umbilicus of sufficient depth and good morphology, with minimal scarring. The cone-shaped flap is useful for attaining these goals.

INDICATIONS

There have been several reports in the literature on umbilical reconstruction or umbilical plasty using skin grafts or local flaps, or both (1–5). Features common to all these reports concern the planar elements of the reconstruction, involving grafts or flaps that are combined in a complex fashion. As the umbilicus is a three-dimensional construction, it is desirable to reconstruct the lateral walls with flaps, so that the umbilicus

will retain its depth over time. It is also desirable to minimize suturing.

The cone-shaped flap technique utilizes a single flap or a combination of two flaps, to form the three-dimensional structure of a circular cone, with a single or double suture line. Postoperative scarring that appears on the body surface is in an inconspicuous, single, straight line. The shape generally preferred for umbilical reconstruction is longitudinal, and attaining such a shape is easier with this procedure. The technique can be used not only for umbilical defects, but also for protrusion and umbilical herniation (6).

FLAP DESIGNS AND OPERATIVE TECHNIQUE

Type 1 (Fig. 1)

Design a triangular flap with its apex oriented in a cranial direction in the umbilical region to be reconstructed or where the umbilicus is absent. After making a skin incision, the fatty tissue immediately below the flap should be preserved. To form a conical flap with point D at its apex, bring points B and C together, and maintain the position of these points with a suture. In

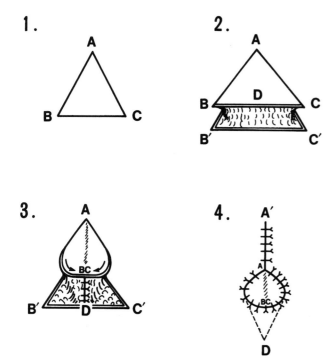

FIG. 1. Diagram of type 1 procedure. A triangular flap is formed into a conical flap and advanced toward the caudal side. (From Itoh, Arai, ref. 6, with permission.)

addition, stitch point D and line BC together. The subcutaneous fatty tissue caudal to the site of the flap should be thoroughly removed, and an advancement flap taken toward the caudal side, to affix point D of the flap to the abdominal wall. Suture points A'-A-BC together with the skin at this location, so that the umbilicus will have the proper longitudinal length.

Type 2 (Fig. 2)

Design a rhombic flap in the umbilical region to be reconstructed or, in the absence of the umbilicus, a triangular flap with the left and right sides adjacent to the umbilical region. As in the type 1 procedure, separate the flap from the surrounding tissue, while preserving continuity at the bottom of the flap. Deeply resect the subcutaneous fatty tissue at point D, and affix point D to the abdominal wall. Close the donor site directly with sutures, from the ends to the center, with the conical flap buried subcutaneously. An incision should be made directly above and perpendicular to the sutured region, to hold the upper end of the incision together with point A of the buried flap. Suture the bottom end to point BC of the flap, to form an umbilicus with its major axis pointing upward (Figs. 3 and 4).

CLINICAL RESULTS

Both types of the procedure were used in 9 patients, all with good results. With the type 1 technique, the possibility of longitudinal hypertrophic scarring is greater. However, with patients requiring flaps within the umbilical area, the type 1 procedure may be desirable, as postoperative scarring can be aligned with the longitudinal furrow that is formed at the bottom of the umbilicus.

SUMMARY

Umbilical reconstruction can be carried out by forming a circular cone with a flap that is anchored to the abdominal wall. The procedure depends on a three-dimensional structure with a single or double suture line; the reconstructed umbilicus retains its depth over a long period of time.

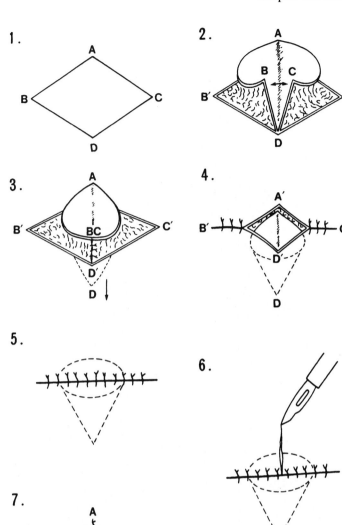

1.

2.

3.

4.

5.

6.

7.

FIG. 2. Diagram of type 2 procedure. A rhombic flap is formed into a conical flap, and the donor site is closed with sutures from the end to the center, with the flap buried subcutaneously. An incision perpendicular to the suture line is carried out, and the reconstructed umbilicus is formed. (From Itoh, Arai, ref. 6, with permission.)

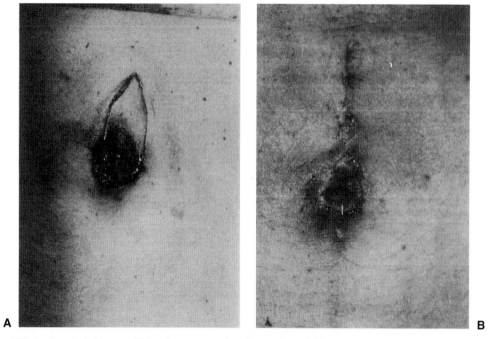

FIG. 3. Case 1. A 40-year-old female patient with endometriosis of the umbilicus. **A:** A triangular flap is designed in the upper region of the tissue defect. **B:** Reconstructed umbilicus 2 weeks postoperatively.

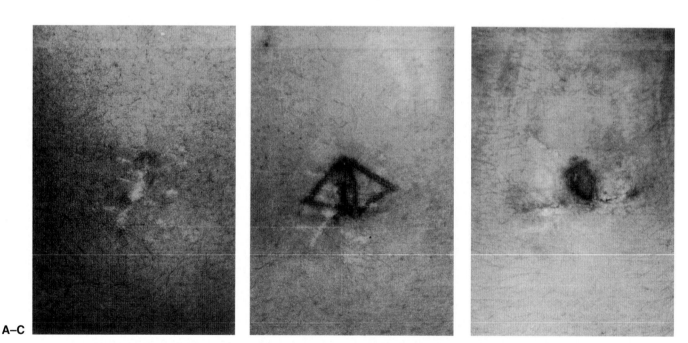

FIG. 4. Case 2. A 21-year-old female patient presenting with a cicatrized umbilical defect subsequent to omphaloceleplasty at birth. **A:** The umbilical region with old scarring. **B:** A rhombic flap is designed. **C:** Reconstructed umbilicus 10 months postoperatively. (From Itoh, Arai, ref. 6, with permission.)

References

1. Baroudi R. Umbilicoplasties. *Clin Plast Surg* 1975;2:431.
2. Borges AF. Reconstruction of the umbilicus. *Br J Plast Surg* 1975;28:75.
3. Kirianoff TG. Making a new umbilicus when none exists. *Plast Reconstr Surg* 1978;61:603.
4. Apfelberg DB, Maser MR, Lash H. Two unusual umbilicoplasties. *Plast Reconstr Surg* 1979;64:268.
5. Jamra FA. Reconstruction of the umbilicus by a double V-Y procedure. *Plast Reconstr Surg* 1979;64:106.
6. Itoh Y, Arai K. Umbilical reconstruction using a cone-shaped flap. *Ann Plast Surg* 1992;28:335.

CHAPTER 407 ■ EXPANSION OF VAGINAL LINING BY GRADUATED DILATION

T. R. BROADBENT

The tissues of the vaginal area are soft and distensible. This is clearly evident in the dilated, stretched tissues at the time of a normal delivery. It is reasonable to assume that these same tissues could be stretched, elongated, or dilated with gradual external pressure, and such is the case.

INDICATIONS

Almost all patients with congenital vaginal atresia, with tissues unscarred by trauma, tumor, or previous surgery, should first be treated by dilation (1). Surgical construction of a vagina can certainly be done by skin grafting (2,3), but it involves hospitalization, discomfort, and scarring of graft donor area and vaginal tract. Of prime concern is the difficult hygiene problem of offensive odor that is present for life. Every patient with an absent vagina is entitled to construction of a vaginal tract by dilation, a painless office and home nonoperative procedure. Should this fail, surgery and grafting are always available.

ANATOMY

The external genitalia are normal in these patients, including the labia and secretions from Bartholin's glands. Sexual intercourse is therefore quite possible and quite normal, requiring no artificial lubrication. However, a lubricant is recommended for the first month of sexual activity.

TECHNIQUE

At some time in the management of the patient with an absent vagina, a consultation with her and her partner or family is important. Everyone must understand the procedure and the goals. It is of equal importance to have a private consultation with the patient, during which her anatomy can be discussed and, by palpation and with a mirror, she can see the normal anatomy, but with the absence of a vagina. Between the rec-

tum and urethra and between the labia, there is always a dimple—soft, pink, and shiny—where the vaginal opening should be (Fig. 1). Once this is identified, the patient will know where to put pressure with the dilators.

Beginning with the smallest dilator and with adequate lubrication (Fig. 2) gentle pressure is placed on the dimple in a pulsing in-and-out fashion (Fig. 3). Pain should not be produced, but there should be enough pressure to make it discernible if the tissue is to be stretched. Bleeding should not be produced; an unpleasant, uncomfortable, or bleeding episode should always be avoided. At the time of the first visit, the physician can move from the first to at least the third or even perhaps the fourth dilator within a half hour.

It is then important to have the patient herself put this dilator in and out of the very new and shallow vagina, so that she knows it will work, that something positive has happened. The patient then is quite aware of the fact that with a little more effort, more can happen (Figs. 4 and 5).

The patient should be lying on her back with a large pillow under her shoulders and a small pillow under her hips to tilt the vagina forward and to bring her arms far enough down so that the dilator can be pushed in the right direction. If the dilator is tilted backward, it will be pushing toward the rectum. This will not only be uncomfortable, but it will be only partially successful in stretching the vaginal area. If the dilator is tilted too far anteriorly, it will be pressing on the urethra and, again, can cause irritation and be less effective in producing a vaginal tract.

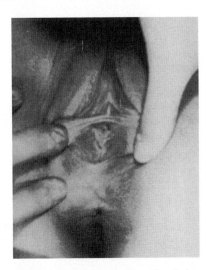

FIG. 1. Congenital vaginal agenesis. Note dimple between normal labia where vaginal orifice would normally be.

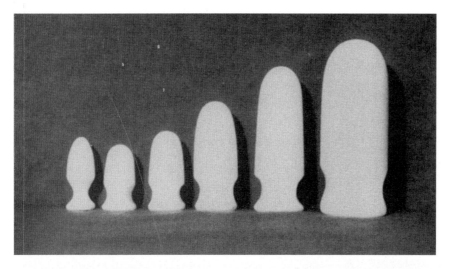

FIG. 2. Set of graduated dilators. (Courtesy of McGhan Medical, 700 Ward Drive, Santa Barbara, CA 93111.)

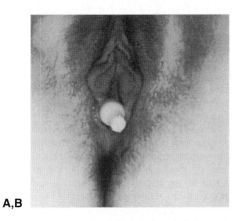 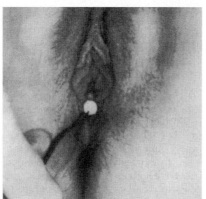

A,B

FIG. 3. Vaginal agenesis. Progressive pressure dilation with a no. 3 dilator. **A:** Dilator placed on vaginal orifice dimple. **B:** Dilator pushed into the tissue.

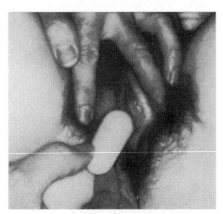 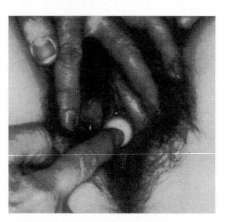

A,B

FIG. 4. Vaginal agenesis. Progressive pressure dilation with a no. 5 dilator. **A:** Placement of dilator. Note that it should not angle posteriorly to the rectum or anteriorly to the urethra. **B:** Dilator pressed into new vaginal tract.

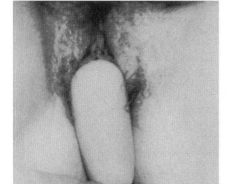 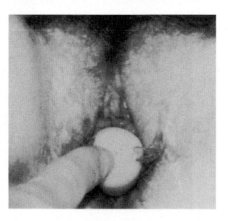

A,B

FIG. 5. Vaginal agenesis. Progressive pressure dilation with a no. 6 dilator. **A:** Before entry. **B:** After entry into new dilated vaginal tract. The patient is ready for sexual activity.

After the first visit, the patient is instructed to carry out the mechanical dilation by pressure 15 minutes twice a day. This is to be done with a clock, for the time always seems longer than it really is. In the evening, after having completed this exercise, the patient is instructed to place the largest dilator that can be accommodated into the vagina and then to assume a sitting position on a hard surface. This can be a desk top or a hard chair.

There is never any difficulty in obtaining diameter in the vagina, only in obtaining depth. Sitting on the dilator with pressure up into the vaginal tract helps a great deal to achieve this. To sit on the dilator on a soft cushion would defeat the purpose, since there would not be any pressure directed through the dilator into the dome of the vaginal tract. The patient is instructed to do the dilation in an in-and-out and side-to-side fashion 15 minutes twice a day and to sit on a dilator 10 minutes a day.

A vaginal tract that will accommodate satisfactory sexual activity can be formed in 6 to 8 weeks, although most patients are advised that it may take 3 months. Once sexual activity has been assumed, the dilators no longer need to be used. Since these patients are somewhat anxious about the effectiveness of sexual activity, they are advised to use some external lubrication to begin with. Most do so only a few times, and all patients have discontinued use of a lubricant after 1 month.

The dilators are washed with ordinary soap and water after each use, and normal bathing is all that is required as far as care of the genitalia is concerned. The patient should be encouraged to check with her physician whenever she has any concerns to ensure a gradual, progressive program.

CLINICAL RESULTS

Fourteen of 15 patients with congenital atresia of the vagina have had a vagina successfully constructed by progressive graduated dilation. One failure represented a patient unwilling to spend the time or effort to accomplish what would have been possible. All patients have appeared to be normal adult females in body habitus and secondary sexual characteristics, with development of the breasts, vulvar labia, and body hair pattern.

The success of the procedure rests heavily on the willingness of the physician to spend enough time with the patient, to educate her about her own anatomy, and to gain her confidence in a very private matter. The patient must be assured of success by partial successful dilation during the first visit when the dilators are used. Motivation is important, and anticipated sexual activity is the prime motivator.

Dilation is started 3 months before anticipated use of the vagina. Patients and parents often want to start earlier because of their emotional stress over the absence of a vagina. In addition, no one knows when marriage or use of the vagina may be imminent. However, disappointment is likely if the vagina is not used once dilated. Sexual activity continues the dilation; without it, manual dilation one or two times a week is probably indicated, although this remains to be proven. Recoil of a dilated vagina may not occur or, if it does, may not be significant. At any rate, redilation of an unused vagina has been observed to be very easy and rapid.

These patients do not have a hygiene problem with odor and dryness (such as with a skin-grafted vagina), and the mucosa looks normal and pink and is soft and resilient. There have been no contractures, and although the vaginal vault can look a bit flat or shallow, sexual intercourse has been satisfactory. A large vaginal speculum can be passed into the vaginal tract after the dilation described above.

SUMMARY

Expansion of the vaginal lining by graduated dilation is probably the simplest and most effective way to permit normal sexual intercourse in patients with congenital vaginal atresia.

References

1. Broadbent TR, Woolf RM. Congenital absence of the vagina: reconstruction without operation. *Br J Plast Surg* 1977;30:118.
2. Castanares S. Plastic construction of the artificial vagina in congenital total absence. *Plast Reconstr Surg* 1963;32:368.
3. McIndoe AH. The treatment of congenital absence and obliterative conditions of the vagina. *Br J Plast Surg* 1950;2:254.

CHAPTER 408 ■ VAGINAL MUCOSAL FLAPS

A. WEISS, JR.

Vaginal mucosal flaps can be very useful in reconstruction of the female perineum following vulvectomy (1). This procedure is frequently used in the treatment of Bowen's disease, which most commonly occurs in women under 50 years of age (2,3). The resulting introital stenosis can be quite disabling sexually. The standard vulvectomy procedure currently in vogue

requires a clitorectomy for closure. This produces a further loss of sexual response.

The use of vaginal mucosal flaps obviates the need for clitorectomy and provides a technique for treatment and prevention of introital stenosis that has been much more satisfactory than the standard method of treatment using skin grafts (4,5).

INDICATIONS

Vaginal mucosal flaps have several advantages over skin grafts:

1. Amputation of the clitoris is not required in order to establish a satisfactory bed for a graft.
2. A split-thickness skin graft dressing requires an indwelling catheter for periods of 7 to 10 days, which is not required in this procedure.
3. The period of immobilization is reduced to only a few hours.
4. The perineum does not require fastidious cleansing, since these local tissues are fairly resistant to the bacteria encountered in that area.
5. The donor site is not a source of pain or scar formation because it is in a graft, and it is well camouflaged because it is hidden within the vagina.
6. Late complications of maceration and abnormal changes in the graft are not present because the mucosal tissue is normally accustomed to this environment.

Because this flap is well innervated and vascularized, it frequently has excellent sensitivity, and it has been found to be most useful in the reconstruction of the perineum following vulvectomy.

ANATOMY

The blood supply of this flap originates primarily from the vaginal arteries that enter the lower lateral region of the vaginal wall. These arteries anastomose freely with the uterine and rectal plexi. The veins follow a similar pattern of distribution. As a result of this excellent vascular supply, survival of this flap is not a problem.

The nerve supply is derived from the branches of S2, S3, and S4 by means of the internal pudendal nerve. It likewise enters from a lower lateral distribution, which in these patients frequently produces a flap that retains excellent sensibility.

FLAP DESIGN AND DIMENSIONS

The planning of the flap is easily accomplished, since the blood supply is excellent and the tissue is very elastic. Up to one-half of the vaginal circumference may be used with primary closure, and the remaining tissue subsequently will stretch to provide a normal functional vagina.

Flaps measuring up to 6 cm in width and 12 cm in length have been moved without difficulty. The base of the flap is best placed as near the introitus as possible to allow for maximal rotation. The flap, when taken almost to the cervix, will easily reach and resurface the entire clitoral area (Fig. 1).

OPERATIVE TECHNIQUE

The operative procedure is most easily performed with the patient in the lithotomy position. The use of epinephrine 1:200,000 injected locally has been found to reduce the intraoperative bleeding significantly without any decrease in flap survival. If present, an old scar should be completely excised and the original deformity recreated in secondary procedures. Care must be taken not to damage the urethral sphincter.

It is important to elevate some of the submucosa of the vaginal wall with the flap, since the blood supply originates from within the submucosal layer. The base of the pedicle should not be extensively dissected in order to preserve adequate blood supply to the flap. The vaginal flap is then rotated and sutured into place. Closure is almost always possible without tension, since the flap tissues are very distensible (Fig. 2).

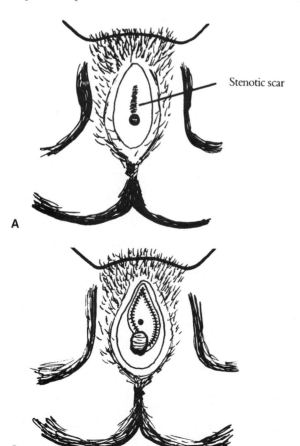

A

Stenotic scar

C

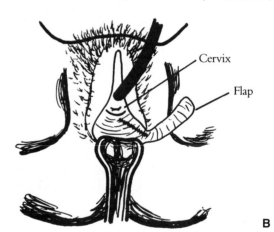

Cervix

Flap

B

FIG. 1. A: Lithotomy position demonstrating the stenosed introitus secondary to scar contracture. **B:** The scar must be excised to recreate the original deformity. A Foley catheter is frequently used to protect the urethra. The flap is demonstrated. **C:** The flap sutured into the defect, relieving the stenosis and allowing for more normal contour. Note that the clitoris is easily covered with a flap of this size.

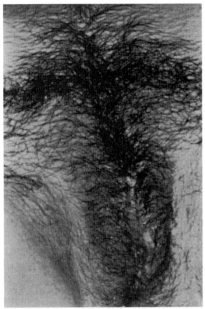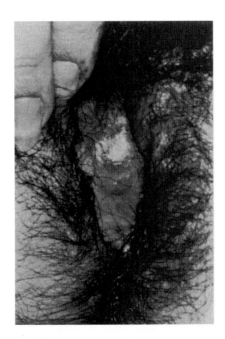

A,B

FIG. 2. Final result. **A:** The stenosis is released and there is no evidence of contracture or tension around the area. **B:** The exposed vaginal mucosal flap results in relatively normal appearing labia.

A topical antibiotic ointment, such as bacitracin, is then applied three times daily for 10 days, at which time dilations of the introitus are begun. Either a biologic or prosthetic dilator may be used with success.

CLINICAL RESULTS

Long-term follow-up has shown a normal-appearing introitus without any recurrence of stenosis.

SUMMARY

Vaginal mucosal flaps have several advantages over standard methods for coverage of vulvectomy wounds.

References

1. Weiss AW Jr. A new method of perineal reconstruction following vulvectomy. *Plast Reconstr Surg* 1980;65:824.
2. Abell MR, Gosling JRG. Intraepithelial and infiltrative carcinoma of vulva: Bowen's type. *Cancer* 1961;14:318.
3. Rutledge RN, Sinclair M. Treatment of intraepithelial carcinoma of the vulva by skin excision and graft. *Am J Obstet Gynecol* 1968;102:806.
4. Delgado G. Plastic procedures in cancer of the lower genital tract. *Am J Obstet Gynecol* 1978;131:775.
5. Shaw W. *Shaw's textbook of operative gynecology*, 4th Ed. New York: Churchill-Livingstone, 1976.

CHAPTER 409 ■ MEDIAL THIGH SKIN FLAPS FOR REPAIR OF VAGINAL STENOSIS

A. I. PAKIAM

Vaginal stenosis can vary from the simpler introital strictures to those which are deeper and involve large segments of the vagina. The minor problems can be safely dealt with by local transposition flaps with good results (1). However, the more extensive varieties, which can amount to a virtual obliteration of the canal, present a far greater challenge to the ingenuity and technical capabilities of the surgeon.

INDICATIONS

In the Western world, most severe cases of vaginal stenosis are due to trauma to the pelvis and perineum, overzealous repair of the anterior and posterior vaginal walls for the treatment of cystocele and/or rectocele (especially if severe infection is a complication), and stenosis following radiotherapy and/or surgery for neoplasia.

Conversely, in the underprivileged parts of the world, vaginal stenosis is more likely to be due to tropical diseases such as severe lymphogranuloma and also may follow prolonged obstructed labor and poor obstetrical management. Female circumcision is practiced in many parts of the world to cure infertility or to punish infidelity (2). The result of this may be vulval adhesions of varying severity. In some Middle Eastern countries, the deliberate insertion of crude rock salt into the vagina results in virtual obliteration of the cavity by severe scarring. Several methods are available to treat vaginal stenosis.

Dilation

Conservative treatment by continual dilation has succeeded in creating a useful skin-lined pouch. Nonoperative therapy has the advantage of unscarred tissue (3,4).

Split-Thickness Skin Grafts

If skin grafts are to be used, the scar excision must be complete to achieve any degree of success. A second stage is often necessary because of the severe bleeding encountered. Thick split-thickness skin grafts are placed some 7 to 10 days later, after the initial packing has been removed. Even under ideal conditions, the "take" of the graft is difficult to achieve, owing to problems of immobilization. Indeed, if the initial graft succeeds, the problem of having to wear a dilator continually to prevent subsequent graft contracture makes great demands on the patient. The eventual result is often inadequate and disappointing (5–9).

Full-Thickness Grafts

This method diminishes subsequent graft contracture, and the use of a dilator may be avoided. However, graft survival is more difficult to achieve technically, owing to the same problems that beset thinner skin grafts.

Local Flaps

The problems associated with grafts can be overcome by the use of bilateral, partially deepithelialized medial thigh flaps.

Groin flaps, although tempting because of their axial pattern of vasculature, may distort the external genitalia (10–19).

FLAP DESIGN AND DIMENSIONS

The flaps are proximally based, and the proximal part is deepithelialized with a skin-graft knife. Sufficient normal skin is left at the tip of the flap to cover the defect created by dissection of each lateral vaginal wall. The dimensions of the flap vary according to the defect. A typical flap measures 15 cm in length and 5 to 6 cm in width.

The deepithelialized portion of the flap aids in maintaining the viability of the tip of the flap. Indeed, a completely deepithelialized local flap may be extremely useful in the repair of vesicovaginal or rectovaginal fistulas, since the dermis provides a greatly needed blood supply to the repaired area.

OPERATIVE TECHNIQUE

The patient is placed in the lithotomy position, and excision of the scar from the lateral walls of the vagina is carried out. Dissection is avoided over the anterior and posterior walls in order to avoid damage to the urethra, bladder, and rectum, particularly if the cause of the stenosis has been an overzealous repair of a cystocele and/or a rectocele.

The flaps are rotated through 180 degrees and inserted through a subdermal tunnel into the vaginal cavity, where they are sutured. Care is taken to ensure that there is no dangerous kinking of the flap and that the tunnel through which it is migrated is not tight (Fig. 1). The donor site is closed in layers after wide undermining, with a gap left at the base of the flap, in order to avoid constriction. A later secondary adjustment to the base of the flap to remove the dog-ear and relieve intertrigo has so far not been necessary (Figs. 1 and 2).

CLINICAL RESULTS

Patients operated on have demonstrated stenoses close to the introitus. The length of the stenosed segment has varied between 1 and 2.5 cm, the narrowest of which would barely

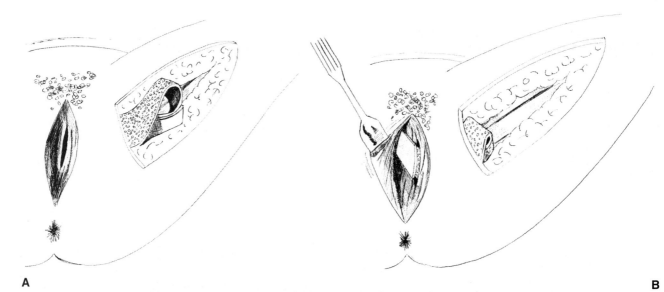

A   B

FIG. 1. A: Illustration showing the flap being migrated into the subdermal tunnel. B: The distal surface (with intact skin) is sutured to the vaginal lateral wall defect. Kinking of the deepithelialized base must be avoided.

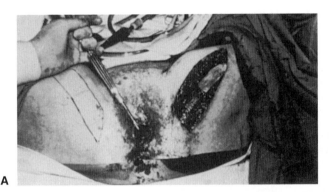
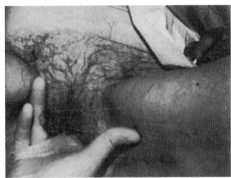

A   B

FIG. 2. A: Operative views showing the design of the thigh flaps and the deepithelialized portion at the base of the flap on the left thigh. **B:** Postoperative view 6 months later showing a cavity that will admit two fingers for a distance of 10 cm. Note the linear scar on the medial side of the left thigh, after the wound was closed primarily.

admit the tip of a hemostat. All patients have achieved good results, the longest follow-up being 3 years, with no recurrence noted. The use of dilators has not been necessary.

SUMMARY

Medial thigh skin flaps can be used to repair vaginal stenoses, especially those near the introitus.

References

1. Pakiam AI. Repair of posttraumatic vaginal stenosis using local thigh flaps. *Br J Plast Surg* 1980;33:54.
2. Iregbulem LM. Postcircumcision vulval adhesions in Nigerians. *Br J Plast Surg* 1980;33:83.
3. Frank RT. The formation of an artificial vagina without operation. *Am J Obstet Gynecol* 1938;35:1053.
4. Woolf RM. Congenital absence of the vagina: reconstruction without operation. *Br J Plast Surg* 1977;30:118.
5. Abbé R. New method of creating a vagina in a case of congenital absence. *Med Rec NY* 1898;54:836.
6. Counsellor VS. Congenital absence of the vagina. *JAMA* 1948;136:861.
7. McIndoe AH, Bannister JB. An operation for the cure of congenital absence of the vagina. *Br J Obstet Gynaecol* 1938;45:490.
8. McIndoe AH. Treatment of congenital absence and obliterative conditions of the vagina. *Br J Plast Surg* 1950;2:254.
9. Whitely JM, Parrott MH, Rowland W. Split-thickness skin graft technique in the correction of congenital or acquired vaginal atresia. *Am J Obstet Gynecol* 1964;89:377.
10. Conway H, Stark RB. Construction and reconstruction of the vagina. *Surg Gynecol Obstet* 1953;97:573.
11. Simmons RJ, Millard DR. Reconstruction of a functioning vagina following radiation therapy for cancer of cervix. *Surg Gynecol Obstet* 1961;112:761.
12. West JT, Ketcham AS, Smith RR. Vaginal reconstruction following pelvic exenteration for cancer or postirradiation necrosis. *Surg Gynecol Obstet* 1964;118:788.
13. Williams EA. Congenital absence of the vagina: a simple operation for its relief. *Br J Obstet Gynaecol* 1964;71:511.
14. Williams EA. Vulva-vaginaplasty. *Proc R Soc Med* 1970;63:40.
15. Song IC, Cramer MS, Bromberg BE. Primary vaginal reconstruction after pelvic exenteration. *Plast Reconstr Surg* 1973;51:506.
16. Morley GW, Lindenauer SM, Youngs D. Vaginal reconstruction following pelvic exenteration: surgical and psychological considerations. *Am J Obstet Gynecol* 1973;116:996.
17. Schellhas HF, Fidler JP. Vaginal reconstruction after total pelvic exenteration using a modification of the Williams' procedure. *Gynecol Oncol* 1975;3:21.
18. Magrina JF, Masterson BJ. Vaginal reconstruction procedures following radical pelvic surgery. *J Kansas Med Soc* 1981;82:61.
19. Magrina JF, Masterson BJ. Vaginal reconstruction in gynecological oncology: a review of techniques. *Obstet Gynecol Surg* 1981;36:1.

CHAPTER 410 ■ VULVOPERINEAL FASCIOCUTANEOUS FLAP FOR VAGINAL RECONSTRUCTION

F. GIRALDO

EDITORIAL COMMENT

These are good flaps for vaginal reconstruction based, we believe, on the same vessels as the pudendal flaps described by Joseph and Wee (Chap. 411).

Partial or complete vaginal reconstruction for both acquired and congenital abnormalities is a challenging problem. In recent years, flaps based on the terminal vessels of the internal pudendal artery have been useful (1–6). A recently-designed pedicled vulvoperineal fasciocutaneous flap, supplied by the external branches of the superficial perineal vessels, has been used successfully for the reconstruction of congenital vaginal agenesis (7).

INDICATIONS

The vulvoperineal flap has been used for vaginoplasty in the Mayer-Rokitansky syndrome. There are potential applications for partial and complete vaginal reconstruction in other congenital anomalies, including testicular feminization and masculinized adrenogenital syndromes, as well as in cases of male-to-female transsexualism. The flap is reliable and can also be used for reconstruction of acquired perineal and vaginal defects secondary to trauma or postoncologic resection. Important advantages include flap security and reliability, with well-established vascularization beneath the lateral border of the labia majora, and a sensitive flap due to the innervation of its posterior two-thirds.

It is not indicated for reconstructive purposes when its design is laterally extended to the inguinal fold, in those cases in which malignant neoplasia affects the vulva or lower vagina and there is the presence or possibility of lymphatic spreading.

The vulvoperineal flap can be based on a deepithelialized or adipofascial pedicle; an island flap is not advocated because of the difficult dissection and isolation of the superficial perineal artery in the fat of the ischiorectal space.

ANATOMY

The perineal region is a relatively neglected area anatomically and requires further definitive clarification. A cadaveric study (8) of the blood supply to the skin and fascia of the anterior perineal region, labia major, and adjacent labial integuments (Fig. 1) in 15 female cadavers led to some new and specific findings. The two principal pedicles providing the major blood supply to the anterior perineal region include an anterior pedicle—the deep external pudendal artery (DEPA), which issues from the femoral artery. This vessel crosses from the deep plane to a subcutaneous location, piercing to the longus adductor muscle aponeurosis about 8 to 10 cm from the pubis symphysis. It then runs along the surface of the adductor muscle aponeurosis, giving off both abdominal and perineal branches 4 to 6 cm distant from the pubis symphysis. The perineal branch or anterior labial artery goes medially to nourish the soft tissues of the superior third of the labia majora and adjacent integuments.

Another principal pedicle is a posterior pedicle—the superficial perineal artery (SPA), a direct branch of the internal pudendal artery, which emerges from Alcock's canal at the ischium. The SPA divides into an internal branch, the internal posterior labial artery, constantly present and closely related to the bulboclitoridean muscle, and an external branch, the external posterior labial artery, located near the ischioclitoridean muscle root and coursing through the anterior perineal region under the lateral border of the labia majora.

A supraaponeurotic intralabial plexus is integrated by multiple anastomoses between the different arterial afferences included in the stromal tissue of the labia majora and immediately adjacent skin, over the adductor and perineal aponeuroses.

The course of the superficial perineal nerve closely follows the internal branch of the SPA. When it crosses over the perineal superficial transverse muscle, it divides into subcutaneous rami, which sensitively innervate the posterior two-thirds of the labia majora.

FLAP DESIGN AND DIMENSIONS

The vulvoperineal fasciocutaneous flap is designed in a vertical, rectangular fashion, centered over the lateral border of the labia majora, nourished by the terminal vessels of the SPA, and posteriorly based on the anterior perineal triangle base (perineal superficial transverse muscle) between the anus

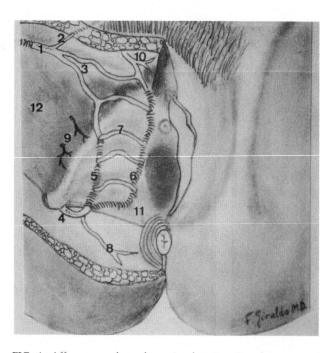

FIG. 1. Afferent vessels to the perineal region. *1* = deep external pudendal artery (DEPA); *2* = abdominal branch of the DEPA; *3* = perineal branches of the DEPA; *4* = superficial perineal artery (SPA); *5* = external branch of the SPA; *6* = internal branch of the SPA; *7* = supraaponeurotic intralabial plexus; *8* = perineal superficial transverse artery; *9* = adductor musculocutaneous perforators; *10* = abdominal-wall vascular anastomosis; *11* = perineal aponeurosis; *12* = adductor aponeurosis. (From Giraldo et al., ref. 8, with permission.)

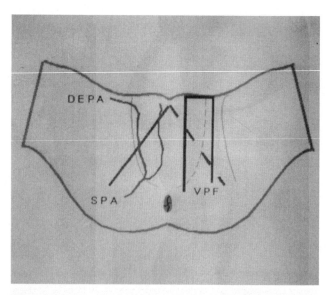

FIG. 2. Diagram of anatomy and design of the vulvoperineal flap. *DEPA* = deep external pudendal artery; *SPA* = superficial perineal artery; *VPF* = vulvoperineal flap in a vertical-rectangular orientation centered on the lateral border of the labia majora. The anterior half contains the adductor aponeurosis and the posterior half, the perineal aponeurosis (refer to text).

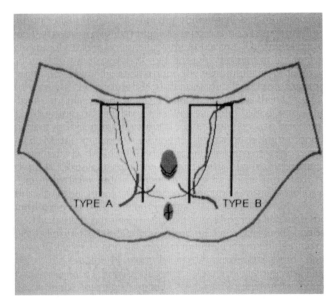

FIG. 3. Diagram of types of vulvoperineal fasciocutaneous flaps (refer to text).

and the ischial tuberosity. This design allows for a perfectly-defined vascularization system following the major axis of the flap—the lateral border of the labia majora—which is formed principally by the anastomotic circuit between the external branches of the SPA (external posterior labial arteries) and the perineal branches of the DEPA (external anterior labial arteries).

The posterior half of the flap (under the ischiopubic bony rami) is integrated by the superficial and medial (Colles' fascia) perineal aponeuroses, including the SPA and subcutaneous rami of the superficial perineal nerve, presenting a fasciocutaneous pattern of vascularization. The anterior half of the flap (over the ischiopubic bony rami) includes the adductor aponeurosis as a "continuation" of the perineal aponeurosis and supraadjacent soft tissues, presenting a direct cutaneous pattern of vascularization (Fig. 2).

Following the classification of fasciocutaneous flaps established by Cormack and Lamberty (9), we defined two types of vulvoperineal flaps. Type A, one-third of all our anatomic dissections, is vascularized by small perforators at its base, arising from the SPA orientated with the long axis of the flap, with a predominantly vertical direction of the intralabial plexus at the deep fascia level. In Type B flaps, two-thirds of all our anatomic dissections, the blood supply depends on a simple, sizeable, and consistent external posterior labial artery arising from the superficial perineal vessels (Fig. 3).

Although we have utilized vulvoperineal flaps measuring 8 to 9 × 3 cm for complete vaginal reconstruction in the Mayer-Rokitansky syndrome, larger flaps are available, always bearing in mind the experience of authors who have reported similar perineal artery flaps.

OPERATIVE TECHNIQUE

The technique is basically the same as originally reported (7,10), apart from a few important modifications (Fig. 4). After establishing a sterile field and inserting a Foley catheter in the bladder, the first step consists of a 2.5- to 3.0-cm U-shaped incision in the vestibular mucosa and submucosal compact tissue across the region of the dimple, 1 cm under the urethral meatus, and extended transversely to the labia minora.

The second step is the formation of the rectovesical space by means of blunt digital dissection between the bladder and rectum. A relatively bloodless cleavage plane is found, except for a critical zone over the anterior rectal wall, about 2 to 3 cm distant from the approach incision. Absolute hemostasis is obtained with the use of electrocautery and packing, to ensure a successful take of the flaps.

At a third step, a 3-cm wide and 8- to 10-cm long rectangular vulvoperineal flap is outlined vertically, with the longitudinal axis centered over the lateral border of the labia majora. After this, the flap is elevated at the lateral and superior margins, thereby identifying and transecting the anastomosis between the SPA and the DEPA included in the subcutaneous tissue over the aponeurosis of the adductor muscles. The adductor longus aponeurosis is incised and elevated, to preserve the vascular structures, and the flap is dissected anterior to posterior until the ischiopubic bony rami. At this important anatomic reference point, the insertions of the adductor aponeurosis must be detached by means of sharp dissection, thus entering over the superficial perineal muscles. The posterior half of the flap is carefully elevated by blunt dissection with a cotton ball.

At the fourth step, the flaps are transposed through subcutaneous tunnels beneath the posterior zone of the retained labia majora, from the donor site to the rectovesical space. The left vulvoperineal flap is rotated counterclockwise 90 degrees beneath the labial skin bridge; the right flap is rotated 90 degrees clockwise.

At the fifth step, a 7-mm strip of the flap pedicle is deepithelialized beneath the labial skin bridge and sutured. The donor site is closed by direct approximation.

The sixth step consists of the formation of the neovaginal pouch by approximating in sequence the medial, distal, and lateral margins of the flaps, with vertical mattress sutures using 3-0 Dexon. We leave the adductor and perineal aponeuroses free of sutures, thus facilitating the capacity for vulvoperineal skin distension. Additionally, a closed suction drainage system is left at the rectovesical space and exteriorized through the skin of an ischiorectal fossa.

Finally, as a seventh step, the tubed neovagina is then transposed into the cavity, but the apex is not sutured at the back. The skin margins of the vaginal pouch are then sutured to the anterior and posterior vestibular borders and to adjacent labial skin with 4-0 chromic sutures, avoiding a circular closure at the new introitus. The neovaginal pouch permits the introduction of four big sheets of tulle and antibiotic ointment, and this packing is secured into position by two 2-0 nylon sutures over a tie bolster, between both sides of the labia minora.

The mean operative time for the procedure is 2.5 hours. Postoperatively, the patient must rest in bed at least 2 days, and a urinary catheter is maintained for 1 week. The closed suction drainage system is usually removed on the third postoperative day. Cefoxitine and clindamicine are prescribed for 1 week. The tulle is removed on the seventh postoperative day.

CLINICAL RESULTS

Between 1991 and 1995, six female patients, varying in age from 16 to 22 years (mean: 18 years), with Mayer-Rokitansky syndrome, have been treated with bilateral vulvoperineal fasciocutaneous flaps for complete vaginal reconstruction. All patients were operated on by the same surgical team (gynecologic and plastic surgeons). The early postoperative period included a hospital stay of about 9 to 11 days (mean: 10 days); the closed suction drainage system was removed on the third postoperative day, with a mean blood collection of 100 cc. The Foley catheter was removed on the seventh postoperative day,

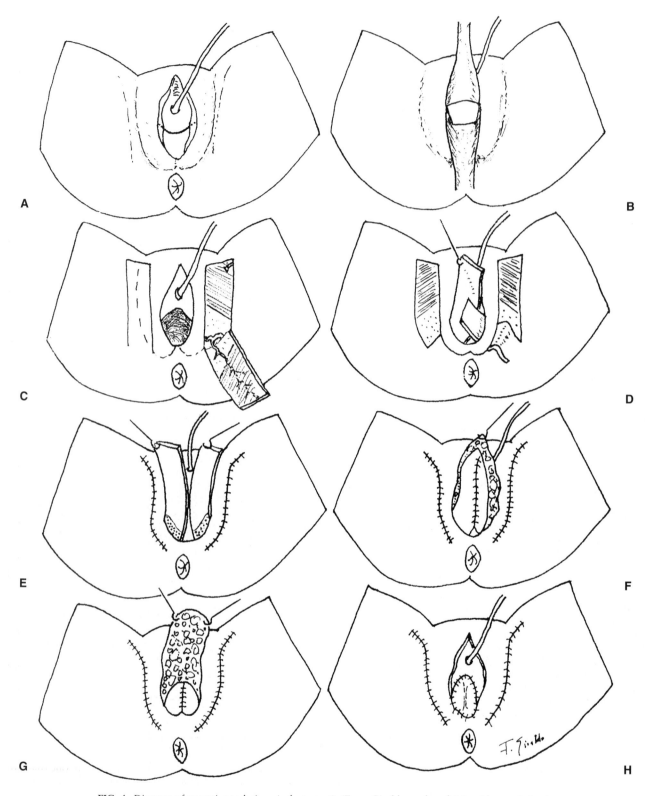

FIG. 4. Diagram of operative technique (refer to text). (From Giraldo et al., ref. 10, with permission.)

with no urinary or wound infections. The early postoperative course was afebrile, and patients experienced moderate postoperative perineal pain over 48 hours, without ileus. The first two patients treated with metronidazole experienced vomiting during the first 48 hours after surgery; at present, we are using clindamicine successfully.

The endovaginal packing was removed on the seventh postoperative day without analgesics, and visual exploration of the endoneovagina showed a healthy and viable artificial vagina with adequate measurements. Labial edema was a minor complication. All the patients considered their reconstructions to have had satisfactory cosmetic results. Patients who have a partner (the first two in the series) reported adequate sexual relationships with no difficulties; intercourse with the use of lubricants was possible 3 to 4 weeks postoperatively. No urinary infection or urethral-anal incompetence were noted. Problems secondary to the reconstruction, such as the need for meticulous hygiene for 6 months postoperatively, were minor.

Endovaginal examination performed by adult speculum showed adequate dimensions and no complications, such as epidermic cysts, local infections, introital strictures, neovaginal stenosis, or mechanical lesions. Persistent hair within the vagina was finer and more dispersed in the younger patients (16 to 17 years of age); in a patient with the longest follow-up (4 years), cutaneous methaplasia and incipient hairy atrophy, most dispersed on the left hemivagina, were verified. Depth and width were measured carefully and without pressure, by means of the number of fingers that could be introduced. In all cases, bidigital vaginal examinations were possible until the indicis PIP joint was passed.

SUMMARY

Paired vulvoperineal fasciocutaneous flaps have been used for complete vaginal reconstruction in six patients with Mayer-Rokitansky syndrome. Results have been encouraging.

References

1. Morton KE, Davies E, Dewhurst J. The use of fasciocutaneous flaps in vaginal reconstruction. *Br J Obstet Gynaecol* 1986;93:970.
2. Hagerty RC, Vaughn TR, Lutz MH. The perineal artery axial flap in reconstruction of the vagina. *Plast Reconstr Surg* 1988;82:344.
3. Dumanian GA, Donahoe PK. Bilateral rotated buttock flaps for vaginal atresia in severely masculinized females with adrenogenital syndrome. *Plast Reconstr Surg* 1992;90:487.
4. Wee JT, Joseph VT. A new technique of vaginal reconstruction using neurovascular pudendal-thigh flaps: a preliminary report. *Plast Reconstr Surg* 1989;83:701.
5. Woods JE, Alter G, Meland B, Podratz K. Experience with vaginal reconstruction utilizing the modified Singapore flap. *Plast Reconstr Surg* 1992;90:270.
6. McIndoe AH, Banister JB. An operation for the cure of congenital absence of the vagina. *J Obstet Gynaecol Br Empire* 1938;45:490.
7. Giraldo F, Gaspar D, Gonzalez C, et al. Treatment of vaginal agenesis with vulvoperineal fasciocutaneous flaps. *Plast Reconstr Surg* 1994;93:131.
8. Giraldo F, Mora MJ, Solano A, et al. Anatomic study of the superficial perineal neurovascular pedicle: implications in vulvoperineal flap design. *Plast Reconstr Surg* 1997;99:100.
9. Cormack GC, Lamberty BGH. A classification of fasciocutaneous flaps according to their patterns of vascularization. *Br J Plast Surg* 1984;37:80.
10. Giraldo F, Solano A, Mora MJ, et al. The Malaga flap for vaginoplasty in the Mayer-Rokitansky-Kuster-Hauser syndrome: experience and early-term results. *Plast Reconstr Surg* 1996;98:305.

CHAPTER 411 ■ NEW TECHNIQUE OF VAGINAL RECONSTRUCTION USING NEUROVASCULAR PUDENDAL-THIGH FLAPS

V. T. JOSEPH AND J. T. K. WEE*

EDITORIAL COMMENT

This is an excellent and reliable technique. The location of the vessels is tricky but easily learned. Most of the other local techniques of vaginal reconstruction are based on Dr. Wee's original description of the vessels.

The neurovascular pudendal-thigh flap is a useful one that can reliably reconstruct the vagina in congenital and acquired conditions. The technique is simple, safe, and reliable, with no stents or dilators required. The reconstructed vagina has a natural angle and is sensate, and donor-site scarring in the groin is inconspicuous.

INDICATIONS

Previous attempts to reconstruct the vagina (1–11) suffered from a variety of disadvantages, including the necessity of stenting, an unphysiologic angle of the reconstructed vagina,

* Deceased.

the precarious vascularity of some flaps, and donor-site morbidity. Cadaveric studies (12) of the blood and nerve supply of the perineum, medial groin, and upper thigh led to the design of the neurovascular pudendal-thigh flap, which enables reconstruction of an innervated vagina with skin flaps that have a robust and reliable blood supply. The technique is superior to previously available methods. It is simple, safe, and reliable. No stents or dilators are needed, and the reconstructed vagina has a physiologic angle for intercourse and is sensate. Donor-area scars in the groin are well hidden.

However, in squamous cancers of the vulva and lower third of the vagina, there is a high possibility of lymphatic spread to the groin; in such cases, it may be prudent to avoid the pudendal-thigh flap, as its use would then be tantamount to using potentially malignant tissue for reconstruction.

The procedure is not limited to vaginal reconstruction: it may be used for the closure of difficult perineal wounds and fistulas, especially after irradiation. In males, it may be used to reconstruct the scrotum or penis.

ANATOMY

The internal pudendal artery supplies the perineum by means of its first branch, the inferior rectal artery, which courses through the anal region, and then by means of the perineal artery, which enters the superficial perineal pouch at the base of the perineal membrane. The perineal artery, after giving off the transverse perineal artery, continues on as the posterior labial arteries. The posterior labial arteries anastomose with branches of the deep external pudendal artery, as well as the medial femoral circumflex artery and the anterior branch of the obturator artery over the proximal part of the adductor muscles (Figs. 1–3).

The main anastomoses are with the deep external pudendal artery. Hence, by a process of "capture" of adjacent territory of the deep external pudendal artery, the posterior labial arteries extend to the femoral triangle. This is the vascular basis of the pudendal-thigh flap, which is nourished by this direct cutaneous system of arteries. The deep fascia and the epimysium over the proximal part of the adductor muscles underlying the flap should be included in the flap, to prevent injury to the direct cutaneous arteries when the flap is elevated (Fig. 4). The veins closely follow the arterial supply.

The posterior region of the labia majora is supplied medially by the posterior labial branches of the perineal nerve from

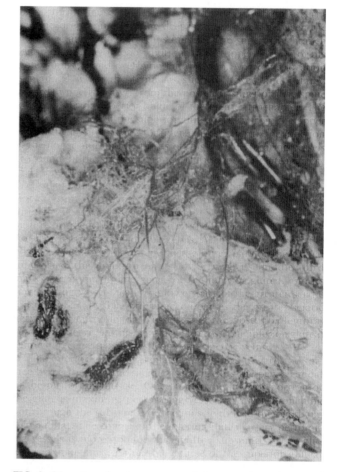

FIG. 2. Dissection showing anastomosis between the main arterial trunks in the groin. (From Wee and Joseph, ref. 12, with permission.)

the pudendal nerve. Laterally, the perineum is supplied by the perineal rami of the posterior cutaneous nerve of the thigh. The anterior region of the labia majora is an indeterminate area of mixed innervation, supplied by the pudendal, ilioinguinal, and genitofemoral nerves.

The posterior part of the pudendal-thigh flap retains its innervation from the posterior labial branches from the

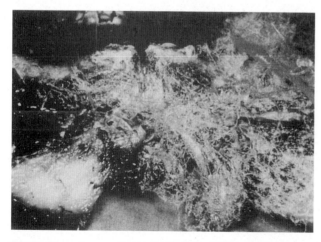

FIG. 1. Corrosion cast demonstrating arterial anastomosis around the thigh and pudendal region. (From Wee and Joseph, ref. 12, with permission.)

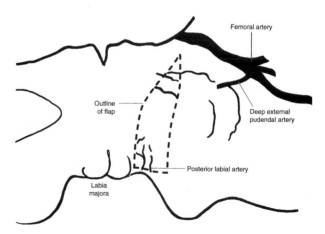

FIG. 3. Diagrammatic illustration of arterial supply of the pudendal-thigh flap. (From Ehrlich RM, Alter GJ, eds. *Reconstructive and plastic surgery of the external genitalia.* Philadelphia: WB Saunders Co., 1996, with permission.)

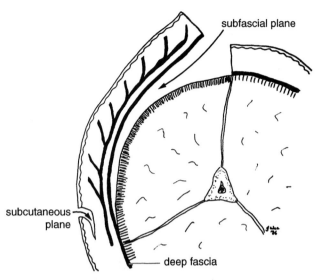

FIG. 4. The subfascial plane in which the flap is elevated. (From Wee, Joseph, ref. 12, with permission.)

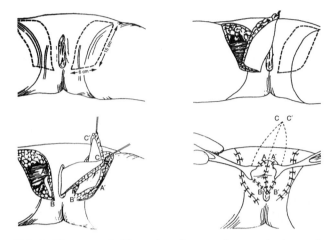

FIG. 5. Diagrammatic illustration of progressive steps in the surgical procedure for pudendal-thigh flap vaginal reconstruction. (From Ehrlich RM, Alter GJ, eds. *Reconstructive and plastic surgery of the external genitalia*. Philadelphia: WB Saunders Co., 1996, with permission.)

pudendal nerve, as well as from the perineal rami of the posterior cutaneous nerve of the thigh when it is elevated. The anterior part of the flap near the medial corner of the femoral triangle, supplied by nerve twigs of the genitofemoral and ilioinguinal nerves, may be denervated in the process of elevation. Hence, sensation would be retained only in the lower part of the reconstructed vagina.

FLAP DESIGN AND DIMENSIONS

A skin flap measuring 15 × 6 cm, with its posterior skin margin at the level of the posterior end of the introitus, can be raised as a skin island borne on a subcutaneous pedicle supplied by the posterior labial arteries (Fig. 3). It can be transposed through 70 degrees to meet its counterpart from the opposite side, forming a cul-de-sac in the midline. By raising the flap with the deep fascia of the thigh and the epimysium of the adductor muscles, an additional barrier is created, which prevents inadvertent damage to the neurovascular structures of the flap. It is probable that the addition of the layer of fascia may confer improved vascularity on the flap, as in a type A fasciocutaneous flap (13).

The flap is essentially horn-shaped, with the flare of the horn at its base. It is planned lateral to the hair-bearing area of the labia major and centered on the crease of the groin. The base of the flap is marked transversely at the level of the posterior end of the introitus. In the adult, the base can be 6 cm wide. This will allow direct closure of the donor site without much undermining. The flap can measure up to 15 cm in length and still remain safe. This places the tip of the flap in the femoral triangle. The dimensions of the flap can be made proportionally smaller in prepuberal females. A flap 15 × 6 cm is safe in adults, since it is arterialized throughout its length by the posterior labial and deep external pudendal arteries (Fig. 5).

In congenital cases, the plane between the base of the bladder and the rectus has to be created. A Foley catheter in the bladder and a finger or Hegar dilator in the rectum would facilitate the development of this plane and avoid visceral injuries. In ablative cancer resection, the lower marginal incision to remove the vagina usually ends as a circumferential incision at the mucocutaneous junction with the labia minora. The posterior skin margin of the flap is sutured to the opposite margin and also to this circumferential incision at the mucocutaneous junction.

OPERATIVE TECHNIQUE

The patient is placed in a lithotomy position with the legs in stirrups. The bladder is catheterized. The abdomen is prepared to allow simultaneous laparotomy or pelvic exenteration. A narrow transverse drape at the level of the pubis separates the abdomen from the perineum.

The incision, beginning at the tip of the flap, is deepened through skin and subcutaneous tissue down to deep fascia on two sides, except for the posterior margin of the flap. The subfascial plane is developed, raising the epimysium of the adductor muscles with the deep fascia. The deep fascia is tacked to the skin flap to prevent shearing. The flap is elevated until the posterior skin margin is reached. The margin is incised through dermis to subcutaneous tissue to a depth of 1.0 to 1.5 cm, and then undermined in a plane parallel to the skin for a distance of about 4 cm posteriorly (Fig. 6). This enables the flap to be transferred through 70 to 90 degrees, to meet its counterpart in the midline, and to allow the posterior skin margin of the flap to be sutured to the labia minora. This is

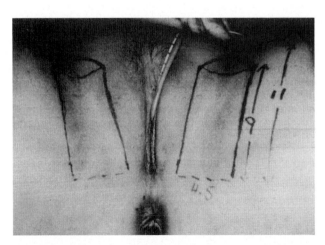

FIG. 6. Vaginal atresia: outline of flaps for reconstruction. (From Ehrlich RM, Alter GJ, eds. *Reconstructive and plastic surgery of the external genitalia*. Philadelphia: WB Saunders Co., 1996, with permission.)

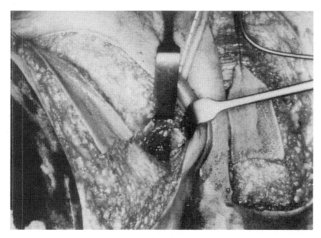

FIG. 7. Flap margins demarcated. Labial attachment divided, showing tunnel for cross-passage of flap. (From Ehrlich RM, Alter GJ, eds. *Reconstructive and plastic surgery of the external genitalia.* Philadelphia: WB Saunders Co., 1996, with permission.)

effected by elevating the labia off the pubic rami and the perineal membrane.

At this plane of elevation of the labia off the periosteum of the pubic rami and the peroneal membrane (in order to tunnel the flaps), there is no danger of denervating the labia, as the posterior labial nerves have already entered the labial fat pad far behind posteriorly. The clitoral nerves are also in no danger, because they do not pass through the superficial perineal pouch, but instead course through the deep perineal pouch to reach the clitoris.

The flaps are tunneled under the labi (Fig. 7). The posterior suture line where both flaps meet is completed first, with the flaps everted through the introitus. After the tip is reached, the anterior suture line is then begun. The tip of the cul-de-sac is then invaginated and anchored to the curve of the sacrum in the totally exenterated pelvis, by taking a large bite of periosteum with nonabsorbable sutures (Fig. 8). Correspondingly, the tip of the new vagina may be anchored to the rectum or bladder in anterior or posterior partial exenterations. In congenital cases, the tip of the new vagina may be moored to whatever pelvic structures are suitable, e.g., to uterine rudiments. The opening of the vagina is sutured to the mucocutaneous edge of the labia minora. Drains are inserted into the cavity containing the vagina, as well as flap donor sites. The

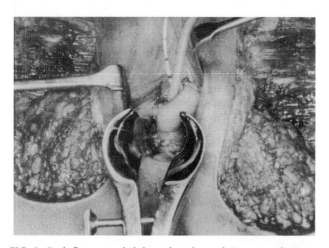

FIG. 8. Both flaps tunneled through and apex being sutured. (From Ehrlich RM, Alter GJ, eds. *Reconstructive and plastic surgery of the external genitalia.* Philadelphia: WB Saunders Co., 1996, with permission.)

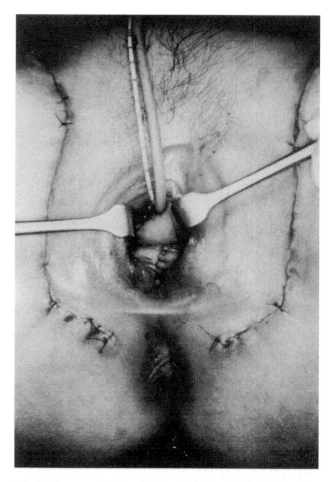

FIG. 9. Flaps sutured together to create neovagina. Donor areas closed by primary suture. (From Ehrlich RM, Alter GJ, eds. *Reconstructive and plastic surgery of the external genitalia.* Philadelphia: WB Saunders Co., 1996, with permission.)

patient is kept in bed with thighs adducted, until healing occurs. Urinary catheter drainage is continued throughout.

Only the lower part of the flap can be seen through the introitus for its circulation to be monitored postoperatively (Fig. 9). Photoplethysmography may be used to monitor the deeper part of the flap, if desired. Attempts at monitoring the flap by cutting the dermis with a #15 blade to elicit bleeding, would cause pain because the flaps retain their innervation.

CLINICAL RESULTS

In a preliminary small series of three patients, there were no complications, even as experience with the technique was being accumulated. This illustrates the robustness and intrinsic viability of the flaps. Reconstruction of a stable, skin-lined vagina was achieved, with no vaginal contraction. No stenting or dilatation was required to maintain the dimensions of the reconstructed vagina, unlike the situation with some other techniques. In contrast to other procedures utilizing the gracilis myocutaneous flap, even at its most reliable use, there was no incidence of flap necrosis.

The pudendal-thigh flap is very robust, with a reliable blood supply. There have been no problems with flap survival in our limited series. Among advantages of this procedure are the following. (1) This is a simple technique that can be completed in 2 or 2.5 hours with little blood loss. (2) The blood supply of the flaps is reliable and leads to early wound healing.

(3) No stents need be maintained, since the reconstructed vagina is stable. (4) The introduction of well-vascularized flap tissue into the pelvic cavity after exenteration aids in obliterating dead space, leading to primary healing of the exenterated cavity. (5) The angle of inclination of the vagina is physiologic and natural. (6) The linear scars of the donor sites are well-hidden in the groin crease and perineum; no thigh wounds need to be made to raise the flaps or harvest skin grafts. (7) The reconstructed vagina is sensate and retains the same innervation of erogenous zones of the perineum and upper thigh.

SUMMARY

The neurovascular pudendal-thigh flap procedure can be used reliably to reconstruct the vagina in congenital and acquired conditions.

References

1. Goldwyn RM. History of attempts to form a vagina. *Plast Reconstr Surg* 1977;59:319.

2. Frank RT. The formation of an artificial vagina without operation. *Am. J Obstet Gynecol* 1938;35:1053.
3. McIndoe A. The treatment of congenital absence and obliterative conditions of the vagina. *Br J Plast Surg* 1949;2:254.
4. Williams EA. Congenital absence of the vagina: a simple operation for its relief. *J Obstet Gynaecol Br Commonwealth* 1964;71:511.
5. McCraw JB, Massey FM, Shanklin KD, Horton CE. Vaginal reconstruction with gracilis myocutaneous flaps. *Plast Reconstr Surg* 1976;58:176.
6. Heath PM, Woods JE, Podratz KC, et al. Gracilis myocutaneous vaginal reconstruction. *Mayo Clin Proc* 1984;59:21.
7. Lagasse LD, Berman ML, Watring WG, Ballon SC. The gynecologic oncology patient: restoration of function and prevention of disability. In: L McGowan ed. *Gynecologic Oncology*. New York: Appleton-Century-Crofts, 1978;398.
8. Lacey PM, Morrow CP. Myocutaneous vaginal reconstruction. In: Morrow CP, Smart GE, eds. *Gynecologic oncology*. Berlin: Springer-Verlag, 1986. P. 255.
9. Wheeless CR. Vulvar-vaginal reconstruction. In: Coppleson M, ed. *Gynecologic oncology: fundamental principles and clinical practice Vol. 2*. Edinburgh: Churchill Livingstone, 1981, 933.
10. Song R, Wang X, Zhou G. Reconstruction of the vagina with sensory function. *Clin Plast Surg* 1982;9:105.
11. Wang TN, Whetzel T, Mathes SJ, Vasconez LO. A fasciocutaneous flap for vaginal and perineal reconstruction. *Plast Reconstr Surg* 1987;80:95.
12. Wee JTK, Joseph VT. A new technique of vaginal reconstruction using neurovascular pudendal-thigh flaps: a preliminary report. *Plast Reconstr Surg* 1989;83:701.
13. Dibbell DG. A fasciocutaneous flap for vaginal and perineal reconstruction (Discussion). *Plast Reconstr Surg* 1987;80:103.

CHAPTER 412 ■ "SHORT" GRACILIS MYOCUTANEOUS FLAPS FOR VULVOVAGINAL RECONSTRUCTION

J. T. SOPER

EDITORIAL COMMENT

The use of the short skin paddle over the proximal portion of the gracilis myocutaneous flap unquestionably increases flap viability, since the skin paddle is notoriously unreliable on the distal third of the muscle. Described in another chapter (Chapter 422), the transverse orientation of the skin island over the gracilis muscle will provide for a longer island of skin.

In the short gracilis flap modification of the classic long gracilis flap, the dominant vascular pedicle supplying the gracilis muscle is deliberately sacrificed, and a smaller myocutaneous unit is developed from the medial thigh.

INDICATIONS

The long gracilis flap has been used for a variety of complex pelvic reconstructions (1–7). In a modified short gracilis flap (7,8), a smaller skin island is developed and the primary vascular pedicle is deliberately sacrificed. Direct comparisons of reconstructions using both long and short gracilis flaps have revealed no increase in flap loss or other flap-specific complications with the use of the short flap (7–9). The short flap can be considered merely a modification or variation of the long flap, and both forms are often used by the reconstructive surgeon.

Currently, the short flap is our preference, when a gracilis myocutaneous flap is used for neovaginal reconstruction after pelvic exenteration. We are reluctant to use this flap, if there has been hypogastric or obturator artery ligation or chemoradiation delivered to the groin, situations that would theoretically impair the vascularity of the short flap.

ANATOMY

The thin, strap-like gracilis muscle is the most medial adductor of the thigh. It originates from the pubic tubercle and runs posterior to the adductor longus, to insert into the medial tibial plateau.

The gracilis muscle derives its major blood supply from a vascular perforator from branches of the medial femoral circumflex artery. This supports a large territory of skin extending along the medial thigh and into the distal third of the thigh posterior to the adductor longus. The dominant vascular pedicle is constant in location, entering the deep gracilis muscle, with paired venae comitantes and nerve approximately 6 to 8 cm distal to the pubic tubercle, after passing between the adductor longus and brevis muscles (Fig. 1). An accessory blood supply, derived from anastomotic terminal branches of the obturator and pudendal arteries, enters within the proximal 1 to 3 cm of the gracilis muscle (Fig. 1). These accessory vessels are not as well-defined as the dominant vascular pedicle, but they can support the short gracilis myocutaneous flap for pelvic reconstructions.

FLAP DESIGN AND DIMENSIONS

The gracilis flap can be rotated either anteriorly or posteriorly within a wide arc of rotation, allowing the flap to be deployed for anterior vulvar or groin reconstruction, neovaginal formation, or repair of posterior vulvar and perineal defects. The arc of rotation of the classic flap is around the mobilized dominant vascular pedicle, while the short flap is rotated around the origin of the muscle from the pubic tubercle. If a classic long gracilis flap is developed, the proximal muscle can be divided to facilitate rotation but, usually, there is sufficient mobility so that division of the muscle is not necessary. Furthermore, division of the proximal muscle deprives the flap of its secondary blood supply.

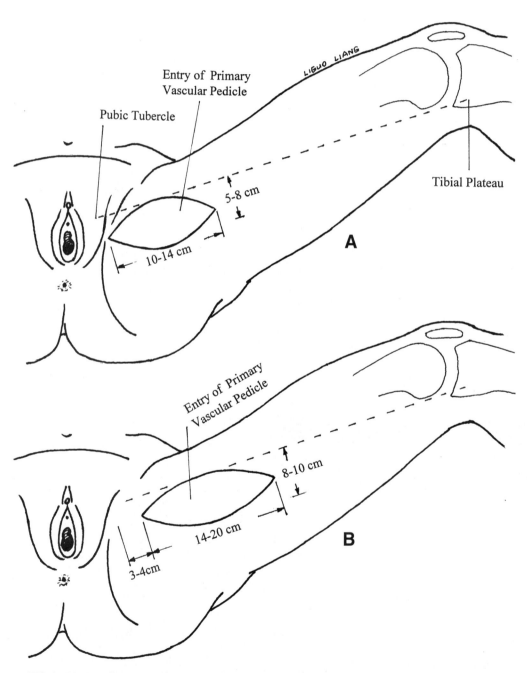

FIG. 1. Diagram showing comparison of the size and location for short (A) and long (B) gracilis flap skin islands. Skin for the island should be harvested posterior to a line from the pubic tubercle to the medial tibial plateau.

OPERATIVE TECHNIQUE

The patient is positioned in the modified Whitmore position, using Allen stirrups with the hips abducted approximately 45 degrees and flexed slightly. The medial thighs are prepped to the knees, to allow access to the full skin island, if needed. A guideline is drawn on the medial thigh from the pubic tubercle to the medial tibial plateau, along the margin of the adductor longus muscle. The skin island supplied by the gracilis will be located posterior to this line. A 10- to 14-cm long × 5- to 8-cm wide ellipsoid skin island centered over the proximal gracilis muscle will be used for the short flap, with the proximal margin located at the crural fold (Fig. 2).

A full-thickness incision is made along the anterior and distal margins of the skin island through the fascia (Fig. 1). It is important that the incision be either straight to the fascia or slightly flared at its base, so that the skin will not be undermined and lose vascularity. The skin is loosely anchored to the fascia with temporary interrupted sutures, to prevent shearing of the fat away from the underlying fascia during manipulation of the flap. The belly of the gracilis muscle is identified at the distal margin of the flap, posterior to the adductor longus. It is isolated and divided. The remainder of the full-thickness incision is completed around the margin of the skin island through the fascia.

The gracilis is mobilized from its bed with sharp and blunt dissection. It is important to work from the distal tip of the flap toward the origin, so that the dominant vascular pedicle can be identified and preserved, if desired (Fig. 3). The dominant vascular pedicle enters the deep anterior belly of the gracilis approximately 6 to 8 cm from the pubic tubercle, emerging from underneath the belly of the adductor longus muscle. With its paired venae comitantes, it is easily distinguished from the loose areolar tissue between the muscles. The nerve usually enters with, or just proximal to, the dominant vascular pedicle. If a classic long flap is to be used, the pedicle is mobilized; if a short flap is to be used, the pedicle is cross-clamped, divided, and ligated (Fig. 3). The nerve can usually be spared, to provide muscular innervation and sensibility to the skin island in the short flap, but may be sacrificed. The remainder of the gracilis flap is mobilized to its origin. In a short flap, the 2 to 3 cm of the proximal gracilis muscle should not be aggressively skeletonized, so that small accessory vessels are not stripped away from the muscle.

For neovaginal construction, a subfascial tunnel is constructed to the vaginal introitus with sharp and blunt dissection. The tunnel should allow passage of the gracilis flap freely without pressure. Bilateral flaps are rotated posteriorly through the tunnels and allowed to hang freely between the patient's legs. The neovaginal tube is constructed by approximating the skin edges with interrupted absorbable sutures.

When unilateral or bilateral flaps are used for vulvar reconstructions, the flaps are rotated either anteriorly or posteriorly, depending on the defect, without use of the subfascial tunnels. The muscle is anchored to the deep tissues of the defect with loose interrupted sutures, and the skin approximated with interrupted absorbable sutures.

The thigh incisions are irrigated and closed in layers over closed suction drains. Patients are allowed to ambulate within 24 to 48 hours after surgery.

CLINICAL RESULTS

Patients receiving the gracilis flap for pelvic reconstruction have undergone radical surgery, often with prior irradiation or combined chemoradiation; any analysis of complications

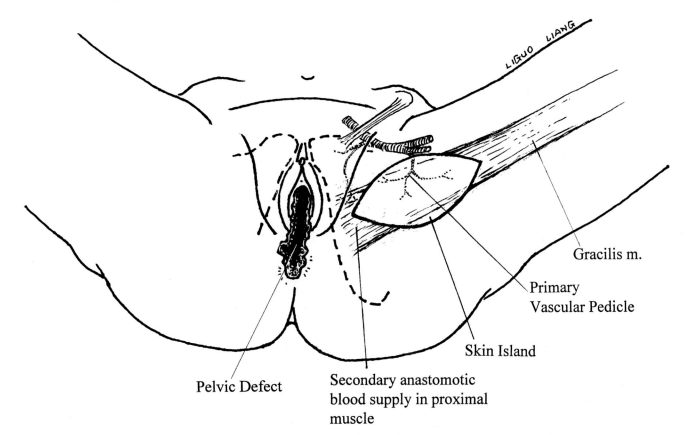

FIG. 2. The skin island for the "short" gracilis flap is harvested by incising the anterior margin first, to facilitate identification of the gracilis muscle. Relationships of primary and secondary blood supplies to the gracilis muscle are schematically illustrated.

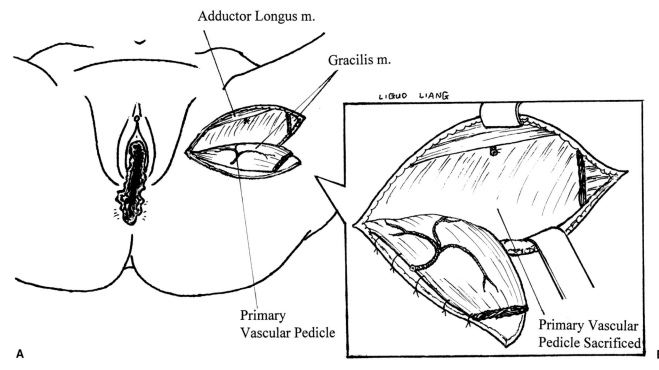

FIG. 3. After developing the skin island dividing the distal gracilis muscle, the flap is elevated from the medial thigh. The primary vascular pedicle is identified (**A**), entering the muscle 7 to 8 cm from its origin. Although this vascular pedicle is preserved in the long flap, it is deliberately sacrificed (**B**) in the short gracilis flap.

should recognize the morbid nature of these procedures. If gracilis flaps are used during an exenteration, the neovaginal reconstruction can be performed by a second team, without interrupting the abdominal procedure.

Flap-specific complications can be arbitrarily divided into those related to the donor site and those involving the flap specifically. In our experience, patients with short gracilis flaps tend to have fewer donor-site infections or hematomas than those who receive long gracilis flaps (9). Additionally, patients with short flaps have smaller medial-thigh scars than those with long flaps. However, these donor-site complications are usually only minor inconveniences, rather than major sources of morbidity.

Complications involving the flap include introital stenosis, neovaginal prolapse, flap loss, and indirect complications of rectovaginal fistula formation caused by tissue pressure upon a rectosigmoid anastomosis. Stenosis of the vaginal introitus is observed in approximately 9 percent of patients, occasionally requiring operative revision in women who desire intercourse, but it is also a relatively minor complication. Avoidance of a circular introital scar and proper planning at the time of neovaginal formation can usually prevent this complication. Overall, approximately 47 percent of our patients are sexually active after gracilis flap reconstruction (9).

Neovaginal prolapse has been observed more frequently in patients receiving the classic long gracilis flap than in those with short gracilis flap neovaginas after exenteration (10); in our experience, prolapse after exenteration occurs in only 3 percent of patients (9). This relatively low incidence is probably related to a compulsive effort to fit the neovagina snugly within the pelvic crater, and to anchor it to the sacral hollow, symphysis, and/or levator plate.

Flap loss of varying degrees is observed in approximately 10 to 20 percent of patients with gracilis flaps, ranging from minor loss of skin and subcutaneous tissue from the tips or margins of the flaps, to complete loss of one or both myocuta-

neous units (1–10). Flap loss of less than 50 percent of the flap is usually considered only a minor inconvenience. Patients in this category are treated with dilute peroxide irrigation until there is a good base of granulation tissue. The muscle usually survives, and a functional neovagina or vulvar reconstruction results after muscle reepithelialization.

Loss of more than 50 percent of the flap usually requires operative debridement. Total loss of the myocutaneous unit frequently occurs in these patients, often resulting in chronic vaginal stenosis or other pelvic complications. We analyzed factors associated with the loss of gracilis myocutaneous flaps in 22 women with classic long flaps and in 24 with short flaps for pelvic reconstruction (9). The incidence of major flap loss was 14 and 17 percent, respectively, a nonsignificant difference.

Considering various clinical and operative factors, only performance of a gracilis flap neovagina, in conjunction with pelvic exenteration combined with rectosigmoid anastomosis, was significantly associated with major flap loss, compared to other exenterative procedures or other types of radical pelvic procedures. It is possible that pressure on the myocutaneous unit from surrounding tissue compromises venous return or blood flow into the flap. Similarly, a myocutaneous flap might jeopardize healing of a rectosigmoid anastomosis. It has been reported (5) that two of three patients in a series receiving gracilis flaps under these conditions developed major flap loss and rectovaginal fistula. Use of a single gracilis flap, a smaller flap such as the bulbocavernosus myocutaneous flap, or a rectus myocutaneous or myoperitoneal flap might avoid these complications, when neovaginal reconstruction is performed in conjunction with rectosigmoid anastomosis.

SUMMARY

The short gracilis flap modification can be successfully utilized for complex pelvic reconstructions. Analysis of flap-specific complications indicates that the risk of loss for a gracilis neo-vagina is increased, when the procedure is performed following pelvic exenteration with rectosigmoid anastomosis, compared to total pelvic exenteration or other radical pelvic reconstructions.

References

1. McCraw JB, Masey, FB, Shanklin, KD, et al. Vaginal reconstruction with gracilis myocutaneous flaps. *Plast Reconstr Surg* 1976;58:176.
2. Becker DW, Massey FM, McCraw JB. Myocutaneous flaps in reconstructive pelvic surgery. *Obstet Gynecol* 1979;54:178.
3. Morrow CP, Lacey CG, Lucas WE. Reconstructive surgery in gynecologic cancer employing the gracilis myocutaneous pedicle graft. *Gynecol Oncol* 1979;7:176.
4. Berek JS, Hacker NF, Lagasse LD. Vaginal reconstruction performed simultaneously with pelvic exenteration. *Obstet Gynecol* 1984;63:318.
5. Lacey CG, Stern JL, Feigenbaum S, et al. Vaginal reconstruction after exenteration with use of gracilis myocutaneous flaps: the University of California at San Francisco experience. *Am J Obstet Gynecol* 1988;158:1278.
6. Cain JM, Diamond A, Tourimi HK, et al. The morbidity and benefits of concurrent gracilis myocutaneous graft with pelvic exenteration. *Obstet Gynecol* 1989;74:185.
7. Copeland CJ, Hancock KC, Gershenson DM, et al. Gracilis myocutaneous vaginal reconstruction concurrent with total pelvic exenteration. *Am J Obstet Gynecol* 1989;160:1095.
8. Soper JT, Larson D, Hunter VJ, et al. Short gracilis flaps for vulvovaginal reconstruction after radical pelvic surgery. *Obstet Gynecol* 1989;74:823.
9. Soper JT, Rodriguez G, Berchuck A, et al. Long and short gracilis flaps for vulvovaginal reconstruction after radical pelvic surgery: comparison of flap-specific complications. *Gynecol Oncol* 1995;56:271.
10. Soper JT, Berchuck A, Creasman WT, et al. Pelvic exenteration: factors associated with major surgical morbidity. *Gynecol Oncol* 1989;35:93.

CHAPTER 413 ■ RECONSTRUCTION OF THE VAGINA USING THE MODIFIED "SINGAPORE" FLAP

J. E. WOODS, P. YUGUEROS, AND W. J. KANE

EDITORIAL COMMENT

This flap also demonstrates the reliability of the circulation to the perineal area and its usefulness for vaginal reconstruction.

A modification of the originally described (1) Singapore flap for vaginal reconstruction is a single-stage procedure, with excellent flap reliability, simplicity, and a relatively brief time required to carry out the procedure.

INDICATIONS

There are various techniques for reconstructing the vagina. We have concluded that the simplest and most acceptable approach in our hands is a modification of the flap originally described by Wee and Joseph (1), which we have modified (2). This modification involves a single-stage procedure with excellent flap reliability and the potential for normal or near-normal function, with minimal donor-site morbidity and technical simplicity.

ANATOMY

Pudendal thigh flaps are based on the posterior labial arteries, which are a continuation of the perineal artery. These arteries anastomose with branches of the deep external pudendal artery, as well as the medial femoral circumflex artery, and the anterior branch of the obturator artery over the proximal portion of the adductor muscle. When elevated, the posterior portion of the flap retains innervation from the posterior labial branches from the pudendal nerve, as well as from the perineal rami of the posterior cutaneous nerve of the thigh. Thus, the flaps may be expected, at least in their proximal portions, to be partially sensate (1).

FLAP DESIGN AND DIMENSIONS

The flaps, which are designed to measure 15×6 cm, are raised bilaterally in the groin crease just lateral to the labia majora, and include the deep fascia and the epimysium of the adductor muscles, to avoid inadvertent damage to the neurovascular structures. The base of the flap is located at the level of what would be the normal posterior margin of the vaginal introitus, before its disruption by surgery.

OPERATIVE TECHNIQUE

While the flaps were originally designed and used as island flaps (1), because so many patients have had previous heavy radiation and multiple procedures, as well as concomitant intraoperative irradiation, we simply divide the labia posteriorly, allowing them to retract forward, avoiding any possible

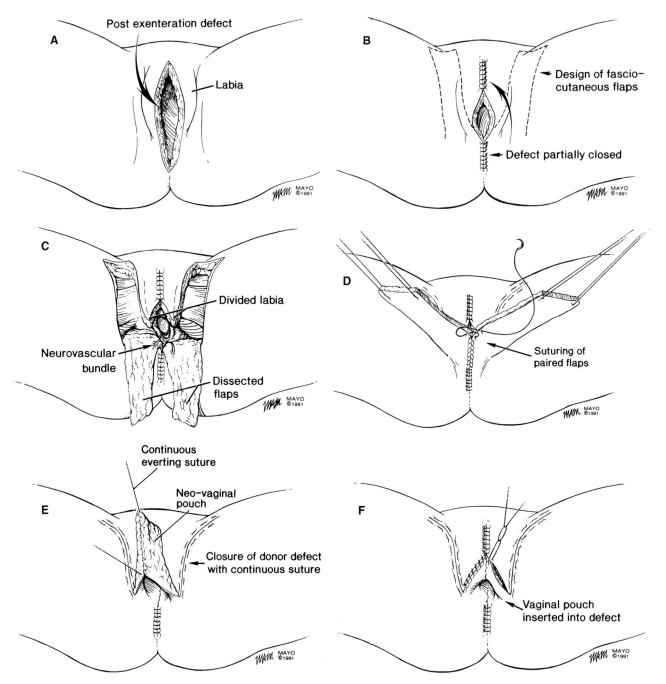

FIG. 1. Diagrammatic representation of vaginal reconstruction using the modified Singapore flap. **A:** Exenteration defect prior to reconstruction. **B:** Partial suturing of defect with 6- × 15-cm flaps straddling the inguinal crease. **C:** Flaps elevated at the subfascial level, with division of the labia posteriorly, to allow easy insetting of the neovagina without incision of the skin at the base of the flaps. **D:** Initial suturing of the flaps is carried out to evert the flap edges into the neovagina, avoiding burial of the dermis. **E:** The completed pouch prior to insetting. Note preliminary closure of the donor defects. **F:** Nearly completed suturing of neovagina after insetting. (From Woods et al., ref. 2, with permission.)

flap compromise, and allowing for optimal insetting. This permits easy suturing and insetting of the pedicle flaps, with some minimal aesthetic loss that has not appeared to be a concern of patients. Figure 1A–F illustrates the technique diagrammatically and photographically.

After the flaps have been elevated, they are sutured together with moderately long-lasting absorbable sutures, and they provide a pouch that is ample for normal intercourse. Once the pouch is completed, it is invaginated into the cavity, which may require partial closure after a total exenteration. The remnants of the portions of the flap remaining outside the cavity are sutured to the wound margins, to provide completion of the repair.

Since this procedure is often done at the time of total or partial exenteration, and the gynecologic surgeon is continuing intraabdominal surgery concomitantly with our repair, we have provided a nonabsorbable suture attached to the apex of the pouch, which is then fixed by the intraabdominal surgeon to the sacrum or adjacent structures. A Vaseline-coated pack is placed in the vagina with an external tag to allow easy removal, and a T-binder is used to maintain the pack within the cavity. The pack may be changed on a daily basis after the second postoperative day, and helps to maintain the position of the vagina, with the T-binder in place, during the initial several weeks of healing. This minimizes the probability of prolapse, when the apex of the pouch cannot be fixed in the pelvis.

We prefer to use absorbable sutures in areas where suture removal at a later date will occasion a great deal of discomfort, utilizing 2-0 or 3-0 Vicryl in the suturing of the pouch.

CLINICAL RESULTS

In 31 patients in whom this procedure was carried out, many of them under adverse circumstances after extensive ablative procedures and both previous and intraoperative irradiation, only one flap failure occurred, and this was in an extremely heavily-irradiated patient. We have experienced dehiscence and other wound complications occasionally, but these have been related almost totally to extensive ablative procedures and irradiation, rather than to the flap itself. Of course, function varies with the patient's age and degree of debilitation from extensive radiation and chemotherapy. We have performed the procedure in irradiated patients who have received radiotherapy to the inguinal and perineal regions, but do so with some caution, as this has been the only situation in which we have seen flap failure. Even with a history of radiation, if there are not extensive stigmata signifying radiation damage, we have carried out the procedure without significant morbidity.

There have been some problems with stenosis at the neointroitus, but these can be minimized by the use of dilators once healing has occurred or, occasionally, by a small Z-plasty type of procedure.

SUMMARY

This single-stage procedure, a modification of the Singapore flap, has been very useful in cases of vaginal reconstruction. The flaps are reliable and technically simple, with the potential for normal or near-normal function, and minimal donor-site morbidity.

References

1. Wee JT, Joseph VT. A new technique of vaginal reconstruction using neurovascular pudendal-thigh flaps: a preliminary report. *Plast Reconstr Surg* 1989;83:701.
2. Woods JE, Alter G, Meland B, Podratz K. Experience with vaginal reconstruction utilizing the modified Singapore flap. *Plast Reconstr Surg* 1992;90:270.

CHAPTER 414 ■ RECTUS ABDOMINIS FLAPS IN VAGINAL AND PELVIC RECONSTRUCTION

G. R. TOBIN

Rectus abdominis flaps and their variations are readily adaptable to all types of exenterative pelvic surgery, to reconstruction of all patterns of vaginal resection, and to defects of the groin, external pelvis, vulva, and perineum (1–4).

INDICATIONS

Radical pelvic resection of the vagina and endopelvic organs creates exceptionally difficult reconstructive challenges that are well-served by the distally-based rectus abdominis muscle-skin flap carrying an inversely-tubed epigastric skin paddle to form a neovagina. None of the other described techniques of vaginal reconstruction (5–8) provides as much volume of well-vascularized tissue to defects that are usually irradiated. In addition to restoring sexual function, rectus abdominis flaps block entry of the bowel into the pelvis, revascularize the irradiated pelvic-cavity wall, and lessen the incidence of pelvic infection, fistulae, and chronically-open perineal wounds. Even when intercourse will likely not be resumed postoperatively, the patient receives the benefit of pelvic filling with well-vascularized tissue to lessen infections and healing complications.

The flap was developed specifically for vaginal reconstruction in the radical pelvic resection defect (1), although it can be varied and used in other conditions of vaginal absence. It has become the choice of many experienced surgeons for oncologic reconstruction, because it provides a highly reliable vaginal replacement, while also filling the endopelvic defect with well-vascularized tissue. The excellent perfusion of the flap revascularizes the defect and reduces the incidence of postoperative pelvic infections, while the bulk of the flap and muscle pedicle serves to block bowel herniation.

When male patients having abdominal-perineal resection or exenteration would benefit from the bulk and revascularization provided by this flap, the flap is deepithelialized to the deep dermal level and placed in the pelvic space without being tubed. If a skin paddle is required for perineal closure, an appropriately-sized island is left on the distal paddle beyond the deepithelialized portion and inset into the perineal defect.

Additional advantages of the flap result from its exceptional versatility in paddle design and placement. Following a

supralevator extenteration, flaps from the thigh or groin (7,8) must be passed around the retained vaginal cuff through a difficult dissection. With the rectus abdominis flap, the distal end is simply joined to the vaginal cuff at the cut end. With some rectal and posterior vaginal-wall resections for rectal lesions, the bladder and anterior vaginal wall can be retained. In these cases, the paddle is designed with dimensions appropriate to the resection and inset along the margins of the retained anterior vagina, without complete tubing. If partial vulvectomy is required with the vaginectomy, the distal end of the flap is enlarged and opened onto the perineum in a trumpet-like fashion (see Fig. 4C).

Circumstances in which the flap is not indicated include transection of the muscle and vascular pedicle by previous incision. Deep inferior epigastric vessel ligation probably also precludes use of the flap. The most distal of the segmental collateral vessels entering the posterolateral surface of the muscle are usually preserved in transfer, and these could theoretically supply the flap in the absence of the deep inferior epigastric vessels, but I am not aware that this has yet been established. Another reservation is in reconstruction of vaginal agenesis when the abdomen is unscarred (Rokitansky-Kuester-Hauser syndrome and related conditions). Since a less conspicuous donor-site scar is preferable to a long vertical scar, design of the flap with a transverse skin paddle placed just below the umbilicus, as in the paddle used for TRAM-flap breast reconstruction (9), provides a more acceptable donor-site scar for this group of patients, if vaginal reconstruction with flap tissue is preferred over skin grafts and stents (Abbe-McIndoe technique) (10,11).

ANATOMY

The anatomic features relevant to the rectus abdominis muscle-skin flap are shown in Fig. 1A. The rectus abdominis

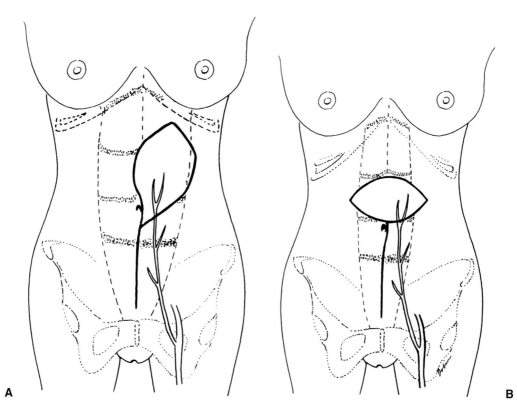

FIG. 1. Cutaneous paddle designs of rectus abdominis flaps for reconstruction showing the relationship of the paddle to the muscle, vascular pedicle, laparotomy incision, and surface landmarks. **A:** Diagram of the most frequently used design, with a vertical paddle axis aligned with the muscle. **B:** Diagram of the transverse paddle, which can be used to lessen tissue bulk in the deep pelvis. (From Tobin et al., ref. 2, with permission.)

muscle-skin flap is based on either of the paired rectus abdominis muscles spanning the abdominal wall from the ventral thoracic cage to the pubis on either side of the linea alba. The dense rectus sheath fascia encases the upper three-quarters of the muscle, but the posterior rectus sheet is absent distal to the linea arcuata.

The blood supply to the upper muscle is the superior epigastric vessels, which are divided in transfer of this flap. These are a continuation of the internal mammary vessels and run on the deep surface of the muscle. The overlying epigastric skin is supplied by cutaneous perforators from the muscle, which pass through the anterior rectus sheath.

The blood supply of the distal muscle is the deep inferior epigastric vessels, which originate from the external iliac vessels near the inguinal ligament, and run on the deep surface of the distal muscle. Cutaneous perforators from this portion of the muscle supply the hypogastric abdominal skin, which is also supplied by the superficial inferior epigastric vessels that run in a parallel pattern in the subcutaneous tissue.

The deep inferior and superior epigastric vascular systems are joined by anastomic vessels across a vascular watershed in the mid-portion of the muscle near the umbilicus. This allows the entire muscle-skin unit to receive a vascular supply from either end. For example, this flap carries an epigastric skin paddle supplied by cutaneous perforators from the upper muscle, across the vascular watershed from the deep inferior epigastric vascular pedicle. This mirrors the vascular supply of the TRAM flap used for breast reconstruction, in which hypogastric skin is carried by cutaneous perforators from the lower muscle supplied across the watershed from the superior epigastric pedicle (9).

The muscle also receives a collateral vascular supply from segmental vessels that accompany the motor nerves entering the posterolateral border of the muscle. In transposition of this flap, most of these are divided to permit transfer, but the most caudal one or two can usually be preserved in vaginal reconstruction. More distal transfers require dividing all of them.

FLAP DESIGN AND DIMENSIONS

The full cutaneous territory of the flap extends vertically from the costal margin to the pubis, and horizontally from lines defined by the ipsilateral anterior superior iliac spine and contralateral mid-inguinal line. Therefore, the cutaneous paddle can be designed in a wide variety of patterns within this area and can be placed anywhere along the course of the muscle. The most common cutaneous paddle design for vaginal reconstruction is a wide vertical ellipse centered over the upper half of the muscle, extending from just below the umbilicus to just below the costal margin, and approximately 20 to 25 cm long (Fig. 1A). The paddle width is related to the intended luminal diameter by the formula within, an 11-cm-wide paddle provides a luminal diameter of about 3.5 cm. If needed, substantially greater paddle widths of up to three times this size can be reliably carried, when placed within the vascular territory described above.

An alternative cutaneous paddle design that is occasionally useful is a transversely-oriented ellipse placed just above or just below the umbilicus (Fig. 1B). The half of the ellipse forming the proximal neovagina is centered over the muscle, and the half of the ellipse forming the distal neovagina extends either medially across the mid-line (as in Fig. 1B), or laterally toward the flank. This allows the distal neovagina to be made much less bulky when the endopelvic passage is narrow and bulk is unwanted, such as in vaginectomies with bladder preservation and colonic pull-through for low rectal anastomosis. Placement of the transverse paddle above the umbilicus better protects the usual stoma sites, while placement of the

paddle first below the umbilicus leaves a lower scar profile and can be used if stomas are not needed.

Deepithelialized, untubed paddles are used in males when the benefits of well-vascularized tissue bulk are desired without a vaginal reconstruction. If needed, a distal skin island can be preserved and inset into the perineal defect.

OPERATIVE TECHNIQUE

The steps of the operative technique are demonstrated in Figs. 2–4. Following incision of the skin paddle, a corresponding island of the underlying anterior rectus sheath is incised. This fascial island can be made narrower than the overlying skin paddle, to permit direct closure of the remaining anterior rectus sheath. A 0.5- to 1.0-cm-wide strip of anterior rectus sheath adjacent to the linea alba, and another lateral strip of anterior rectus sheath 3 to 4 cm wide, are left in situ (Fig. 2A–C) for subsequent direct closure of the anterior fascial layer.

The muscle is transected at the level of the skin-paddle cephalic end, and the superior epigastric vessels are divided. The skin paddle and muscle pedicle are then elevated from the underlying posterior rectus fascia by sequential division of the segmental neurovascular pedicles that enter the lateral muscle border. This is continued only until the flap is sufficiently mobilized to reach the recipient site. Distal to the skin paddle, the anterior rectus sheath is left in situ and attached to the overlying hypogastric skin and subcutaneous tissue, to provide abdominal-wall structure following flap transfer.

Subsequent to flap elevation, the vaginal pouch is formed by inverse tubing of the skin paddle. This is done with the flap transposed distally onto the groin region surface, which allows a second surgical team to construct a urinary conduit and colostomy while the vagina is simultaneously being formed. The lateral margins and periumbilical apex of the paddle are sutured to each other, to form a pouch closed on one end with the skin on the inside (Fig. 3). The flap is then passed through the distal mid-line peritoneal incision into the pelvis, and the open end of the vaginal pouch is inset into the vaginal cuff or perineal defect, to form a neo-introitus (Fig. 4A–D).

Following placement of colostomy and urinary conduit stomas, the abdominal donor site and the lower abdomen are closed directly. At the skin-fascial paddle donor site, the lateral and medial strips of the anterior rectus sheath may be sutured together, to provide a second layer of fascial closure over the intact posterior rectus sheath. Occasionally, these fascial margins cannot be completely approximated due to excess tension; they are then simply inset into the underlying posterior rectus sheath. This method of fascial inset without anterior sheath closure was used routinely in the initial group of patients reconstructed with this flap (1); no hernias or fascial bulges occurred at the fascial donor site. However, the theoretic potential for donor-site weakness led us to leave fascial margins and to close the anterior rectus sheath whenever possible (2,3).

Distal to the umbilicus, the mid-line anterior rectus-sheath incision is closed by suturing it to the linea alba over the transposed muscle pedicle (Fig. 1A). The skin-paddle donor site is closed directly in continuity with the laparotomy incision by direct approximation of the elliptical margins. Closed suction drains are used at both donor and recipient sites. Stents or dilation of the neovagina are not needed postoperatively.

CLINICAL RESULTS

We have used the rectus abdominis flap in reconstruction of radical pelvic resections in over 100 cases since 1983 (1–3).

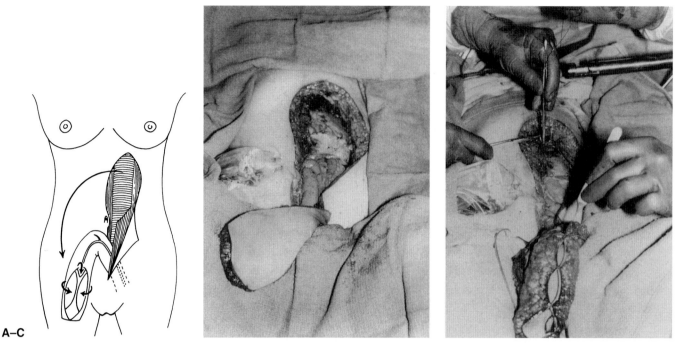

A–C

FIG. 2. Demonstrating steps of the operative procedure. **A:** Schema of a vertical flap transposition from the abdominal field to the groin region for formation of the vaginal pouch, which allows simultaneous construction of the urinary conduit and colostomy. (From Tobin et al., ref. 2, with permission.) **B:** Flap transposition in a patient showing the flap and donor site. **C:** Formation of the neovagina by inverse tubing of the paddle and closure of the anterior rectus sheath in process.

Our experience with the flap in vaginal reconstructions has been substantially more favorable than with gracilis flaps (7,12,13) or any other method that we used previously.

Advantages of rectus abdominis reconstructions are many. First, the obliteration of the residual endopelvic space and the exclusion of bowel allowed by the bulk of the flap and location of the pedicle are far superior to any other flap. Second, rectus abdominis flaps are far more reliable than gracilis flaps (7,12). The gracilis flap has one of the highest incidences of flap loss, and the rectus abdominis has one of the lowest (14). Third, a single flap restores the vaginal pouch, compared with bilateral flaps that are required by the gracilis and several other flap reconstructions. Fourth, the rectus abdominis donor site closes in continuity with the laporotomy incision and avoids additional donor sites on the thighs, which are

occasionally sensitive (13). Fifth, surface quality is excellent, and stents or dilators are not required to maintain neovaginal luminal dimensions. Finally, revascularization of irradiated pelvic wounds is provided by the excellent vascularity of the flap, and the incidence of infection after radical pelvic surgery when this flap is used has fallen dramatically from that occurring before its introduction.

In our cases to date, we have had only one complete flap loss, which occurred in a heavy smoker whose iliac artery was severely narrowed and occluded postoperatively. There was one other significant partial paddle loss, a 30 percent loss, successfully treated by skin grafting the muscle bed. There was one partial prolapse. We have had no donor-site hernias or bulges, and we have not used any prosthetic patches to reinforce the donor site.

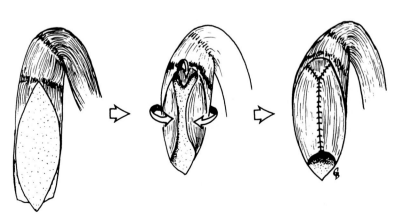

FIG. 3. Inverse tubing method of the skin paddle used to create a vaginal pouch. (From Tobin et al., ref. 2, with permission.)

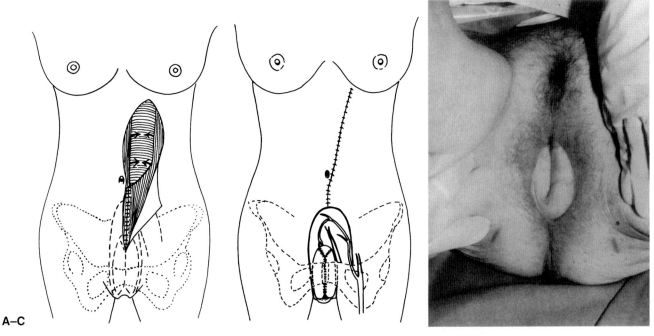

A–C

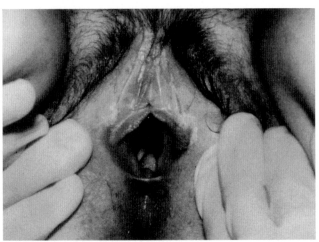

D

FIG. 4. Closure of the donor defect after inset of neovagina and stomas. **A:** Diagram illustrating direct closure of the anterior rectus fascia donor site above the umbilicus (*arrows*) and abdominal-wall closure below the umbilicus by suture of the anterior rectus fascia to the linea alba. **B:** Direct closure of the cutaneous donor site in continuity with the laparotomy. **C:** Neovagina and vulva reconstructed in a patient who had a simultaneous exenteration and vulvectomy. **D:** Neovagina reconstructed in a patient who had a supralevator exenteration. The introitus and a short vaginal cuff were preserved. (Fig. 4A and B from Tobin et al., ref. 2, with permission.)

SUMMARY

The distally-based rectus abdominis muscle-skin flap is a highly reliable, versatile technique for vaginal reconstruction, endopelvic revascularization, and reconstruction of large defects of the pelvic exterior, lower abdomen, groin, or perineum. The procedure is recommended over other methods of vaginal reconstruction for radical pelvic resections.

References

1. Tobin GR, Day TG. Vaginal and pelvic reconstruction with distally based rectus abdominis myocutaneous flaps. *Plast Reconstr Surg* 1988;81:62.
2. Tobin GR, Pursell SH, Day TG. Refinements in vaginal reconstruction using rectus abdominis flaps. *Clin Plast Surg* 1990;17:705.
3. Tobin GR. Pelvic, vaginal and perineal reconstruction in radical pelvic surgery. *Surg Oncol Clin North Am* 1994;3:397.
4. Shepherd JH, Van Dam PA, Jobling TW, Breach N. The use of rectus abdominis myocutaneous flaps following excision of vulvar cancer. *Br J Obstet Gynaecol* 1990;97:1020.
5. Goldwyn RM. History of attempts to form a vagina. *Plast Reconstr Surg* 1977;59:319.
6. Doering DL, Bosscher JR, Tobin GR. Pelvic reconstructive surgery. In: Shingleton HM, et al., eds. *Gynecologic oncology: current diagnosis and treatment.* Philadelphia: WB Saunders, 1996;486–502.
7. McCraw JB, Massey FM, Shanklin KD, et al. Vaginal reconstruction with gracilis myocutaneous flaps. *Plast Reconstr Surg* 1976;58:176.
8. Hurwitz DJ, Dweibel PC. Gluteal thigh flap repair of chronic perineal wounds. *Am J Surg* 1985;150:386.
9. Hartrampf CR, Scheflan M, Black PW. Breast reconstruction with a transverse abdominal island flap. *Plast Reconstr Surg* 1982;69:216.
10. Abbé R. New method of creating a vagina in a case of congenital absence. *Med Rec* 1898;54:836.
11. McIndoe A. Treatment of congenital absence and obliterative conditions of the vagina. *Br J Plast Surg* 1950;2:254.
12. Heath PM, Woods JE, Podratz MD, et al. Gracilis myocutaneous vaginal reconstruction. *Mayo Clin Proc* 1986;59:21.
13. Massey FM. Vulvovaginal reconstruction following radical resection. *Clin Obstet Gynecol* 1986;29:617.
14. Mathes S, Nahai F. Muscle and myocutaneous flaps. In: Goldwyn RM, ed. *The unfavorable result in plastic surgery: avoidance and treatment,* 2nd ed. Boston: Little, Brown, 1984;111.

CHAPTER 415 ■ TRANSPELVIC RECTUS ABDOMINIS FLAP RECONSTRUCTION OF DEFECTS FOLLOWING ABDOMINAL-PERINEAL RESECTION

S. S. KROLL

EDITORIAL COMMENT

It is important to divide the rectus muscle completely, rather than to use the muscle as a point of pedicle attachment. The vasculature is extramuscular in the inferior portion and will leave a much smaller opening in the perineal reflection than is required by passing the muscle through.

Defects left after abdomino-perineal resection (APR) of rectal cancers are often very slow to heal secondarily, particularly if radiotherapy has been administered. An effective method of achieving a healed wound is to transfer an inferiorly-based rectus abdominis myocutaneous flap to the perineum through the pelvis immediately following the APR (1).

INDICATIONS

The most common indication for this procedure is an APR for treatment of rectal cancer (Fig. 1). The flap is most useful for previously irradiated patients, but can also be used in non-irradiated patients in order to achieve primary healing and to keep the bowel away from the perineum, if the patient needs subsequent radiotherapy. Variations of the procedure can also be used for vaginal reconstruction (2), and for the reconstruction of defects following radical removal of the sacrum for treatment of advanced sarcomas.

ANATOMY, FLAP DESIGN AND DIMENSIONS

The flap is a standard vertical rectus abdominis myocutaneous flap based on the deep inferior epigastric vessels (Fig. 2) (3,4).

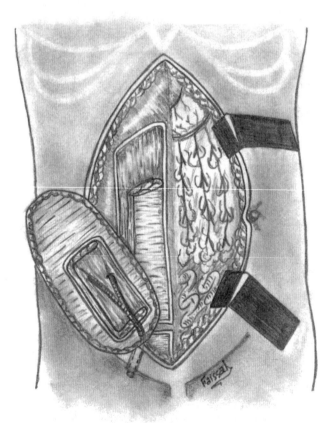

FIG. 2. Diagram showing required horizontal incision made in the posterior rectus sheath near the pedicle origin, so that the sheath does not kink the pedicle where it turns into the pelvis.

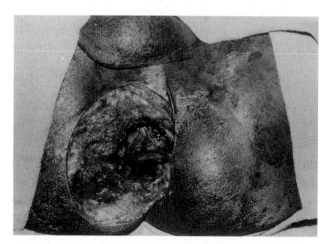

FIG. 1. A large defect after abdomino-peroneal resection for treatment of rectal carcinoma. (From Kroll et al., ref. 1, with permission.)

1188

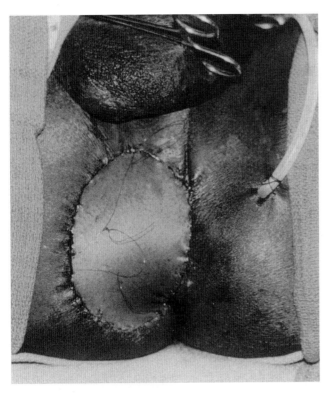

FIG. 3. After passing the flap through the pelvis, the flap tip is brought out in the perineum to repair the skin defect. (From Kroll et al., ref. 1, with permission.)

The flap tip should be extended past the costal margin to increase the potential arc of rotation, should that be necessary. The random portion over the rib cage should extend laterally, parallel to the ribs and following the direction of the underlying blood vessels. Flap width will depend on abdominal skin laxity, but is always at least 8 cm, usually more.

OPERATIVE TECHNIQUE

An inferiorly-based rectus abdominis myocutaneous flap is elevated in the usual manner (3) on the side opposite the planned colostomy. The inferior part of the flap (closer to the pedicle) is deepithelialized, so that the exposed skin paddle will come from the upper abdomen. The rectus muscle insertion on the pubis is usually not detached, to protect the pedicle against excessive traction. The flap is transferred through the pelvis into the perineal defect, and the area of exposed skin is marked. The flap is brought back up to the abdomen, to deepithelialize the remaining skin that will be buried, then passed back to the perineum, where it will remain permanently. The posterior rectus sheath is released with a horizontal incision to avoid restriction of the pedicle, which might otherwise impede vascular flow and lead to partial flap loss.

In the perineum, the flap skin paddle can be used to reconstruct missing vaginal wall or external skin (Fig. 3). If no skin is required, the entire flap can be deepithelialized and buried in the pelvis, to provide needed bulk and to be a source of non-irradiated tissue to improve healing.

Once the flap has been delivered to the perineum, the general surgeon returns to perform the colostomy, if one is required. After that has been completed, the abdomen is closed. The superior part of the posterior rectus sheath is closed to the midline fascia with heavy running suture. (I use No. 1 Novafil, but Prolene or nylon will work fine.) The posterior sheath inferior to the horizontal release is left open, so that the pedicle will not have any interference. The anterior sheath is closed from top to bottom in two layers, using the same heavy running suture (5). The subcutaneous wound is closed over a drain using 2-0 Vicryl for Scarpa's fascia and 3-0 buried Vicryl for the dermis. Sutures or staples are used for the skin, depending on the surgeon's preference. Because of the skin sacrifice, the umbilicus will be displaced to one side, while the colostomy placed through the opposite (usually the left) rectus abdominis muscle will be drawn to the mid-line.

CLINICAL RESULTS

The blood supply to the flap is generally good and, barring a technical error, flap necrosis is uncommon unless the surgeon has forgotten to release the posterior rectus sheath near the origin of the deep inferior epigastric vessels, as described above. Similar to post-TRAM-flap surgery, ventral hernias or bulges can occur, if the fascial repair has not been meticulous (5). Wound dehiscence in the perineum occurs occasionally, but is generally a self-limiting problem. Seromas can also develop, particularly if the wound has not been adequately drained.

SUMMARY

The transpelvic rectus abdominis flap is a relatively simple, reliable, and effective way to bring non-irradiated tissue into the lower pelvis or perineum. It is particularly useful for immediate repair of defects created by APR, but difficult to perform later. It should be considered whenever an APR must be performed in an irradiated wound, especially if a large defect is anticipated.

References

1. Kroll SS, Pollock R, Jessup JM, Ota D. Transpelvic rectus abdominis flap reconstruction of defects following abdominal-perineal resection. *Am Surg* 1989;55:632.
2. Tobin GR, Day TG. Vaginal and pelvic reconstruction with distally based rectus abdominis myocutaneous flaps. *Plast Reconstr Surg* 1988;73:734.
3. Mathes SJ, Nahai F. *Clinical atlas of muscle and musculocutaneous flaps.* St. Louis: Mosby, 1979.
4. Mathes SJ, Nahai F. *Clinical applications for muscle and musculocutaneous flaps.* St. Louis: Mosby, 1982.
5. Kroll SS, Marchi M. Comparison of strategies for preventing abdominal-wall weakness after TRAM flap breast reconstruction. *Plast Reconstr Surg* 1992;89:1045.

CHAPTER 416 ■ PENILE SKIN FLAP FOR VAGINAL RECONSTRUCTION IN MALE TRANSSEXUALS

R. MEYER

Transsexualism has been recognized as a serious gender disorder (1). Once there were very few surgeons who would undertake the transformation of male genitals into those of the opposite sex. Today, more surgeons are challenged by these operations, and such surgeons work concurrently with psychiatrists and endocrinologists.

The method I present is used to create a neovagina in the male transsexual using the penile skin as an island flap for vaginal lining (2–4). The labia are shaped with scrotal skin using two Z-plasties; a small bud of corpus cavernosum covered by innervated glans skin substitutes for a clitoris. This method has the double advantage of needing only one intervention and of providing a very satisfying aesthetic and functional result (Fig. 1).

INDICATIONS

There have previously been four different techniques used to form a vulva and a vagina in the male transsexual: (1) invagination of the penile skin as an anteriorly based flap, (2) use of a full-thickness penile skin graft for the vaginal lining, (3) use of a split-thickness skin graft for vaginal lining, scrotal and penile skin forming only the labia, and (4) use of penile skin as a posteriorly based flap. With the previous invagination of penile skin as an anteriorly or posteriorly based flap, a second intervention was needed to resect the redundant scrotal skin and to shape the labia. Surgeons using this two-stage procedure wished to avoid cutting through the skin at the base of the flap in order not to jeopardize the blood supply of the penile skin.

I am proposing a fifth technique: Using a penile skin flap to construct a neovulva and neovagina, I perform a one-stage aesthetic and functional procedure. Since I cut through the skin and not through the subcutaneous tissue, I still maintain sufficient vascularization.

FLAP DESIGN AND DIMENSIONS

In my one-stage procedure, the penile skin is invaginated as an island flap. I perform ablation of the corpora cavernosa, castration, and plastic construction of a neovagina in the same procedure.

My technique consists of forming a cavity between the bladder and the rectum to receive invaginated penile skin. In order to obtain an anterior convergence of the labia in front of a newly built clitoris at the base of the amputated corpora cavernosa, I perform a very superficial Z-plasty in the lower inguinal zone bilaterally. By removing a large amount of scrotal skin on both sides of the new vaginal introitus and at the perineal commissure, in addition to the bilateral anterior Z-plasty, I cut the skin practically all around the penile flap. The flap, deprived of any cutaneous continuity, remains connected to surrounding tissue only by a dense subcutaneous vascular layer that ensures its blood supply. Thus the penile flap becomes a subcutaneous island flap (Fig. 2). In the last few years I have added a construction of a sensitive clitoris to my

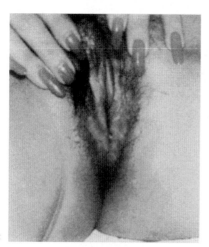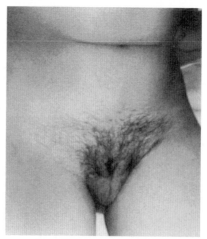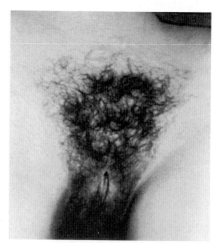

A–C

FIG. 1. A–C: Three representative cases showing late results.

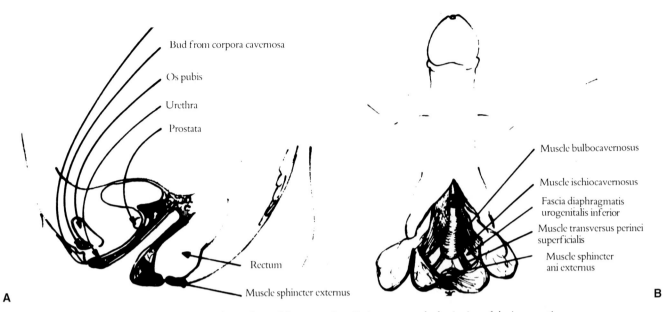

FIG. 2. **A:** The anatomic relationships of the neovagina. **B:** Anatomy at the beginning of the intervention.

procedure. For that purpose, I combine my method of invaginating the penile skin with the technique of Eldh (5), which is included in his two-flaps procedure using penile and scrotal skin sutured together. In this technical addition, the neurovascular bundle of the penis is dissected free together with a part of the glans and brought to the site of a neoclitoris through a slit in the skin.

OPERATIVE TECHNIQUE

After placing a urinary catheter in position, the first step consists of dissecting the penile skin, together with the skin of the glans, from the corpora cavernosa and the corpus spongiosum through an 8-cm midline incision in the posterior part of the scrotum (Fig. 3). I leave as much as possible of the subcutaneous penile blood supply, preserving the perineal arteries and veins (see Fig. 2). At this point a dorsal part of the glans, which is attached to the dissected neurovascular bundle, is trimmed

to achieve a suitable size and is shaped to simulate the clitoris. It is brought out by means of a slit in the penile skin some centimeters anterior to the urethral meatus. The neurovascular pedicle is placed in a gentle curve under the penile flap in order to avoid kinking. The preserved part of the preputial skin is used to create a hood by suturing these edges to the edges of the slit. The proximal segment of the corpus spongiosum is dissected free from the corpora cavernosa before proceeding to their ligature and transection at their base. The two remaining stumps of the corpora are sutured together in the midline to construct a small, erectile neoclitoris.

Bilateral orchiectomy is the next step. The spermatic cords and accompanying vessels are sectioned at the level of the inguinal ring, and suture ligatures are applied to their stumps. The penile flap is then pulled downward, and a horizontal incision is made at its anterior base at the proper location of the new orificium urethrae. Together with the previously inserted catheter, the urethra is passed through this hole, trimmed to a new adequate length, and its free edges are sutured to the skin.

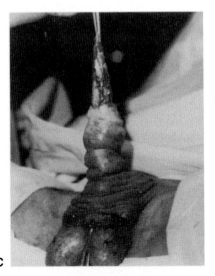
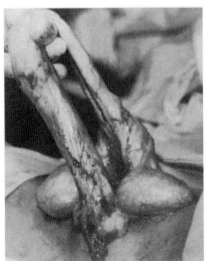
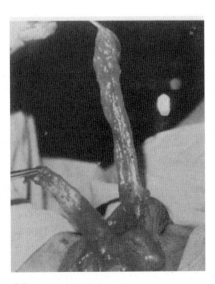

FIG. 3. **A:** Intraoperative view at the beginning of the procedure. **B:** Dissection of the corpora cavernosa from the penile skin. **C:** The corpora cavernosa fully separated from the penile skin.

Formation of the new vaginal cavity is begun by a horizontal incision in the perineum. I transect the fascia diaphragmatis urogenitalis inferior (Denonvillier's), cut the rectourethral muscle and levator ani muscle in the midline, and enlarge the vaginal introitus created this way by blunt dissection between the bladder and rectum, following the urethra up to the prostate (Fig. 4). The inverted penile skin is then pushed into the new vaginal cavity and held in position by packing with an ointment-treated gauze roll only or by a rubber foam mold in a condom. The posterior base of the penile flap is trimmed and sutured to perineal skin, while the redundant scrotal skin is removed.

To give a natural appearance to the labia majora, a bilateral Z-plasty is performed in the lower inguinal zone. The anterior branches converge in front of the site of the neoclitoris, which is emphasized by folding the skin of the glans with pinching mattress sutures. Beneath, a budlike prominence has been shaped from the remaining tissue of the corpora cavernosa (Fig. 5). A Penrose drain is inserted into the perineal cavity on each side. The urethral catheter and the vaginal packing are removed between the fifth and seventh postoperative days. An inflatable silicone obturator is then inserted and used without interruption for 2 to 3 months (Fig. 6).

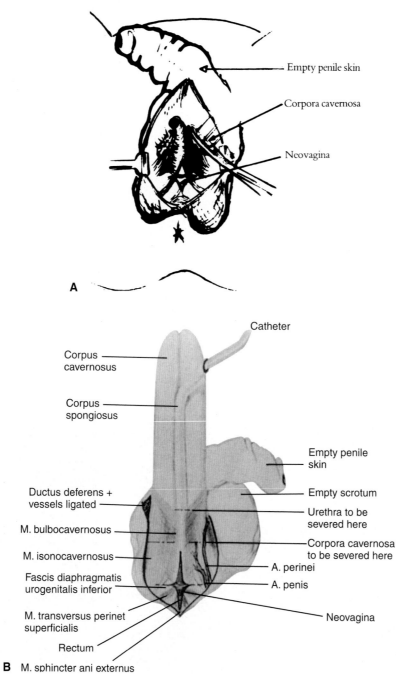

FIG. 4. A,B Anatomy after resection of the corpora cavernosa. **C:** Intraoperative view of the new vaginal space ready to receive the invaginated penile skin. *(Continued)*

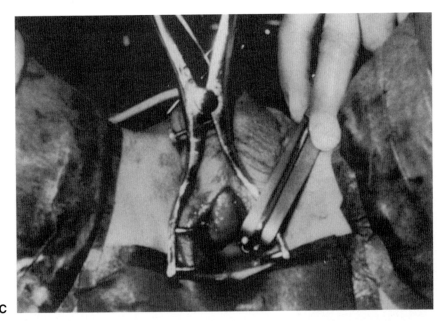

FIG. 4. *Continued.*

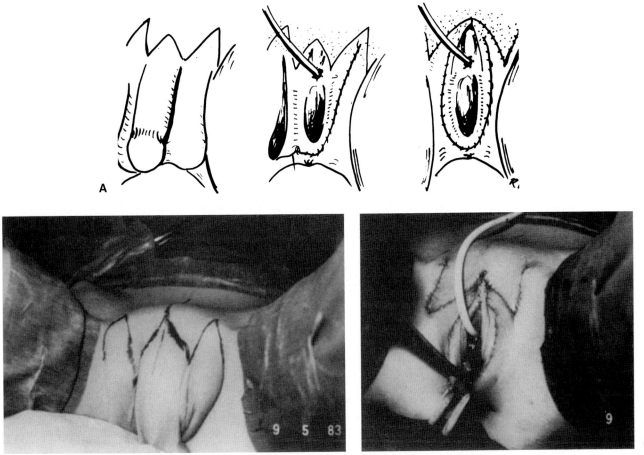

FIG. 5. **A,B:** The bilateral Z-plasties performed in the lower inguinal zone to give a natural appearance to the labia majora. The anterior branches converge in front of the site of the neoclitoris obtained from the remaining tissue of the corpora cavernosa and innervated parts of the glans. **C:** The end of the procedure.

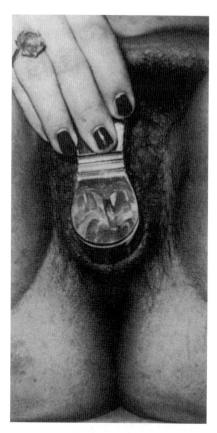

FIG. 6. One month postoperatively. Control with a Plexiglas obturator.

CLINICAL RESULTS

My experience with 85 operated patients shows that the subcutaneous vascular supply of the penile island flap is quite adequate. When a split-thickness skin graft is used for vaginal lining and the scrotal and penile skin is used only for labial reconstruction, one encounters the disadvantages of all split-thickness skin procedures. With the use of a full-thickness penile skin graft for the vaginal lining, the hazard of a poor "take" is even greater. In my hands, full-thickness skin grafts

have been useful for enlarging, and especially for deepening, the neovagina secondarily in cases of insufficient caliber and length.

Since the vulva is tailored by extensive resection of scrotal skin and bilateral Z-plasties, only three patients needed a secondary aesthetic correction. I have observed two strictures of the new urethral meatus. In one patient, however, a retracted meatus was corrected surgically after 3 months. In four patients, a rectovaginal fistula that needed secondary closure appeared later in the postoperative course. This probably occurred as a result of pressure from the obturator.

Of my 85 operated male transsexuals, 6 are married as females. A great number of these patients also desire additional operations, such as augmentation mammaplasty, rhinoplasty, blepharoplasty, laryngoplasty, and voice change.

In the last 18 years, among patients who consulted me for surgical treatment of gender identity problems, only about 20 percent underwent surgery. This reflects not only the difficulty of diagnosis, but also the fact that although surgery seems currently to be the only efficient therapeutic procedure for the true transsexual, expected social integration fails in many instances. It is therefore very important to continue postoperative psychiatric treatment to ensure ultimate success. A functionally and aesthetically satisfactory operative procedure represents only the beginning of a new life.

SUMMARY

A subcutaneous island skin flap created from the penis can be effectively used in a one-stage procedure to create a neovagina. It obviates the problems associated with both skin grafts and procedures that involve more than one stage.

References

1. Edgerton MT. Transsexualism: a surgical problem. *Plast Reconstr Surg* 1973;52:74.
2. Meyer R, Boscovic D. Problem of transsexualism. *Atti del Simposio de Chirurgia Riparatrice dell'Uretra*, Ban, 1970.
3. Meyer R, Kesselring UK. Dio Neubildung eines aeusseren weiblichen Geschlectsapparates beim Transsexuellen. In 13. *Jahrestagung der Deutschen Gesellschaft fuer Plastische and Wiederherstellungschirurgie, September 1975, Stuttgart,* Stuttgart: Thieme-Verlag, 1977.
4. Meyer R, Kesselring UK. Der maennliche Transsexualismus. *Gynaekol Rundsch* 1978;18:96.
5. Eldh J. Construction of a neovagina with preservation of the glans penis as a clitoris in male transsexuals. *Plast Reconstr Surg* 1993;91:985.

CHAPTER 417 ■ RECTOSIGMOID FLAP FOR VAGINAL RECONSTRUCTION

S. K. KIM AND K. J. PARK

Many methods are used for vaginoplasty, including the split-thickness skin graft, full-thickness skin graft, and inverted penile skin flap. However, these procedures are not entirely satisfactory in cases of reconstructed vaginal stenosis, inadequate vaginal length, or poor lubrication. The small intestine, ascending colon, and sigmoid colon can be used in an intestinal flap procedure. The authors have modified a previously described method in which a loop of rectosigmoid is isolated, closed at one end, and brought down on its vascular pedicle as a neovagina, and then anastomosed to the perineum. The reconstructed vagina has good tactility, adequate size, rare cavity constriction, and natural internal lubrication.

INDICATIONS

The female external genitalia are composed of the clitoris, labia majora and labia minora, and vagina. In reconstruction, the most important aim is to reconstruct a vagina with normal sexual function. Rectosigmoid flap vaginoplasty (1) is considered the best choice in the case of congenital vaginal atresia (Mayer-Rokitansky-Küster-Hauser syndrome), male-to-female transsexual patients who have received penectomy and orchiectomy, female pseudohermaphroditism, vaginal defect after ablation of cervical cancer, and vaginal trauma (2).

ANATOMY

The blood supply of the rectosigmoid intestinal flap is based on the superior hemorrhoidal artery from the inferior mesenteric artery (Fig. 1). Innervation of the flap is from the autonomic system, with sympathetic (inferior mesenteric and hypogastric nerve) and parasympathetic components (hypogastric plexus).

FLAP DESIGN AND DIMENSIONS

A transverse Pfannenstiel incision is made along the lines of skin cleavage just above the symphysis. The upper skin flap is dissected from the underlying rectus muscles, and the usual midline incision of the muscles and peritoneum is made. After exploration of the abdomen with a self-retaining retractor, and beginning in the left lateral gutter along Toldt's line, mobilization of the sigmoid colon is begun. After dissection of the medial peritoneum of the sigmoid colon, the avascular plane between the visceral fascia and parietal fascia of the rectum is dissected with electrocautery. The critical point of these procedures is the protection of the superior rectal vessels from any injury or trauma.

After dissection of the peritoneum in the Douglas pouch, the anterior dissection of the rectum is performed to below 2 to 3 cm of peritoneal reflection. After full mobilization of the rectosigmoid, transections of the rectum and mesorectum are

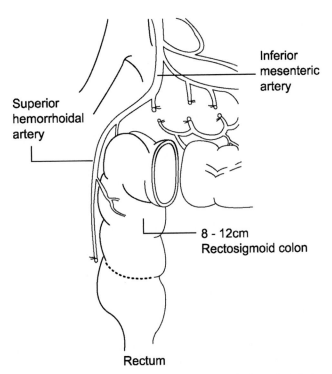

FIG. 1. The intestinal anatomy and arterial supply from the inferior mesenteric and superior hemorrhoidal arteries. A 12- to 14-cm length of rectosigmoid is resected, and the superior hemorrhoidal artery is retained.

1195

made. Although mesorectal transection can be safely performed with electrocautery, the superior rectal artery and vein are best ligated for prevention of accidental bleeding during the procedures of the perineal team. The rectum is transected with a linear stapler after mesorectal dissection. The bleeding of the distal rectal stump can be secured with simple interrupted absorbable sutures or packing of gauze. The bleeding of the proximal rectal stump (distal end of the rectosigmoid flap) can be safely controlled with electrocautery. The next important step is the preservation of the vascular arcades after several ligations of mesenteric vasculature. In these procedures, surgeons should pay careful attention to preserve not only the superior rectal vessels for the rectosigmoid flap, but also vascular arcades or marginal vessels for the sigmoid colon.

A 12- to 14-cm segment of the rectosigmoid is isolated with the vascular pedicle. The proximal side of rectosigmoid flap is closed with staples or continuous absorbable suture. The final step of the abdominal operation is completed by performing the colorectal anastomosis, using the intraluminal stapler (end-to-end or side-to-end), without tension between the sigmoid colon and distal rectal stump (Fig. 1). The rectosigmoid flap is brought down through the peritoneal opening to the perineal introitus by using Allis forceps.

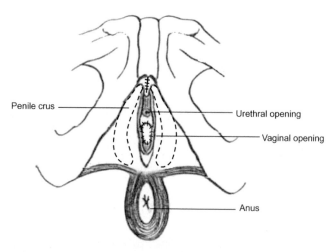

FIG. 2. A vaginal cavity made by incising the transversus perinei superficialis muscle between the bulbus spongiosus of the penis and rectum. The remaining distal penile crus are sutured to each other and then placed on the anterior portion of the urethral orifice.

OPERATIVE TECHNIQUE

The current operation is performed with a two-team approach by plastic and general surgeons. The general surgery team isolates the rectosigmoid intestinal flap, and the plastic surgery team makes the vaginal cavity through a dissection between the penis and rectum in transsexual patients. In other patients, we create sufficient length and width of the vaginal cavity through the opening of the obstructed vagina. The blood supply of the rectosigmoid intestinal flap is based on the superior hemorrhoidal artery from the inferior mesenteric artery. Innervation of the flap is from the autonomic system, with sympathetic (inferior mesenteric and hypogastric nerve) and parasympathetic components (hypogastric plexus). When isolating the rectosigmoid intestinal flap, we resect a 12- to 14-cm length of rectosigmoid, keeping the superior hemorrhoidal

artery, and then perform end-to-end or side-to-end anastomosis between the remaining sigmoid colon and rectum, by using an intraluminal stapler (Proximate ILS; Ürünler, Ankara, Turkey). The proximal portion of the rectosigmoid flap is closed with 3-0 Vicryl suture.

In patients with an intact penis and scrotum, we execute penectomy and orchiectomy, and then construct a urethral opening at the proper site. Clitoroplasty using the penile glans is performed in patients who desire a clitoris. However, most do not want this, because a constructed clitoris is unsatisfactory in shape, so we suture the remaining distal penile crura to each other and attach them to the anterior portion of the urethral orifice for substitution of a clitoris (Fig. 2). This procedure offers patients excellent sexual sensitivity. The bulbospongiosus muscle is stripped of the bulky urethral portion and used to augment the new labia majora.

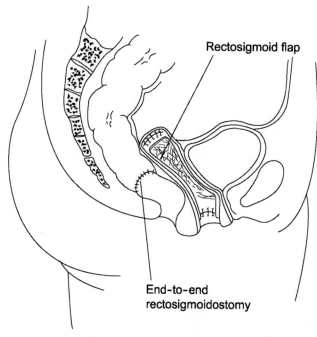

FIG. 3. The position of the new vagina and the suture line. The segment usually does not run all the way down to the perineum. Skin flaps are generally necessary to form the lower vaginal segment.

In the orchiectomy, we remove the testes and epididymis but preserve the spermatic cord and surrounding tissues to form sufficient volume in the labia majora. For penectomy patients, we create a vaginal cavity by incising the transversus perinei superficialis muscle and fibrous connections. Bundles of puborectalis and rectovesicalis muscles must be cut to create a cavity of sufficient size. After complete blunt dissection of the Denonvilliers fascia (septum rectovesicale), we transfer the prepared rectosigmoid flap to the new vaginal cavity through the peritoneal opening of the peritoneal reflex region. We then suture the end of the rectosigmoid flap to the skin of the new vaginal orifice (Fig. 3). One or two Silastic drains are placed inside the new vaginal wall through the vaginal orifice, and a suction drain (Hemovac, Zimmer, Milan, Italy) is inserted in the abdominal cavity. A sponge packing (Merocele; Urban and Fischer Verlag, Munich, Germany) is inserted in the new vaginal cavity for snug approximation of the rectosigmoid flap and the surrounding tissue.

CLINICAL RESULTS

The cosmetic and functional results of rectosigmoid vaginoplasty were excellent. The reconstructed vagina revealed a mean vaginal cavity depth and width of 13 cm and 3.8 cm, respectively (2). Postoperatively, all patients could enjoy sexual intercourse with orgasm (2,3). Complications were relatively rare, but excessive mucus discharge (3,4), constriction of the vaginal orifice (3), abdominal pain, vaginal bleeding during intercourse, and constipation were complications in the early postoperative period in some patients (2). The rectosigmoid vaginoplasty was safe, and the rate of satisfaction was also very high.

After examining patients who underwent rectosigmoid vaginoplasty, we analyzed the results by follow-up study. The reconstructed vaginas were of adequate size for sexual intercourse, and the cosmetic configuration was good, with rare malodor. All patients were able to have intercourse, and none experienced vaginal stenosis.

SUMMARY

Rectosigmoid vaginoplasty is considered very safe because the resultant cosmetic configuration and function are well maintained over the long run. Especially for transsexual patients, who have received penectomy and orchiectomy, congenital vaginal atresia patients, and those with vaginal injury after removal of malignant tumor of the uterus, rectosigmoid vaginoplasty is considered the best choice.

References

1. Baldwin JF. The formation of an artificial vagina by intestinal transplantation. *Ann Surg* 1904;40:398.
2. Kim SK, Park JH, Lee KC, et al. Long-term results in patients after rectosigmoid vaginoplasty. *Plast Reconstr Surg* 2003;112:143.
3. Darai E, Toullalan O, Besse O, et al. Anatomic and functional result of laparoscopic-perineal neovagina construction by sigmoid colpoplasty in women with Rokitansky's syndrome. *Human Reprod* 2003;18:2454.
4. Moudouni S, Koutani A, Attya AI, et al. The use of isolated sigmoid colon segment for vaginal replacement in young adults. *Urol Nephrol* 2004;30:567.

CHAPTER 418 ■ BILATERAL SUPEROMEDIAL THIGH FLAPS FOR PRIMARY RECONSTRUCTION OF THE VULVA

B. HIRSHOWITZ

The bilateral superomedial thigh flap can be raised and transferred to reconstruct either the vulva or the scrotum without recourse to delay procedures.

INDICATIONS

The main application of the flap so far has been in patients following radical excision of the vulva for malignancy (1,2). See Chapter 436 for flap use in scrotal defects.

ANATOMY

The superomedial thigh skin flap is a probable arterial flap with ample blood supply derived from three main sources (3) (Fig. 1):

1. The deep external pudendal artery—a direct cutaneous artery—is a branch of the femoral artery lying deep to the fascia lata, which it pierces on the medial side of the thigh.

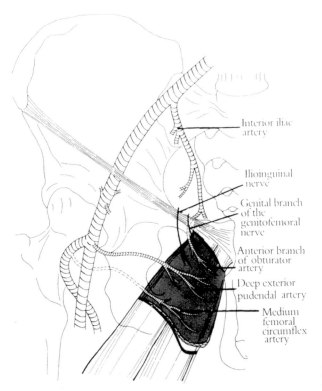

FIG. 1. Schematic diagram of the superomedial thigh flap with its probable arterial and nerve supply.

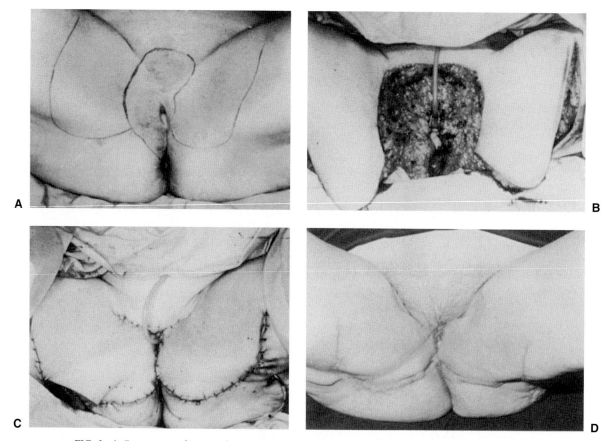

FIG. 2. A: Recurrence of Paget's disease of vulva. The outlines for the wide reexcision and the adjacent thigh flaps are shown. B: A large defect resulted from the excision. Both flaps have been raised. C: Suturing of the flaps has been almost completed. Part of the right donor site has been left for delayed suturing because of tension. D: Reconstructed vulva 3 months postoperatively.

2. The anterior branch of the obturator artery, which is itself a branch of the anterior trunk of the internal iliac artery, curves downward along the anterior margin of the obturator foramen and supplies the gracilis and adductor muscles and the overlying skin.
3. The medial femoral circumflex artery, which supplies muscular branches to the gracilis and adductor muscles and is a musculocutaneous artery, arises from either the femoral or profunda femoral artery.

The use of superomedial thigh flaps ensures virtual normal sensation, since both the genital branch of the genitofemoral nerve and the ilioinguinal nerve are likely to be retained with these flaps. This fact may have importance for the erotic propensity of the vulva and scrotum.

FLAP DESIGN AND DIMENSIONS

With the patient in a lithotomy position, the flap is outlined adjacent to a scrotal or labial defect. The base of the flap overlies the adductor longus muscle, while distally the flap reaches lateral to the perineum. The width of the flap roughly corresponds to the width of the defect. Its shape is rectangular, but in the case of a smaller defect, it can be curved inward laterally.

OPERATIVE TECHNIQUE

The flap is raised off the underlying fat distally and, more proximally, off the fascia lata covering the origin of the gracilis and adductor longus muscles. Blunt dissection is used to free the flap as its base is approached, and care is taken to avoid damaging any large perforating vessels.

Vulvar reconstruction commences with approximation of the proximal part of the medial flap margins to reform the subpubic area. This is followed by suturing the flaps together in the region of the perineal body, and last, the flap margins are sutured to the mucosa around the urinary meatus and vaginal orifice. However, during final suturing, some readjustment of the suture line may be necessary.

Primary closure of the donor site is undertaken when the defect is small and, in elderly subjects, when the skin is lax. With the larger defect, closure of part of the donor site in its inferolateral aspect may be delayed (Fig. 2C) or a skin graft may be applied. Primary closure of the donor site under undue tension may cause embarrassment to the flap circulation.

CLINICAL RESULTS

The viability of the flap before its medial transposition can be confirmed by intravenous fluorescein, but in 14 flaps raised so far (for both scrotal and vulvar defects), no compromise to the circulation was encountered.

SUMMARY

The superomedial thigh skin flap has proven a reliable method of resurfacing large vulvar defects.

References

1. Rutledge FN, Sinclair M. Treatment of intraepithelial carcinoma of the vulva by excision and graft. *Am J Obstet Gynecol* 1968;102:806.
2. Delgado G. Plastic procedures in cancer of the lower genital tract. *Am J Obstet Gynecol* 1978;131:775.
3. Har-Shai Y, Hirshowitz B, Marcovich A, et al. Blood supply and innervation of the supermedial thigh flap employed in one-stage reconstruction of the scrotum and vulva—an anatomical study. *Ann Plast Surg* 1984;13:504.

CHAPTER 419 ■ V-Y ADVANCEMENT MYOCUTANEOUS GRACILIS FLAP FOR RECONSTRUCTION OF THE VULVA

I. J. PELED AND Y. ULLMANN

Vulvar reconstruction is sometimes necessary following mutilating surgical procedures. The V-Y advancement myocutaneous gracilis flap combines the advantages of the V-Y principle and the muscle flap.

INDICATIONS

Reported methods for vulvar reconstruction have included direct suture, skin grafts, and flap plasty (1,2). The gracilis myocutaneous flap (3) has been used mainly as a rotation island flap (4), and V-Y advancement flaps are commonly used as cutaneous flaps. Myocutaneous flaps have been reported for use in ischial and sacral pressure sores (5) and anal reconstruction (6). The V-Y advancement myocutaneous gracilis flap combines the advantages of the V-Y principle and the muscle flap. It can be used for reconstruction of the vulva following vulvectomy, with and without lymphadenectomy, and after direct trauma.

ANATOMY

The created skin triangles are random flaps supplied by perforators coming from the underlying gracilis muscle. The gracilis is a type II muscle, with the medial femoral circumflex branch of the profunda femoris artery being the main pedicle. There are usually two to three vascular pedicles, with the superior one dominant. Division of the muscle in the distal third of the thigh enables the upward mobility of this myocutaneous flap.

FLAP DESIGN AND DIMENSIONS

With the patient in the lithotomy position, unilateral or bilateral (Fig. 1A) triangles are drawn on the inner aspect of the thigh overlying the gracilis muscle; the triangles are based at the created defect, with the width of the flap the same as the

width of the defect. The apex of the triangle, which is 30 to 45 degrees, reaches the junction of the lower and middle thirds of the medial thigh.

OPERATIVE TECHNIQUE

The skin is incised following the markings until the gracilis muscle is reached. The muscle is divided distal to the apex of the skin triangle, thus allowing complete mobility of the musculocutaneous flap(s) (Fig. 1A and B). The proximal insertion of the gracilis in the pubis does not interfere with the proximal advancement of the flap although, in some patients, it may be divided for better release. The flap is sutured to the remaining vaginal mucosa, and the donor area is closed in a V-Y advancement fashion (Fig. 1C and D).

One flap can easily close the entire defect and, by splitting the base of the triangle, the contralateral side can be reached. When bilateral flaps are raised, some redundancy in the skin is allowed; this can be used to simulate the labia majora.

CLINICAL RESULTS

We have used this procedure for reconstruction after radical vulvectomy and bilateral lymphadenectomy. Most of the

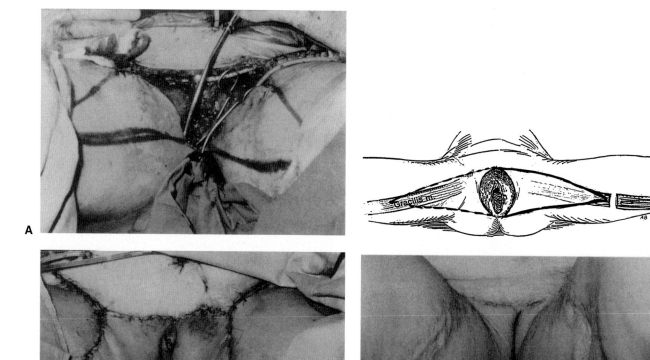

FIG. 1. A 58-year-old female patient after radical vulvectomy and bilateral lymphadenectomy. **A:** Triangular flaps drawn on both sides of the defect, above the gracilis muscle. **B:** Schematic representation of the division of the gracilis muscle. **C:** Result at the end of the procedure. The flaps are sutured to the remaining vaginal mucosa. **D:** At 1 year postoperatively. (From Peled, ref. 8, with permission.)

patients had bilateral flaps fabricated, but some of them had very satisfactory results with the unilateral flap. The technique combines the reliability of myocutaneous flaps with the simplicity and usefulness of V-Y advancement island flaps (7,8). By using this procedure for reconstruction of the vulva, we have obtained satisfactory results, with only very minor complications of delayed wound healing.

SUMMARY

Reconstruction of the vulva with V-Y advancement triangular island myocutaneous gracilis flaps is safe and simple to perform. It combines the reliability of myocutaneous flaps with the simplicity of the V-Y advancement principle, yielding very good results with relatively scarce minor complications.

References

1. Korlof B, Nylen B, Tillinger KG, Tjernberg B. Different methods of reconstruction after vulvectomies for cancer of the vulva. *Acta Obstet Gynecol Scand* 1977;58:411.
2. Nahai F. Muscle and musculocutaneous flaps in gynecologic surgery. *Clin Obstet Gynecol* 1981;24:1277.
3. McCraw TB, Massey FM, Shanklin KH, Horton CE. Vaginal reconstruction with gracilis myocutaneous flaps. *Plast Reconstr Surg* 1976;58:176.
4. Soper JT, Rodriguez G, Berchuck A, Clarke-Pearson DL. Long and short gracilis myocutaneous flaps for vulvovaginal reconstruction after radical pelvic surgery: comparison of flap-specific complications. *Gynecol Oncol* 1995;56:271.
5. Wingate GB, Friedland TA. Repair of ischial pressure ulcers with gracilis myocutaneous island flaps. *Plast Reconstr Surg* 1978;62:245.
6. Peled IJ, Manny J, Wexler MR, Luttwak EM. The triangular island skin flap for the treatment of anal ectropion. *Dis Colon Rectum* 1984;27:33.
7. Peled IJ, Wexler MR. The usefulness and versatility of V-Y advancement flaps. *J Dermatol Surg Oncol* 1983;9:1003.
8. Peled IJ. Reconstruction of the vulva with V-Y advanced myocutaneous gracilis flaps. *Plast Reconstr Surg* 1990;86:1014.

CHAPTER 420 ■ GLUTEAL THIGH FLAP FOR RECONSTRUCTION OF PERINEAL DEFECTS

R. L. WALTON, D. J. HURWITZ, AND J. BUNKIS

EDITORIAL COMMENT

This is an excellent flap and its reliability is dependable as one elevates the skin and underlying fascia over the posterior thigh. If designed as an innervated flap, it may give rise to most uncomfortable dysesthesias.

The cutaneous territory of the descending branch of the inferior gluteal artery provides an excellent source of sensate coverage for defects of the perineum (1–5).

INDICATIONS

The gluteal thigh flap is an extremely reliable flap for providing closure of groin, perineal, sacral, trochanteric, and ischial defects. It represents a significant alternative to muscle or musculocutaneous flaps, particularly in the ambulatory patient. There is no functional defect imposed by its use.

Its inherent nerve supply can be used to provide sensibility over critical pressure areas, with minimal donor-site morbidity. By incorporating the posterior fascia lata (femoral fascia), the gluteal thigh flap has been used in the support and closure of perineal hernias.

ANATOMY

Theoretically, the skin of the entire posterior thigh can be elevated as an axial cutaneous flap. The inferior gluteal artery is a terminal branch of the dorsal parietal division of the internal iliac artery. It exits the pelvis between the piriformis and coccygeus muscles through the lower portion of the sciatic foramen and descends in the interval between the femur and tuberosity of the ischium. In its course beneath the gluteus maximus muscle, the inferior gluteal artery gives off multiple perforating branches to this muscle which then supply the skin of the inferior buttock (3,6).

Just proximal to its emergence from the inferior margin of the gluteus maximus muscle, the artery anastomoses with the obturator and medial femoral circumflex arteries and sends several deep branches to the hamstring muscles. It then extends along the midline of the posterior thigh deep to the posterior femoral fascia (posterior fascia lata) from the ischium to the popliteal region.

There is considerable anatomic variation in the size of the inferior gluteal artery. The cutaneous territory of the posterior thigh probably has a dual blood supply (Fig. 1)—that arising from a subfascial plexus created by the descending branch of the inferior gluteal artery and a fascial plexus lying above the deep fascia that is fed by musculocutaneous perforators of the femoral and obturator arteries or the inferior gluteal artery. To a variable degree, both vascular systems

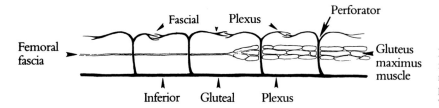

FIG. 1. Dual blood supply of the gluteal thigh flap. The subfascial plexus is supplied by the inferior gluteal vessels, and the fascial plexus is supplied by musculocutaneous and fascial perforating vessels.

feed a plexus of vessels just superficial to the deep fascia. A poorly developed inferior gluteal artery may be inadequate as the sole nutrient support for an island pedicle flap, and in such instances, proximal perforating vessels of the femoral system must be preserved.

In part, the venous drainage from the gluteal thigh flap parallels its arterial supply. Usually, several venae comitantes accompany the descending branch of the inferior gluteal artery in the thigh. In the proximal thigh, one vein may course medially through the subcutaneous tissue to drain into the saphenous vein. More often, the veins continue beneath the gluteus maximus muscle to join the internal iliac system. In addition, there is a parallel superficial venous system above the posterior femoral fascia in the subcutaneous tissue. This system forms multiple anastomoses with surrounding muscle perforators superior, medial, and lateral to the cutaneous territory. Peninsular flaps in this region rarely demonstrate venous congestion due to insufficient collateral drainage. Island flaps, however, may be prone to develop this complication unless the descending inferior gluteal vascular pedicle is fully developed and included in the flap.

The gluteal thigh flap is innervated by the posterior femoral cutaneous nerve (Fig. 2). This nerve is composed of several fascicles that emerge from the sciatic foramen with the inferior gluteal vessels. The fascicles then converge to form the main trunk of the nerve. This juncture is located near a point midway between the ischium and the greater trochanter. The nerve then extends axially down the posterior thigh below the femoral fascia to the popliteal fossa. It is intimately associated

with and lies medial to the descending branch of the inferior gluteal artery.

The cutaneous territory of the posterior femoral cutaneous nerve is represented by the S1–S3 dermatomes and extends superiorly from a line joining the ischium and the greater trochanter, laterally to the posterior border of the tensor fasciae latae, medially from a line joining the ischium to the medial femoral condyle, and inferiorly to the popliteal fossa.

FLAP DESIGN AND DIMENSIONS

Island pedicle modifications of this flap can reach further and provide a more tailored closure. The dissection, however, is technically more difficult and carries the risk of injury to the vascular pedicle.

The thickness of the gluteal thigh flap may vary from 2 to 12 cm. Thicker flaps are more common in females and obese males. While thick flaps are more cumbersome and difficult to transpose, they may be advantageous in providing padding over pressure points in denervated extremities; a thin flap may be unsatisfactory for these purposes.

In the ambulatory patient, sacrifice of the posterior femoral cutaneous nerve poses no major sensory deficit. It is important, however, to inform the patient of possible numbness along the posterior thigh and popliteal region.

Centered over its axial vessels, the flap may measure up to 34 cm in length and 15 cm in width. The flap can be trans-

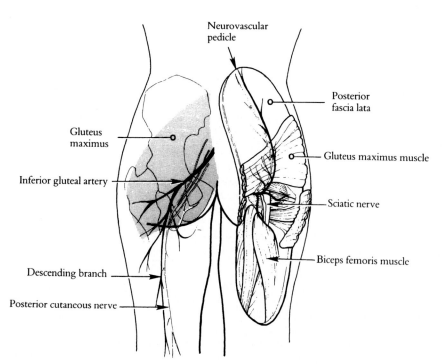

FIG. 2. Flap anatomy. The inferior gluteal artery exits the sciatic foramen beneath the piriformis and courses beneath the gluteus maximus muscle (shaded). At the inferior border of the gluteus maximus, the artery gives off several deep branches to the hamstrings. In approximately two-thirds of patients, it continues down the posterior midline of the thigh beneath the femoral fascia as the descending branch. The posterior femoral cutaneous nerve emerges from the sciatic foramen as several fascicles that converge at the inferior border of the gluteus maximus to form the main trunk of the nerve. The nerve then descends down the posterior midline of the thigh medial to the descending branch of the inferior gluteal artery. The right side of the diagram depicts the anatomic relationships of important structures after flap elevation.

posed with the gluteus maximus muscle as a compound mus-culocutaneous flap or transferred alone as a direct cutaneous arterialized flap (3,4).

The gluteal thigh flap is designed over the central axis of its neurovascular pedicle (Fig. 3). This is located midway between the greater trochanter and the ischial tuberosity and is perpendicular to the gluteal crease. Doppler assessment is quite helpful in precise identification of the proximal position of the inferior gluteal artery in the buttock. Beyond the gluteal crease, however, the course of the descending branch of this vessel is difficult to determine by this method.

The point of rotation of the flap (Fig. 4) varies according to the demands for coverage. In peninsular flaps, the cone of rotation absorbs up to one-third of the flap's length—this fact must be considered in planning. Generally, one chooses a point of rotation that is located midway between the greater trochanter and the ischial tuberosity. If an axial extension incorporating the gluteus maximus muscle is contemplated, the point of rotation can be extended to the sciatic foramen, which is approximately 5 cm above the ischial tuberosity. This maneuver increases the potential reach of the flap. In island pedicle modifications, the sciatic foramen can serve as the pivot point of the flap, extending its reach to the sacrum, groin, and deep perineal regions.

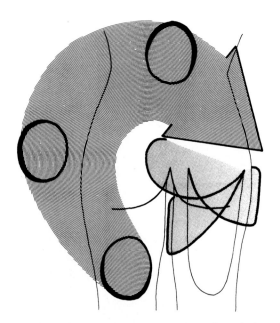

FIG. 4. Arc of rotation. The gluteal thigh flap will reach the pubis, deep perineum, sacrum, and ischium medially. Laterally, the flap reaches the greater trochanter and the anterior superior iliac spine. Island pedicle modifications (left side) have an extended reach because they lack a cone of rotation.

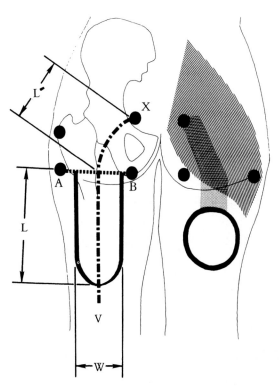

FIG. 3. Flap design. The flap is designed over the central axis of the inferior gluteal artery and the posterior femoral cutaneous nerve (left side of diagram). These originate at the sciatic foramen (X), which lies approximately 5 cm above the ischial tuberosity. The artery and nerve cross the gluteal crease at a point midway between the greater trochanter and ischial tuberosity. (A, B). The neurovascular pedicle then courses down the midline of the posterior thigh. Flap width (W) may vary between 6 and 15 cm, and flap length may reach 34 cm or to within 8 cm of the popliteal fossa. The length (reach) of the flap (L) can be extended (L') by splitting the gluteus maximus muscle and using this muscle as the proximal base of the flap (compound musculocutaneous flap). Island pedicle modifications (right side of diagram) may incorporate the gluteus muscle or only the neurovascular pedicle, depending on the size of the descending branch of the inferior gluteal artery.

OPERATIVE TECHNIQUE

After the appropriate design is chosen and oriented over the posterior thigh, an incision is made along the inferior margin of the flap through the deep fascia. Careful identification of the posterior femoral cutaneous nerve is important to determine the level of dissection, as well as proper flap orientation. Just lateral to the nerve, the inferior gluteal vessels are usually found encased in fat. The vessels and nerve are divided and then freed from their attachments to the underlying muscles by sharp dissection. Extreme care should be exercised during this part of the dissection, since it is quite easy to elevate the flap off its neurovascular pedicle.

As the dissection proceeds proximally, the deep fascia is divided medially and laterally until the inferior margin of the gluteus maximus muscle is reached. Several large femoral perforators will be encountered proximally, and these should be divided if they interfere with transposition of the flap. If more length is needed, the gluteus maximus muscle can be split medial and lateral to its neurovascular pedicle and included as the proximal base of the flap (Fig. 5A). The sciatic nerve lies just lateral and deep to the root of the vascular pedicle and receives one or two large branches from its proximal aspect. These branches should be preserved in the ambulatory patient.

In perineal wounds, there is often a skin bridge separating the flap from the recipient defect. This bridge can be incised to accommodate the flap, or a subcutaneous tunnel can be created. In either case, the flap can be deepithelialized in any part for subcutaneous insertion (Fig. 5B). At the base of a peninsular flap, backcuts are often necessary to facilitate transposition and insetting.

In most cases, the donor defect can be easily closed in primary fashion. If the width of the flap exceeds 7 to 10 cm, however, it may be necessary to close the defect with a split-thickness skin graft.

When using an island flap, the initial dissection is carried out as described for the peninsular flap (Fig. 6A). If the descending

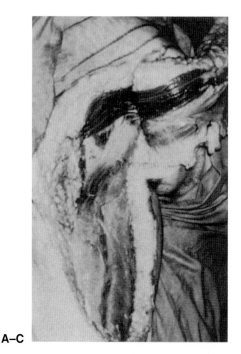
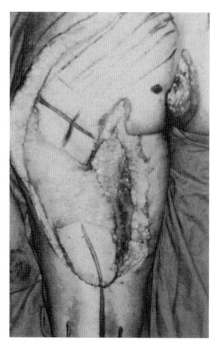
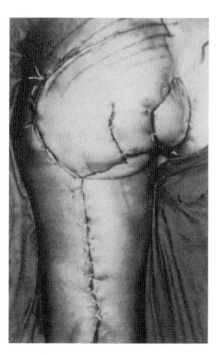

A–C

FIG. 5. Elevation of the flap. **A:** After elevation of the flap, the gluteus maximus muscle can be detached from its insertion and split if additional length is needed. **B:** The flap may be deepithelialized in any part for transfer through subcutaneous tunnels or to fill large defects. **C:** The flap transposed to a perineal defect. Donor sites less than 7 to 10 cm wide can be closed primarily.

branch of the inferior gluteal artery is readily identified and has a palpable pulse at the proposed proximal margin of the flap, then a careful subfascial dissection of the neurovascular pedicle is performed to its root. At the level of the inferior border of the gluteus maximus muscle, the pedicle will give off several large branches. These branches are divided after careful identification of the main vascular trunk. Numerous vascular perforators will

be encountered as the pedicle is dissected from the undersurface of the gluteus maximus muscle, requiring attentive care in dissection. In one-third of patients, the inferior gluteal vessels will not be palpable, and skeletonization of the pedicle may be hazardous. In these situations, it is important to preserve the deep fascia proximal to the skin island and incorporate the deep fascia, the overlying subcutaneous tissue, and a portion of the glu-

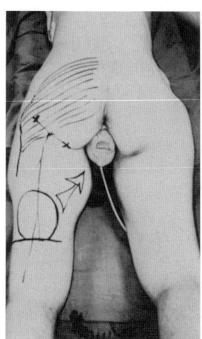
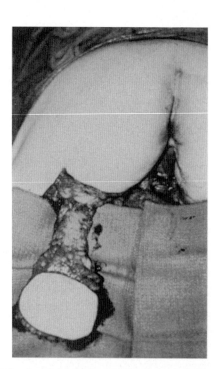
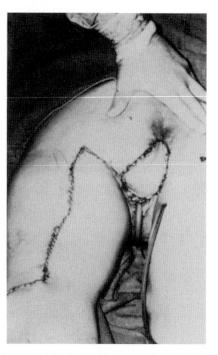

A–C

FIG. 6. **A:** Perineal hernia following abdominal-perineal resection. **B:** After reduction of the hernia, the fascial rim of the defect is patched with fascia lata (upper right). A gluteal island flap is elevated on its neurovascular pedicle. **C:** The flap is transposed to the perineal defect.

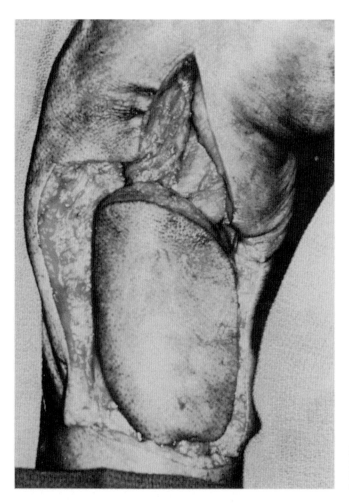

FIG. 7. If the descending branch of the inferior gluteal artery is poorly developed, the proximal deep fascia, subcutaneous tissue, and inferior portion of the gluteus maximus muscle are used as a composite pedicle.

teus maximus muscle as a composite pedicle (Fig. 7). This maneuver will ensure adequate perfusion of the skin island. In some situations, it may be advantageous to detach the gluteus maximus muscle from its origin to accommodate the mechanics of transposition. The flap is then transferred to the recipient defect.

When transposing island pedicle modifications of the flap, one must avoid twisting, kinking, or traction of the neurovascular pedicle. This is particularly important when the rotation exceeds 90 degrees. The subcutaneous tunnel through which the flap passes also must be large enough to avoid constriction of the vascular pedicle.

CLINICAL RESULTS

We have employed the inferior gluteal thigh flap for closure of 60 wounds in 46 patients. There have been two flap failures. One was due to failure to recognize that the inferior gluteal artery was already thrombosed. The other loss, in an attempted free flap, was due to venous thrombosis. Partial loss (including superficial epidermal slough) was noted in three flaps. Of these, one was secondary to hematoma, and the second was due to venous congestion in a severely skeletonized island pedicle modification. The third flap lost the distal 4 cm as a result of wound infection. Two flaps have dehisced (ischial, trochanteric defects) with pseudobursa formation; in both these cases, wound hematoma was identified as the underlying cause. Two more flaps had delayed healing due to partial dehiscence. One wound infection was encountered

24 hours postoperatively and was manifested by cellulitis of the flap (*Streptococcus spp.*). This resolved with intravenous antibiotics. One patient experienced dysesthesia in an island pedicle flap transferred to close a trochanteric defect. This was attributed to tethering of the nerve from a tight closure, a complication that could have been avoided by planning a longer flap.

SUMMARY

The inferior gluteal artery skin flap can be used as either a standard or island flap to cover significant perineal defects. Fascia can be included to repair hernial defects.

References

1. Hurwitz DJ. Closure of a large defect of the pelvic cavity by an extended compound myocutaneous flap based on the inferior gluteal artery. *Br J Plast Surg* 1980;33:256.
2. Le Quang C. Two new free flaps developed from aesthetic surgery: II. The inferior gluteal thigh flap. *Aesthet Plast Surg* 1980;4:159.
3. Hurwitz DJ, Swartz WM, Mathes SJ. The gluteal thigh flap: a reliable, sensate flap for the closure of buttock and perineal wounds. *Plast Reconstr Surg* 1981;68:521.
4. Walton R. The inferior gluteal thigh flap. In: Mathes S, Nahai F, eds. *Clinical applications for muscle and musculocutaneous flaps.* St. Louis: Mosby, 1982.
5. Hurwitz DJ, Walton RL. Closure of chronic wounds of the perineal and sacral regions using the gluteal thigh flap. *Ann Plast Surg* 1982;8:375.
6. Haertsch P. The surgical plane in the leg. *Br J Plast Surg* 1981;34:464.

CHAPTER 421 ■ GRACILIS MUSCLE AND MUSCULOCUTANEOUS FLAPS TO THE PERINEUM

F. R. HECKLER

The gracilis muscle and musculocutaneous units are therapeutic mainstays for dealing with clinical problems requiring reconstruction of the perineum, genitalia, medial thigh, groin, perirectal area, and lower buttock (see Fig. 1).

The gracilis muscle, whether used as a simple muscle or compound musculocutaneous flap, has all the features classically enumerated in describing favorable muscle-flap donor sites. (1) Transfer of the muscle to a new site leaves no noticeable residual functional loss in the donor leg. (2) The skin segment available in the musculocutaneous flap is considerable in size, but the donor defect can be closed primarily. Donor-site scars, located as they are on the upper inner thigh, are relatively inconspicuous. (3) The vascular pedicle is consistent in location, easily dissected, and of sufficient size and length to be attractive for free microvascular transfer. (4) The single motor nerve is likewise easily accessible and may be divided without denervating adjacent leg muscles, making the gracilis useful in distant transfers for reanimation of paralyzed areas.

INDICATIONS

The gracilis musculocutaneous unit and muscle flap are well suited for reconstruction of defects in the perineum. When bulk is required, such flaps may be used alone or in combination.

The highly vascular nature of these flaps assists wound healing in the adverse bacteriologic environment of the perineum and has been successful even in heavily irradiated fields. Gracilis flaps have been used in the closure of persistent perineal sinuses (1–4), repair of perineal hernias after pelvic exenteration (5), and closure of massive postoperative or postirradiation perineal defects (6,7) (see Figs. 4, 5, and 8).

Gracilis flaps have been used for correction of intractable vaginal prolapse (8). Several authors report success using gracilis muscle transfer to substitute for a flaccid rectal sphincter (9–12), whether the dysfunction is neurologic or traumatic in etiology.

The vagina (13,14) can be reconstructed using bilateral gracilis musculocutaneous flaps, and the use of unilateral flaps for hemivaginectomy or partial vaginectomy also has been reported. Reconstruction is preferably performed immediately following extirpative surgery, allowing primary wound closure, easier postoperative management, and markedly diminished postoperative morbidity (see Fig. 5). Additionally, neovaginal reconstruction allows the patient to retain a more normal self-image and the functional potential for sexual intercourse. Postoperative examination for tumor recurrence in the pelvis is facilitated.

Fistulas between bladder, urethra, rectum, vagina, and skin can cause major morbidity. The majority of such fistulas can be repaired using local tissues. Great problems exist, however,

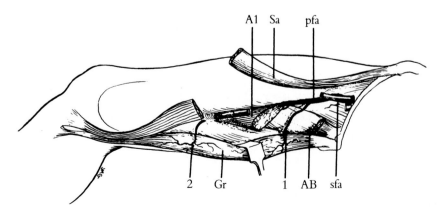

A1 Sa pfa

2 Gr 1 AB sfa

FIG. 1. Medial thigh anatomy as related to the gracilis flap. The dominant vascular pedicle passes between the adductor longus (Al) and adductor brevis (AB) muscles to reach the gracilis 8 cm distal to the pubic tubercle. The secondary distal pedicles enter the muscle at the junction of its middle and distal thirds [Sa, sartorius (cut); pfa, profunda femoris artery; sfa, superficial femoral artery; 1, dominant gracilis vascular pedicle; Gr, gracilis muscle; 2, distal vascular pedicle from superficial femoral). (From Heckler, ref. 14, with permission.]

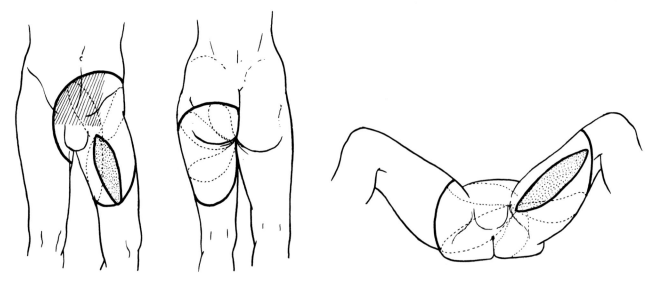

FIG. 2. Areas of use for gracilis muscle and musculocutaneous flaps. The functional arcs of rotation for the gracilis muscle and musculocutaneous flaps are outlined. The shaded area in the suprapubic region is covered with difficulty by the gracilis musculocutaneous flap, since a full 180-degree rotation is required. Excessive kinking of the vascular pedicle may occasionally result. This area is reached easily by the gracilis muscle flap, which may simply be turned over rather than rotated. (From Heckler, ref. 14, with permission.)

when fistulas occur in irradiated fields, when there is fistula recurrence after standard surgical repair, when the fistula is of unusual magnitude, and when local tissues are inadequate in quantity for use in repair. Under such conditions, the use of distant, well-vascularized gracilis flaps has proved to be most effective (4,14–17) (see Figs. 6 to 8).

A number of authors have reported additional uses for gracilis muscle and musculocutaneous flaps. They have been used for subtotal penile reconstruction in sickle cell patients (18), total penile reconstruction (19–23), scrotal reconstruction (24), and groin and vulva repair (2,17,25).

ANATOMY

The gracilis muscle is part of the adductor muscle group in the medial thigh (Fig. 1). It is the most superficial muscle of this group, originating from the medial segment of the inferior pubic ramus and lower half of the symphysis pubis. The muscle belly is flattened in configuration and runs distally, lying between the sartorius and adductor longus anteriorly, the adductor magnus on its deep surface, and the semimembranosus posteriorly. It ends in a rounded tendon that passes behind the medial femoral condyle to insert on the medial surface of the upper end of the body of the tibia.

The gracilis receives its vascular supply through a single dominant proximal artery and two or three more distant minor pedicles. The dominant proximal vessel is derived from the profunda system, usually as a branch of the medial femoral circumflex artery. It approaches between the adductor longus and adductor brevis muscles, entering the deep aspect of the gracilis 8 to 10 cm distal to the pubic tubercle. This artery is accompanied by paired venae comitantes. Each of the vessels has a diameter ranging from 1.2 to 1.9 mm.

At the junction of the middle and distal thirds of the gracilis, there are usually one or two additional vascular pedicles entering the muscle. These vessels are branches of the superficial femoral artery and are about one-third the size of the dominant proximal pedicle. An additional minor branch of the obturator artery enters the gracilis near its origin.

The motor nerve of the gracilis is an anterior branch of the obturator nerve. The nerve accompanies the proximal dominant vascular pedicle, entering the muscle near the entrance of the artery. Both motor and sensory fibers are present, but transferred skin sensation in the gracilis musculocutaneous flap is modest at best.

FLAP DESIGN AND DIMENSIONS

The gracilis musculocutaneous territory consists of the segment of medial thigh skin directly overlying the *proximal two-thirds* of the gracilis muscle and varying amounts of adjacent skin (Figs. 2 and 3). Because the gracilis is a long, narrow

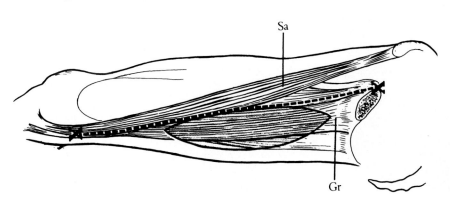

FIG. 3. Gracilis musculocutaneous territory. A straight line is drawn between the adductor longus tendon at the pubic tubercle (x) and the tendon of the semitendinosus (x). The gracilis musculocutaneous territory lies completely posterior to this line (Sa, sartorius; Gr, gracilis). (From Heckler, ref. 14, with permission.)

muscle, it is quite possible to locate the skin island improperly, which will result in skin necrosis.

A straight line is first drawn on the skin between the easily palpated adductor longus origin at the pubic tubercle and the semitendinosus tendon at the knee. The line should be drawn on the medial thigh skin *prior* to putting the patient in the lithotomy position, since in postures where the knee is flexed, the lax gracilis migrates somewhat posteriorly and topographic skin landmarks may be unreliable. This is particularly true in obese patients and patients with loose skin. The line should be drawn with the patient supine and with the leg straight and slightly abducted.

The skin paddle should be designed *posterior* to the line. For practical purposes, a skin island can usually be relied on with maximum dimensions of 8 cm in width and 22 cm in length.

The survival of the skin overlying the distal third of the muscle is less reliable. Several possible reasons have been suggested for this. (1) The sartorius in the distal thigh partially overlies the gracilis, separating it from the overlying skin. (2) The majority of musculocutaneous perforators emerging from the gracilis are located proximally, with few, if any, distally. (3) Approximately 60 percent of cadaver dissections will demonstrate a direct cutaneous branch of the superficial femoral artery that at least partially supplies the skin in the area. Regardless of which factor is primarily causative, wide clinical experience indicates that the skin overlying the distal third of the muscle should not be included in the gracilis musculocutaneous flap. If the clinical situation demands inclusion of this skin, the area should be carefully evaluated with intravenous fluorescein prior to flap inset (26).

OPERATIVE TECHNIQUE

Gracilis Muscle Flap

Since no skin paddle is planned, the skin incision may run the full length of the thigh. The saphenous vein and nerve will be seen during the initial skin reflection and should be preserved. The gracilis is easily identified, particularly in the distal thigh, where its rounded tendon is seen lying between the obliquely longitudinal muscle fibers of the sartorius anteriorly and the wider, flat fascial expansion of the semimembranosus posteriorly.

Dissection proceeds from distal to proximal. The gracilis tendon is circumferentially dissected and divided. Dissection in a proximal direction is in an essentially bloodless plane and proceeds rapidly. All vascular pedicles to the gracilis approach from an anterior direction and enter the muscle on its deep surface. The minor, more distal pedicles are ligated as they are encountered. The adductor longus is retracted as the proximal half of the gracilis is dissected, allowing easy identification of the major neurovascular pedicle.

Absolute skeletonization of the vessels is usually not necessary and adds some element of risk in terms of vessel spasm or injury. The dominant vascular pedicle is the center of the functional arc of rotation of the flap, and further dissection adds only minimally to its functional reach.

The flap is transferred to the planned recipient site through either a subcutaneous or submuscular tunnel, depending on the circumstances. This tunnel must be of appropriate dimensions to preclude vascular compression of the muscle pedicle. The donor site is closed primarily in layers over a suction drain.

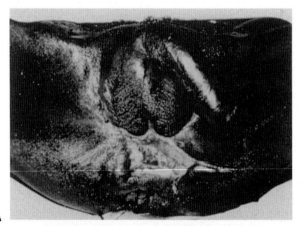

A

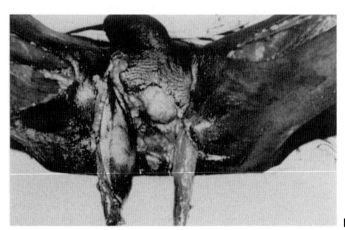

B

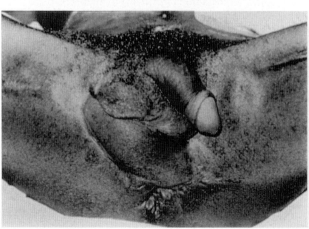

C

FIG. 4. Patient with massive perineal fistulas and sinuses from inflammatory bowel disease. **A:** The perineal defect communicates with a large rectocutaneous fistula, as well as a large urethrocutaneous fistula. Preliminary diverting colostomy and suprapubic cystostomy have been performed. **B:** Gracilis muscle and musculocutaneous flaps dissected and delivered to perineum. Muscle flap will be applied to help seal urethroperineal fistula following closure. Muscular portion of musculocutaneous flap will be applied to seal rectoperineal fistula following rectal closure, and skin will then be used to resurface area. **C:** Result 6 months postoperatively at time of colostomy closure.

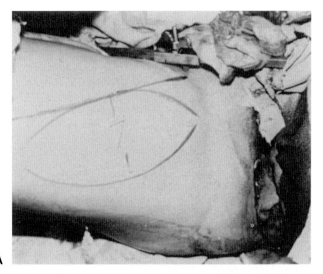
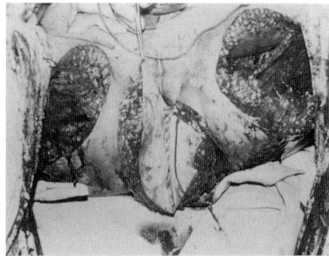

A

B

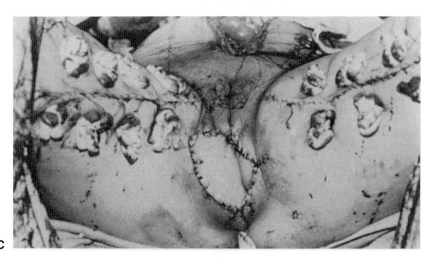
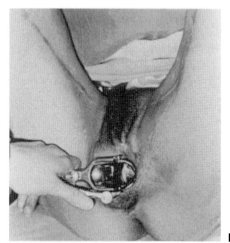

C

D

FIG. 5. Vaginal reconstruction with bilateral gracilis musculocutaneous flaps. **A:** Gracilis musculocutaneous flap designed on thigh for use in primary vaginal reconstruction following pelvic exenteration. **B:** Bilateral gracilis musculocutaneous flaps tunneled to perineum. Posterior suture line already in place for formation of vaginal pouch. **C:** Vaginal pouch completely inset. Distal ends of gracilis musculocutaneous flaps form neovaginal apex, while proximal ends form neovaginal orifice. Abdominal surgery with formation of ileal loop bladder and permanent colostomy progresses simultaneously with vaginal reconstruction. **D:** Reconstructed vagina easily admits full length of vaginal speculum. (From Heckler, ref. 14, with permission.)

Gracilis Musculocutaneous Flap

It is easiest to begin the dissection *distal* to the skin paddle by first incising longitudinally along the topographic line for a short distance. Initial dissection can then be carried out for localization of the gracilis without concern for separating the cutaneous portion of the flap from the muscular portion. The rounded gracilis tendon is found just above the knee, lying between the obliquely directed sartorius fibers and the flat semimembranous fascial expansion.

The gracilis tendon should be circumferentially dissected and then placed under tension. The skin-paddle design must then be reexamined to ensure that it has been properly located, centered over the longitudinal axis of the gracilis muscle. Improper location of the skin-paddle design and subsequent partial separation of the skin and muscle components of the musculocutaneous unit are, in my opinion, the most common causes of failure in use of this flap.

Once correctness of flap design is ensured, dissection proceeds rapidly. The gracilis tendon is transected, and the skin-island incisions are deepened to fascial level. Dissection proceeds in the avascular fascioareolar plane between the adductor longus and gracilis. The more distal, minor vascular pedicles of the gracilis are divided as they are encountered. The adductor longus is retracted anteriorly, and the critical dominant proximal pedicle of the gracilis is easily seen running between the adductor longus and brevis, entering the gracilis 8 cm distal to the pubic tubercle.

The skin edges are temporarily sutured to the muscle to prevent inadvertent disruption of the important musculocutaneous perforating vessels, and the gracilis is dissected free posteriorly by dividing the semimembranosus fascia.

The proximal vascular pedicle is the center of the functional arc of rotation of the flap, and further dissection of the muscle proximal to the major pedicle is therefore generally of no benefit. Incision and elevation of the gracilis fascia proximally may occasionally be of aid in allowing easier rotation and relocation of the flap.

The donor site is closed primarily over a suction drain. Some tension is invariably present, but I have not needed to resort to skin grafting the donor site in any of my patients, and scars have been acceptable.

General Perineal Reconstructions

When highly vascular flaps with bulk are needed to fill defects that have considerable depth, it is occasionally helpful to fill such perineal cavities with a gracilis muscle flap and then to cover the surface with a gracilis musculocutaneous flap from the opposite side (Fig. 4).

Correction of Intractable Vaginal Prolapse

In this condition, bilateral gracilis muscle flaps may be developed and tunneled behind the posterior vaginal wall. The tendons are each sutured to the opposite adductor longus tendon under considerable tension. It has been reported that gracilis muscles transferred in such a fashion provide reliable dynamic support for the lax vaginal wall (14).

Anal Sphincter Reconstruction

Voluntary control of gracilis motor function must be present. The gracilis muscle is mobilized, tunneled to the perineum, and passed circumferentially around the rectum. It is then sutured to the opposite ischial periosteum. The gracilis is not normally synergistic with the rectal sphincters, and considerable postoperative bowel habit rehabilitation is required.

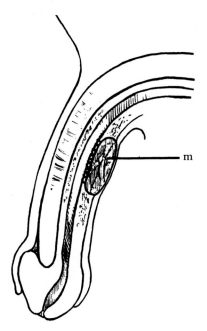

FIG. 6. Muscle flap for urethrocutaneous fistula repair. The urethra is reconstituted by closing the remaining urethral tissue or with local turnover flaps. If local tissue is inadequate, the urethra may be reconstructed with a skin graft tubed over an indwelling catheter. The muscle flap is tunneled subcutaneously to the repair site and interposed between the urethral repair and the overlying skin closure. If skin cover is inadequate, a skin graft is placed on the outside of the muscle (m) in preference to using a musculocutaneous flap, which is too bulky. (From Heckler et al., ref. 16, with permission.)

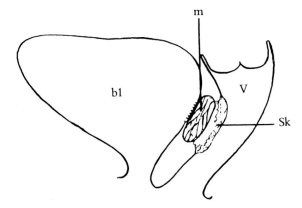

FIG. 7. Closure of vesicovaginal fistula with gracilis musculocutaneous flap. The muscle or musculocutaneous flap is interposed between the bladder and vaginal suture lines. The flap also can be interposed between the rectum and vagina if this is the site of the fistula. If there is a vaginal mucosal deficit, the musculocutaneous flap is chosen to supply additional skin (bl, bladder; m, gracilis muscle; Sk, cutaneous portion of gracilis muscle flap; v, vagina). (From Heckler, ref. 14, with permission.)

Vaginal Reconstruction

The patient is in the lithotomy position (Fig. 5). Bilateral gracilis musculocutaneous flaps are elevated and passed through generous subcutaneous tunnels to the perineum. Here, the neovagina is constructed, suturing the flaps to each other in pouchlike fashion, skin side in. The neovaginal pouch is deposited into the perineopelvic defect, with the distal ends of the flaps becoming the neovaginal apex and the proximal flaps becoming the vaginal orifice. A vaginal vault approximately 15 cm in depth results, with no tendency toward late contraction and no need for obturation.

Urethrocutaneous Fistulas

It is safest to perform definitive fistula closure when local tissue reaction has regressed and infection is well controlled (Fig. 6). To this end, initial temporary urinary diversion, fistula debridement, and urethral marsupialization are performed. Definitive repair is usually done 4 to 6 months later.

The gracilis muscle is dissected and passed subcutaneously to the base of the penis. The musculocutaneous flap is too bulky for inclusion in penile urethral repair. Therefore, if additional skin is required, a skin graft is applied to the transferred muscle. Mucosal closure of the fistula is carried out, and the transferred muscle is sutured over the mucosal suture line in watertight fashion. If inadequate mucosa for urethral reconstitution is present, a skin graft is tubed over the urethral catheter and the muscle is then applied. Skin closure over the muscle is performed using carefully mobilized local tissues or a skin graft.

Vesicovaginal, Rectovaginal, and Rectocutaneous Fistulas

Local infections and acute tissue reaction must first be controlled. This requires diversion of the urinary stream. A preliminary diverting colostomy is, likewise, advisable for management of rectovaginal or rectocutaneous fistulas (Fig. 7).

A transvaginal approach will usually allow adequate exposure for excision of the fistula tract and mucosal closure,

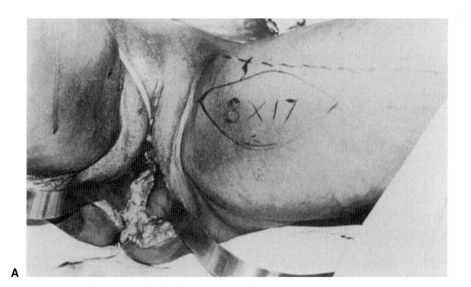

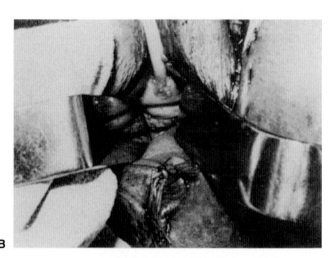

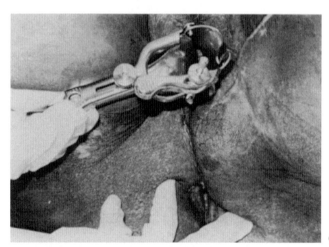

FIG. 8. Hemivaginal reconstruction for necrosis of posterior vaginal wall and large rectovaginal fistula following therapeutic irradiation. **A:** Patient with necrosis of posterior vaginal wall and large rectovaginal fistula following pelvic irradiation. Previous diverting colostomy has been performed. Excision of fistulous tract and remaining posterior vaginal wall has been carried out. Unilateral gracilis musculocutaneous flap designed on inner thigh. **B:** Reconstruction of rectum has been performed using available local mucosa. Cutaneous portion of gracilis musculocutaneous flap reconstitutes posterior vaginal wall (seen between retractors), and gracilis muscle is interposed between vaginal mucosal reconstitution and rectal reconstruction. **C:** Vaginal reconstruction allows easy and full access with vaginal speculum, and rectal muscle is sutured over the bowel closure to seal it off, and the skin segment allows tension-free skin closure.

although a transabdominal approach may occasionally be required. The gracilis muscle flap is employed if remaining vaginal mucosa is adequate for tension-free closure; otherwise, the musculocutaneous flap is used (Fig. 8).

The muscle flap is dissected and tunneled to the fistula site in the usual manner and is interposed between the rectal or bladder closure and the vaginal suture line. If the musculocutaneous flap is used where there is a lack of vaginal tissue, it is best to dissect a skin paddle somewhat in excess of the size of the apparent defect. Delivering excess tissue to the site of the fistula repair allows accurate trimming and precise fitting of the flap to the defect. Extending the thigh donor incision proximally through the labia also will help greatly in accurate insetting of the flap in the tight confines of the vagina.

In correction of major rectocutaneous fistulas, excision of considerable amounts of perianal or perineal skin is often required, owing to extensive fistulization, induration, and infection. Here, the musculocutaneous flap is most useful. After debridement and closure of the enteral wall, the gracilis muscle is sutured over the bowel closure to seal it off, and the skin segment allows tension-free skin closure.

CLINICAL RESULTS

My own clinical experience with gracilis flaps has been acquired from surgery performed on 53 patients. There were 20 unilateral flaps and 33 bilateral flaps, for a total of 86 flaps. Forty-two musculocutaneous flaps were used, with the remainder being simple muscle flaps. None of the flaps has failed. This success rate is particularly gratifying because the gracilis musculocutaneous flap seems to have gained some notoriety for relative lack of reliability.

SUMMARY

I feel that with proper care in flap design and dissection, gracilis muscle and musculocutaneous flaps are quite reliable. They remain useful and versatile tools in the armamentarium of the reconstructive surgeon who is called on to repair difficult wounds in the perineum.

References

1. Bartholdson L, Hulten L. Repair of persistent perineal sinuses by means of a pedicle flap of musculus gracilis. *Scand J Plast Reconstr Surg* 1975;9:74.
2. Bostwick J III, Hill HL, Nahai F. Repairs in the lower abdomen, groin, or perineum with myocutaneous or omental flaps. *Plast Reconstr Surg* 1979;63:186.
3. Baek SM, Greenstein A, McElhinney AJ, Aufses AH Jr. The gracilis myocutaneous flap for persistent perineal sinus after proctocolectomy. *Surg Gynecol Obstet* 1981;153:713.
4. Ward MW, Morgan BG, Clark CG. Treatment of persistent perineal sinus with vaginal fistula following proctocolectomy for Crohn's disease. *Br J Plast Surg* 1982;69:228.
5. Bell JG, Weiser EB, Metz P, Hoskins WJ. Gracilis muscle repair of perineal hernia following pelvic exenteration. *Obstet Gynecol* 1980;56:377.
6. Page CP, Carlton PK Jr, Becker DW. Closure of the pelvic and perineal wounds after removal of the rectum and anus. *Dis Colon Rectum* 1980;23:2.
7. Sorosky JI, Bass DM, Curry SL, Hewett WJ. Gracilis myocutaneous flap as a life-saving procedure in control of necrosis following radiotherapy and radical surgery for pelvic malignancy. *Gynecol Oncol* 1982;13:405.
8. Dibbell DG. Dynamic correction of intractable vaginal prolapse. *Ann Plast Surg* 1979;2:254.
9. Pickrell K, Masters F, Georgiade M, et al. Rectal sphincter reconstruction using gracilis muscle transplant. *Plast Reconstr Surg* 1954;13:46.
10. Landeen JM, Habal MB. The rejuvenation of the anal sphincteroplasty. *Surg Gynecol Obstet* 1979;149:78.
11. Kalisman M, Sharzer LA. Anal sphincter reconstruction and perineal resurfacing with a gracilis myocutaneous flap. *Dis Colon Rectum* 1981;24:529.
12. Maruyama Y, Ohnishi K, Hashimura C. Functional reconstruction of anal constriction using a gracilis musculocutaneous flap. *Acta Chir Plast* 1983;25:76.
13. McCraw JB, Massey FM, Shanklin KD, et al. Vaginal reconstruction with gracilis myocutaneous flaps. *Plast Reconstr Surg* 1976;58:176.
14. Heckler FR. Gracilis myocutaneous and muscle flaps. *Clin Plast Surg* 1980;7:27.
15. Graham JB. Vaginal fistulas following radiotherapy. *Surg Gynecol Obstet* 1965;120:1019.
16. Heckler FR, Aldridge JE Jr, Somprasong S, Jabaley ME. Muscle flaps and musculocutaneous flaps in the repair of urinary fistulas. *Plast Reconstr Surg* 1980;66:94.
17. Larson DL, Bracken RB. Use of gracilis musculocutaneous flap in urologic cancer surgery. *Urology* 1982;19:148.
18. Heckler FR, Dibbell DG, McCraw JB. Successful use of muscle flaps on myocutaneous flaps in patients with sickle cell disease. *Plast Reconstr Surg* 1977;60:902.
19. Orticochea M. The musculocutaneous flap method: an immediate and heroic substitute for the method of delay. *Br J Plast Surg* 1972;25:106.
20. Orticochea M. A new method of total reconstruction of the penis. *Br J Plast Surg* 1972;25:347.
21. Hester TR, Hill HL, Jurkiewicz MJ. One-stage reconstruction of the penis. *Br J Plast Surg* 1978;31:279.
22. Wheeless CR, McGibbon B, Dorsey JH, et al. Gracilis myocutaneous flap in reconstruction of the vulva and female perineum. *Obstet Gynecol* 1979;54:97.
23. Persky L, Resnick M, Desprez J. Penile reconstruction with gracilis pedicle grafts. *J Urol* 1983;129:603.
24. Westfall CT, Keller HB. Scrotal reconstruction utilizing bilateral gracilis myocutaneous flaps. *Plast Reconstr Surg* 1981;68:945.
25. Parkash S. The use of myocutaneous flaps in block dissections of the groin in cases with gross skin involvement. *Br J Plast Surg* 1982;35:413.
26. McCraw JB, Myers B, Shanklin KD. The value of fluorescein in predicting the viability of arterialized flaps. *Plast Reconstr Surg* 1977;60:710.

CHAPTER 422 ■ TRANSVERSE GRACILIS MUSCULOCUTANEOUS FLAP

N. J. YOUSIF, H. S. MATLOUB, R. KOLACHALAM, B. K. GRUNERT, AND J. R. SANGER

EDITORIAL COMMENT

The transverse reorientation of the skin flap has allowed far greater survival than trying to base the, flap along the length of the muscle. Survival is based on the anatomic dissection showing the transverse nature of the blood supply to the overlying skin.

The transverse gracilis musculocutaneous flap can be utilized both for filling smaller osseous cavities and for coverage of soft-tissue deficits. A transverse cutaneous paddle follows the direction of the blood vessels, rather than that of the muscle fibers, allowing for maximum cutaneous perfusion, simplifying the dissection, and limiting the effects of skin mobility seen in traditional flap patterns.

INDICATIONS

The traditional concept that the blood supply to the muscles and their overlying skin could be considered nearly synonymous (1–4) implied that complete muscle survival would naturally result in complete survival of all the overlying skin. The gracilis muscle did not always conform to that supposition. Previous vertical orientation of the skin component of the gracilis musculocutaneous flap (5–13), because of skin

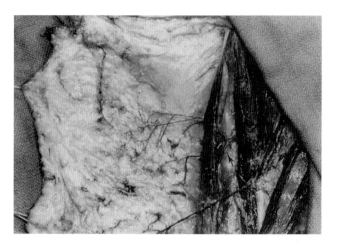

FIG. 1. A left lower extremity after elevation of the cutaneous flap. Two large musculocutaneous branches from the proximal pedicle (*arrow*) of the gracilis muscle divide in the anterior subcutaneous tissue after they exit the muscle. (From Yousif et al., ref. 14, with permission.)

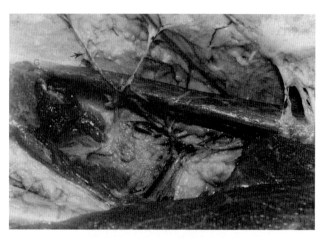

FIG. 3. In this dissection of a right lower extremity, a large septocutaneous branch (*arrow*) is seen dividing into anteriorly- and posteriorly-directed vessels. In the dissection, no large musculocutaneous branches were noted from the proximal pedicle of the gracilis muscle (G). (From Yousif et al., ref. 14, with permission.)

mobility, often allowed for elevation outside the skin territory of the muscle perforators. Recent anatomic studies and analysis of the musculocutaneous vessels of the gracilis (14) reveal a strong transverse tendency of the musculocutaneous vessels and demonstrate that only a small portion of the gracilis muscle is necessary to encompass all the musculocutaneous or septocutaneous perforators from the proximal pedicle.

ANATOMY

Cadaveric anatomic and latex injection studies have determined that the cutaneous vessels of the gracilis consistently connect to the surrounding cutaneous vessels through dynamic interarterial gateways (14) (Figs. 1–3). This allows

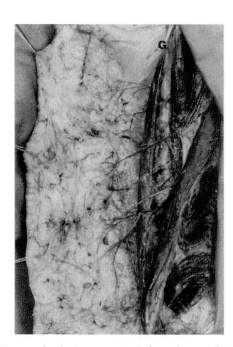

FIG. 2. Segmental subcutaneous vessels from the superficial femoral artery are noted to perfuse the skin over the middle portion of the gracilis muscle (G). (From Yousif et al., ref. 14, with permission.)

extension beyond the anatomic vascular territory in both transverse and vertical directions (Fig. 4). The proximal pedicle enters the gracilis muscle 10 ± 2 cm below the pubic tubercle. The dissections identify both septocutaneous and musculocutaneous perforators from the proximal gracilis pedicle. These branches have a pronounced tendency to travel in a transverse direction, supplying the cutaneous territory over the adductor longus and sartorius anteriorly, and extending for >5 cm beyond the posterior margin of the gracilis muscle (Fig. 5). This allows a transverse design of the gracilis musculocutaneous flap, such that the vascular perforators are invariably included in the cutaneous portion of the flap.

FLAP DESIGN AND DIMENSIONS

When transversely oriented, the cutaneous paddle follows the direction of the blood vessels, rather than that of the muscle fibers, and is centered over the main pedicle, i.e., about 10 cm below the pubic tubercle. This allows for maximum cutaneous perfusion by matching the cutaneous axis to that of its blood supply. The design also simplifies the dissection, allowing more secure placement of the preoperative outline of the cutaneous paddle, and limiting the variability due to skin mobility in the traditional flap pattern (11–13). The anterior limit of the ellipse shape may overlie the surface marking of the superficial femoral artery, and the posterior limit is the posterior midline of the thigh. The width of the cutaneous segment is determined by the amount of skin in the upper medial thigh that would allow direct closure. Flaps have been transferred measuring 25×10 cm, with complete cutaneous survival. Another advantage is that the location of the final scar may be more hidden.

SUMMARY

The musculocutaneous perforators from the proximal pedicle of the gracilis muscle tend to orient themselves in a transverse direction. This allows for a transverse orientation of the cutaneous paddle of the gracilis muscle and provides a flap that can be utilized for reconstructions that fill smaller osseous cavities and restore soft-tissue losses.

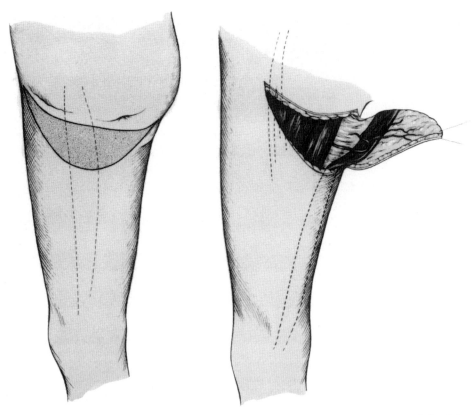

FIG. 4. Design of the transverse gracilis flap centers the cutaneous paddle over the main pedicle of the gracilis muscle. (From Yousif et al., ref. 14, with permission.)

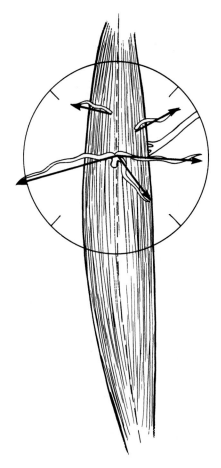

FIG. 5. The cutaneous perforators from the proximal pedicle of the gracilis muscle were characterized by vectors beginning at their origin, following their course, and ending at the point where the vessel terminated in the subdermal plexus. (From Yousif et al., ref. 14, with permission.)

References

1. Tansini I. Sopra it nuovo processo di amputatzione della mammella. *Gazetta Med Ital* 1906;57:141.
2. Bakamjian VY, Littlewood M. Cervical skin flaps for intraoral and pharyngeal repair following cancer surgery. *Br J Plast Surg* 1964;17:191.
3. Owens N. A compound neck pedicle designed for repair of massive facial defects: formation, development, and application. *Plast Reconstr Surg* 1955;15:369.
4. Orticochea M. The musculocutaneous flap method—an immediate and heroic substitute for the method of delay. *Br J Plast Surg* 1972;25:106.
5. Mathes SJ, McCraw JB, Vasconez L. Muscle transposition flaps for coverage of lower extremity defects: anatomic considerations. *Surg Clin North Am* 1974;54:1337.
6. McCraw JB, Massey FM, Shanklin MD, Horton DE. Vaginal reconstruction with gracilis myocutaneous flaps. *Plast Reconstr Surg* 1976;58:176.
7. Vasconez L, Bostwick J III, McCraw JB. Coverage of exposed bone by muscle transposition and skin grafting. *Plast Reconstr Surg* 1974;53:526.
8. McCraw JB, Dibbell DG, Carraway JH. Clinical definition of independent myocutaneous vascular territories. *Plast Reconstr Surg* 1977;60:341.
9. Mathes SJ, Nahai F. *Clinical atlas of muscle and musculocutaneous flaps.* St. Louis: C. V. Mosby, 1979.
10. Mathes SJ, Nahai F. Classification of the vascular anatomy of muscles: experimental and clinical correlation. *Plast Reconstr Surg* 1981;67:177.
11. Labanter HP. The gracilis muscle flap and musculocutaneous flap in the repair of perineal and ischial defects. *Br J Plast Surg* 1980;33:95.
12. Harii K, Ohmori K, Toni S. Free gracilis muscle transplantation with microneurovascular anastomoses for the treatment of facial paralysis. *Plast Reconstr Surg* 1976;57:133.
13. Webster MHC, Soutav DS. Gracilis. In: *Practical guide to free tissue transfer.* London: Butterworths, 1986. Pp. 104–107.
14. Yousif NJ, Matloub HS, Kolachalam R, et al. The transverse gracilis musculocutaneous flap. *Ann Plast Surg* 1992;29:482.

CHAPTER 423 ■ LOCAL SKIN FLAPS OF THE PENIS

C. E. HORTON AND I. B. KAPLAN

EDITORIAL COMMENT

The use of local tissue, particularly in this specialized area, is always preferable to the use of outside flaps or skin grafts.

The function of the penis as a conduit for urine and sperm, as well as its erectile capability for sexual activity, requires that it be covered with pliable, well-vascularized skin. Skin loss causing superficial genital scars can usually be repaired with skin grafts of varying thickness. However, when underlying structures, most commonly the urethra, need reconstruction, the area of surgery must be covered with normal, pliable, well-vascularized skin in the form of flaps.

INDICATIONS

Tissue defects of the penis may be congenital or acquired. Acquired conditions include trauma, acute or chronic infections, premalignant or malignant conditions, and burns that can cause structural loss in the genital area. By far the majority of local flaps for reconstruction of the penis and urethra have been presented in the voluminous literature dealing with the repair of congenital anomalies of the genital area, viz., hypospadias and epispadias.

To date, more than 300 procedures have been described for the repair of hypospadias—the majority of them using some form of local skin flaps for construction of the urethra and coverage of the penile shaft after release of chordee. Urethral fistulas continue to be the most common complication of hypospadias surgery, and repair of these and other acquired fistulas constitutes the most common reason for the use of local penile flaps.

Because of the laxity of penile skin and its favorable blood supply, local flaps, either alone or in combinations, can be ingeniously devised to repair and cover most penile defects. It is perhaps simplest to classify local penile flaps as (1) scrotal, (2) penile shaft, (3) glanular, and (4) preputial.

OPERATIVE TECHNIQUE

Scrotal Flaps

The scrotum is a convenient source of the flaps for the penis and perineum, and possible flap designs are boundless. Scrotal hair-bearing skin (1) has been abandoned as a means of urethral reconstruction because of accumulations of calcareous deposits on the hairs, with the potential for obstruction and infection.

Scrotal flaps have been used as coverage of the ventral surface of the penis after urethroplasty (2–6) (Figs. 1, 2). Scrotal advancement (7) and transposition flaps (8) (Fig. 3) have long been used for coverage of the base of the denuded penis.

A bipedicle scrotal flap (9) (Fig. 4) can be used to cover the entire penile shaft. The penis is buried in a bed under the scrotal skin, and the glans is extruded through a buttonhole placed in the dependent portion of the sac. At a second procedure, the penis is freed from its scrotal bed by bilateral incisions diverging from the glans. The scrotal flap now adhering to the dorsolateral penile shaft is closed along its ventral aspect, a Z-plasty being incorporated to interrupt the linear closure.

Transposed flaps of scrotal dartos muscle (Fig. 5) have been used by the senior author to reinforce suture lines over repaired urethral fistulas. The advantages of scrotal flaps include the ease and rapidity with which they can be elevated, the fact that they are directly adjacent to the penis, and that the scrotal donor site can be closed primarily without difficulty. Ideally, scrotal flaps should be used for the base of the penis, and not distally.

The disadvantages of scrotal flaps relate to the unsightly cosmetic appearance of the rugose hairy skin on the penile shaft and to the torsional effect that larger flaps produce on the erect organ. Additionally, these flaps will not reach the penile tip without much difficulty.

Penile Shaft Flaps

One-stage hypospadias repairs (10–15) using penile shaft skin flaps based on the hypospadic meatus have achieved recent popularity (12–14). In one technique (Fig. 6), a lateral flap of ventral skin based on the meatus and extending distally onto the inner surface of the prepuce is tubed over a catheter and brought out to the penile tip. A subcutaneous "mesentery" can be left to vascularize the urethral flap along its length.

The "flip-flap" procedure (14,15) (Fig. 7) involves the construction of a new distal urethra from a triangular flap of skin based on the meatus and "flipped" distally to form the ventral and lateral sides of the urethra, the roof being completed by a V-shaped glanular flap.

Penile Shaft Flaps for Repair of Urethral Fistulas

Penile urethral fistulas have taxed the ingenuity of surgeons for decades. Various local flaps have been described both for

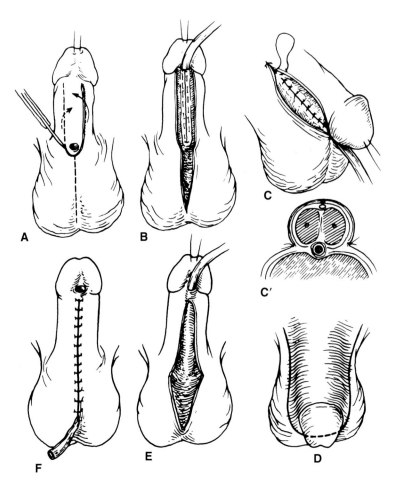

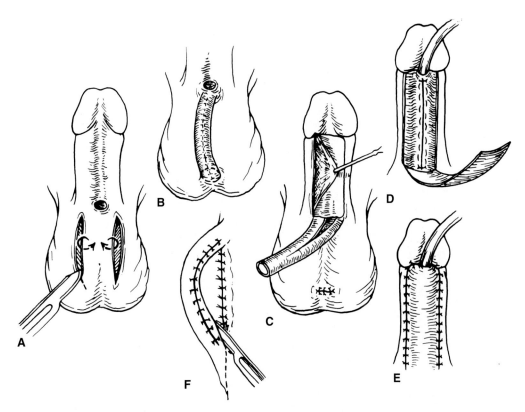

FIG. 1. A–F: Cecil-Culp coverage of ventral urethra with scrotal flaps after urethral reconstruction.

FIG. 2. A–F: Wehrbein-Smith urethroplasty with tubed scrotal flap.

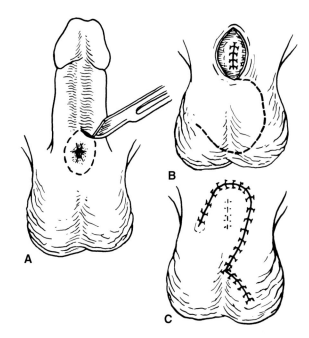

FIG. 3. A–C: Scrotal transposition flap.

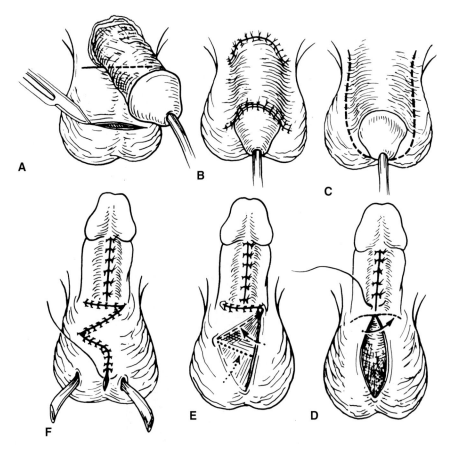

FIG. 4. A–F: Bipedicle scrotal flap.

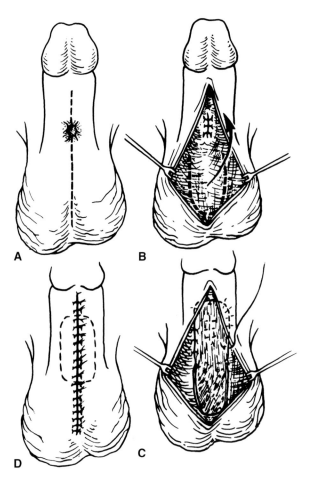

FIG. 5. **A–D:** Dartos flap transposed to cover repaired ventral urethral fistula.

closure of the fistula itself and for coverage of the repair. Turnover or "hinge" flaps based on the side of the fistula (16) and then flipped over like a trapdoor have been used to place an epithelial lining on the urethral side of the fistula. A dermal flap (17) incorporating an epidermal flap has been designed as a "cork" to plug a fistulous hole in the urethra (Fig. 8).

Various procedures have been described to achieve a two-layer closure over a fistula. After repair of the fistula, a deepithelialized flap is mobilized and advanced from one side of the fistula and covered by a full-thickness flap mobilized from the opposite side.

A turnover flap based on a subcutaneous mesentery adjacent to a strictured urethra has been described (19) (Fig. 9). Recently, a one-stage urethroplasty (20) for urethral strictures has been described using a transverse distal island of penile skin constructed on a subcutaneous pedicle and used as a patch or tube to reconstruct the urethra (Fig. 10).

Transposition/Advancement Flaps and Z-Plasties

The elasticity of the penile skin can be used to cover the distal portion of the penile shaft by the simple expedient of mobilizing the penile skin widely to the base of the penis and then unfurling the tube of rolled back penile skin to cover the distal defect.

Simple rotation flaps can be designed on the penile shaft skin to cover repaired urethral fistulas (16) (Fig. 11). A repaired fistula near the base of the penile shaft is more simply covered with a transposed scrotal flap (16).

Z-plasties can be used to lengthen penile skin and to interrupt linear skin closures between the penile shaft and the scrotum (22) (Fig. 12).

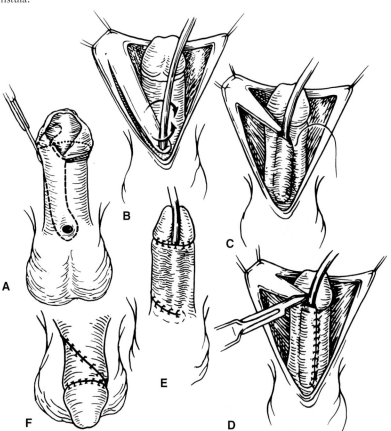

FIG. 6. **A–F:** DesPrez-Persky urethroplasty using ventral penile skin extending onto the inner prepuce as a vascularized flap.

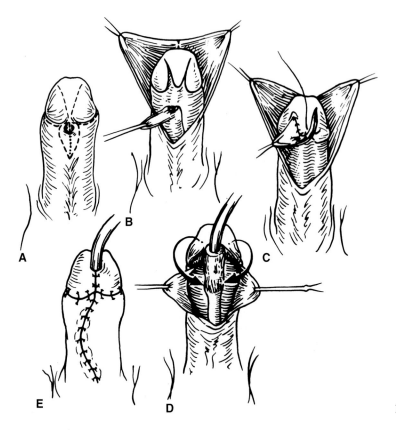

FIG. 7. A–E: Horton-Devine "flip flap."

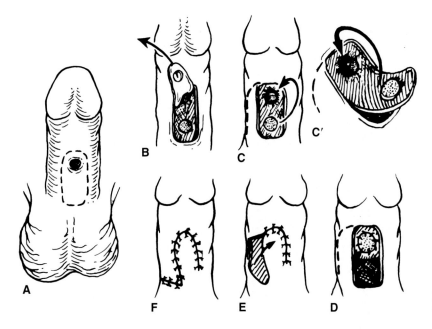

FIG. 8. A–F: Heckler-Mathes dermal flap with epidermal "cork" for urethral fistula repair.

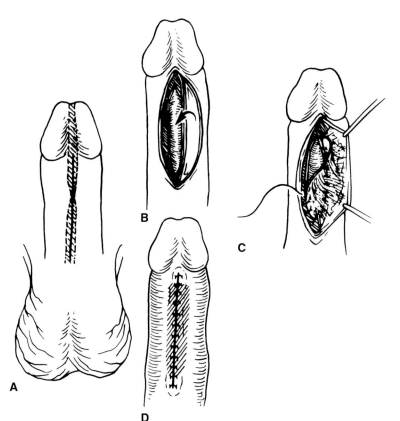

FIG. 9. A–D: Turnover flap based on subcutaneous mesentery.

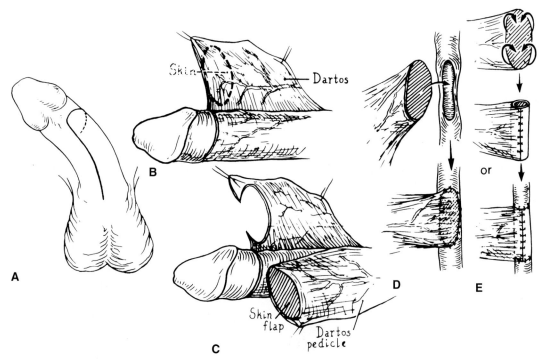

FIG. 10. A–E: Penile skin island flap on subcutaneous dartos pedicle.

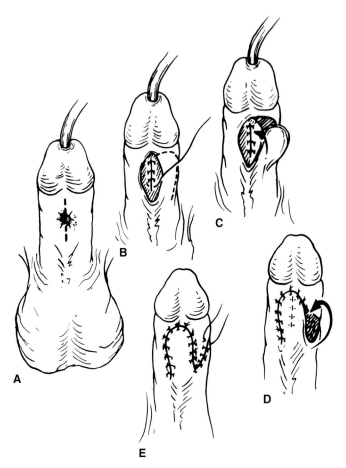

FIG. 11. A–E: Transposition flap to cover repaired shaft fistula.

Glans Flaps

The V-shaped glans flap has been used in both primary hypospadias repair (23) and to correct meatal stenosis, either as a result of previous hypospadias repair or as a result of cicatricial narrowing secondary to local inflammation (Fig. 13). The dorsal roof of the meatus is incised and allowed to spread open, and the V-shaped glans flap is advanced into the dorsal meatotomy incision in a Y-to-V fashion.

The glanular "wing" flaps first described by these authors are used to cover a newly created distal urethra and to reshape the flattened spadelike glans and give it a more normal conical appearance. Prior to this midline glans flap design, meatal

stenosis was a common occurrence when repaired hypospadic urethras were brought to the tip of the penis.

A meatoplasty using a U-shaped skin flap can be taken from the underside of the shaft-glans junction (24) (Fig. 14). After the meatal stricture has been slit open into healthy urethra, the tongue of skin is sewn into the defect.

Preputial Flaps

Flaps of preputial skin are useful for coverage of glans defects (25). The double lining of the prepuce means that the inner surface can still be used when burns and other surface injuries

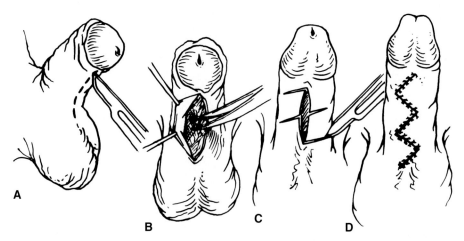

FIG. 12. A–D: Double Z-plasty used to lengthen deficient ventral skin after chordee resection.

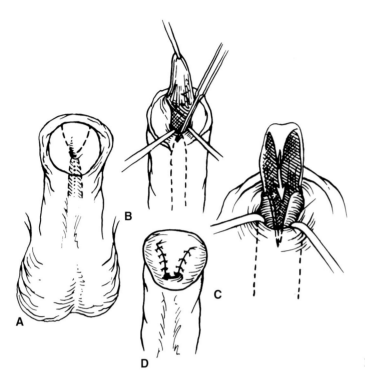

FIG. 13. A–D: V-shaped glans flap for meatal stenosis.

destroy the outer surface. This preputial double lining can be separated into its inner and outer layer quite simply by blunt dissection and can be advanced proximally to cover the entire shaft of the penis in some cases, being sutured to the residual penoscrotal skin or used as an advanced scrotal flap at the base of the penile shaft (26).

Transferring the excess dorsal preputial hood is a well-accepted means of resurfacing the ventral portion of the penile shaft in hypospadias surgery. The preputial skin is extended and brought to the ventral surface either by the buttonhole technique (27,28) or by the longitudinal preputial splitting technique (29), or by simply shifting the unfolded, trimmed preputial skin around the lateral aspect of the penis (30). The lateral transfer technique is especially useful to correct minor degrees of penile torsion in association with distal hypospadias.

The double-layered prepuce has been used to create vascularized flaps for a neourethra and coverage of the ventral penis (31–33).

The "tumble flap" (Fig. 15) uses the central area of the inner leaf of the prepuce, formed into a tube and left attached to the dorsal preputial skin by subcutaneous attachments. A buttonhole flap is used to transfer prepuce, along with the tubed vascularized skin, to the ventral surface of the penis, where it is used to reconstruct the urethra proximal to the tip of the penis.

A transverse preputial island flap (Fig. 16) of the inner preputial skin is separated with a subcutaneous tissue pedicle from the dorsal penile skin and spiraled around to the ventrum.

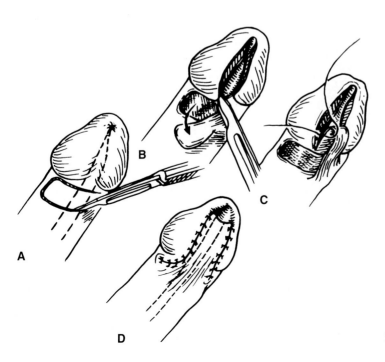

FIG. 14. A–D: U-shaped distal shaft skin flap for meatoplasty.

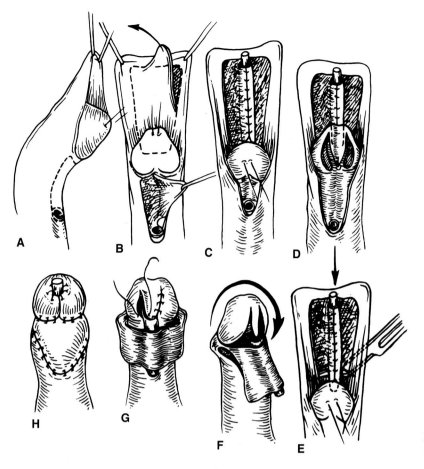

FIG. 15. A–H: Hodgson-Toksu preputial "tumble" flap.

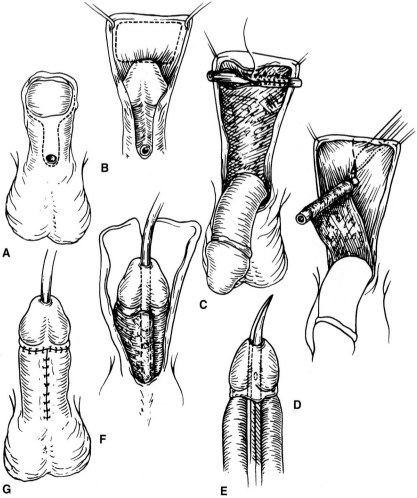

FIG. 16. A–G: Duckett transverse preputial island flap.

This tubed vascularized flap is then anastomosed to the proximal urethra delivered to the tip of the glans by a coring technique and covered by Byars-type preputial flaps.

SUMMARY

The various local flaps available for penile defects have been outlined and their differing indications discussed.

References

1. Rochet B. Nouveau procédé pour refaire le canal pénien dans l'hypospadias. *Gaz Hebd Med Chir* 1899;4:673.
2. Cecil AB. Hypospadias and epispadias: diagnosis and treatment. *Pediatr Clin North Am* 1955;2:711.
3. Culp OS. Experiences with 200 hypospadias: evolution of a therapeutic plan. *Surg Clin North Am* 1959;39:1007.
4. Wehrbein HL. Hypospadias. *J Urol* 1943;50:335.
5. Smith DR. Surgical treatment of hypospadias. *J Urol* 1955;73:329.
6. Arconti JS, Goodwin WE. Use of scrotal skin to cover wound defects in the groin and pubic area. *J Urol* 1956;75:292.
7. Robinson DW, Stephenson KL, Padgett EC. Loss of coverage of the penis, scrotum, and urethra. *Plast Reconstr Surg* 1946;1:58.
8. Horton CE, McCraw JB, Devine CJ, Devine PC. Secondary reconstruction of the genital area. *Urol Clin North Am* 1977;4:133.
9. Cassen PR, Bonnano PC, Converse JM. Penile skin replacement: indications and techniques. In: Heusten JT, ed. *Transactions of the Fifth International Congress of Plastic and Reconstructive Surgeons*. Melbourne, Australia: Butterworth, 1971.
10. Duplay S. De l'hypospadias périnéo-scrotal et de son traitement chirurgical. *Arch Gen Med* 1874;23:513.
11. Browne D. Hypospadias. *J Postgrad Med* 1949;25:367.
12. DesPrez JD, Persky L, Kiehn CL. One-stage repair of hypospadias by island flap technique. *Plast Reconstr Surg* 1961;28:405.
13. Broadbent TR, Woolf R, Toksu E. Hypospadias: one-stage repair. *Plast Reconstr Surg* 1961;27:154.
14. Horton CE, Devine CJ. One-stage repair of hypospadias: a combined approach and plastic procedure. Norwich, NY: Eaton Laboratories, Medical Film Division, 1960.
15. Bevan AD. A new operation for hypospadias. *JAMA* 1917;68:1032.
16. Horton CE, Devine CJ, Graham JK. Fistulas of the penile urethra. *Plast Reconstr Surg* 1980;66:407.
17. Horton CE. Urethral fistulas. In: Horton CE, ed. *Plastic and reconstructive surgery of the genital area*. Boston: Little, Brown, 1973;402.
18. Walker D. Outpatient repair of urethral fistulae. *Urol Clin North Am* 1981;8:582.
19. Orandi A. One-stage urethroplasty. *Br J Urol* 1968;40:717.
20. Quartey JKM. One-stage penile/preputial cutaneous island flap urethroplasty. *J Urol* 1983;129:284.
21. Horton CE, Devine CJ. Chordee without hypospadias. In: Horton CE, ed. *Plastic and reconstructive surgery of the genital area*. Boston: Little, Brown, 1973;384.
22. Arneri V. Reconstruction of the male genitalia. In: Converse JM, ed. *Reconstructive plastic surgery*, 2d Ed. Philadelphia: Saunders, 1977;3907.
23. Horton CE, Devine CJ. Hypospadias. In: Gibson T, ed. *Modern trends in plastic surgery*. London: Butterworth, 1966;268–284.
24. Blandy JP, Tressider GC. Meatoplasty. *Br J Urol* 1967;39:261.
25. Happle R. Surgical treatment of erythroplasia of Queyrat. *Plast Reconstr Surg* 1977;59:642.
26. Bruner J. Traumatic avulsion of the skin of the external genitalia. *Plast Reconstr Surg* 1950;6:334.
27. Theirsch C. Behandlung der epispadias. *Arch Heilkunde* 1869;10:20.
28. Nesbit R. Plastic procedure for correction of hypospadias. *J Urol* 1941; 45:699.
29. Byars LT. Functional restoration of hypospadias deformities. *Surg Gynecol Obstet* 1951;92:147.
30. Horton CE, Devine CJ. Hypospadias. In: Converse JM, ed. *Reconstructive plastic surgery*, 2nd ed. Philadelphia: Saunders, 1977;3857.
31. Hodgson NB. A one-stage hypospadias repair. *J Urol* 1970;104:281.
32. Toksu E. Hypospadias: a one-stage repair. *Plast Reconstr Surg* 1970; 45:365.
33. Duckett JW. Transverse preputial island flap technique for repair of severe hypospadias. *Urol Clin North Am* 1980;7:423.

CHAPTER 424 ■ GLANS SKIN FLAP

G. F. SHUBAILAT

In the treatment of hypospadias and epispadias, the objectives of a good repair are to straighten the penis by correcting the chordee and to reconstruct a neourethra with its external meatus opening at the tip of the conical glans, resulting in a normal-appearing and normally functioning organ (1).

ANATOMY

The dorsal artery of the penis provides most of the blood supply to the cavernous spaces of the spongy glans penis. The rest is derived from the deep artery and the artery to the bulb. Venous drainage is through the unpaired dorsal vein of the penis.

The skin of the glans is supplied by the dorsal nerve of the penis, a branch of the pudendal nerve S2-4. The erectile tissue is supplied by the autonomic cavernous nerves that arise from the lumbar sympathetic ganglia (2).

FLAP DESIGN AND DIMENSIONS

To fulfill the criteria involved in the treatment of hypospadias and epispadias, the use of a V-shaped incision on the glans to develop one midline flap to line one side of the neourethra and two lateral flaps to produce a more conical glans has been described and popularized (3). The flap has been used in a single-stage technique for the primary repair of all types of hypospadias and epispadias (4) and has been

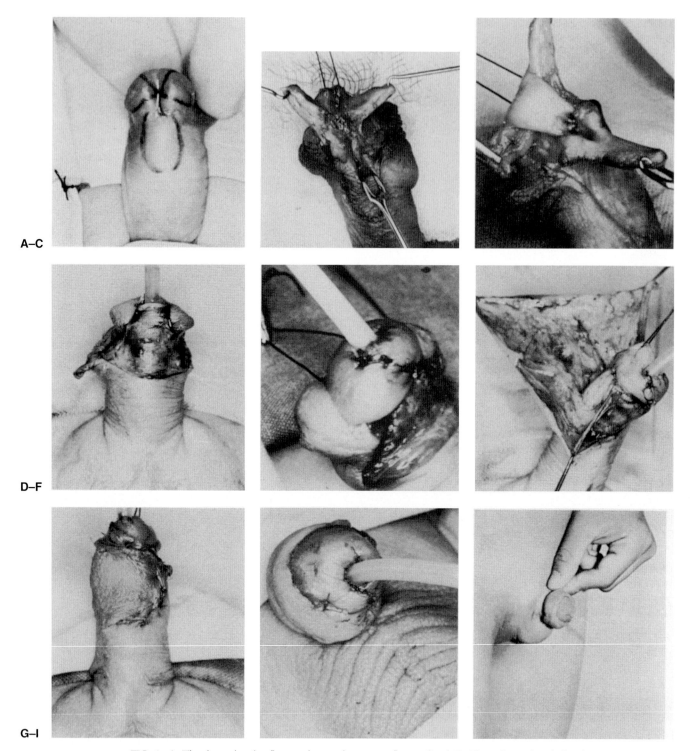

FIG. 1. A: The three glanular flaps and ventral turnover flap outlined. **B:** Flaps elevated and chordee excised. **C:** V-shaped median flap fitted into the dorsal meatotomy. Ventral turnover flap raised. **D:** Turnover flap sutured to both sides of the median flap constructing the neourethra. **E:** The lateral glanular wings interdigitated over the neourethra and sutured together and to the free distal edge of the turnover flap. **F:** The prepuce is unfolded and mobilized. **G:** Prepuce is rotated to cover ventral defect. **H:** Operation completed. **I:** Final result.

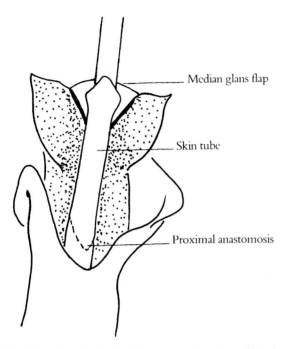

FIG. 2. Glans flap depicted. A free preputial tube graft is shown bridging the defect.

adapted as the final stage of other once-popular multistaged repairs (5).

A triangle is marked with its apex in the midline at the coronal sulcus and its sides diverging distally to a wide base located at the tip of the penis. These markings are made on the ventral skin in hypospadias and on the dorsal skin in epispadias. The coronal sulcus is marked, thus defining two lateral glanular wings (Fig. 1A).

OPERATIVE TECHNIQUE

A traction suture of 4-0 silk is applied to the glans. I have stopped infiltrating with xylocaine and epinephrine. I use a Penrose tube as tourniquet to the base of the shaft to allow me to operate in a bloodless field. Hemostasis is secured at the end of the operation, before final closure of the skin flaps. The two lateral and midline glanular flaps are dissected free. An incision is made in the midline, starting at the coronal sulcus and extending proximally to the existing meatus, splitting it for a distance of 0.5 cm into the urethra. The skin edges are undermined, and any existing fibrous bands causing the

chordee are excised (Fig. 1B). Straightening of the penis is confirmed by inducing a simulated erection (6).

The three flaps are now ready to be incorporated into the different techniques for repair of the various types of hypospadias and epispadias.

The operative steps in distal penile hypospadias repair are depicted in Figure 1C–I. In more severe types of hypospadias, the existing meatus is mobilized to a more proximal position on the shaft, leaving a defect that is too wide for the midline glanular flap to reach. To bridge this defect, in the uncircumcised patient or where there is adequate preputial skin left, I have improved my results and decreased the incidence of stricture and fistula by constructing a vascularized island flap that is tubed and moved ventrally on its vascular pedicle to reconstruct a new urethra in defects up to 5 cm. In the already circumcised patient, a tube of free full-thickness preputial skin is constructed over a catheter splint of appropriate caliber (Fig. 2). The proximal end of the free or vascularized tube is anastomosed obliquely to the existing meatus. Distally, the midline glanular flap is fitted into the seam of the tube like a tongue in a groove. The glanular wings are then approximated over the tube, and the rest of the preputial skin is rotated to cover the ventral skin defect.

The same operative principles apply in the treatment of epispadias (Fig. 3A–C).

In the treatment of distal glanular stricture with resultant proximal fistulas, a secondary ventral turnover flap can be developed to widen and reconstruct the strictured segment and incorporate it with the glanular flaps (Fig. 4A–E). In more proximal strictures a vascularized island preputial patch flap has been very successful and reliable in restoring the normal wide caliber in the strictured segment.

In the least severe type, where an external meatus of adequate caliber opens dorsally at the coronal sulcus of a patulous glans and the absence of chordee is confirmed by simulated erection, the midline glans flap can be modified and used as a bipedicled flap. It is left in continuity with the floor of the existing meatus, and a proximal ventral turnover flap is used to reconstruct the roof of the neourethra (as demonstrated earlier in our treatment of distal glanular urethral strictures with coronal fistulas).

In repairs of distal lesions, the urine is diverted with a silicone Foley catheter through the repair for 2 to 3 days. In more severe types, we discontinued using perineal urethrostomy, and we always use suprapubic Cystocath drainage for 10 days and a perurethral catheter for splintage and as a safeguard standby drainage in case the suprapubic drainage blocks.

The fluffed pressure dressing is soaked off after 2 days. Some surgeons use cold sterile compresses frequently. A urinary antiseptic should be administered while the catheter is in place. Lubrication and dilatation of the new meatus are

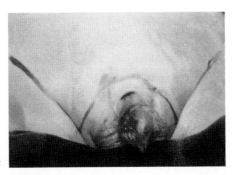
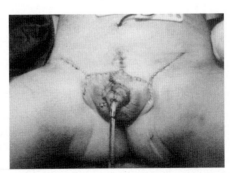
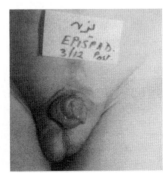

A–C

FIG. 3. Epispadias. A: Preoperative. B: End of one-stage operation. C: A three-month result.

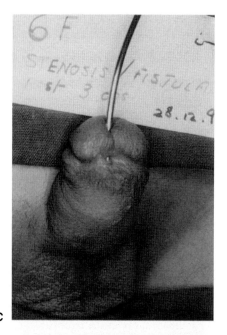
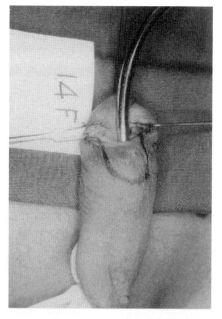
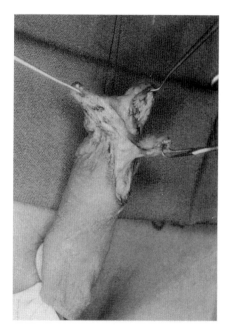

A–C

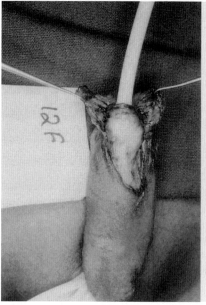
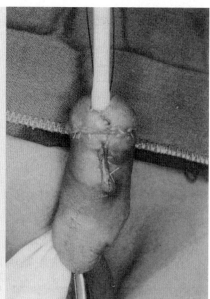

D,E

FIG. 4. A: Distal stricture and fistula. B: Stricture released open. C: Secondary turnover and lateral glanular flaps developed. D: Neourethra constructed over Foley catheter. E: Completed repair.

carried out thrice daily using the nozzle of an ophthalmic antibiotic tube after the removal of the catheter.

CLINICAL RESULTS

In our series of 800 cases with different types of hypospadias where the glans flap was used in one-stage repair, I was the main surgeon in 500 cases. Primary healing was attained in 96% of repairs of distal penile types. Since I have introduced the vascularized preputial island pedicled flap in one-stage repairs of severe types of proximal hypospadias cases as an alternative to a free preputial skin graft, the incidence of strictures and fistulas was reduced from 23% early in the series to 11%. While stricture is a common cause of fistula formation, the latter can occur due to hematoma formation under the very delicate and thin skin causing breakdown of the suture line or sloughing of skin edges. It is my experience that very

few acute fistulas heal spontaneously by reintroducing a catheter. Established fistulas and strictures are preferably repaired after a time lapse of 6 months. Dehiscence of the wound occurred in 3% of our early 62 reported cases. This was either due to a child forcibly pulling out the catheter or due to infection (which we found to be more common in adult cases due to the increased sebaceous and sweat gland activity in the operated areas). Meatal stenosis can be managed by V-Y meatoplasty.

SUMMARY

The glans flap as originally described by Horton and Devine (3) was successfully incorporated into all my techniques of dealing with different types of hypospadias and epispadias and their complications in a large series of patients over the last 23 years.

References

1. Shubailat GF, Ajluni NJ. Experience with the glans flap operation for distal penile hypospadias. *Plast Reconstr Surg* 1978;62:546.
2. Gardner E, Gray DJ, O'Rahailly R. In: Temer H, ed. *Anatomy*. Philadelphia: Saunders, 1975;503.
3. Horton CE, Devine CJ. Hypospadias. In: Gibson T, ed. *Modern trends in plastic surgery*. London: Butterworth, 1966;268–284.
4. Horton CE, Devine CJ, Adamson JE, Carraway JH. Hypospadias, epispadias and exstrophy of the bladder. In: Grabb WC, Smith JW, eds. *Plastic surgery*. Boston: Little, Brown, 1979;855–868.
5. Bialas RF, Horton CE, Devine CJ. The adaptability of the glans flap in hypospadias repair. *Plast Reconstr Surg* 1977;60:416.
6. Horton CE, Devine CJ. Simulated erection of the penis with saline injection: a diagnostic maneuver. *Plast Reconstr Surg* 1977;59:670.

CHAPTER 425 ■ PREPUCE SKIN FLAP

R. HAPPLE

EDITORIAL COMMENT

In an uncircumcised penis, the prepuce is a ready source of local flap material that can be used for a variety of purposes.

The prepuce skin flap, as described in this chapter, is unique because it need not be moved from its natural position and consequently has no pivot point. This flap serves to cover large defects of the glans penis and is especially suitable for the surgical treatment of penile precancerous lesions. The prepuce skin flap can obviously be used only if the foreskin is still present. However, in view of the fact that precancerous lesions of the penis very seldom occur in circumcised men, this problem rarely arises.

INDICATIONS

The prepuce skin flap is used mainly in the treatment of erythroplasia of Queyrat (1) (Fig. 3) or Bowen's disease (2) (Fig. 4). Moreover, patients suffering from lichen sclerosus et atrophicus of the penis may be relieved of pain and discomfort by use of this flap technique (3). However, if one of these diseases has involved the urethral meatus, other operative measures are required in combination with this flap.

FLAP DESIGN AND DIMENSIONS

The extent of the area to be excised is first outlined on the glans penis. The prepuce is then stretched over the glans, and the flap is outlined in correspondence to the expected defect on the glans (Fig. 1A and B), with its base running parallel to the coronary sulcus. The remaining circumference of the external part of the prepuce is resected following the coronary sulcus.

OPERATIVE TECHNIQUE

The flap is raised by blunt dissection from the internal part of the prepuce (Fig. 1C), and the prepuce is removed by resecting its internal part along the coronary sulcus. The excision of the lesion on the glans is made next (Fig. 1D), and the defect is covered by the prepared skin flap. The remaining wound edges are sutured along the coronary sulcus (Fig. 1E).

If the entire surface of the glans has to be reconstructed, the flap comprises the total circumference of the external part of the prepuce. In this case, triangular incisions are made at the distal part of the flap in order to adapt it to the conical shape of the glans.

If a penile precancerosis has extended to the adjacent surface of the foreskin, the prepuce skin flap can be raised in the same way as described before, because the external and internal parts of the prepuce can easily be separated by blunt dissection (Fig. 2).

A great deal of oozing is prevented by preliminary infiltration of the glans with a solution containing a vasoconstrictive drug.

CLINICAL RESULTS

The success rate of this flap is very high, provided meticulous hemostasis has been maintained. In my experience, patients do not suffer any functional deficit after this operation, even after removal of the entire surface of the glans. Apparently, sexual function does not depend on the presence of the normal skin of the glans penis.

SUMMARY

The prepuce skin flap is an ideal source of tissue in resurfacing defects of the glans penis.

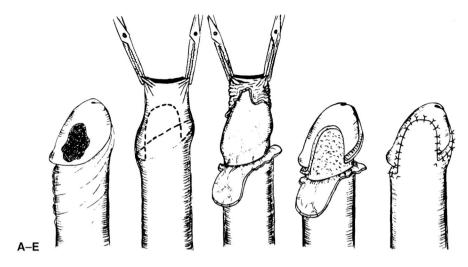

A–E

FIG. 1. A–E: Closure of a defect of the glans by means of a prepuce skin flap.

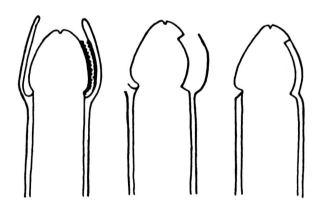

FIG. 2. Removal of a precancerous lesion involving the glans and the adjacent surface of the internal part of the prepuce.

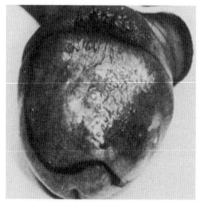
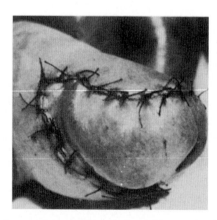
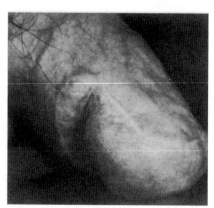

A–C

FIG. 3. Prepuce skin flap for the treatment of erythroplasia of Queyrat. **A:** The defect is outlined on the glans. **B:** The flap is sutured onto the defect, and the remaining wound edges are closed along the coronary sulcus. **C:** Final result.

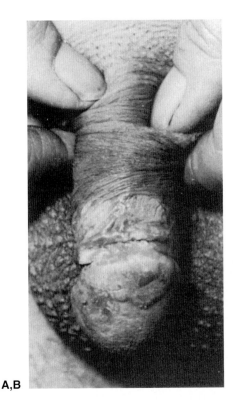
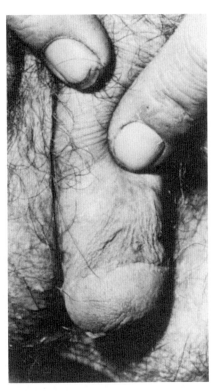

A,B

FIG. 4. Prepuce skin flap for the treatment of Bowen's disease involving adjacent areas of the glans and the prepuce. **A:** Prior to surgery. **B:** Final result.

References

1. Happle R. Surgical treatment of erythroplasia of Queyrat. *Plast Reconstr Surg* 1977;59:642.

2. Happle R. Zur operativen Behandlung des Morbus Bowen an der Glans penis. *Hautarzt* 1972;23:125.
3. Happle R. Chirurgische Behandlung des Lichen sclerosus et atrophicus penis. *Dermatol Monatsschr* 1973;159:975.

CHAPTER 426 ■ DEEPITHELIALIZED OVERLAP SKIN FLAP OF THE PENIS

E. D. SMITH

A penile skin flap is sutured over a deepithelialized flap to provide a strong cover for both primary hypospadias repair (1–4) and closure of fistulas (5,6). This procedure also avoids superimposing another suture line over the urethral closure.

In many techniques of repair, the suturing of the outer skin involves edge-to-edge apposition. This is a potentially weak junction, especially if, in addition, that suture line is superimposed over a deeper line of urethral closure.

INDICATIONS

Except for enlarging the distal glanular orifices, for which only meatotomy and hemicircumcision are suitable, this technique can be used to repair any degree of hypospadias.

FLAP DESIGN AND DIMENSIONS

In the overlap technique, skin closure is achieved by the apposition of two raw surfaces together, produced by shaving of skin from one side (full thickness) and overlapping the flaps

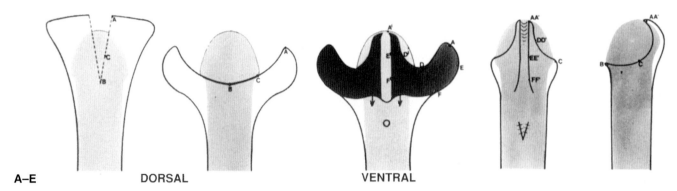

A–E   DORSAL   VENTRAL

FIG. 1. **A–E:** First stage of repair, including skin transfer, correction of chordee, and meatotomy (see text for description). (From Smith, ref. 1, with permission.)

like a double-breasted suit. Tissue adherence by granulation tissue repair is very rapid and solid, depending as it does on a broad surface of good vascularity. Further, the flat plate of overlapping skin has two laterally placed suture lines, so that suture lines are not superimposed.

The preliminary transfer of preputial skin right to the tip of the glans in the first stage ensures that the urethral tube will be constructed by a single epithelium in continuity, without any "break" or anastomosis between changes of epithelium from one section to another (as occurs in techniques involving buried strips, free grafts, or pedicle tubes for part of the length only). Such preliminary transfer also provides sufficient skin for a firm overlap of deepithelialized layers over the whole length of the repair.

There are no skin appendages (hair follicles or sweat glands) in preputial or penile skin, so the dermis will not reepithelialize beneath the double layer. The principle of overlapping skin could be applied to the final stages of any number of techniques (4).

OPERATIVE TECHNIQUE

The hypospadias repair is performed in two stages. The objective of the first stage is twofold: (1) the correction of all elements of chordee, and (2) the transfer of the prepuce to the tip of the ventral surface of the glans to establish viable skin for the subsequent urethral reconstruction. The second stage involves fashioning a complete skin tube to the tip of the penis, supported by overlapping skin layers and denuded of epithelium on one side to allow "double breasting" of raw surfaces.

First-Stage Repair

When the patient is 3½ years of age, the first stage of the repair is performed (Fig. 1). First, the dorsal prepuce is cut longitudinally to the coronal groove (Fig. 1A). The preputial flaps are denuded of their inner layer (which is discarded) and rotated from the dorsal to the ventral side (Fig. 1B).

An area on the glans on either side of the central blind groove is denuded of epithelium to beyond the tip of the glans (Fig. 1C). At this point, the two raw areas are joined by a transverse incision (line with arrows in Fig. 1C), which allows total release of all the penile skin and access to all the elements contributing to chordee (skin release, Buck's fascia, and central chordee band).

Chordee elements may extend well proximal to the orifice. After this is completed, the preputial flaps are sutured dorsally and laterally (points *B* and *C* in Fig. 1E) into the coronal

groove. As seen ventrally, the dark areas represent the inner, denuded surface of the prepuce.

The preputial flaps are then applied ventrally to the glans and sutured right to the tip distally (*AA′, EE′,* etc.). Proximally, the skin flaps join the midline to compensate for any deficiency of skin after correction of the chordee (Fig. 1D). A liberal meatotomy is performed. The extent of the mobilized and sutured prepuce is illustrated (Fig. 1E).

Figure 2 shows the end result of the first stage ventrally. The penis is straight, and there is continuous skin from the orifice to the tip of the glans. No catheter is used.

Second-Stage Repair

Three months after the first stage has been completed, the second phase of the repair is undertaken (Fig. 3). A deep

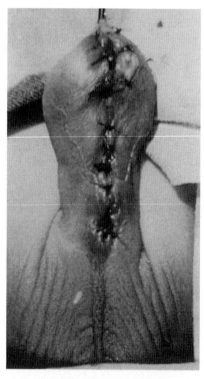

FIG. 2. The end result of the first stage, with solid skin continuously from urethral orifice to tip of glans penis. (From Smith, ref. 3, with permission.)

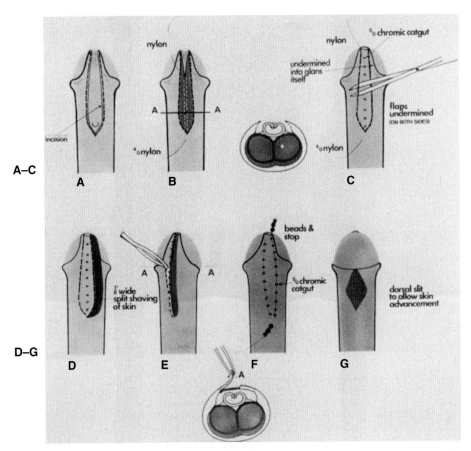

FIG. 3. A–G: The second stage of repair (see text for description). The deepithelialization is shown in parts D through F. (From Smith, ref. 1, with permission.)

ventral U-shaped incision is made from the penile orifice to the tip of the glans, producing a thick layer of skin (Fig. 3A). This central strip should be 12 mm wide. A complete skin tube is fashioned by inverting the raw edges and bringing them together (*AA*) with continuous 4-0 nylon sutures placed over a temporary no. 10 or 12 French catheter (Fig. 3B). The needle should not penetrate the skin, only the subcutaneous tissue.

Further support for this tube is provided by interrupted 5-0 chromic catgut sutures, drawing more subcutaneous and fascial sutures over the primary suture line (Fig. 3C). The lateral skin flaps are undermined, and a deep incision is made on either side of the tube, halfway through the glans. This maneuver allows the tube to slip into the substance of the glans, which is closed over the tube as the outer layers of skin are being overlapped (Fig. 3E, F).

A 3-mm-wide strip of skin is then shaved from one lateral flap to provide a raw surface (Fig. 3D). This is accomplished, using scissors, by creating two or three narrow strips that commence proximally. The first strip should commence laterally, not at the medial edge (Fig. 4A).

The medial edge of the shaved skin is then sutured beneath the opposite flap, commencing at the level of the coronal groove (Fig. 3E). This suture line is not superimposed on the primary suture line of the skin tube, which is now completely covered by the skin flap (Fig. 4B, C).

Subsequently, the opposite flap is swung over the raw area and sutured (*AA*), including the glans tissue at the glans level, in order to project the skin tube into the substance of the glans (Fig. 3F). Tissue adherence of the denuded areas is very strong, and no suture lines are superimposed. If there is tension, a dorsal relieving incision is made (Fig. 3G). Finally, a suprapubic stab cystotomy (not illustrated) is performed for urinary diversion for a period of 12 days.

Use in Fistula Closure

The principle of the overlap flaps also may be applied to the repair of a hypospadias fistula (5,6). The edges of the fistula are excised, and the urethral mucosa is first closed separately with inverting 5-0 chromic catgut sutures. The penile skin is undermined, and one side is "shaved" for at least 3 mm beyond either end of the fistula. The skin is then overlapped to bring the raw flaps together.

CLINICAL RESULTS

Of 480 repairs performed, the rate of postoperative fistula formation was 2.3 percent.

SUMMARY

The principle of a deepithelialized overlap flap has been a major contribution to the prevention and treatment of fistulas in hypospadias repairs.

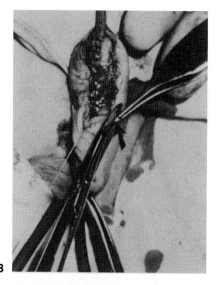
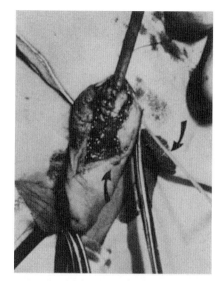

A,B

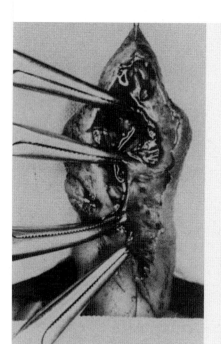
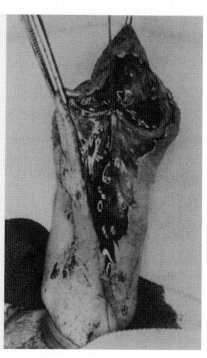
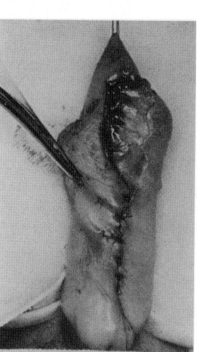

C–E

FIG. 4. **A:** Creation of the "shaved" area on one side. A small strip is commenced proximally (arrow) with scissors. This first strip should commence laterally, not on the medial edge. **B:** A skin strip is excised and discarded (upper arrow). The lower arrow shows the raw surface of the first strip. Two or three further strips are then excised, until the full width of raw area is achieved. **C:** The shaved lateral flap (artery forceps used only to obtain the photograph). **D:** Medial edge of shaved area sutured (5-0 chromic catgut) beneath opposite lateral flap, covering the primary urethral tube. **E:** Opposite lateral flap brought over the shaved area. (**A** and **B** from Smith, ref. 3, with permission. **C** through **E** from Smith, ref. 1, with permission.)

References

1. Smith ED. A deepithelialized overlap flap technique in the repair of hypospadias. *Br J Plast Surg* 1973;26:106.
2. Smith ED. Multiple-stage hypospadias repair. In: Whitehead ED, Leiter E, eds. *Current operative urology.* Hagerstown, MD.: Harper & Row, 1984.
3. Smith ED. Hypospadias. In: Holder TM, Ashcroft KW, eds. *Pediatric surgery.* Philadelphia: Saunders, 1980.
4. Belman AB. The Broadbent hypospadias repair. *Urol Clin North Am* 1981; 8:483.
5. Walker RD. Outpatient repair of urethral fistulae. *Urol Clin North Am* 1981;8:573.
6. Lau JTK, Ong GB. Double-breasted technique for the repair of urethral fistulas after hypospadias surgery. *Br J Urol* 1982;54:111.

CHAPTER 427 ■ INGUINAL SKIN FLAP FOR URETHRAL RECONSTRUCTION

S. ZENTENO ALANIS

Obtaining adequate function in urethral reconstruction of congenital or acquired defects presents multiple problems. None of the techniques currently described is ideal. Urethral reconstruction has been undertaken using flaps, pedicle tubes, free grafts, or combined methods (1–10). Seeking to avoid the disadvantages of the various procedures, I have been using a technique that employs a tubed flap to reconstruct urethral segments (11).

INDICATIONS

The advantages of this technique are as follows:

1. Because of flap elasticity, tissues do not suffer retraction, as they do in free grafts.
2. If the anastomoses are done as indicated, it is possible to avoid severe strictures.
3. The skin of this region is hairless.
4. There is ample tissue to reconstruct sizable defects in the urethra.
5. There is no need for grafting in the donor area.

FLAP DESIGN AND DIMENSIONS

A flap is designed in the inguinoscrotal area measuring 10 to 12 cm long and about 4 to 5 cm wide. The base of the flap should be placed as close as possible to that part of the urethra which is to be reconstructed (Fig. 1).

OPERATIVE TECHNIQUE

To ensure survival of the flap (which should be as thin as possible), a surgical delay is necessary. After 3 weeks, the distal end is detached and the flap is tubed with the skin inside, using a no. 24 French catheter (see Fig. 3C and D). The end of the flap is turned down to the proximal (or distal, depending on the preoperative plan) segment of the urethra, which has been partially dissected, and an anastomosis is performed (see Fig. 3D). This procedure is done by creating triangular flaps on each end and imbricating them (Fig. 2), or else by using a Z-plasty procedure to avoid the stricture produced by a circular scar.

Three to 4 months later after a urethrogram, the base of the tubed flap is dissected (Fig. 3E) and carried to the distal (or proximal) segment of the urethra. An anastomosis is performed using the same technique described above (Fig. 3F). In both stages, the donor area is closed by direct approximation of the edges, taking advantage of the mobility of tissue in the scrotal area (Fig. 3G).

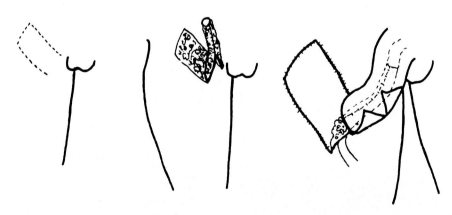

FIG. 1. Diagrammatic representation of the inguinal skin flap used for urethral reconstruction. The distal end of the flap can be anastomosed to either the proximal or distal urethral defect, depending on the defect and the design of the flap.

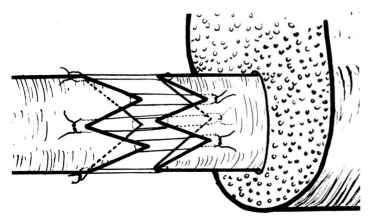

FIG. 2. Diagrammatic representation of the triangular flaps created at the site of the anastomoses that are used to prevent circular scar contractures.

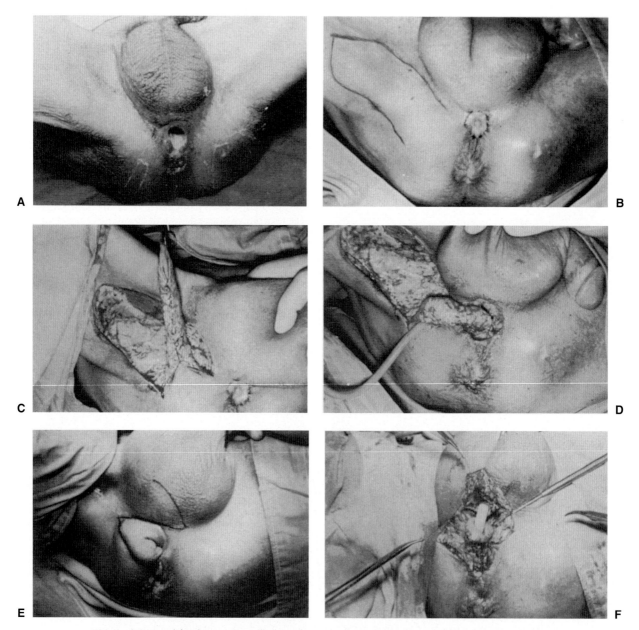

FIG. 3. A: Perineal fistula accounting for loss of urethra segment. **B:** Design of the inguinal flap. **C:** Tubed urethral flap with skin surface on the inside. **D:** Tubed flap anastomosed to proximal urethra, with a Foley catheter in place. Donor area of tube closed by direct approximation. **E:** Design for second stage. **F:** Intraoperative view of distal urethral anastomosis. *(Continued)*

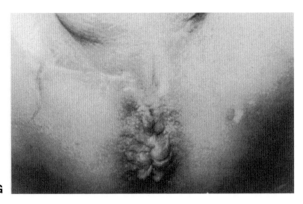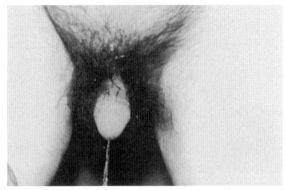

FIG. 3. *Continued.* **G:** Final perineal appearance. **H:** Patient during micturition.

SUMMARY

A tubed inguinal skin flap has several advantages as a technique for urethral reconstruction.

References

1. Johanson B. Reconstruction of the male urethra in stricture. *Acta Chir Scand [Suppl.]* 1953:176.
2. Pressman D, Greenfield LD. Reconstruction of the perineal urethra with a free full-thickness skin graft from the prepuce. *J Urol* 1953;69:677.
3. Marshall VF, Spellman RM. Construction of urethra in humans by free grafts of mucosa from urinary bladder. *Plast Reconstr Surg* 1957;20:423.
4. Lapidas J. Simplified modification of Johanson urethroplasty of deep bulbous urethra. *J Urol* 1959;82:115.
5. Turner-Warwick RT. A technique for posterior urethroplasty. *J Urol* 1960;83:416.
6. Webb H, Campbell J, Grindley J, Erich J. Use of the Z-plastic procedure in urethra-urethral anastomosis. *Ann Surg* 1963;157:579.
7. Wood-Smith DP. Hypospadias: some historical aspects and the evolution of methods of treatment. In: Converse JM, ed. *Reconstructive plastic surgery.* Philadelphia: Saunders, 1964;2010.
8. Kishev S. Surgical restoration of the penile urethra. *Plast Reconstr Surg* 1964;33:47.
9. Ardelyi R. Substitution of a total traumatic defect of urethra. *Acta Chir Orthop Trauma (Czech)* 1966;33:364.
10. Cowan RJ, Sullivan LD. Experiences with perineal urethroplasty for stricture. *Plast Reconstr Surg* 1968;41:137.
11. Zenteno Alanis S. An innovation in total penis reconstruction. *Plast Reconstr Surg* 1969;43:418.

CHAPTER 428 ■ TUBED ABDOMINAL SKIN FLAP FOR PENILE RECONSTRUCTION

J. M. NOE

The use of a vertical midline lower abdominal tubed flap turned inside out so that the abdominal skin forms an internal tunnel, with a split-thickness skin graft used for the exterior of the inverted tube, allows a phallus-like structure to be constructed in only two stages without excessive morbidity and with cosmetic and psychologic objectives achieved (1,2).

INDICATIONS

Historically, the major methods for reconstructing a penis have developed largely from war injuries (3–15). Other causes of loss or absence of the penis have been burns, cancer, infections, metabolic or vascular derangement, punitive ablation, or congenital abnormality. The flap described in this chapter has been used almost exclusively for the construction of male genitalia for the female-to-male transsexual.

The object of any method of reconstruction is a penis that is satisfactory psychologically, cosmetically, and physiologically. No attempt was made to meet all these reconstructive objectives, but only the psychologic and cosmetic objectives

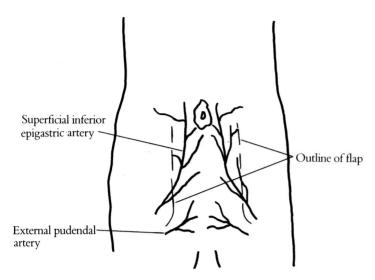

Superficial inferior epigastric artery

Outline of flap

External pudendal artery

FIG. 1. The blood supply of the tubed abdominal flap.

and that part of the physiologic objective concerned with producing a rigid penis, so that coitus is possible with a temporary implant (1). No attempt was made to construct a urethra in the transsexual, because the difficulties and complications outweigh the benefits of being able to stand while urinating.

In this situation, there is little place for a permanent prosthesis in the construction of a penis. In a movable organ without sensation that is obtained when an abdominal tubed flap is used, extrusion of any permanent implant is likely (16). Therefore, a removable prosthesis, inserted at the time of intercourse, best overcomes the problem.

No claim is made of providing an organ that serves as an area of genital stimulation. Because the tubed flap has a very coarse, tough sensation, the clitoris is neither amputated nor is its sensibility compromised; it continues to serve its sexual function.

ANATOMY (17)

The midline tubed abdominal flap is largely supplied by musculocutaneous perforating vessels from the deep inferior epigastric artery, except for the base of the flap, which is supplied by the external pudendal artery (Fig. 1). When the flap is raised, the perforating vessels from the deep inferior epigastric artery are divided. In the second stage, when the superior pedicle is cut free, all the blood supply is from the external pudendal system; the flap is then a random flap based on this blood supply.

OPERATIVE TECHNIQUE

There are two stages to the procedure: (1) a bipedicle vertical midline lower abdominal tubed flap is constructed, and (2) the upper end of this tube is cut loose and the glans penis is constructed. At this second stage, a hysterectomy and bilateral salpingo-oophorectomy can be performed. A hysterectomy should not be done prior to the first stage, to prevent either the midline or the Pfannenstiel incision from interfering with the blood supply to the tubed flap.

First Stage

Two incisions are made 8 to 9 cm apart, extending from the umbilicus to the area of the pubic symphysis, to create a verti-

cal tube (Fig. 2). These incisions are carried down through the skin and subcutaneous tissue until Camper's areolar fascia is identified. Camper's fascia is then undermined (after it is incised in a vertical direction parallel to the incisions on the skin), and a tubed flap is then created with the abdominal skin inside. Camper's fascia is sutured together around the outside of this tube.

A split-thickness skin graft taken from a hairless area is wound around the tube. The skin graft is placed in a spiral fashion, so that no longitudinal scars are created. A thick, potentially hair growing split-thickness skin graft (to simulate pubic hair) is also placed at the base of the inferior pedicle to provide extra skin for use in the second stage and to allow the tube to bend downward 180 degrees to the genital area.

The flap donor site is closed under tension. Scrub sponges "cored" out have been used as part of the dressing to support the tubed flap in its new position.

When all the wounds are well healed and the blood supply is sufficient to nourish the tube from its lower pedicle, the second stage is done.

Second Stage

Releasing the upper end of the tube, fashioning the tip to construct a glans and corona, and fusing the labia majora (as needed to create a scrotal appearance) are accomplished during the second stage. A hysterectomy and bilateral salpingo-oophorectomy also can be performed, going through the midline scar created when the donor site of the flap was closed.

A transverse elliptical incision is made around the upper pedicle of the tube, going through it to release that end of the tube from the abdomen. The glans penis is then constructed, after removing excess subcutaneous tissue. The corona is fashioned by using epidermal-to-dermal stitches to create an overlap of local skin.

By leaving the lining skin tube open at both the proximal and distal ends, it is possible to maintain better hygiene within this tunnel. The tunnel within the tube also facilitates the use of a temporary, custom-made T-shaped baculum, which is inserted through the proximal opening of the tunnel (at the base of the constructed penis) (Fig. 3). It provides rigidity for intercourse. The insert rests on the pubic symphysis, so that an "erection" can be transmitted from this bony area outward through the penis. Conversely, external pressure on the tip can be transmitted back to the clitoral area, affording some stimulation there.

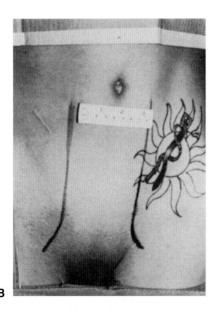
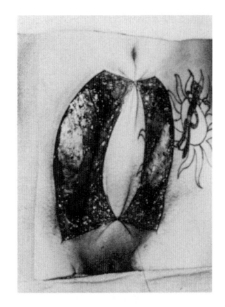

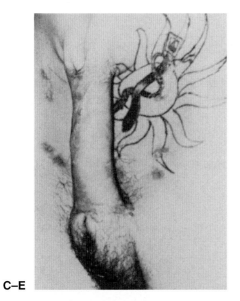
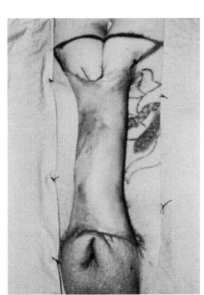
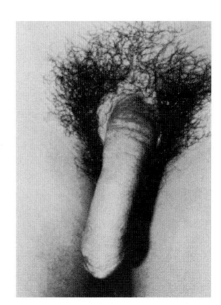

FIG. 2. A: Flap outlined in lower abdomen. **B:** Incisions down to Camper's fascia. **C:** Healed flap. Note that the split-thickness skin graft was placed in spiral fashion. **D:** Incision for second stage. **E:** Representative example. (From Noe et al., ref. 1, with permission.)

A,B

C–E

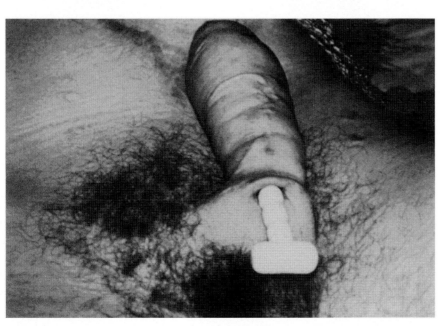

FIG. 3. Baculum in place in inner tube.

The labia majora are fused in the midline to create a scrotum. Each labium is incised in its midline, hemostasis is obtained, and then a three-layer closure from side to side (consisting of the posterior epithelium, the subcutaneous tissue, and the anterior epithelium) is performed. The inferior end is left open to facilitate hygiene and permit urination.

No attempt is made to amputate the clitoris nor to interfere in any way with its sensibility.

Third Stage (Optional)

An optional third stage in phalloplasty for transsexuals is the placement of testicular prostheses into the labia (17,18). Hair-bearing labial flaps have been transposed to the suprapubic area to accomplish additional release of the phallus and more closely to simulate the male escutcheon (19).

CLINICAL RESULTS

Between 1966 and 1978, 48 female-to-male transsexual patients underwent surgery with the midline abdominal tubed method at the Stanford Gender Dysphoria Program (19,20). There were 154 operative procedures performed on 48 patients. Fifty-eight percent of these patients had one or more complications. Obesity, previous abdominal surgery with abdominal scars, and acne were frequently associated with these complications. Forty-two percent of the complications were in the first stage, 19 percent in the second stage, and 30 percent in the third stage. Graft loss requiring regrafting was the largest complication in the first stage, followed by tube dehiscence.

SUMMARY

The vertical midline lower abdominal tubed flap, used with a split-thickness skin graft, allows a phallus-like structure to be constructed in only two stages.

References

1. Noe JM, Birdsell D, Laub DR. The surgical construction of male genitalia for female-to-male transsexuals. *Plast Reconstr Surg* 1974;53:511.
2. Noe TM, Sato R, Coleman C, Laub DR. Construction of male genitalia: the Stanford experience. *Arch Sex Behav* 1978;7:297.
3. Bogaras N. Ueber die voile plastische Wiederherstellung eines zum Koitus faehigen Penis. *Zentralbl Chir* 1936;63:1271.
4. Blum V. A case of plastic restoration of the penis. *J Mt Sinai Hosp* 1938; 4:506.
5. Frumkin AP. Reconstruction of the male genitalia. *Annu Rev Soviet Med* 1944;2:214.
6. Gillies HD, Millard DR. Congenital absence of the penis. *Br J Plast Surg* 1948;1:8.
7. McIndoe A. Deformities of the male urethra. *Br J Plast Surg* 1948;1:29.
8. Farina R, Frier EG. Total reconstruction of the penis. *Plast Reconstr Surg* 1954;14:351.
9. Morales PA, O'Connor JJ, Hotchkiss RS. Plastic reconstructive surgery after total loss of the penis. *Am J Surg* 1956;92:403.
10. Munawar A. Surgical treatment of the male genitalia. *J Int Coll Surg* 1957; 27:352.
11. Gelb J, Malament M, LoVerme S. Total reconstruction of the penis. *Plast Reconstr Surg* 1959;24:62.
12. Fleming JP. Reconstruction of the penis. *J Urol* 1970;104:213.
13. Orticochea M. A new method of total reconstruction of the penis. *Br J Plast Surg* 1972;25:347.
14. Hoopes JE. Surgical correction of the male external genitalia. *Clin Plast Surg* 1975;1:325.
15. Puckett CL, Montie JE. Construction of male genitalia in the transsexual using a tubed groin flap for the penis and a hydraulic inflation device. *Plast Reconstr Surg* 1978;61:523.
16. Evans AT. Buried-skin-strip urethra in tube pedicle phalloplasty. *Br J Plast Surg* 1963;16:280.
17. Rea CE. The use of testicular prosthesis made of Lucite with a note concerning the size of the testis at different ages. *J Urol* 1943;49:727.
18. Noe TM, Laub DR, Schulz W. The external male genitalia: the interplay of surgery and mechanical prosthesis. In: Meyer J, ed. *Clinical management of sexual disorders*. Philadelphia: Williams & Wilkins, 1976.
19. Dubin BJ, Sato RM, Laub DR. Results of phalloplasty. *Plast Reconstr Surg* 1979;64:163.
20. Laub DR, Dubin BJ. Gender dysphoria. In: Grabb WC, Smith JW, eds. *Plastic surgery*, 3rd ed. Boston: Little, Brown, 1979;883.

CHAPTER 429. Tubed Groin Skin Flap and Microsvascular Free Flap Phalloplasty

C. L. Puckett

www.encyclopediaofflaps.com

Online
Chapter

CHAPTER 430 ■ RADIAL FOREARM FREE FLAP FOR PENILE RECONSTRUCTION

C. K. HERMAN, A. S. HOSCHANDER, AND B. STRAUCH

EDITORIAL COMMENT

This is an excellent and most elegant method for penile reconstruction, providing the ability to micturate standing up, return of erogenous sensibility, and the possibility of stiffness, usually done as a second operative procedure approximately 1 year later. The editors recommend the use of a temporary arteriovenous fistula between the saphenous vein and the femoral artery, which will facilitate revascularization of the forearm flap. For patients who have a considerable amount of hair on the forearm, one should consider laser hair removal for two or three sessions to prevent a hairy neourethra.

The radial forearm free flap has been successfully used for single-operation total penile reconstruction for more than two decades. First described as an alternative to nonmicrosurgical procedures by Chang and Hwang in 1984 (1), this fasciocutaneous flap has evolved into the most effective method of near-total or total phallic reconstruction. A number of modifications have led to improved functionality and cosmesis (2–7). Historical methods of reconstruction, including local tube flaps and myocutaneous flaps, have demonstrated significant drawbacks, including absent or minimal sensation. The radial forearm free flap allows a sensate (both erogenous and tactile) reconstruction, with a non- or minimally hair-bearing neophallus, and potential for the addition of an erectile or semirigid prosthesis to enable coitus.

INDICATIONS

Major deformities of the penis requiring phallic reconstruction can occur secondary to trauma, neoplasm, or infection. Congenital absence of the penis is seen in male patients with micropenis and male pseudohermaphroditism, as well as in female patients with gender dysphoria. The goals of phalloplasty include a reliable and durable reconstruction, a sensate neophallus, urethral integrity to allow voiding while standing, and adequate rigidity or erectile function to allow penetration. The radial forearm free flap is one of many microsurgical and nonmicrosurgical options available for total phallic reconstruction. Use of the radial forearm free flap should be reserved for cases in which total or near-total phallic reconstruction is required.

The radial forearm flap is based on a neurovascular pedicle with adequate length to reconstruct the penis. The fasciocutaneous radial forearm free flap receives its blood supply from the radial artery, a branch of the brachial artery. The radial forearm free flap may be considered among the first-line surgical therapies for total penile reconstruction.

ANATOMY

As noted, the fasciocutaneous radial forearm free flap receives its blood supply from the radial artery, a branch of the brachial artery. The radial artery vascular supply perfuses the fasciocutaneous flap via cutaneous perforating vessels that course through a thin intermuscular septum and the antebrachial fascia. These perforating vessels most commonly arise from the proximal and distal thirds of the radial artery; the middle third rarely contributes perforating branches. The cephalic vein or basilic vein or both provide venous drainage of the flap. The medial and lateral antebrachial cutaneous nerves constitute the neurosensory component of the flap, with enhanced dermatomal sensation in the distal forearm corresponding to the glans component of the reconstruction. The structural component of the flap includes the volar forearm skin, subcutaneous adipose tissue, and deep fascia.

FLAP DESIGN AND DIMENSIONS

Several modifications of the original design by Chang and Hwang (1) have been described (3,4,6,7). The central concept pervades all techniques: a radial forearm fasciocutaneous flap that is relatively hairless along its ulnar border. The radial forearm free flap is created with a width of approximately 13 cm and a length of approximately 12 cm. The basic flap design consists of three separate areas: the neourethral area, the external skin covering, and an intervening deepithelialized area. The neourethra is located along the ulnar portion (area A) (Fig. 1). The neourethra should be 2 to 3 cm in width and is positioned on the ulnar side of the flap, which is generally less hair-bearing. Bordering the neourethra radially is a segment of tissue measuring 0.5 to 1 cm (area B) that will require deepithelialization. Lateral to area B is an area measuring 8 to 10 cm that will become the outer surface of the neophallus (area C). A small tongue flap, centered at the distal end of this segment, will form the orifice of the distal urethra.

OPERATIVE TECHNIQUE

The flap is first outlined on the patient's nondominant forearm (2). The perfusion of the superficial palmar arch by the ulnar artery should be assessed with a preoperative Allen test, by ultrasonic Doppler flowmeter testing, or by arteriography. The Allen test is generally considered sufficient for this purpose.

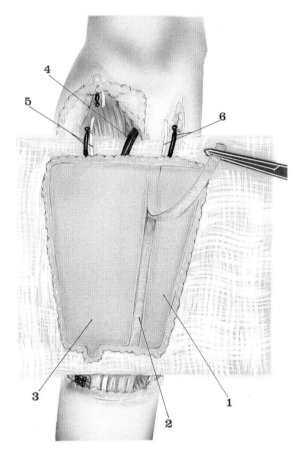

FIG. 1. Elevation of flap and deepithelialization of Area *B*. 1. Area (*A*); 2. area (*B*);3. area (*C*); 4. radial artery and veins; 5. cephalic vein and lateral cutaneous nerve of the forearm; 6. basilic vein and medial cutaneous nerve of the forearm.

A pneumatic tourniquet is applied with elevation exsanguination. Initially, the area radial to the neourethra (area *B*) is deepithelialized. The radial vascular bundle, found at the lateral edge of the flexor carpi radialis tendon, is then identified at the distal lateral portion of the flap and dissected. Laterally, at the edge of the flap, the cephalic vein is isolated and ligated. The ulnar incision is then made and carried down deep to the fascia. The dissection continues radially until it reaches the thin intermuscular septum, which contains the septocutaneous perforating vessels of the radial artery. This dissection is carried out from distal to proximal. The basilic vein and the medial cutaneous nerve of the forearm are located at the proximal medial border of the flap and can be ligated and raised with the flap. Next, the radial portion of the flap is raised from the brachioradialis medially. The muscle is retracted laterally, and the radial vascular bundle connected to the flap is dissected from the distal edge of the flap to its origin from the brachial artery.

Again, the septocutaneous perforators are preserved in the intermuscular septum. During this dissection, it is important to identify and preserve the superficial branch of the radial nerve. This nerve can be found as it courses with the cephalic vein and pierces through or travels beneath the brachioradialis tendon. The cephalic vein and lateral cutaneous nerve of the forearm are identified in the groove between the brachioradialis and biceps muscles. At this point, the vein and nerve are isolated and ligated. The cephalic vein may be dissected proximally for additional length, if necessary. Once the flap is completely raised and is being perfused and drained only by the

radial artery and its venae comitantes, the tourniquet is released, and the distal radial artery is clamped while perfusion of the hand is assessed. When adequate perfusion of the hand is confirmed, the distal radial vascular bundle can be ligated (Fig. 1).

The creation of the neophallus begins with rolling of the neourethra (area *A*) over a urinary catheter, with the epidermis positioned internally, and suturing it to the medial side of the deepithelialized portion of the flap (area *B*) (Fig. 2). The shaft of the neourethra is then created by wrapping the lateral area (area *C*) around the neourethra with the epidermis positioned externally. The lateral, radial border of the flap is sutured to the lateral portion of the deepithelialized area (Fig. 3). The distal edges of areas *A* and *C* are sutured to each other to create the orifice of the neourethra (Fig. 4).

The recipient site may be prepared by a separate team during flap elevation. Recipient-vessel preferences may vary, including the inferior epigastric vessels, vein grafts to the femoral vessels, and saphenous vein. Our preferred technique is as follows. The saphenous vein is dissected in the thigh, and approximately 20 cm of vein is harvested. The saphenous vein is left attached to the femoral vein, and the free end is anastomosed to the femoral artery. creating a temporary loop arteriovenous fistula. The site of attachment should be prepared at the site of the native phallus, but if no native phallus exists, an incision should be made over the pubic symphysis. The recipient nerves should be located at this time. It is preferable to isolate the dorsal penile (or clitoral) branches of the pudendal nerve; if these are not found, the pudendal nerves may be used. The thigh incision may be extended medially to the

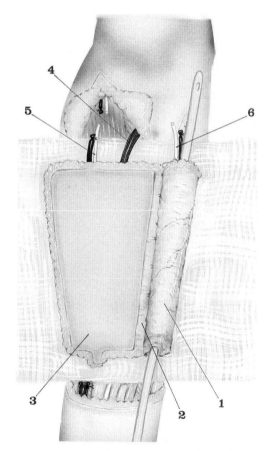

FIG. 2. Creation of neourethra over a catheter. 1. Area (*A*); 2. area (*B*) 3. area (*C*); 4. radial artery and veins; 5. cephalic vein and lateral cutaneous nerve of the forearm; 6. basilic vein and medial cutaneous nerve of the forearm.

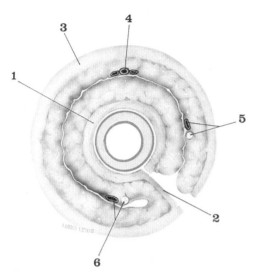

FIG. 3. Cross-sectional view. 1. Area (*A*) 2. area (*B*) 3. area (*C*) 4. radial artery and veins; 5. cephalic vein and lateral cutaneous nerve of the forearm; 6. basilic vein and medial cutaneous nerve of the forearm.

recipient bed to improve blood flow from the vein grafts to the neophallus.

The neophallus is now detached from its radial vascular pedicle in the forearm and transferred to its new location. The neophallus should be secured to the recipient bed with tacking sutures. The catheter is now inserted into the bladder, and a primary anastomosis between the flap's neourethra and the native urethra is made. The saphenous vein loop is now bisected. The venous limb is anastomosed to the cephalic vein, and the arterial limb is anastomosed to the radial artery. The paired pudendal nerves are anastomosed to the medial and lateral cutaneous nerves of the forearm. The neophallus is now completely sutured to the recipient bed, and the remainder of the incisions are closed. Finally, a suprapubic catheter is placed to divert urine away from the healing urethral anastomosis. The urinary catheter is left in place from 10 days to 4 weeks, at which point a retrograde urethrogram or a voiding trial may be performed.

The donor site is closed by approximating the forearm muscle to cover any exposed tendons. A split-thickness skin graft is then used to cover the donor site. Flap viability should be assessed hourly, by using standard assessment techniques, such as capillary refill, color, turgor, and pulse checks via palpation or Doppler analysis.

Many modifications to this flap have been made since its original design in 1984. Some of these modifications have created the possibility of increasing the length of the phallus and the ability to add a prosthesis, as well as different designs for a more aesthetically pleasing corona. It is our preference to provide rigidity to the shaft by incorporating an irradiated human costal cartilage graft. This operation generally is performed at least 1 year after the initial reconstruction, when adequate protective sensation is present. Other techniques to achieve rigidity also can be used, including various inflatable penile prosthetic devices.

CLINICAL RESULTS

Reconstruction of the penis has been accomplished by many methods, including both microsurgical and local flaps, with the radial forearm free flap providing the most reliable results. Cheng et al. (5) studied 136 patients who had undergone vari-

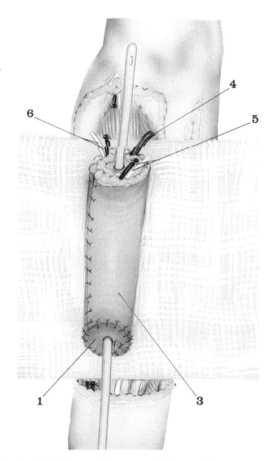

FIG. 4. Radial forearm flap prepared for transfer to recipient area. 1. Area (*A*) 2. area (*B*) 3. area (*C*); 4. radial artery and veins; 5. cephalic vein and lateral cutaneous nerve of the forearm; 6. basilic vein and medial cutaneous nerve of the forearm.

ous methods of penile reconstruction. Of these patients, 93 had penile reconstruction by using the radial forearm flap, with 13 (14%) patients experiencing a major complication. The main complications of this flap are the formation of fistulae (10%) and urethral strictures (3%), as well as partial flap necrosis (6.5%). Complete flap loss occurred in one case and required a new flap from the contralateral forearm. The radial forearm flap was described as having an appropriate thickness and texture as well as having hairless skin. Additionally, the flap is reported as having good erogenous and tactile sensation, with tactile sensation returning to the flap within 6 months for those who underwent nerve coaptation. Erogenous sensation returned in 81% of patients, allowing generation of an orgasm in the majority of cases. The appearance of the neophallus is acceptable, and micturition can be achieved while standing. The major disadvantage of this flap is the donor-site deformity, but this is usually tolerated well under the circumstances that warrant a total penile reconstruction.

SUMMARY

The construction and reconstruction of a neophallus by using the radial forearm free flap is aesthetically acceptable and widely functional. This technique can achieve both protective and erogenous sensation, as well as the ability to micturate while standing. Many congenitally male patients will regain the ability to achieve orgasm and ejaculate with appropriate stimulation. The addition of a penile prosthesis allows pleasurable and successful coitus.

References

1. Chang TS, Hwang WY. Forearm flap in one-stage reconstruction of the penis. *Plast Reconstr Surg* 1984;74:251.
2. Strauch B, Yu HL. *Atlas of microvascular surgery: anatomy and operative approaches.* Stuttgart: Thieme, 1993;318.
3. Gottlieb LJ, Levine LA. A new design for the radial forearm free-flap phallic construction. *Plast Reconstr Surg* 1993;92:276.
4. Gilbert DA, Williams MW, Horton CE, et al. Phallic innervation via the pudendal nerve. *J Urol* 1988;41:160.
5. Cheng KX, Hwang WY, Aie AE, et al. Analysis of 136 cases of reconstructed penis using various methods. *Plast Reconstr Surg* 1995;95:1070.
6. Hu ZQ, Hyakusoku H, Gao JH, et al. Penis reconstruction using three different operative methods. *Br J Plast Surg* 2005;58:487.
7. Rashid M, Sarwar SU. Avulsion injuries of the male external genitalia: classification and reconstruction with the customised radial forearm free flap. *Br J Plast Surg* 2005;58:585.

CHAPTER 431 ■ ULNAR FOREARM FLAP FOR PHALLIC RECONSTRUCTION

D. A. GILBERT

EDITORIAL COMMENT

(Chapters 431–434) There are now multiple methods of reliable canal reconstructions utilizing microvascular techniques. Each of the authors claims significant advantages for each of their own techniques, and they are probably all correct. All of these flaps work for reconstruction of the penis. However, the biggest problem is the location of the recipient vessels. A solution to this problem of recipient vessels is the use of the saphenous vein plugged info the femoral artery, creating a temporary A-V fistula. The fistula is then brought into the perineal area, divided, and a large artery and vein are available for attachment to the penile reconstruction.

The microsurgical free forearm flap has become the mainstay of modern phallic reconstruction (1,2). Such reconstructions have classically depended on the radial forearm flap. However, the flap may also be based on the ulnar artery (3), providing a thin, malleable, non-hirsute, sensate flap that can be sculpted to the patient's needs.

INDICATIONS

Phallic reconstruction should ideally: (1) be a one-stage microsurgical procedure that can be reliably reproduced; (2) have both tactile and erogenous sensibility; (3) be created with a competent neourethra that allows voiding while standing; (4) have enough bulk to tolerate insertion of a prosthetic stiffener to allow for successful intromission; (5) be aesthetically acceptable to the patient and his partner; (6) grow through childhood to an acceptable adult size; and (7) be associated with acceptable donor-site morbidity.

Early reconstructions often failed because of the multiple procedures involved or because of fistulae, strictures, or hair in the urethra. More important, the final product lacked sensation and had a poor aesthetic appearance. The development of microsurgical techniques allowed for selection of distant flaps, the transfer of free tissue, and the coaptation of nerves from the donor flap to recipient nerves in the perineum.

Indications for total phallic reconstruction include posttraumatic loss, female-to-male transsexual surgery, developmental micropenis, exstrophy/epispadias deformities, and sickle cell disease.

Drawbacks of the ulnar forearm flap include the obvious donor-site deformity on the forearm, possible cold intolerance in the ipsilateral hand, potential loss of function, and hirsutism in many patients (including female-to-male transsexuals on testosterone therapy). Although the ulnar aspect of the forearm is often relatively hairless and can be used to construct the urethra, subsequent hair growth inside the neourethra is not only unsightly but, more serious, excess hair possibly promotes bacterial colonization and calculus formation. To date, we have not had any patients who have experienced complications with postoperative cold intolerance or permanent ulnar nerve injury in the donor hand.

ANATOMY

The ulnar forearm flap is vascularized by the ulnar artery and its paired venae comitantes (Fig. 1). The caliber and length of the ulnar artery are superior to those of the radial artery. The ulnar artery arises as a continuation of the brachial artery, and then runs distally to the ulnar wrist. The artery is covered proximally by the long flexors, and distally by skin, subcutaneous tissue, and the flexor carpi ulnaris. Within the distal forearm, two predictable vascular pedicles

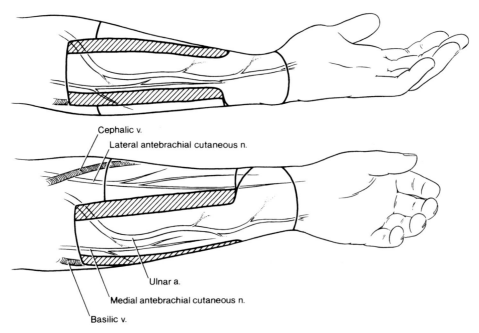

FIG. 1. "Cricket bat" centered over the ulnar aspect of the forearm. (From Gilbert et al., ref. 6, with permission.)

from the ulnar artery to the flap are identified. The largest one is usually found at the mid-forearm level, where the ulnar artery lies deep between the flexor digitorum superficialis and the flexor carpi ulnaris. The second perforator is located distally between the proximal perforator and the wrist.

The antebrachial fascia invests the forearm musculature and the ulnar artery in a firm sheet that separates the muscles from each other and from overlying veins and nerves. The proximal forearm fascia is pierced by nerves, arteries, and veins that run superficially through the premuscular fascia to the overlying skin. The veins include the cephalic, basilic, and medial antebrachial. The cephalic vein runs proximally from the wrist over the radial side of the forearm, collecting tributaries from the volar and dorsal forearm. The basilic vein begins over the dorsal-ulnar wrist, and runs proximally to the ulnar side of the elbow. The medial antebrachial vein runs from the volar-ulnar wrist to the side of the elbow. All these veins communicate with or receive tributaries from the median cubital vein.

The lateral antebrachial nerve is the anatomic continuation of the musculocutaneous nerve arising at the elbow, entering the antebrachial fascia deep to the cephalic vein, and dividing into anterior and dorsal branches that provide sensation to the radial-volar and dorsal areas of the forearm.

The medial antebrachial nerve lies medial to the brachial artery in the upper arm, and then pierces the antebrachial fascia, to run distally and superficially with the basilic and other antebrachial veins. This nerve divides into anterior and ulnar branches, to innervate the ulnar-volar and dorsal-ulnar forearm.

FLAP DESIGN AND DIMENSIONS

All prospective patients undergo a standard preoperative assessment that includes an Allen's test, to evaluate and confirm "two-vessel patency" in the upper extremity. Should there be any doubt concerning the vascular integrity of either forearm vessel, patients undergo upper-extremity angiogra-

phy. Inherent to candidacy for surgery is the ability to tolerate an extended microvascular procedure.

Phallic flap dimensions are planned to accommodate each patient's specific anatomic needs regarding the urethral and outer-shaft width and length. In preteen and adolescent patients, the phallus assumes a somatic growth rate—not a "genital growth rate"—following transfer, and phallic size must be planned to accommodate the disparity (4).

The quality of subcutaneous fat is also assessed in the forearm of each patient. Those with thicker subcutaneous fat have a larger diameter reconstruction that requires added width for outer-shaft coverage, in which there is a great deal of subcutaneous adipose tissue. In some cases, we achieved shaft coverage using a split-thickness skin graft; the cosmetic results were amazingly good.

Our present design incorporates the original Biemer triple skin design and includes a fourth distal island "neoglans" (5,6). This island, a distal continuation of the neourethral island, is rotated proximally over deepithelialized distal shaft skin, to create a pseudoglans and palpable step-off at the coronal sulcus. The urethral component is at least 3.5 cm wide.

OPERATIVE TECHNIQUE

Deepithelialization is completed on the urethral borders between the urethra and the lateral skin flaps, and over the distal skin flaps adjacent to the neoglans. Elevation of the forearm flap is begun after the ulnar artery is determined to be anatomically normal by Doppler examination.

The ulnar artery and its venae comitantes are identified and ligated distally. The ulnar nerve is identified and left in its bed. From laboratory dissections and clinical experience, we have found that the forearm fascia can be dissected into two layers. The thicker deep antebrachial fascia is left intact on the forearm musculature, while a thinner superficial layer is elevated within the flap. Over the vascular pedicle, the plane of dissection is directed through the deep investing muscle fascia, to incorporate the ulnar artery and venous branches. During dissection of the vascular pedicle, the ulnar

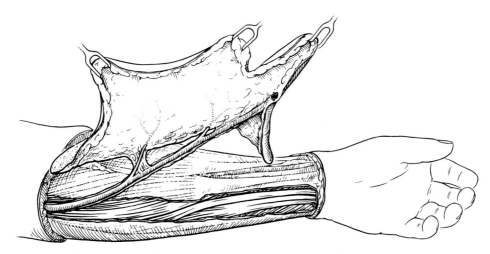

FIG. 2. Flap elevated on ulnar vessels. (From Gilbert et al., ref. 6, with permission.)

artery is gently separated from the ulnar nerve along its length. The dorsal sensory branches of the ulnar nerve are preserved (Fig. 2).

The ulnar artery is then dissected proximally to its origin from the brachial artery. When the full length of the ulnar artery is required, a counterincision in the deep fascia between the brachial radialis or the flexor superficialis provides exposure of the bifurcation of the brachial artery. It is important to identify the anterior interosseous nerve when dissecting the ulnar artery beneath the flexor superficialis muscles. Transient loss of "pinch" can occur, if traction is placed on this nerve.

Numerous veins are often encountered at the proximal forearm, but we favor the basilic and cephalic veins for anastomosis. Their diameter is similar to the recipient saphenous vein. If additional vascular egress is required, we anastomose the donor vena comitans and the recipient inferior epigastric vena comitans. Depending on the flap design, we try to preserve one of the major superficial veins in the forearm. Although the flap donor site has transient postoperative swelling, we have not experienced any chronic postoperative edema.

The lateral and medial antebrachial nerves are dissected in the forearm, usually close to the cephalic and basilic veins, respectively.

Construction of the neophallus is begun while the flap is still perfusing on the forearm. The neourethra is tubed with a two-layer closure, usually with a running locked suture, to achieve a more watertight seal (Figs. 3, 4). The phallic shaft is crafted by suturing the lateral flaps to each other in a "clamshell" fashion. Finally, the neoglans is formed by rotating the glans paddle proximally, to create an appropriate conically-shaped neoglans configuration (Figs. 5, 6).

Prior to the microsurgical transfer, the length and diameter of the donor and recipient vessels are estimated. The recipient inferior epigastric artery is anastomosed to the donor artery. If the epigastric artery is absent, a venous fistula is created, using a saphenous-vein interposition graft between the femoral artery and the adjacent saphenous vein. This fistula is cut in half, thereby creating a saphenous-vein interposition graft that serves as a conduit between the "recipient" femoral and "donor" ulnar arteries, as well as venous egress.

A urethral anastomosis is then carried out between the neourethra and native urethra. Where possible, this anastomosis is completed with a two-layer closure of long-term absorbable suture. A gracilis muscle is often elevated and rotated over the urethral anastomosis for added vascularity at the anastomotic site. The gracilis can be modified and, where necessary, skin grafted to mimic a neoscrotum.

The venous anastomoses and nerve coaptation are then completed.

When distal branches of the pudendal nerve cannot be located, dissection is carried out to identify the pudendal nerve more proximally (at the exit from Alcock's canal). Alternatively, a nonerogenous recipient nerve can be used. We have used the ilioinguinal, genitofemoral, saphenous, hypogastric, and gracilis nerves to achieve phallic sensation.

The final step is to cover the forearm flap donor site with a split-thickness skin graft. Some advancement of the surrounding skin interface is attempted, to diminish the size of the

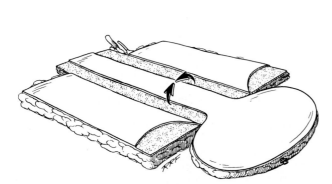

FIG. 3. Neourethra planned closure. (From Gilbert et al., ref. 6, with permission.)

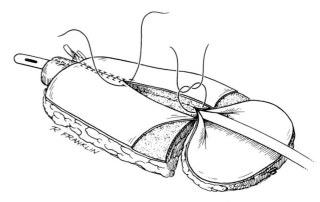

FIG. 4. Skin closure over neourethra. (From Gilbert et al., ref. 6, with permission.)

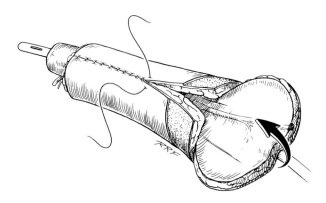

FIG. 5. Over surface closed and glans planned to be closed. (From Gilbert et al., ref. 6, with permission.)

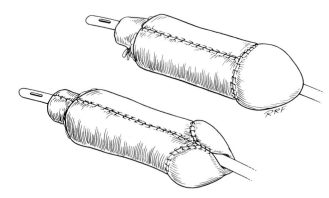

FIG. 6. All wounds are sutured anteriorly and posteriorly. (From Gilbert et al., ref. 6, with permission.)

donor site. A thick (20/1000 to 25/1000 of an inch) split-thickness skin graft is harvested from the thigh and applied to the forearm. By preserving the forearm antebrachial fascia, we find the donor site is smooth and bloodless, and readily accepts the skin graft. More recently, we have used full-thickness skin grafts harvested from the groin bilaterally, to cover the donor site. A nonadherent dressing and custom splint are then placed on the forearm.

Postoperatively, a custom splint is constructed to shield the penis. The splint encircles the phallus and rests on the pubis. It is secured, so that no pressure can be applied from the sides or from the top. The penis is kept in an erect position.

CLINICAL RESULTS

We have gradually modified our approach to phalloplasty, with the goals of improved function and aesthetic results. Over the past 2 years, we have completed 21 ulnar-based forearm microsurgical phalloplasties, with no failures. The youngest patient in this group was 6 years of age, and the oldest was 40 years of age (mean age: 24.3 years). Of the 21 phalloplasties, three patients required reoperation to relieve arterial thrombi. All of these arterial thrombi occurred in cases where a saphenous-vein interposition graft was used between the recipient femoral artery and the donor ulnar artery. One thrombus occurred 12 days after phallic reconstruction. All thrombi were successfully removed, and the flaps survived with a combination of surgical thrombectomies, injection of intraarterial urokinase, and replacement of the saphenous-vein interposition grafts.

Three patients had postoperative urethral stenosis that required internal urethrotomy to correct. Four patients had

postoperative urethrocutaneous fistulae, of which one resolved spontaneously, one was successfully closed with an intraoral mucosal graft, and the two others await fistula repair.

Fourteen of the 18 patients had nerve coaptation to branches of the pudendal nerve. Two patients had coaptation to genitofemoral nerves, one to the ilioinguinal nerve, and one patient awaits nerve coaptation.

Fourteen patients claim a return of postoperative sensibility. Five patients have had successful insertion of a penile prosthesis.

SUMMARY

Recent modifications in forearm phalloplasty with ulnar forearm flaps have been described. These modifications have improved overall phallic function and aesthetic results, and have provided acceptable outcomes at the forearm donor site.

References

1. Chang TS, Hwang WY. Forearm flap in one-stage reconstruction of the penis. *Plast Reconstr Surg* 1984;74:251.
2. Gilbert DA, Horton CE, Terzis JK, et al. New concepts in phallic reconstruction. *Ann Plast Surg* 1987;18:128.
3. Lovie MJ, Duncan GM, Glasson DW. The ulnar artery forearm flap. *Br J Plast Surg* 1984;37:486.
4. Gilbert DA, Jordan GH, Devine CJ Jr, et al. Microsurgical forearm "cricket-bat-transformer" phalloplasty. *Plast Reconstr Surg* 1992;90:711.
5. Beimer E. Penile construction by the radial arm flap. *Clin Plast Surg* 1988;15:425.
6. Gilbert DA, Schlossberg SM, Jordan GH. Ulnar forearm phallic construction and penile reconstruction. *Microsurgery* 1995;16:314.

CHAPTER 432 ■ PREFABRICATED LATERAL ARM FLAP FOR PENILE RECONSTRUCTION

R. K. KHOURI, P. PELISSIER, AND V. M. CASOLI

Excellent long-term results in penile reconstruction have been achieved with a prefabricated free flap, using a lateral arm/proximal forearm donor site. The procedure consists of prefabricating a neourethra by inserting a tubed, full-thickness skin graft in the lateral arm flap a few months prior to phalloplasty reconstruction.

INDICATIONS

One of the primary goals of phalloplasty is the creation of a urinary conduit that will allow the patient to void in a standing position. However, for the neophallus to be fully functional, it must look like a phallus, be rigid enough to allow sexual intercourse, and have ample sensation for protection and erotic stimulation. These goals have been achieved with a prefabricated lateral arm free flap (1). The lateral arm, with an extension to the proximal forearm (see chapter on the proximal forearm flap), is preferred, because it has a greater bulk when the flap is tubed. It can recover excellent sensibility, and it leaves a less conspicuous donor-site scar than the radial forearm flap.

ANATOMY

Excellent erogenous and protective sensation can be achieved by coapting the easily identified posterior cutaneous nerves of the arm and forearm to the clitoral or penile nerves. The constant anatomy of the lateral arm makes flap elevation quite straightforward (2,3). The upper arm has a moderately thick subcutaneous tissue layer and, consequently, its use results in greater bulk when the flap is tubed.

FLAP DESIGN AND DIMENSIONS AND OPERATIVE TECHNIQUE

The lateral arm allows for a substantial tissue length of up to 30 cm, and 10 to 12 cm in circumference, making it the best option for simultaneously incorporating a neourethra alongside a permanent inflatable prosthesis. When compared to flaps that incorporate bone or a rigid implant, the inflatable prosthesis allows a patient to control the degree of rigidity in the neophallus. In addition, it is much easier to repair a fistula while the tubed flap has no functional role in the arm and has ample available surrounding tissue than when the tube is isolated as a penis and must function as a urinary conduit. When compared with a radial forearm phalloplasty, the donor-site scar on the lateral arm has less morbidity and is easier to hide with clothing.

The prefabrication requires two stages.

First Stage

A large, full-thickness skin graft is harvested from a hairless area, such as the flank or groin. This graft, which should measure approximately 4 cm in width and 23 cm in length, is carefully tubed, epithelial side in, around a #24 or #26 French Silastic catheter. We then embed this construct into the superficial subcutaneous tissue of the lateral arm, along the axis of the intermuscular septum (Fig. 1). The graft remains in place for 3 to 5 months, until it matures and contraction is complete. The take of the graft is monitored with a flexible fiberoptic endoscope. If there is any breakdown, or if there is less than complete take of the graft, additional grafting is performed under local anesthesia, and more lateral arm tissue can be mobilized. During this period, the patient carries the Silastic catheter inside the lateral arm as a stent for the graft and removes it daily, to irrigate the new embedded epithelial conduit with water.

Second Stage

The flap is elevated according to the design shown in Fig. 2. After preparing the recipient site and dividing the vascular pedicle of the flap, the neophallus is tubed around an inflatable permanent prosthesis, with the prefabricated urethra oriented along the ventral surface. The distal quarter of the flap, which is 1 to 1.5 cm wider than the portion used to form the penile shaft, is fashioned into a glans. This allows for the creation of a penis 18 cm long and 11 to 12 cm in circumference (Fig. 3).

To lengthen the native meatus in transsexuals, the prefabricated neourethra is anastomosed to a labia minora flap tubed around a bladder catheter, and additional tissue from the labia

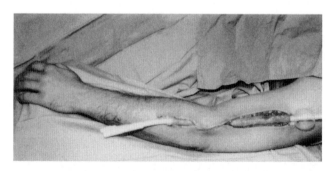

FIG. 1. A full-thickness skin graft is tubed around a #26 French Silastic catheter, with the epithelial surface facing the catheter. The whole construct is buried subcutaneously along the longitudinal axis of the lateral arm flap.

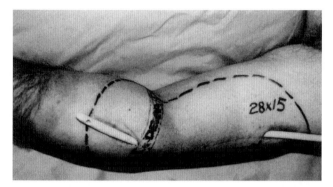

FIG. 2. The lateral flap is planned: the proximal part of the flap will become the penile shaft, and the distal part will be used to construct the glans.

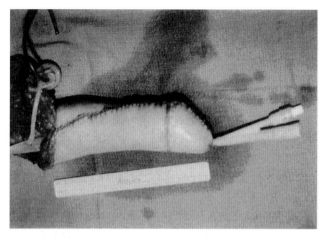

FIG. 3. Prior to insert, the skin flap is tubed around an inflatable penile prosthesis; a #20 French Silastic catheter is placed through the neourethra.

minora is mobilized and drawn over the anastomotic site, to provide extra padding.

We coapt the posterior cutaneous nerves of the arm and forearm to the left and right dorsal penile nerves (or clitoral nerves in transsexuals). We anastomose the posterior radial collateral vessels with the inferiorly mobilized inferior epigastric vessels. The reservoir of the permanent inflatable prosthesis is finally positioned in a pocket beneath the rectus abdominis muscle, and the pump is placed in the scrotum (or inside the labia majora in transsexuals). The lateral arm donor site is closed with a skin graft.

CLINICAL RESULTS

We have a minimum of 4 years' follow-up (range: 4 to 5 years) on four female-to-male transsexuals. The same procedure was performed for each patient. Following the creation of an epithelialized conduit in the upper arm, we confirmed good complete epithelialization with a fiberoptic laryngoscope in all but one patient. This patient required turn-down local flaps to restore epithelial continuity of the tube. After the second-stage transfer, primary healing occurred in all patients. The bladder catheter was removed in the third postoperative week, and all patients were able to void in a standing position.

However, all patients developed fistulas and strictures in the perineal area. These were repaired with local turn-over flaps from the perineal skin, and from the excess tissue brought down with the generous design of the neophallus. All the fistulas healed promptly, following the local surgical pro-

cedures, and the patients were able to void from a standing position without leakage and with a forceful stream.

Inflation of the prosthesis was allowed at 6 months. At 1 year, sensation had returned over the entire neophallus, and intercourse was allowed. At a minimum of 4 years' follow-up, the patients were satisfied with the function and cosmetic appearance of their penises, and all were free of complications.

SUMMARY

The prefabricated lateral arm free flap has provided excellent long-term results, with no exposure of the inflatable prosthesis, and with all patients reporting sexual performance and the ability to void while standing.

References

1. Young VL, Khouri RK, Lee G, Riolo Nemecek J. Advances in total phalloplasty and urethroplasty with microvascular free flaps. *Gun Plast Surg* 1992;19:927.
2. Katsaros J, Schusterman M, Beppu M, et al. The lateral upper arm flap: anatomy and clinical applications. *Ann Plast Surg* 1984;12:489.
3. Brandt KE, Khouri RK. The lateral arm/proximal forearm flap. *Plast Reconstr Surg* 1993;92:1137.

CHAPTER 433 ■ RADIAL FOREARM FLAP FOR PENILE RECONSTRUCTION

L. J. GOTTLIEB, L. A. LEVINE, AND L. S. ZACHARY

The radial forearm free flap was initially selected for penile reconstruction, as it is a thin, potentially sensate, minimally hair-bearing flap, with enough flexibility for its design to incorporate a vascularized urethra (1). Since its initial description, several modifications in the flap technique have emerged (2–8), some of which are described below.

INDICATIONS

Patients with severe penile deformities, regardless of cause (congenital or traumatically acquired, infection, or malignancy), or those who have suffered penile loss or mutilation, are potential candidates for reconstruction using the radial forearm free flap. Gender dysphoria patients may become candidates for penile construction, if they meet the guidelines established by the Harry Benjamin International Gender Dysphoria Association.

Attention must be given to the patient's level of expectation and the ability to deal with potential complications and significant donor-site scars.

ANATOMY

The neurovascular fasciocutaneous radial forearm free flap includes the volar forearm skin with its underlying adipose tissue, the medial and lateral antebrachial cutaneous sensory nerves, the basilic and cephalic veins, and the deep fascia. All of these are connected to the radial artery and its venae comitantes by a thin, intermuscular septum that contains cutaneous perforating vessels. A set of four or five perforating vessels emerges from the proximal and distal thirds of the radial artery. Rarely are significant perforators found in the middle third of the artery (Fig. 1).

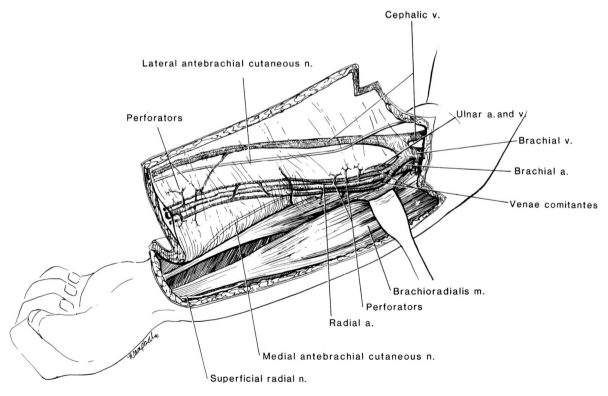

FIG. 1. Anatomy of the fasciocutaneous radial forearm flap. (From Cohen, ref. 9, with permission.)

FLAP DESIGN AND DIMENSIONS

The flap is designed with a centrally-located neourethra in continuity with a neoglans. This design avoids a circumferential meatal suture line without sacrificing length and leads to an improved result.

The dimensions of the flap depend on the patient's needs and desires, as well as the size of the forearm and amount of subcutaneous tissue present. The width of the flap should vary directly with the amount of subcutaneous tissue present. While a width of 13 cm was initially described for penile reconstruction, we have found this to be inadequate for tubing the flap and allowing closure without tension. Additionally, the flap length of 10 cm initially described is generally unsatisfactory for successful intromission. In most cases, our flap dimensions are a minimum of 15 × 17 cm. The size of the wrist may limit flap width distally, where it must be tapered to 13–14 cm (Fig. 2). In situations in which the native urethra ends in the perineum, the length of the neourethra may be safely increased to 25 cm, by designing a proximal extension just above the elbow.

OPERATIVE TECHNIQUE

The non-dominant arm is generally chosen as the donor site. A preoperative Allen test should be performed on all patients for whom a radial forearm flap is being considered. Arteriograms are unnecessary. The patient is placed supine on the operating table, with the non-dominant arm extended on an arm board. Transsexuals and men with perineal urethrostomies are placed in the lithotomy position during the "recipient-site preparation" portion of the case. Other patients may be positioned supine in a "frog-leg" position.

The design of the flap is outlined on the volar aspect of the forearm. The arm should not be shaved. This allows markings for the planned neourethra to be made reliably on the portion of the volar forearm with the least amount of hair. At this time, it is helpful to outline the course of the radial artery and the major veins. After the extremity is moderately exsanguinated with an Esmarch bandage, a sterile tourniquet is inflated to 250 mmHg.

Two strips of skin, each 1 cm wide, on either side of the planned centrally-positioned neourethra, are deepithelialized from the proximal edge of the flap to within 2.5 to 3 cm of the distal portion. Deepithelialization should be continued around the proximal end of the planned neourethra (not shown in the diagram in Fig. 2). The ulnar side of each of these strips is

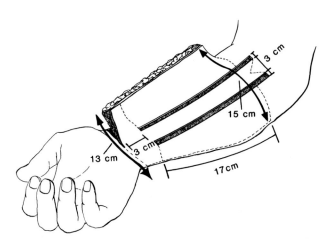

FIG. 2. Flap design and dimensions. (From Cohen, ref. 9, with permission.)

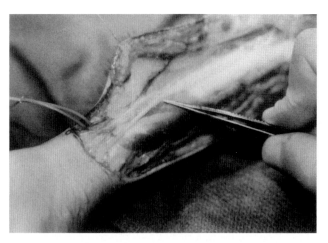

FIG. 3. Sensory branch of the radial nerve at the wrist after it passes beneath the brachioradialis tendon. (From Cohen, ref. 9, with permission.)

incised into the subcutaneous layer. The most distal portion of the flap, which overlies the radial artery, is then incised. The radial artery and its venae comitantes are identified at the wrist and isolated with vessel loops.

An incision is made along the radial border of the flap and carried down through the deep fascia. The dissection then proceeds ulnarly beneath this layer and stops at the thin intermuscular septum, which contains the septocutaneous perforating vessels. The surgeon must be careful to identify and preserve the superficial branch of the radial nerve as it pierces through or beneath the brachioradialis tendon and courses close to the cephalic vein at the wrist (Fig. 3).

The proximal incision is now made, care being taken to identify and preserve the cephalic vein. The medial and lateral antebrachial cutaneous nerves are identified, dissected an additional 3 to 4 cm proximal to the skin paddle, tagged with 7-0 Prolene, and divided.

Next, the ulnar border of the flap is incised and elevated radially beneath the deep fascia. The cutaneous perforating vessels of the ulnar artery should be ligated and divided. This dissection is continued until the ulnar side of the intramuscular septum containing the septocutaneous perforators of the radial artery is encountered.

At this time, the radial artery and its venae comitantes are elevated from their bed from distal to proximal, with careful mobilization of the ulnar edge of the brachioradialis muscle radially. Muscular branches are ligated or coagulated with a bipolar electrocautery. The arterial dissection is continued proximally until the bifurcation of the brachial artery is reached.

The dissection of the proximal venae comitantes proceeds until the two veins coalesce into one. If this dissection is continued more proximally (this often requires an incision in the antecubital fossa skin overlying the cephalic vein), the venae comitantes (which have now coalesced) join the cephalic vein via the profundus cubitalis vein. This extra dissection makes it possible for one large vein to drain not only the superficial cephalic system, but also the venae comitantes (10) (Fig. 4). At this point, full-thickness transverse incisions are made connecting the distal portion of the centrally-placed neourethral skin with the radial and ulnar edges of the flap (Fig. 5).

The tourniquet is released, the flap is perfused, and hemostasis is achieved. The flap is now attached only by the radial vascular bundle. Small vascular clamps are applied to the distal radial vascular bundle, and the perfusion of the hand is examined. Only after an adequate ulnar blood supply to the

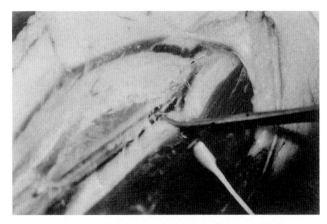

FIG. 4. Venous anatomy of the flap. Note coalescence of venae comitantes (hemostat), which then join the cephalic vein via the profundus cubitalis vein (*arrow*), crossing above the lateral antebrachial nerve. (From Cohen, ref. 9, with permission.)

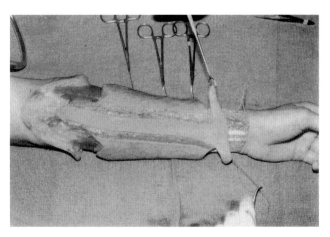

FIG. 5. Flap elevated, ready to be tubed.

hand has been assured is the distal radial vascular bundle clamped, ligated, and divided.

The portion of the flap forming the central neourethra is then tubed over a 12-French Silastic urinary catheter. This is a four-layer closure. Initially, neourethral skin is secured to neourethral skin centrally. The free edge of the ulnar deepithelialized strip is flipped over and secured over this suture line. The radial deepithelialized strip is then advanced and secured, and the volar shaft skin is then closed (Fig. 6). The flap is now turned over and the dorsal skin closure is performed.

The "wings" of the neoglans are trimmed to the appropriate shape and rolled back on the shaft. The distal portion of the shaft that will be under the rolled-back neoglans is deepithelialized (Fig. 7A, B). The neoglans is then secured in its rolled-back position with full-thickness nylon mattress sutures. The constructed neophallus is left on the arm, attached to its proximal vascular pedicle, until the recipient site has been prepared (Fig. 8).

During flap elevation, a separate team prepares the pubic site and the recipient vessels and nerves. Approximately 20 cm of saphenous vein is harvested from the thigh and is left attached to the femoral vein at the fossa ovalis. The divided

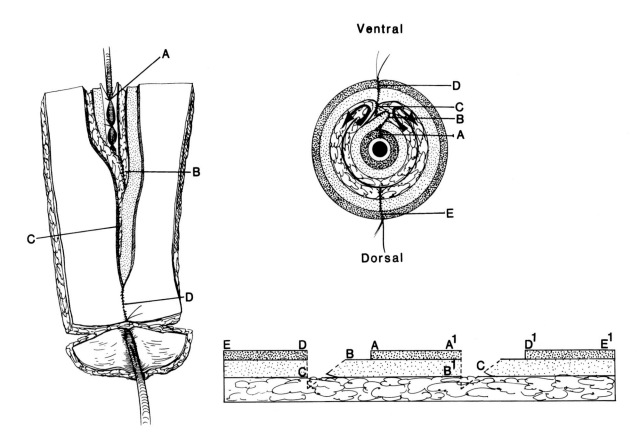

FIG. 6. Four-layer closure of neourethral tube. **A:** Neourethral skin edges. **B:** Ulnar deepithelialized edge closed over layer A. **C:** Radial deepithelialized edge closed over layer B. **D:** Closure of volar shaft skin. **E:** Closure of dorsal skin. (From Cohen, ref. 9, with permission.)

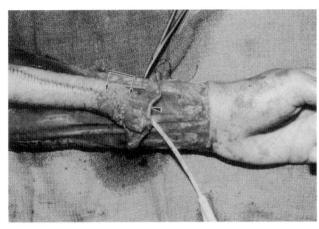
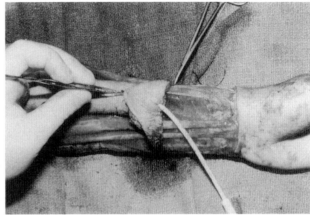

A   B

FIG. 7. Construction of neoglans. **A:** *Arrowhead* on unfolded extension of flap ("wings") that will form the neoglans. Distal shaft (*between connected arrows*) is deepithelialized. **B:** "Wings" that will form the neoglans folded back over shaft. (From Cohen, ref. 9, with permission.)

end of this saphenous vein graft is then anastomosed to the femoral artery, using microsurgical techniques and loupe magnification, to create a temporary loop arteriovenous fistula. This is allowed to flow until the flap is ready for transfer.

If no penile remnant is present, an incision is made over the pubic symphysis. If a portion of the native phallus exists, a degloving incision is designed. The dorsal penile (or clitoral in transsexuals) branches of the pudendal nerve should be isolated. If no nerves are apparent, dissection is continued toward the perineum, and the pudendal nerves are identified as they emerge from Alcock's canal and travel along the inferior ramus of the pubis.

It is our practice to connect the incision used for the saphenous vein harvest to the flap recipient-bed incision, thereby preventing compression, torquing, or kinking of the vein grafts.

The fully-constructed neophallus is detached from the arm, transferred to the pubic area, and secured in place with tacking sutures. Before the proximal radial artery is ligated and divided, 5000 units of heparin are given intravenously by the anesthesiologist.

When a primary urethral anastomosis is possible, an end-to-end two-layered spatulated anastomosis with 4-0 absorbable sutures is performed, after the Foley catheter within the flap is passed through the native urethra into the bladder. The sutures should not traverse the lumen, to reduce the possibility of fistula formation.

The saphenous vein loop is divided, and the cephalic vein is anastomosed end-to-end to the venous limb of the saphenous loop with 8-0 nylon under the operating microscope. This is followed by end-to-end anastomosis of the radial artery to the arterial limb of the saphenous loop with 8-0 nylon.

Epineural microneurorrhaphies between the paired pudendal nerves and the medial and lateral antebrachial cutaneous nerves are performed with 9-0 nylon (Fig. 9).

The remaining wounds about the proximal shaft of the neophallus and femoral vessels are now closed (Fig. 10). A percutaneous suprapubic catheter is placed, to ensure adequate urine drainage away from the healing neourethra. The postoperative dressing incorporates a large Styrofoam (coffee) cup to keep the neophallus supported in the early postoperative period.

The ulnar artery is usually the dominant vessel supplying the palmar arch. The absence of postoperative vascular compromise or cold intolerance has made vascular reconstruction of the radial artery unnecessary. The forearm muscles in the bed of the flap donor site are approximated together and over any exposed tendons with absorbable sutures, to minimize contour irregularities. A split-thickness skin graft, harvested from the hip or thigh, is then applied to this muscular bed. A long arm splint is used to immobilize the elbow, wrist, and fingers.

Perioperative antibiotics and low-dose aspirin are used in all cases. Intravenous antibiotics are discontinued on the second postoperative day, and suppressive oral antibiotic coverage is begun, which continues until the urethral and suprapubic catheters are removed. Low-dose aspirin is continued indefinitely.

Flap viability is assessed by clinical examination, i.e., skin color, turgor, and capillary refill, as well as hourly pulse checks by palpation or with a bedside Doppler probe.

Sequential pneumatic lower-extremity compression boots are used on the first few postoperative days when the patient is confined to bed. Physical therapy for the donor upper extremity begins once the initial dressings are removed on the 7th to 10th postoperative day. Xeroform is applied to the graft and an Ace wrap is applied to the hand and forearm. A compressive garment and wrist splint are then fashioned; the splint is worn an additional 2 weeks and the garment is worn for 3 to 6 months.

Urine is preferentially drained via the suprapubic catheter, allowing the urethral catheter to be capped. The reduces tension on the neophallus and meatus. In the third to fourth postoperative week, a retrograde urethrogram can be performed, by inserting a small catheter alongside the indwelling urethral catheter. The urethral catheter may be removed, if there is no

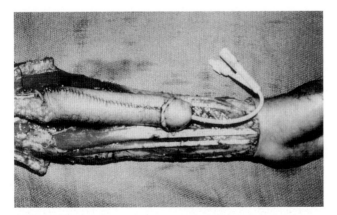

FIG. 8. Constructed neophallus attached to arm by vascular pedicle. (From Cohen, ref. 9, with permission.)

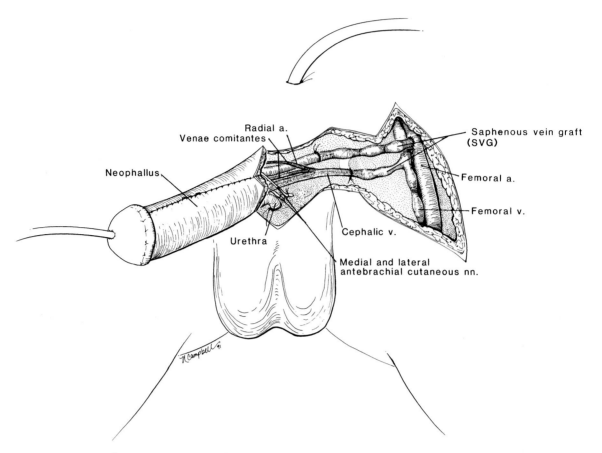

FIG. 9. Schematic representation of urethral and neurovascular connections. (From Cohen, ref. 9, with permission.)

evidence of extravasation or fistula. The suprapubic tube may be removed 1 to 2 days after normal micturition is established.

CLINICAL RESULTS

Sensation in the neophallus is tested by subjective light touch and biothesiometry. The neophallus is insensate for the first month postoperatively, and therefore careful positioning of both neophallus and urinary catheter is necessary to avoid inadvertent pressure injury. Most patients have recovered gross tactile sensation at 4 to 6 months. By 6 to 9 months, they are usually able to stimulate the shaft of the neophallus to orgasm, and have biothesiometry threshold measurements three to four times that of their index fingers. It is safe to consider insertion of a penile prosthesis only after protective sensation develops (11). Sexually active patients describe erogenous sensation leading to orgasm.

The modified radial forearm flap design has eliminated the otherwise frequent complication of meatal stenosis. Urethral stone formation has not been a problem in our patients. Complications with the proximal urethral anastomosis, including sinuses, fistulae, and strictures, are relatively uncommon. Most fistulae close spontaneously. Proximal anastomotic suture-line strictures may be treated with internal urethrotomy. In our experience, one or two neodymium-Yag laser or cold-knife urethrotomies, followed by a short period of self-catheterization, have resulted in a stabilized widely-patent urethra. All patients were ultimately able to void standing.

Maintaining a good coronal ridge is difficult. The suturing technique described in Fig. 5 has led to variable long-term results. Adding a strip of tendon or dermis does not appear to

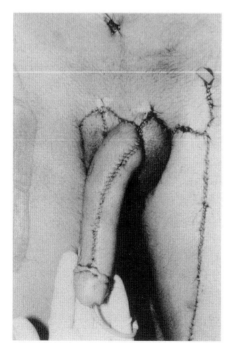

FIG. 10. Neophallus at completion of operation.

help much. Recently, we have been securing the rolled-back portion of the neoglans loosely with sutures, and skin grafting the exposed subcutaneous tissue.

The greatest drawback of the radial forearm flap is the unsightly donor site. The thicker the graft used to close it, the better the aesthetic result. Functional disability of the donor extremity has been rare, although we have had one patient with a radial nerve palsy that resolved, and one patient with postoperative carpal tunnel syndrome that required release. Considering the high quality of penile construction possible with the radial forearm flap, the resultant donor-site scar is usually well-tolerated by patients.

SUMMARY

The radial forearm flap, as part of a cooperative effort among the reconstructive plastic surgeon, urologist, and psychiatrist, allows reconstruction of a neophallus that is aesthetically and psychologically satisfying. The procedure provides protective and erogenous sensation, a neophallus of appropriate size and shape to allow a penile prosthesis permitting successful coitus, and lets the patient void in a standing position through a distal meatus.

References

1. Chang TS, Hwang WY. Forearm flap in one-stage reconstruction of the penis. *Plast Reconstr Surg* 1984;74:251.
2. Meyer R, Daverio PJ, Dequesne J. One-stage phalloplasty in transsexuals. *Ann Plast Surg* 1986;16:472.
3. Koshima I, Tai T, Yamasaki M. One-stage reconstruction of the penis using an innervated radial forearm osteocutaneous flap. *J Reconstr Microsurg* 1986;3:19.
4. Gilbert DA, Williams MW, Horton CE, et al. Phallic innervation via the pudendal nerve. *J Urol* 1988;41:160.
5. Siemer E. Penile construction by the radial arm flap. *Clin Plast Surg* 1988;15:425.
6. Semple JL, Boyd JB. The "cricket bat forearm flap" in one-stage reconstruction of the penis. Presented at the Annual Meeting of the Canadian Society of Plastic Surgery, Pointe-du-lac, Quebec, 1988.
7. Gottlieb LJ, Levine LA. A new design for the radial forearm free flap phallic construction. *Plast Reconstr Surg* 1993;92:276.
8. Trengove-Jones G, Colon LB, Horton C, et al. A new concept in penoscrotal reconstruction: the one-stage free sensory combined radial forearm free flap. Presented at the Annual Meeting of the American Society of Reconstructive Microsurgery, Scottsdale, Arizona, 1992.
9. Cohen M, ed. Mastery of plastic and reconstructive surgery. Boston: Little, Brown, 1994;1401–1407.
10. Gottlieb LJ, Tachmes L, Pkelet RW. Improved venous drainage of the radial artery forearm free flap: use of the profundus cubitalis vein. *J Reconstr Microsurg* 1993;9:281.
11. Levine LA, Zachary LS, Gottlieb LL. Prosthesis placement after total phallic reconstruction. *J Urol* 1993;149:593.

CHAPTER 434 ■ "CRICKET BAT" FLAP: ONE-STAGE FREE FOREARM FLAP PHALLOPLASTY

J. B. BOYD

Since the cricket bat flap (1) relies on transverse folding to separate skin cover from urethra, none of the tissue lies far from the vascular pedicle. The flap is narrow enough to occupy the least hairy portion of the forearm, and the urethra is formed by hairless anterior wrist skin.

The cricket bat modification has been used for penile reconstruction, whether in traumatic, surgical, or congenital cases, and in cases of gender dysphoria. Further modifications in its design permit its use in partial peno-urethral defects and in the treatment of complicated hypospadias.

INDICATIONS

Reliable, one-stage, sensate, peno-urethral reconstruction is ideal for creating a penis in female-to-male transsexuals, and for use after iatrogenic or traumatic loss. Methods based on the original "Swiss roll" technique (2)—where the forearm skin is divided in two by a longitudinal deepithelialized strip, and then rolled in on itself—result in an extremely wide flap with questionable peripheral perfusion and inadequate venous drainage. The fistula rate is high (3), undesirable hairy skin is recruited for the neourethra, and repair of the donor site is a major undertaking.

ANATOMY

The skin of the anterior forearm receives a significant blood supply from the radial artery via perforating septocutaneous vessels passing to the skin along the vascular septum between the brachioradialis and the flexor carpi radialis muscles (Fig. 1). These perforators are plentiful in the distal third of the forearm, but proximally, where tendons give way to muscle bellies, they become sparser. Nevertheless, it is safe to raise a septum-based skin flap anywhere along the course of the radial artery.

After emerging from the septum, the vessels branch laterally and medially, piercing the deep fascia and quickly passing

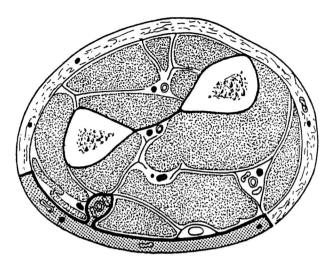

FIG. 1. Section of a radial forearm flap showing disposition of the radial artery, with respect to the vascular septum, the brachioradialis, and the flexor carpi radialis. (From Soutar et al., ref. 4, with permission.)

variations in this basic pattern. Perforating veins connect the superficial veins to the deep system at various points.

Both venous systems are capable of draining the flap alone. Superficial veins are often preferred because of their greater diameter and their independence from the arterial pedicle. However, care should be taken to ensure that the superficial veins have not previously been canalized and undergone partial or complete thrombosis. Whichever vein is selected for draining the cricket bat flap, the surgeon should ensure that the vein occupies the full length of the flap, particularly the distal "handle" portion. Both systems may be combined by preserving the confluence of veins in the proximal forearm.

The median antebrachial cutaneous nerve (C8, T1) enters the forearm in the company of the basilic vein. It soon gives off a number of large anterior branches, which pass down the radial side of the basilic vein and supply the ulnar half of the anterior forearm as far as the wrist. An ulnar branch supplies the ulnar border of the forearm. The lateral antebrachial cutaneous nerve (C5,6) is the forearm continuation of the musculocutaneous nerve. It enters the forearm on the ulnar side of the cephalic vein and, via multiple branches, supplies the radial half of the forearm as far as the wrist, as well as the dorsoradial aspect of the forearm.

to the subdermal plexus. These vessels do not travel far on the surface of the deep fascia; therefore, very little of it needs to be harvested with the flap.

Practically all of the anterior forearm skin can be taken safely. Limits extend from the antecubital fossa to the transverse wrist crease, and from the ulnar border of the forearm to the posterolateral aspect of the radial border. Beyond these medial and lateral boundaries, the viability of the skin is questionable. Raising a flap of such dimensions would require the entire vascular septum to be preserved.

The radial artery originates a few centimeters distal to the antecubital fossa, and then passes distally along the radial side of the pronator teres, lying between the biceps tendon and the bicipital aponeurosis. It crosses anterior to the pronator teres, just proximal to that muscle's insertion into its tubercle on the lateral surface of the radius. In the distal third of the forearm, it first overlies the flexor pollicis longus, and finally the pronator quadratus. Septocutaneous branches from the radial artery pass along the vascular septum between the brachioradialis and flexor carpi radialis muscles, to supply the skin (Fig. 1).

The radial artery is accompanied by venae comitantes. These vessels are constant, but of variable diameter. Often, they are inconveniently small for microvascular anastomosis. In the region of the bifurcation of the brachial artery, there is a confluence of veins. Here, the venae comitantes of both ulnar and radial arteries communicate with each other, as well as with one or more of the large subcutaneous veins of the forearm. This confluence may be incorporated advantageously with the donor vein of the cricket bat flap.

Classically, there are three major subcutaneous veins in the anterior forearm: the cephalic, the median, and the basilic. The cephalic vein lies on the dorsoradial, and the basilic on the dorsoulnar, aspect of the wrist. At the midforearm level, they pass around their respective borders, and then proceed proximally on the radial and ulnar sides of the anterior forearm. The median vein lies in the midline of the anterior forearm. Just distal to the antecubital fossa, it bifurcates into two: the median cephalic and the median basilic. The former angles radially to join the cephalic, and the latter ulnarly to join the basilic. The cephalic and basilic veins then pass up the arm on either side of the biceps muscle. There are

FLAP DESIGN AND DIMENSIONS

The cricket bat flap consists of a longitudinally-oriented skin paddle in which both the urethral segment and the outer covering portion of the flap lie directly over the radial artery (Fig. 2). The narrow, 3-cm-wide "handle" lies in the anterior wrist. The remaining 9-cm-wide "blade" of the flap will constitute the outer covering of the reconstructed penis and is situated proximally. Each segment of the cricket bat measures approximately 12 cm in length.

A useful modification of this flap is to flare out its distal end to 4 cm. As we shall see, this lessens the risk of stenosis at the urethral anastomotic site.

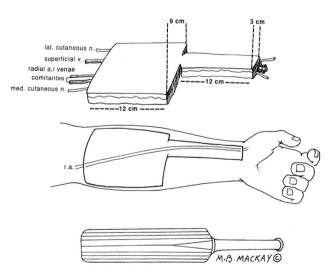

FIG. 2. The cricket bat flap is a longitudinal design in which the radial artery and the venae comitantes run the entire length of the flap. The distal portion of the "handle" may be flared out to 4 cm, reducing the risk of stenosis at the suture line. (From Semple et al., ref. 1, with permission.)

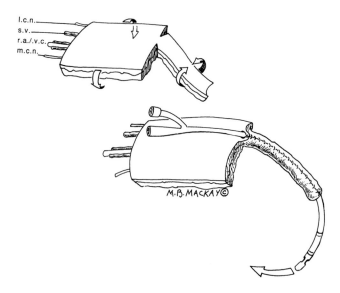

FIG. 3. Once the flap is raised, the distal segment is tubed over a Foley catheter. (From Semple et al., ref. 1, with permission.)

OPERATIVE TECHNIQUE

The flap is designed slightly off-center. This has two advantages: the risk of vessel kinking is minimized when the flap is folded in on itself; and, during final closure, the two seams are made to lie remote from each other, thus lessening the risk of fistula formation.

The cricket bat flap is elevated like any other radial forearm flap (5), but the median and lateral cutaneous nerves of the forearm are included for sensory reinnervation. The proximally-based pedicle provides a 3- to 4-cm length of radial artery and accompanying veins for anastomosis with recipient vessels.

Once the flap is raised, the distal urethral segment is tubed on a #16 Foley catheter (Fig. 3). It is then anastomosed to the urethral remnant, using a single-layer everting closure of 4-0 Vicryl sutures. The flap is folded back 180 degrees at the junction of the "blade" and "handle" (Fig. 4). The wider "blade" portion of the flap is tubed around the urethral reconstruction and is then sutured to itself on the ventral surface (Fig. 5). Because the flap is folded in half, the length of the penis is limited to half the length of the forearm in total reconstruction.

The most useful recipient vessels are the greater saphenous vein and the deep inferior epigastric artery (DIEA). To obtain a workable pedicle, the saphenous vein is divided half-way down the thigh and turned up into the groin region, where it is anastomosed to the DIEA as an arteriovenous fistula (Corlett loop). The loop is then divided at a convenient point for the donor vessels. The pudendal nerves are located dorsally and are anastomosed to the lateral and medial antebrachial cutaneous nerves.

For the return of sexual function, it is necessary to insert inflatable prostheses. In total reconstructions, the implants should be placed within Dacron sheaths, which are anchored to the pubis for stability. This surgery is best carried out after the return of sensation. To enhance the cosmetic appearance, a glans penoplasty may also be performed.

CLINICAL RESULTS

A typical case of total penile reconstruction is illustrated in Figure 5. The flap is easily modified for management of partial defects or the treatment of complex hypospadias (Fig. 6). Of seven cases carried out, all flaps have survived although one patient returned to the O.R. for revision of a venous anastomosis. There were no partial sloughs of skin or areas of fat necrosis. All patients ultimately passed urine in a continuous stream without fistulous leaks, although temporary fistulae were present in three patients. In each case, the fistula arose at the site of urethral anastomosis and closed with conservative management. One patient developed a urethral stricture at the same location, which responded to simple dilatation. Sensory recovery was surprisingly good, and one individual subsequently fathered a child. Donor-site scars were well-tolerated; tissue expansion was offered to all, and performed on none.

SUMMARY

The cricket bat flap has six main advantages over the "Swiss roll" technique. 1) The flap is well-vascularized throughout,

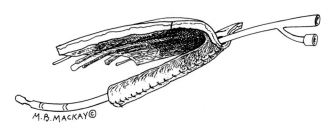

FIG. 4. The flap is then folded back 180 degrees at the junction of the "blade" and the "handle." (From Semple et al., ref. 1, with permission.)

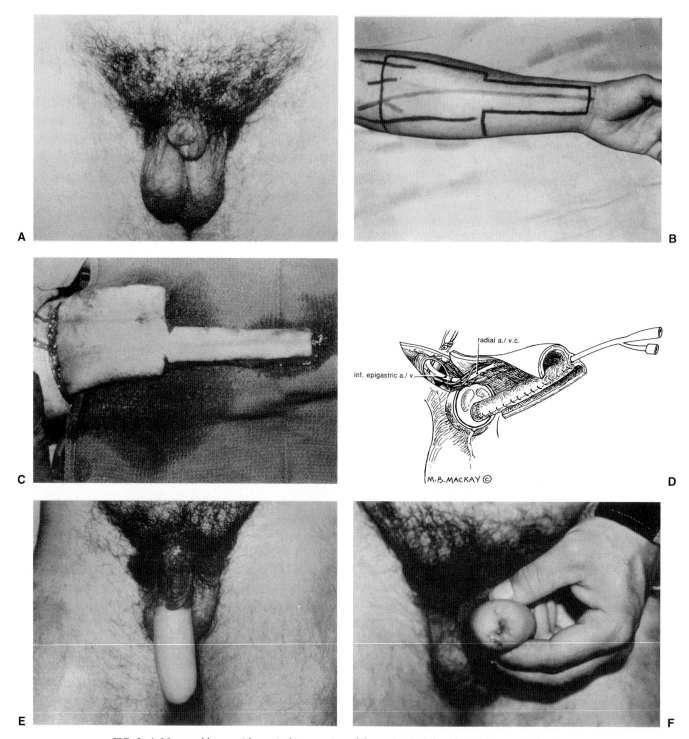

FIG. 5. A 25-year-old man with surgical amputation of the penis was left with a 2-cm stump of corpora and an inadequate urethra. **A:** Preoperative view. **B:** A one-stage free forearm phalloplasty using a cricket bat flap design was planned on the left, non-dominant arm. **C:** The flap elevated, to show the off-center relationship of the "handle" and "blade." **D:** Recipient artery and vein were the deep inferior epigastric vessels (DIEVs) on the right side. Normally, the DIEV is too small at the level at which it needs to be divided. For this reason, we recommend that the greater saphenous vein be pedicled up (refer to text). The pudendal nerves were isolated in the stump and anastomosed to the medial and lateral cutaneous nerves of the forearm. **E:** Postoperative appearance of the penile reconstruction at 6 months. **F:** Postoperative appearance of the meatus. *(Continued)*

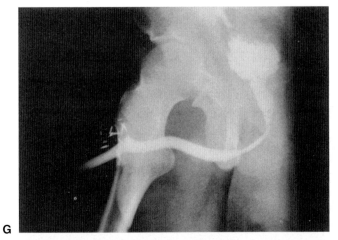

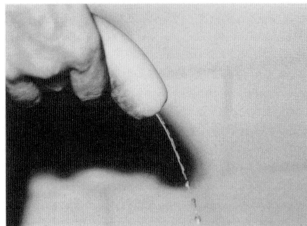

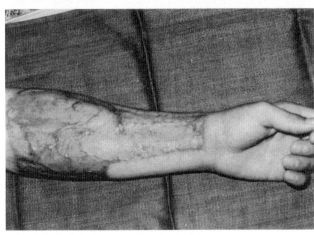

FIG. 5. *Continued.* **G:** Urethrogram showing excellent patency and caliber at the anastomosis. **H:** The patient could void with an excellent stream. **I:** Donor site on left arm. (From Semple et al., ref. 1, with permission.)

with adequate venous drainage. 2) The distal, thin, and hairless portion of the flap is used for urethral reconstruction. 3) Distally, the donor defect is narrow, minimizing tendon exposure. 4) Separation of the suture seams protects against fistula formation. 5) There is no suture line at the urethral opening. 6) The technique may be customized for partial reconstructions.

References

1. Semple JL, Boyd JB, Farrow GA, et al. The "cricket bat" flap: a one-stage free forearm flap phalloplasty. *Plast Reconstr Surg* 1991;88:514.
2. Chang TS, Hwang WY. Forearm flap in one-stage reconstruction of the penis. *Plast Reconstr Surg* 1984;74:251.
3. Matti BA, Matthews RN, Davies DM. Phalloplasty using the free radial forearm flap. *Br J Plast Surg* 1988;41:160.
4. Soutar D. The radial forearm flap: a versatile method for intraoral reconstruction. *Br J Plast Surg* 1985;36:1.
5. Song R, Gao Y, Yu Y, Song Y. The forearm flap. *Clin Plast Surg* 1982;9:21.

CHAPTER 435 ■ SCROTAL FLAP

V. C. LANIER, JR.

Owing to the abundant vascularity, ease of dissection beneath the dartos, and tremendous elasticity, scrotal flaps can cover a vast area without compromising the circulation or the primary use of the scrotal tissue (see Fig. 1).

INDICATIONS

Flaps using scrotal tissue have been employed in the treatment of traumatic injuries (1), hypospadias (2,3), fistulas of the perineum (4), urethroplasties (5), carcinoma of the penis (6), labia reconstruction in transsexual males (7), and pressure sores (8–10).

Avulsive injuries with loss of 50 percent of the scrotum can be managed by elevating the remaining scrotal skin as a large flap and obtaining coverage of both testes (1).

Many variations of the scrotal flap for urethral reconstruction have been reported (2,3). They have been successfully used in reconstruction of the perineal urethra for entities other than hypospadias (4–6).

Conversion of male transsexuals uses the inverted skin of the penis to create a vagina, and the redundant scrotal flaps are used in the construction of the labia. This is described as a two-stage procedure, with the vagina constructed initially, followed by the labia approximately 3 weeks later (7).

Scrotal flaps have been applied to the management of pressure sores of the ischium (8,9) and those of the pubic ramus that are associated with necrosis of the penis (10) (see Fig. 2).

ANATOMY

Scrotal skin is very thin, deeply pigmented, contains hair follicles and sebaceous glands, and is abundantly supplied with elastic tissue and smooth muscle. The median raphe divides the skin into lateral halves from the ventral aspect of the penis to the anus (11).

The dartos lies directly beneath the skin and consists of elastic fibers, connective tissue, and smooth muscle. The dartos is attached to and inseparable from the skin, is free of fat, and contains a generous blood supply. Avulsion of scrotal skin is always associated with a loss of the underlying and intimately attached dartos; testes and spermatic cord are, however, protected by a plane of loose areolar tissue directly beneath the dartos (12,13).

The highly vascularized skin and dartos of the scrotum are supplied by the internal pudendal artery, the superficial external pudendal artery, and the deep external pudendal artery (Fig. 1).

The internal pudendal artery in the male arises from the anterior trunk of the internal iliac and passes through the lesser sciatic foramen about 4 cm above the lower margin of the ischial tuberosity. The artery courses along the inferior ramus of the pubis and terminates as the perineal artery, with its many terminal divisions constituting the posterior scrotal branches. The superficial external pudendal artery arises from the femoral artery and courses medially across the spermatic cord to terminate in the lower abdomen, penis, and scrotum. The deep external pudendal artery arises from the femoral artery and courses deep and medially to the medial aspect of the thigh to terminate in the scrotum by anastomosing with the posterior scrotal branches of the perineal artery, described above.

Venous outflow is through the venae comitantes of the internal pudendal artery and superficial and deep external pudendal arteries into the internal iliac and femoral veins, respectively. The circulation provided by these vessels and the anastomoses within the scrotal skin and dartos

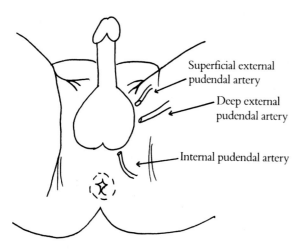

FIG. 1. Arterial circulation to the scrotum.

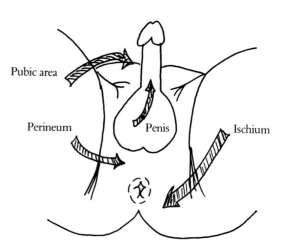

FIG. 2. Rotation arc of scrotal flaps.

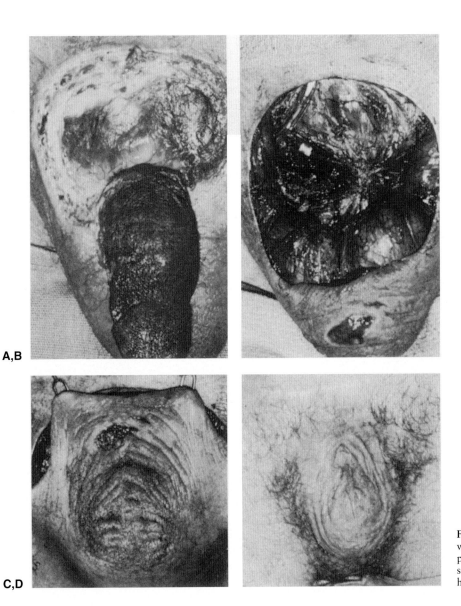

A,B

C,D

FIG. 3. **A:** Pressure sore of anterior pubic ramus with necrosis of penis. **B:** Excision of necrotic penis soft tissue and pubic rami. **C:** Elevation of scrotal flap. **D:** Follow-up at 6 months. Patient has ileal loop urinary diversion.

permit the scrotum to be useful for a variety of pedicle flaps as well as microsurgical repair. A completely amputated penis and scrotum have been successfully replanted using the profunda artery and a dorsal vein of the penis (14).

Lymphatic drainage is into the inguinal and femoral nodes. Scrotal lymphatics do not accompany the pudendal vessels and have no connection with the testes and their tunics (15). Scrotal lymphedema occurs with blockage of the inguinal and femoral nodes.

The scrotum is innervated by the ilioinguinal and external spermatic nerves, which course through the inguinal canal. Entering from the perineum are the pudendal branch of the posterior femoral cutaneous nerve and superficial perineal branches of the internal pudendal nerves.

FLAP DESIGN AND DIMENSIONS

The bilateral circulation permits a circular rotation of the flap to the pubic area anteriorly and the perineal and ischial areas posteriorly, as well as local rotations to the penis (Figs. 2, 3).

SUMMARY

The scrotal skin has an excellent blood supply and can be used to cover various perineal defects.

References

1. Masteri FW. Avulsion of penile and scrotal skin. In: Horton CE, ed. *Plastic and reconstructive surgery of the genital area.* Boston: Little, Brown, 1973; Chap. 29, 451–461.
2. Bouisson MF. Del'hypospadias et de son traitement chirurgical. *Trib Chir* 1861;2:484.
3. Horton CE, Devine, CJ. Jr. Hypospadias. In: Horton CE, ed. *Plastic and reconstructive surgery of the genital area.* Boston: Little, Brown, 1973; Chap. 18, 235–281.
4. Sharma D. Scrotal flap urethroplasty in the primary management of the "watering-can" perineum. *Br J Urol* 1979;51:400.
5. Belman AB. The repair of a congenital H-type urethrorectal fistula using a scrotal flap urethroplasty. *J Urol* 1977;118:659.
6. Jameson RM. Scrotal flap urethroplasty in the treatment of carcinoma of the penis. *Trop Doct* 1976;6:68.
7. Edgerton MT, Bull J. Surgical construction of the vagina and labia in male transsexuals. *Plast Reconstr Surg* 1970;529.
8. Kaplan I. The scrotal flap in ischial decubitus. *Br J Plast Surg* 1972;25:22.
9. Kaplan I. The scrotal flap for ischial decubitus ulcers: a follow-up. *Br J Plast Surg* 1976;29:34.

10. Lanier VC Jr, Neale, HW. Necrosis of penis with decubitus ulcer: debridement and closure with scrotal flap. *Plast Reconstr Surg* 1974;54:609.
11. Lich R Jr, Howerton LW. Anatomy and surgical approach to the urogenital tract in the male. In: Campbell MF, ed. *Urology* Philadelphia: Saunders, 1963; Chap. 1, 37–38.
12. Masters FW, Robinson, DW. The treatment of avulsion of the male genitalia. *J Trauma* 1968;8:430.
13. Millard DR, Jr. Scrotal construction and reconstruction. *Plast reconstr Surg* 1966;38:10.
14. Tamai S. Microsurgical replantation of a completely amputated penis and scrotum. *Plast Reconstr Surg* 1977;60:287.
15. Altchek ED. A modification of the standard technique for repair of scrotal elephantiasis. *Plast Reconstr Surg* 1977;60:284.

CHAPTER 436 ■ MEDIAL THIGH SKIN FLAPS FOR RECONSTRUCTION OF THE SCROTUM

B. HIRSHOWITZ

The bilateral superomedial thigh skin flap can be raised and transferred to reconstruct either the scrotum or the vulva without recourse to delay procedures.

INDICATIONS

The main application so far has been in patients with large loss of scrotal skin in Fournier's gangrene or in a patient with severe scrotal lymphedema (1–4).

ANATOMY

See Chapter 318 for details.

OPERATIVE TECHNIQUE

See Chapter 418 for details of design, flap elevation, and donor-site closure.

With scrotal reconstruction, a saclike form of the new scrotum can be obtained by suturing together the distal margins, as well as some of the lateral margins of the flaps, in the midline. This produces a tightening effect distally, while leaving the central portion of the suture line loose (Fig. 1C).

SUMMARY

Fourteen patients with scrotal and vulvar defects have been reconstructed without flap failure using the bilateral superomedial thigh flap.

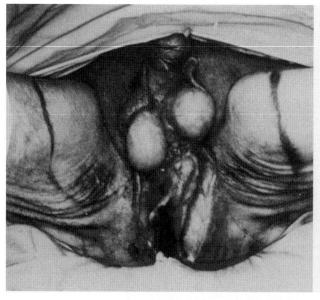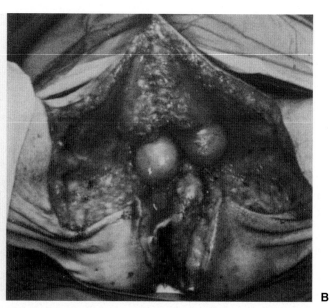

FIG. 1. A: Loss of most of the skin of the scrotum and perineum with exposure of both testes. The proximal half of the ventral surface of the penis is also exposed. The outline of both flaps is shown on the lax proximal thigh skin. **B:** The elevated flaps sutured together in the midline can readily be brought down to cover both testes. *(Continued)*

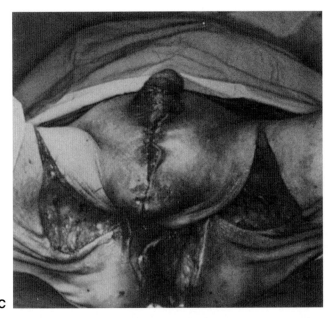 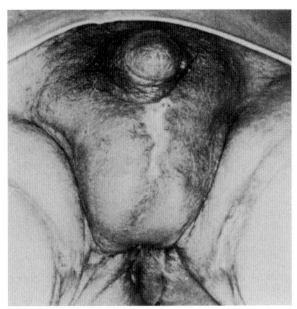

C   D

FIG. 1. *Continued.* C: Both flaps in position before placement of the skin sutures. The skin of the ventral surface of the penis also has been repaired. D: Appearance of the reconstructed scrotum 4 months postoperatively.

References

1. Robinson DW, Stephenson KL, Padgett EC. Loss of coverage of penis, scrotum, and urethra. *Plast Reconstr Surg* 1946;1:58.
2. Millard DR Jr. Scrotal construction and reconstruction. *Plast Reconstr Surg* 1966;38:10.
3. Altchek ED, Hoffman S. Scrotal reconstruction in Fournier's syndrome. *Ann Plast Surg* 1979;3:523.
4. Hirshowitz B, Moscona R, Kaufman T, Pnini A. One-stage reconstruction of scrotum following Fournier's syndrome using a probable arterial flap. *Plast Reconstr Surg* 1980;66:608.

CHAPTER 437 ■ MEDIAL THIGH FASCIOCUTANEOUS FLAP FOR TOTAL SCROTAL RECONSTRUCTION

G. G. HALLOCK

The cutaneous territory of the medial thigh can sustain a long, narrow, fasciocutaneous flap. If the flap is proximally based, a wide arc of rotation is possible, allowing transfer for total scrotal reconstruction (1–5) and other debilitating groin or perineal wounds.

INDICATIONS

Most scrotal defects are acquired, frequently following trauma or iatrogenic sequelae. Coverage of the testicles, without resorting to orchiectomy or burying them in subcutaneous thigh pockets (6), is desirable, but such coverage must also

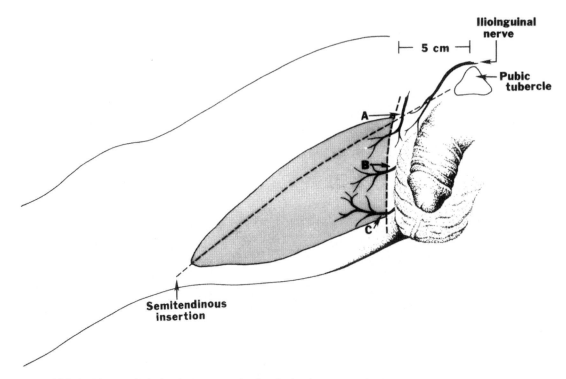

FIG. 1. Diagram depicting the important landmarks for determining the boundaries of the medial thigh fasciocutaneous flap. Although roughly centered over the gracilis muscle, the usual dimensions exceed those of a conventional gracilis musculocutaneous flap. The proximal transverse dotted line must not be violated to preserve the depicted afferent perforators to the fascial plexus. *A,* subcutaneous branch of deep external pudendal artery; *B,* gracilis musculocutaneous perforator; *C,* adductor magnus musculocutaneous perforator. (From Hallock, ref. 4, with permission.)

provide the best possible aesthetic result, to preserve male psychosexual identity. Frequently, the redundant scrotum can be stretched to close small wounds, or a skin graft will suffice (7). However, an unacceptable appearance often results from grafting, or the wound environment is not conducive to ensure adequate graft inosculation. Under such conditions, the medial thigh fasciocutaneous flap may then be a better alternative.

This wide, sensate flap can be taken from a single thigh for single-stage total scrotal reconstruction, while still permitting primary donor-site closure (4,5). In addition, the underlying gracilis muscle always is exposed during this dissection and can be utilized to broaden the potential area of coverage. The flap can also be used for repair of concurrent penile injuries such as urethral fistula (6), where coverage would be mandatory in any case.

ANATOMY

The fascial plexus of the medial thigh receives afferent inflow from direct branches such as the external pudendal vessels or septocutaneous branches of the superficial femoral or medial circumflex femoral arteries, and indirect branches from musculocutaneous perforators of the adductor compartment (1). Several such major perforators are invariably found proximal to a line drawn 5 cm below a parallel line extending from the pubic tubercle to the ischial ramus, which determine the most proximal point for rotation of the medial thigh fasciocutaneous flap (Fig. 1). The greater saphenous vein is found within this area, but can be excluded, as venous outflow paralleling the perforating arteries will still be sufficient.

Since the ilioinguinal nerve accompanies the external pudendal artery to the proximal medial thigh, at least that part of any flap will always be sensate. The distal two-thirds of the medial thigh is innervated by the medial femoral cutaneous nerve, which must be dissected back to its origin from the femoral nerve, if distal flap sensation is desired (2).

FLAP DESIGN AND DIMENSIONS AND OPERATIVE TECHNIQUE

Control of sepsis and adequate debridement must always precede scrotal reconstruction, as this body region is notorious for contamination. Usually, all procedures are facilitated by placing the patient in a lithotomy position.

A line drawn from the pubic tubercle to the insertion of the semitendinous tendon represents the anterior border of this pennant-shaped flap (Fig. 2). The posterior margin usually varies according to skin redundancy, which is determined by squeezing the thigh to simulate primary closure. Often, a flap up to 9 cm in width is possible. The wider the flap, the more likely that collateralization from multiple perforators will be captured, to ensure the safety of a greater flap length. A sharp narrowing of the flap distally toward the knee simplifies donor-site closure. Usually, when longer than 20 cm, this portion will not fluoresce, will be presumed non-viable, and must be discarded.

Elevation begins distally with identification of the deep fascia of the thigh. The fascia is usually retained with the flap, to ensure the integrity of the overlying fascial plexus. A rapid, proximal dissection in a relatively bloodless plane is then possible, stopping 5 cm below the groin crease to preserve the

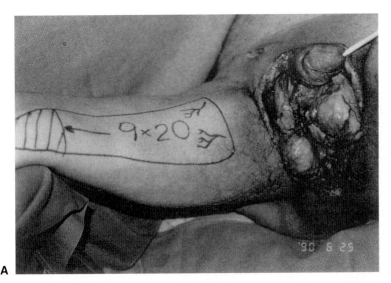
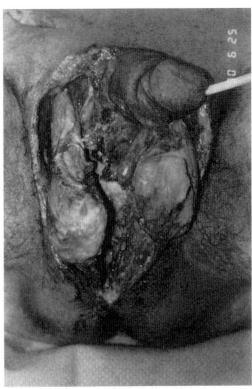

FIG. 2. A massive scrotal and perineal defect with exposed testicles, consequent to debridement for Fournier's gangrene, is seen to the extreme right. A: Outline of a medial thigh fasciocutaneous flap after patient was placed in lithotomy position. Cross-hatched area of the marked flap usually will be discarded, but inclusion facilitates primary donor-site closure. B: Close-up of the same challenging scrotal defect.

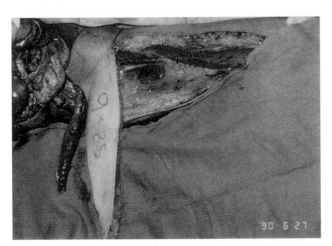

FIG. 3. Since the left groin was less violated by the debridement, the actual medial thigh fasciocutaneous flap was taken from the left thigh. Flap seen here dangling from its proximally-based pedicle at the point of clockwise rotation. The gracilis muscle has also been elevated on its own pedicle, is seen medial to the skin flap, and was used to augment the width of the neoscrotum.

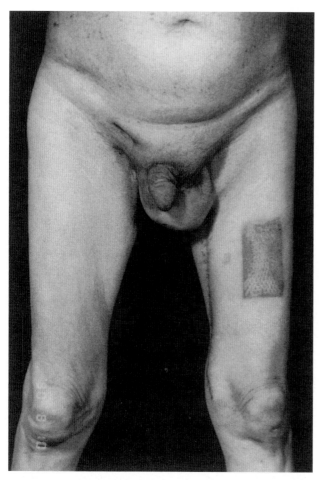

FIG. 4. Appearance 2 months postoperatively, with acceptable scrotal reconstruction, and a linear scar along the medial left thigh the only residue of flap harvesting.

vascular inflow to the flap (Fig. 3). Rotation of the flap as a hammock to cover the testicles and thereby to recreate a scrotum must be accomplished with a tension-free inset. Intravenous fluorescein is routinely administered, to ensure adequacy of circulation to the distal flap, if capillary refill is ambiguous. If necessary, the donor leg is removed from the stirrups and adducted toward the midline, to allow additional removal of distal portions of the flap and to minimize any risk of flap compromise.

If desired, the now exposed gracilis muscle can be divided at its tendinous insertion and rotated to cover the penis or augment potential scrotal coverage. Its proximal elevation will be restrained by the dominant pedicle found entering its medial undersurface, about 8 to 10 cm below the inguinal ligament (8). The single medial thigh donor site for both flaps should easily be closed by primary approximation. A scrotal support is used in the postoperative period until dependent edema subsides.

CLINICAL RESULTS

Although a vascularized flap is not always mandatory for scrotal reconstruction (7), such a choice often results in a superior cosmetic result (Fig. 4) and can better guarantee healing with a minimum of surgical intervention, especially considering the contaminated wound. Bilateral gracilis muscles can be utilized for total scrotal reconstruction, at the expense of violating the two extremities and muscle function, although this is usually expendable (9).

The use of superior (10) or superomedial thigh (11,12) flaps similarly requires bilateral flaps and requires a skin graft for donor-site closure. The omentum (13) and rectus abdominis muscle (14) have also been used, but with the obvious risks of laparotomy or abdominal-wall hernia, respectively. These potential deficits can all be avoided by using a single flap from the medial thigh, based on the recently resurrected fasciocutaneous flap principle (3). A conjoint flap, utilizing the underlying gracilis muscle for further penile (6,8) or scrotal enhancement (4,5), adds to the attributes of this donor region, which can still be closed primarily, causing minimal morbidity.

SUMMARY

When vascularized tissue transfer is required for preservation of testicular function and appearance in total scrotal reconstruction, a local proximally-based medial thigh fasciocutaneous flap is potentially sensate, can be rapidly elevated from a single extremity in a single stage, and leaves virtually no donor-site deficit.

References

1. Cormack GC, Lamberty BGH. The blood supply of thigh skin. *Plast Reconstr Surg* 1985;75:342.
2. Wang N, Whetzel T, Mathes SJ, Vasconez LO. A fasciocutaneous flap for vaginal and perineal reconstruction. *Plast Reconstr Surg* 1987;80:95.
3. Ponten B. The fasciocutaneous flap: its use in soft tissue defects of the lower leg. *Br J Plast Surg* 1981;34:215.
4. Hallock GG. Scrotal reconstruction following Fournier's gangrene using the medial thigh fasciocutaneous flap. *Ann Plast Surg* 1990;24:86.
5. Hallock GG. The chimera flap principle: conjoint flaps. In: Hallock GG, ed. *Fasciocutaneous flaps.* Boston: Blackwell Scientific, 1992;172–180.
6. Heckler FR, Aldridge JE, Songcharoen S, Jabaley ME. Muscle flaps and musculocutaneous flaps in the repair of urinary fistulas. *Plast Reconstr Surg* 1980;66:94.
7. Schaller P, Akcetin Z, Kuhn R, et al. Scrotal reconstruction after Fournier's gangrene with simple skin grafting. *Eur J Plast Surg* 1994;17:261.
8. Heckler FR. Gracilis myocutaneous and muscle flaps. *Clin Plast Surg* 1980;7:27.
9. Westfall CT, Keller HB. Scrotal reconstruction utilizing bilateral gracilis myocutaneous flaps. *Plast Reconstr Surg* 1981;68:945.
10. Tiwari IN, Seth HP, Mehdiratta KS. Reconstruction of the scrotum by thigh flaps. *Plast Reconstr Surg* 1980;66:605.
11. Hirshowitz B, Moscona R, Kaufman T, Pnini A. One-stage reconstruction of the scrotum following Fournier's syndrome using a probable arterial flap. *Plast Reconstr Surg* 1980;66:608.
12. Hirshowitz B, Peretz BA. Bilateral superomedial thigh flaps for primary reconstruction of scrotum and vulva. *Ann Plast Surg* 1982;8:390.
13. Kamei Y, Aoyama H, Yokoo K, et al. Composite gastric seromuscular and omental pedicle flap for urethral and scrotal reconstruction after Fournier's gangrene. *Ann Plast Surg* 1994;33:565.
14. Young WA, Wright JK. Scrotal reconstruction with a rectus abdominis muscle flap. *Br J Plast Surg* 1988;41:190.

CHAPTER 438 ■ PAIRED INGUINAL SKIN FLAPS FOR EPISPADIAS EXSTROPHY REPAIR

C. E. HORTON, C. J. DEVINE, JR., AND N. W. GARRIGUES

The constellation of defects presented by congenital epispadias with bladder exstrophy has been a problem for reconstructive surgeons. Classically, closure of the abdominal defect and genital reconstruction were neglected, while attention was focused on urinary diversion. As advancements in excretory control occurred, attention was drawn to the puzzle of plastic repair of the lower abdomen and genitalia. During recent years, further surgical advancements have offered improved function and better aesthetic appearance in this region. Developing a urinary conduit can no longer be accepted as the single objective in the care of these complex cases.

INDICATIONS

Previous procedures for managing these patients presented numerous disadvantages (1–5). A typical midline closure could divide the escutcheon with a wide hairless scar, frequently tethering the penis to the abdominal wall. Multiple-staged procedures not only produced further morbidity, but often created unaesthetic donor sites. While it may be acceptable to use any available closure in the difficult exstrophy patient, it is in no way acceptable to allow the abnormal escutcheon or the bent penis to remain as permanent, embarrassing results. With this in mind, we have developed a simple, reliable flap with hair-bearing tissue to reconstruct the normal escutcheon, elongate the inferior abdominal wall, and allow penile release.

A great advantage of this approach is the exposure provided for reconstruction of deeper structures. The urethra, corporal bodies, pubic ramus, midline diastasis, and bladder are all made accessible to complete systematic evaluation of the problem. The crura of the corporal bodies can easily be freed from the pubic bone. Release of the chordee, which is particularly important in epispadic patients, is made convenient.

ANATOMY

The vascular supply of these superiorly based flaps is probably from the perforating vessels of both the muscular and pubic branches of the inferior epigastric vessels.

FLAP DESIGN AND DIMENSIONS

Flap design allows excision of unattractive midline scarring. The tissue brought into the suprapubic region is hair-bearing and produces an aesthetic escutcheon. Elongation of the lower abdominal midline mobilizes skin that, in combination with procedures on the deeper structures mentioned above, significantly enhances penile length. The donor defect is a well-hidden inguinal scar.

The paired inguinal skin flaps are W-shaped flaps with each apex extending to a point lateral and inferior to the penis (Fig. 1). Markings are begun at a point inferiorly and laterally to the anterior superior iliac spine and extended inferiorly in the groin crease to a point well below the penile base, usually at a low scrotal level. The marking is then continued superiorly, including a small portion of the scrotum, to the superior penile border, where it is joined by mirrored markings from the opposite groin.

OPERATIVE TECHNIQUE

The flaps are elevated at the subcutaneous level, just superficial to the external oblique aponeurosis. Following repair and release of chordee, corporal bodies, and urethra, the flaps are closed in a V-to-Y fashion. The groin-crease donor site is easily closed without tension as the two flaps are sutured together in the midline (Fig. 2). The flaps may be further rotated to close in a Z configuration. However, this does leave a significant suprapubic skin defect.

Since maximal penile lengthening is desirable, closure of the area must be tension-free. A full-thickness skin graft may be used if the soft-tissue defect is limited to skin only. Typically, however, if a deficit exists, underlying repairs to the deeper structures may necessitate vascularized flaps. We have used an island groin flap tunneled subcutaneously or a rectus femoris musculocutaneous flap to close the created defect.

CLINICAL RESULTS

These simple random flaps have multiple inherent advantages. We have relied on them for reconstruction of 18 patients crippled by epispadias exstrophy. Figures 3 and 4 are characteristic of repair using the paired inguinal skin flaps. Flap loss has not occurred. This may be due to an increased blood supply from the inferior epigastric vessels, caused by the congenital midline diastasis.

SUMMARY

Paired inguinal flaps are reliable random flaps that can be used to great advantage in epispadias exstrophy patients. They allow escutcheon reconstruction by bringing hair-bearing tissue into the congenitally defective and frequently surgically scarred suprapubis. More important, phallic elongation by a single-stage reconstruction is achieved. Excellent exposure for reconstruction of underlying malformed structures is also offered.

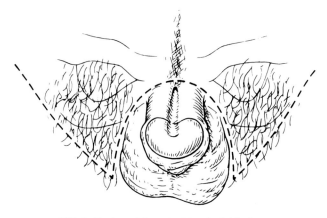

FIG. 1. Design of the paired inguinal skin flaps.

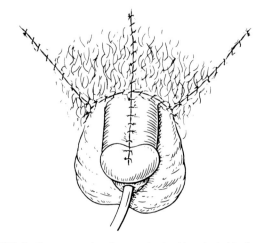

FIG. 2. Reconstructive closure of paired inguinal skin flaps.

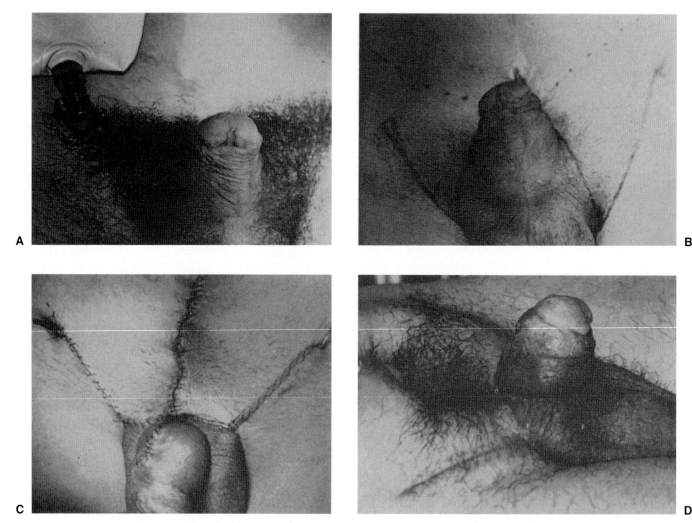

FIG. 3. A–D: An epispadias exstrophy patient with a previous urinary diversion and abdominal wall closure demonstrates significant tethering of the penis within an abnormal escutcheon (A). The paired inguinal skin flaps are designed (B) and transposed (C), allowing full approach to underlying pathology, release of penile tether, enhancement of penile length, and reconstruction of an aesthetic escutcheon (D).

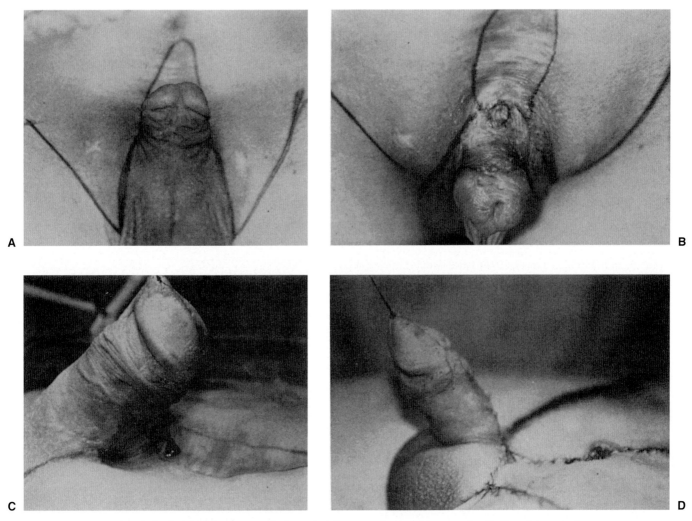

FIG. 4. A–C: An adolescent reveals the typical features of epispadias exstrophy. **D:** Use of the paired inguinal skin flaps allows reconstruction of ventral scarring and diastema, as well as penile release and elongation.

References

1. Simon J. Ectopia vesicae. *Lancet* 1852;2:568.
2. Matthews D. Ectopia vesicae. *Br J Plast Surg* 1958;11:188.
3. Steffensen W, Ryan J, Sinclair E. A method of closure of the abdominal wall defect in exstrophy of the bladder. *Am J Surg* 1956;92:9.
4. Erich J. Plastic repair of the female perineum in a case of exstrophy of the bladder. *Mayo Clin Proc* 1959;34:235.
5. Longacre J, deStefano G, Davidson D. Plastic repair of congenital defects of the ventral body wall with particular reference to exstrophy of the bladder. *Plast Reconstr Surg* 1959;23:260.

CHAPTER 439 ■ RECTUS ABDOMINIS MUSCLE FLAP INCORPORATION INTO BLADDER REPAIR

F. R. HECKLER

Muscle and musculocutaneous flaps have assumed a central role in the reconstruction of difficult wounds in almost all areas of the body. Reports of the use of such flaps within coelomic cavities as adjuncts to visceral repair also have appeared, but to a much lesser extent (1,2). In this context, the rectus abdominis muscle has proven itself, in my practice, to have the potential to aid in successful salvage of difficult urinary bladder closure problems.

INDICATIONS

Bladder defects and wounds, even when relatively extensive, can usually be managed by the standard urologic techniques of debridement, mobilization of remaining healthy bladder wall, and suture closure in multiple layers. Such techniques, combined with temporary bladder decompression using either a transurethral or a suprapubic catheter, usually are followed by a successful outcome, albeit with the accompaniment of a somewhat decreased bladder capacity. However, when additional factors that may contribute to poor wound healing are present, such as prior therapeutic irradiation, severe local scarring, or infection, the introduction of highly vascular, healthy muscle tissue may be an important adjunct to a successful outcome.

ANATOMY

Details of the surgical anatomy of the rectus abdominis muscle are presented in Chapters 362, 363, 364, and 365 and will not be repeated here. Rather, I will concentrate on specific anatomic points pertinent to the transfer of this unit to the urinary bladder.

The paired rectus abdominis muscles run from the pubis below to the costal margins above, enclosed within the fascial rectus sheath. When used as an inferiorly based flap, the vascular pedicle consists of the inferior epigastric artery and vein. These vessels originate from the external iliac artery and vein just prior to their passage beneath the inguinal ligament. The inferior epigastric vessels pass obliquely upward in a preperitoneal plane, penetrate the rectus sheath approximately 8 cm above the pubis, and then course in a cephalic direction along the underside of the muscle. The entire rectus abdominis will survive based on this single arteriovenous pedicle, although only about half this amount is needed for bladder repair.

FLAP DESIGN AND DIMENSIONS

Many of the traumatic defects and pathophysiologic entities in question involve the central suprapubic area, including the pyramidalis muscles and the distal rectus abdominis. The oblique approach of the inferior epigastric vessels and their entry into the rectus sheath at or near the arcuate line generally make the muscle unit available for transfer from one or the other side, despite suprapubic pathology. If doubt about the persistence of an intact inferior epigastric artery exists, a preliminary angiography study will clarify the picture. Alternatively, the vertical midline lower abdominal incision usually used by the urologic member of the reconstructive team will allow preliminary palpation or even direct visualization of the inferior epigastric pedicle, either in its retroperitoneal or its retromuscular course.

OPERATIVE TECHNIQUE

Mobilization of the rectus abdominis is quite straightforward and rapidly accomplished. Either a midline or paramedian skin incision is used, depending on the surgeon's preference and the presence or absence of previous surgical scars on the abdomen (Fig. 1).

The presence of previous low transverse surgical scars (such as Pfannenstiel) does *not* usually preclude the use of the rectus abdominis, since these will normally not have been carried far enough laterally to interfere with the deep inferior epigastric pedicle. Thus, even if the lower rectus has been transected by such an incision, the muscle flap can still be used because the vascular pedicle enters the muscle several centimeters cephalic to the insertion.

The anterior rectus sheath is linearly opened and the rectus muscle is sharply dissected out, care being taken not to avulse it accidentally from the vascular pedicle running immediately deep to it. The muscle is mobilized to the pubis, from which it may be detached, if required, although this is not usually necessary.

The defect in the bladder wall is repaired, and the rectus muscle is applied directly over the bladder suture line with absorbable sutures. The anterior rectus sheath is securely closed, followed by standard wound closure of subcutaneous tissue and skin (Fig. 2).

The need for the addition of pedicled muscular reinforcement of bladder wall repairs is clearly infrequent. However, in certain highly selected patients, it can be the additional

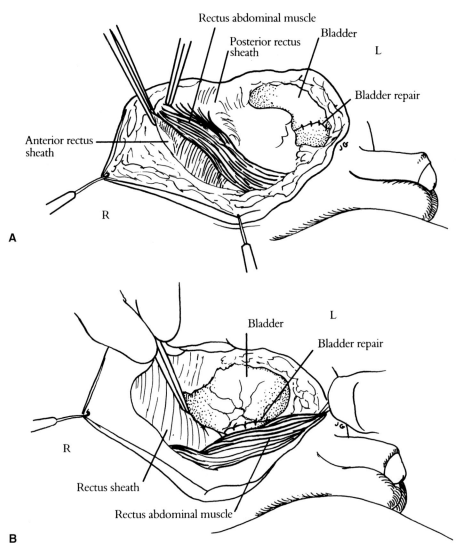

FIG. 1. Anatomic relationships for incorporation of rectus abdominis into bladder repair. A: Inferior rectus sheath is opened either through the anterior or medial edge, with reflection of fascia. The rectus abdominis is mobilized based on its inferior epigastric vascular pedicle. Bladder repair is carried out in standard fashion. B: The rectus abdominis is then rotated inferiorly and medially and sutured directly over the bladder suture line in close apposition to it. (From Heckler et al., ref. 1, with permission.)

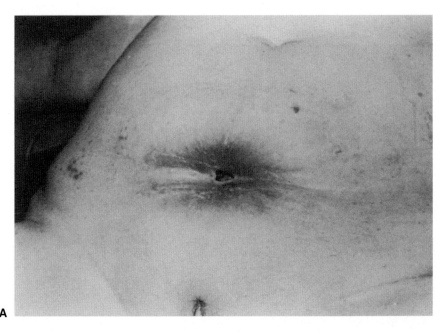

FIG. 2. Rectus abdominis incorporation into a suprapubic vesicocutaneous fistula repair. A: Suprapubic postirradiation ulcer with vesicocutaneous fistula in base. Note that the heavily irradiated area extends laterally to involve both distal segments of the rectus abdominis. *(Continued)*

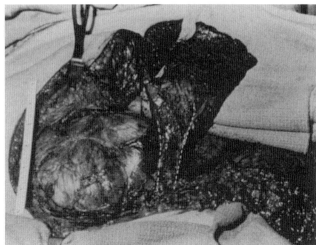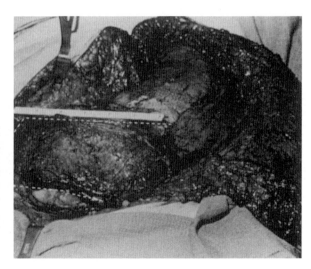

B,C

FIG. 2. *Continued.* **B:** Debridement and bladder mobilization and repair have been carried out. The distal rectus abdominis muscle has been debrided away. Note that the inferior epigastric vascular pedicle (*dotted lines*) approaches obliquely and therefore is still intact. The more cephalic end of the rectus abdominis muscle will be transposed inferiorly and applied to the bladder repair. **C:** The muscle has been rotated inferiorly and is being applied over the bladder repair. In this case, the anterior fascia also has been included to provide distal fascial reconstruction.

ingredient required for overall success. The additional dissection and operating time are quite modest, and the donor-site functional morbidity is minimal.

CLINICAL RESULTS

I have used the rectus abdominis as an aid in bladder repair in six patients, all with success.

SUMMARY

The value of the introduction of healthy, highly vascularized tissues into the healing milieu of wounds whose healing potential is otherwise compromised seems obvious and is a time-honored reconstructive principle (3). In particular, the application of healthy muscle flaps has proved efficacious in obtaining primary healing in a large variety of difficult situations. The incorporation of rectus abdominis muscle flaps into the repair of difficult bladder defects is simply another extension of the principle.

References

1. Heckler F, Aldridge J, Songcharoen S, Jabaley M. Muscle flaps and musculocutaneous flaps in the repair of urinary fistulas. *Plast Reconstr Surg* 1980;66:94.
2. Skef Z, Bellinger M, Blomain E, Ballantine T. Use of the inferior rectus myocutaneous flap for coverage of bladder exstrophy defect. *J Pediatr Surg* 1982;17:720.
3. Brown JB, Fryer M, McDowell F. Permanent pedicle blood-carrying flaps for repairing defects in avascular areas. *Ann Surg* 1951;134:486.

CHAPTER 440 ■ INFERIOR RECTAL ARTERY SPIRAL SKIN FLAP

D. R. MILLARD, JR.

The inferior rectal artery spiral skin flap is an axial-pattern flap that is used to create a skin-lined anal canal. For patients with imperforate anus, it can be used both to prevent and treat rectal mucosal exposure and prolapse (1).

INDICATIONS

Low imperforate anus is a translevator lesion in which the rectum can be brought out to the skin in the anal position without complication using the standard method. In high imperforate anus, the rectum communicates with the bladder, urethra, or vagina above the puborectalis sling of the levator ani muscle and has not descended through the levator sling. Even when the rectum is rerouted through the levator sling (2), pulled through a preserved distal cuff of rectum (3), and simply sutured to a hole in the skin in the anal area, there are complications.

The high percentage of postoperative complications of mucosal ectropion, rectal prolapse, wet bottom, and anal stricture are due to the absence of a distal skin-lined anal canal. After the rectum has been pulled through a hole in the skin in the anal area, skin tension will pull it into ectropion or prolapse,

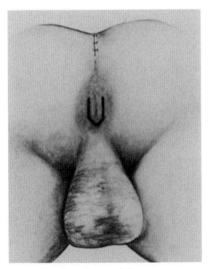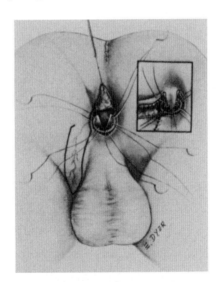

A,B

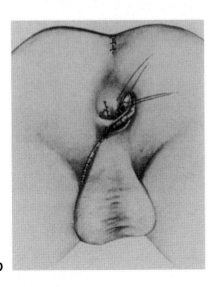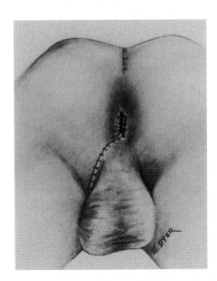

C,D

FIG. 1. A: In primary correction of high imperforate anus, the anal dimple is lifted in a trapdoor flap. (From Millard et al., ref. 1, with permission.) B: The distal rectum has been brought down and released by an incision posteriorly. The spiral flap with the inferior rectal vessels has been marked. Inset: Trapdoor flap let into rectal release. C: Spiral flap donor area closed and flap let into defect between perineal skin and distal end of rectum to create a skin-lined distal anal canal. D: Completed result.

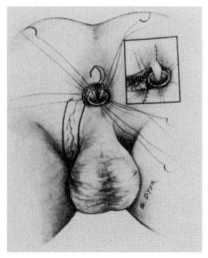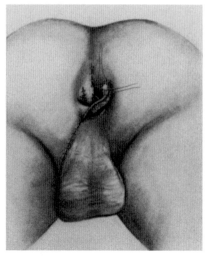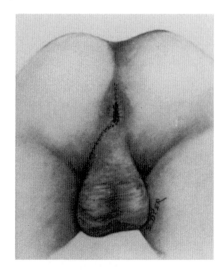

A–C

FIG. 2. **A:** In secondary correction of high imperforate anus, a trapdoor flap cannot be created; there-fore, a small posterior transposition flap is designed. The spiral flap is marked, and the distal rectum is released by posterior incision. **Inset:** Posterior flap transposed 180 degrees into rectal release. **B:** Spiral flap being inserted and donor area closed. **C:** Completion of skin-lined distal anal canal.

and mucosal exposure promotes a flow of mucus. The circular-ity of the anal scar often contracts to produce a stricture.

Surgical attempts to prevent these complications have all been based on the principle of advancement of local skin by flaps from the same axis. This does not alleviate the problem, because the shortage of skin merely causes what has been pulled in to pull out again.

ANATOMY

The flap used to create a skin-lined anal canal is an axial-pattern flap based on the inferior rectal artery.

FLAP DESIGN AND DIMENSIONS

A 1.5 × 5 cm skin flap based at the side of the future anus is taken from the groove between the thigh and the scrotum (Fig. 1B). This flap is taken out of one axis and transposed into a different axis to bring in new skin *without* tension.

In primary cases, a trapdoor flap, based posteriorly, is ele-vated to be inset into the rectal release. In secondary cases, a posterior transposition flap must be designed.

OPERATIVE TECHNIQUE

In primary cases, the usual trapdoor skin flap in the anal area is lifted with its base posterior (Fig. 1A). The distal end of the rectum, rerouted through the levator sling, is brought down the anal canal but sutured short of the external skin by 1.5 cm, thus leaving a raw cuff of the distal anal canal (Fig. 1B). The trapdoor flap is interdigitated across the circular ring of the distal rectum to interrupt the circle (Fig. 1B, inset).

The spiral flap is coiled into the 1.5-cm raw distal anal canal to line it with skin (Fig. 1C). The flap donor area is

sutured without difficulty, and the scar soon becomes unno-ticeable (Fig. 1D).

In secondary cases, the ectropion or prolapse is resected up 1.5 cm from the external skin, leaving the same raw distal anal canal. Since there is no trapdoor flap available, a midline transposition is used to interdigitate across the distal circle of rectum (Fig. 2A, inset). Then the inferior rectal spiral flap is used, as in the primary cases, to line the distal anal canal with skin under no tension (Fig. 2A to C).

CLINICAL RESULTS

By March of 1982 (1), this procedure had been performed in four primary patients and seven secondary patients. The inferior rectal vessels were found to be robust in all 11 patients.

If the colostomy is closed after this anal construction so that the new anal canal will have regular dilatations, there will be no recurrence of the previously common complications.

SUMMARY

The inferior rectal artery skin flap has provided a solution to the problems of constructing an anus in both primary and sec-ondary cases of imperforate anus.

References

1. Millard DR Jr, Rowe MI. Plastic surgical principles in high imperforate anus. *Plast Reconstr Surg* 1982;69:399.
2. Stevens FD, Smith ED, eds. *Ano-rectal malformations in children.* Chicago: Year Book Medical Publishers, 1971;255.
3. Rehbein F. Imperforate anus: experience with abdominoperineal and abdominosacroperineal pull-through procedures. *J Pediatr Surg* 1967; 2:99.

CHAPTER 441 ■ RECONSTRUCTION OF THE ANOPERINEAL AREA WITH THE V-Y ADVANCEMENT TRIANGULAR ISLAND FLAP

I. J. PELED AND Y. ULLMANN

EDITORIAL COMMENT (Chapters 441 and 442)

These are other uses for bilateral V-Y sliding flaps. It is important to determine whether the internal sphincter is working in the anal reconstruction.

The V-Y advancement triangular island flap is described for reconstruction after treatment of anal ectropion. It can be applied after any ablative surgery of the anal area.

INDICATIONS

Tumors of the perianal area may extend into the anal canal, and their resection may leave a large, raw surface in this area. Whitehead deformity or ectropion of the anal mucosa (Fig. 1A), following hemorrhoidectomy, is infrequent but, when present, causes great discomfort, including wet anus, pruritus, bleeding, pain, incontinence, and tenesmus. The treatment consists of excising the everted mucosa and the adjacent skin, and the result, just as after tumor ablation, is a large, raw surface. Leaving this area open for secondary healing, or resurfacing it with skin grafts, may lead to such unwanted consequences as strictures and incontinence.

To avoid these complications and provide resumption of normal sensation in the anal area, it is desirable to use local sensate flaps with intact skin for the reconstruction. Reported procedures have included sliding skin flaps (leaving a raw surface for secondary healing), S-plasty, Limberg flaps (1–3), and muscle flaps such as the gracilis and gluteus maximus (4). The usefulness and versatility of V-Y advancement flaps have previously been reported (5), as well as their application for anal reconstruction (6,7).

ANATOMY

The V-Y advancement gluteal island flap is a random flap that is subcutaneously based on the perforating vessels emerging from the muscle. The gluteus maximus has a dual blood supply from the superior and inferior gluteal arteries, which arise from the internal iliac vessels. Wide lateral undermining of triangular flaps between the dermis and sub-cutaneous tissue allows medial and upward advancement without tension, and does not jeopardize the blood supply to the flap.

FLAP DESIGN AND DIMENSIONS

One or two triangles are drawn on one or both sides of the created defect over the sphincter. The bases are the right and left anal hemicircumference. The height of the triangle(s) is about 8 to 10 cm, so as to obtain an apex of 30 to 45 degrees (Fig. 1B).

OPERATIVE TECHNIQUE

With the patient in the supine position and with elevation and flexion of the hips, the skin, subcutaneous tissue, and fascia of the previously marked triangles are incised perpendicularly, in order to provide two deeply-based island flaps. Undermining is performed lateral to the flaps, in order to free them without interfering with the blood supply. The bases of the triangles are medially advanced and sutured to the mucosa, including the edge of the sphincter, without tension. This medial flap advancement restores the mucocutaneous junction to its proper position inside the anal canal. The donor sites are closed in a V-Y fashion. The mucosa/skin junction is sutured with 3-0 buried absorbable suture, and the rest of the skin with 3-0 nylon (Fig. 1C and D). When the defect involves only a part of the anal circumference, one flap is sufficient to close the defect.

CLINICAL RESULTS

The V-Y advancement principle, applied here to an island musculocutaneous flap, allows great mobility, thus enabling closure of the anal mucosa without tension at the suture line. No recurrences of prolapse or dehiscence have been observed. Using the V-Y principle avoids dog-ears and involves a single-stage surgical procedure. In addition, it is safe, simple, and successful.

SUMMARY

Reconstruction of perianal defects, using one or two medially-advanced triangular island flaps, is an easy and reliable one-stage procedure for resurfacing the anal area with normal and sensate skin.

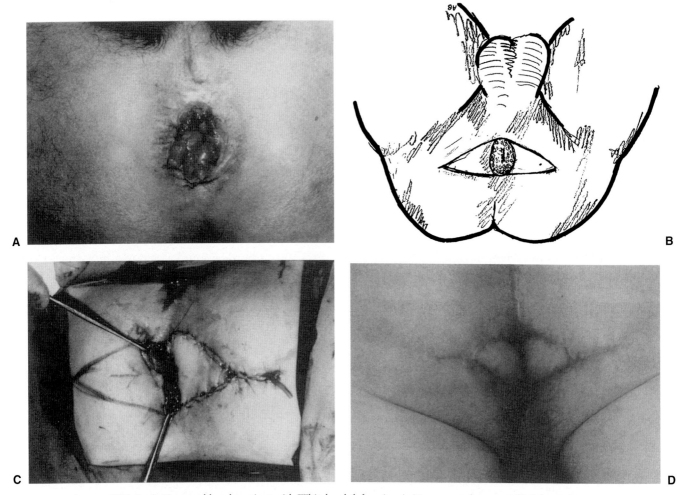

FIG. 1. A 43-year-old male patient with Whitehead deformity. **A:** Note everted mucosa. **B:** Schematic representation of the triangular flap design. **C:** Following wide resection of the everted mucosa seen in Figure 1A, the flap on the left side is proximally advanced and sutured to the remaining anal mucosa. **D:** Both buttocks at 8 months postoperatively are separated, showing no outward retraction of the anal mucosa after the procedure. (From Peled et al., ref. 6, with permission.)

References

1. Rand AA. The sliding skin-flap graft operation for hemorrhoids: a modification of the Whitehead procedure. *Dis Colon Rectum* 1969;12:265.
2. Ferguson JA. Whitehead deformity of the anus: S-plasty repair. *Dis Colon Rectum* 1979;22:286.
3. Kaplan HY, Freund H, Muggia-Sullam M, Wexler MR. Surgical correction of ectropion of the anal mucosa. *Surg Gynecol Obstet* 1982;154:83.
4. Christiansen J. Advances in the surgical management of anal incontinence. *Baillieres Clin Gastroenterol* 1992;6:43.
5. Peled IJ, Wexler MR. The usefulness and versatility of V-Y advancement flaps. *J Dermatol Surg Oncol* 1983;9:1003.
6. Peled IJ, Manny J, Wexler MR, Luttwak EM. The triangular island skin flap for treatment of anal ectropion. *Dis Colon Rectum* 1984;27:33.
7. Sagher U, Krausz MM, Peled IJ. V-Y plasty for perianal reconstruction after resection of tumor. *Surg Gynecol Obstet* 1992;175:31.

CHAPTER 442 ■ ISLAND FLAP ANOPLASTY FOR ANAL CANAL STENOSIS AND MUCOSAL ECTROPION

M. J. PIDALA, F. A. SLEZAK, AND J. A. PORTER

The island flap design has been demonstrated to have distinct advantages over older forms of anoplasty. The operative procedure is presented for treatment of mucosal ectropion and anal canal stenosis.

INDICATIONS

Mucosal ectropion and anal canal stenosis are distinct anorectal abnormalities that have separate etiologies, clinical features, and treatments. Ectropion is most commonly the result of an improperly performed amputative hemorrhoidectomy in which the rectal mucosa has been sutured to the perianal skin. Symptoms include mucous drainage ("wet anus"), pruritus, bleeding, pain, and tenesmus. Treatment is directed toward resection of the prolapsing mucosa and reconstruction of the mucocutaneous junction at the level of the original dentate line.

Anal canal stenosis is most commonly a result of prior hemorrhoidectomy. Other causes include laxative abuse (especially mineral oil), chronic anal fissure, neoplasia, inflammatory bowel disease, and irradiation. Patients often present with constipation, obstipation, pain, bleeding, and narrowed stools. In the more severe forms of anal canal stenosis, the loss of tissue is the underlying pathology that must be addressed.

Anoplasty is a technique used to reconstruct the anal canal and recreate the mucocutaneous junction. It can be used to replace descended mucosa, as seen in ectropion, or to replace fibrous scar tissue, as seen in anal canal stenosis. Since its introduction (1), the island-flap anoplasty has become a popular choice for repair of both (2–10). Compared with earlier forms of anoplasty (3–7,11–17), the island-flap design is simpler, produces less morbidity, and provides an excellent long-term outcome.

FLAP DESIGN AND DIMENSIONS

The shape and design of island flaps have varied among different reports (1,2,8,9,15). The diamond flap, which is recommended, provides a very effective design for the treatment of patients with anal stenosis. A modified V-Y advancement flap has been used for patients with mucosal ectropion. This is similar to the previously described U-shaped flap (1,15). The V-Y design offers more perianal skin to fill the larger defects associated with ectropion, although any shaped flap may be used as long as sufficient skin to cover the anal canal defect with minimal tension is provided. Undermining of the flap should be avoided to prevent destruction of the blood supply and subsequent flap ischemia. The island advancement flap should allow for primary closure of the donor site, to avoid the added discomfort of an open wound.

OPERATIVE TECHNIQUE

For anal canal stenosis, the patient receives a full mechanical bowel preparation including oral antibiotics preoperatively. The morning of the procedure, one dose of an antibiotic is administered intravenously, usually a cephalosporin. Spinal anesthesia is preferred, but local or general anesthesia may be utilized. The patient is placed in the prone jackknife position, with the buttocks taped apart.

A "diamond" flap design is used. A lateral internal sphincterotomy incision is made from the dentate line to the anal verge. If there is a muscular component to the stenotic anal canal, an internal sphincterotomy is performed. A medium-sized Hill-Ferguson retractor usually can be placed into the anal canal at this point, separating the lateral incision and creating a defect to be filled by the advancement flap.

The diamond is outlined with the leading edges at least as long as the original lateral incision. The flap is incised with a scalpel, and the sides are dissected down to the subcutaneous fat. The flap is not undermined. As the flap is advanced into the anal canal, the subcutaneous bands holding the trailing end of the flap are carefully cut. Once fully mobilized, the flap is easily advanced into the anal canal and sutured to the rectal mucosa. The internal sphincter is included in the first sutures to anchor the flap. Suturing is continued around the perimeter of the flap, and the remaining donor site is closed as a straight line.

A contralateral flap is created if there is persistent stenosis following completion of the first flap. The ability to place a medium-sized Hill-Ferguson retractor is a good measure of the adequacy of anal-canal diameter.

For mucosal ectropion, the preoperative preparation, anesthesia, and patient position are similar to those described above for anal stenosis. The initial step in the procedure is excision of the ectropion up to the level of the original dentate line, creating the defect to be filled by the island flap. Bilateral triangular flaps are utilized, as the ectropion is usually circumferential, and each flap provides enough skin to cover one-half the circumference of the anal canal (Fig. 1).

The flaps are mobilized, similar to the above description. They are then advanced into the anal canal and sutured to the rectal mucosa, creating a new mucocutaneous junction (Fig. 2). The internal sphincter is included in this suture line, to anchor the flap and the new dentate line in place. Interrupted 3-0 polyglycolic-acid sutures are continued around the perimeter of the flap. The donor site is closed as a straight line, creating a Y-shaped closure (Fig. 3).

Intravenous antibiotics are administered for 24 hours, followed by a 5-day course of oral metronidazole. The bowels are generally not confined. A regular diet with fiber supplement is

1277

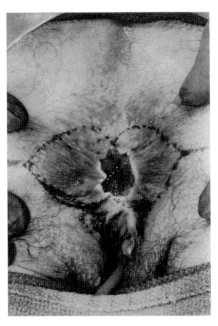

FIG. 1. Bilateral triangular flaps outlined in ink prior to repair. (From Pidala et al., ref. 20, with permission.)

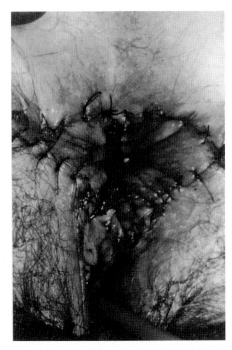

FIG. 3. Intraoperative appearance of anus following primary donor-site closure of bilateral triangular flap anoplasty. (From Pidala et al., ref. 20, with permission.)

begun the morning of the first postoperative day. Stool softeners are used as needed, but liquid stools are to be avoided. Aggressive hygiene is encouraged with the use of a handheld shower head. Sitz baths are avoided for the first few postoperative days to minimize suture-line tension and potential flap dehiscence that might be produced by squatting. The patient is followed in the office until healing is complete (Fig. 4).

CLINICAL RESULTS

Island flap anoplasty was performed in a series of 20 patients with anal canal stenosis and 8 patients with mucosal ectropion (18–20). Perioperative morbidity was minimal, and no flaps were lost to ischemia. The average hospital stay was 3.5 days, and the average length of postoperative follow-up was 36 months. Results were excellent in 91% of these patients who considered their condition to be significantly

improved. No patients believed that their condition had worsened. There were no recurrences of anal stenosis, ectropion, or prolapse, and no patient required subsequent anorectal surgery.

No patients treated for anal stenosis had further pain or bleeding. One-fourth of the patients had persistent constipation. The patients treated for mucosal ectropion had no further mucous drainage or bleeding. One patient who underwent a combined Delorme procedure and anoplasty for ectropion still complained of leakage of stool. All other patients were fully continent.

Complications included five minor wound separations that healed with conservative management, one urinary tract infection with subsequent Clostridium difficile enterocolitis, and one suture-line stricture in a patient undergoing a combined anoplasty and Delorme procedure for mucosal ectropion. This last patient was successfully treated with anal-canal dilatation. There was no flap necrosis in any patient.

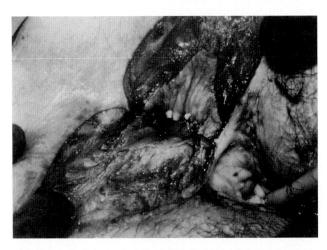

FIG. 2. Bilateral triangular island flaps have been advanced into the anal canal and sutured to the rectal mucosa, creating a new mucocutaneous junction. (From Pidala et al., ref. 20, with permission.)

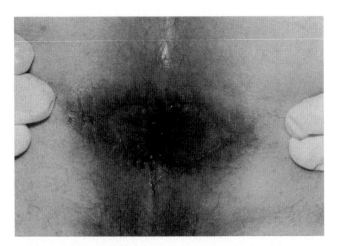

FIG. 4. Appearance of the anus 6 weeks after diamond flap anoplasty. (From Pidala et al., ref. 20, with permission.)

SUMMARY

With its simplicity of construction, maintenance of maximal blood supply, and minimization of suture-line tension, the island flap anoplasty offers a more satisfactory repair when compared to traditional pedicle skin flaps.

References

1. Caplin DA, Kodner, IL Repair of anal stricture and mucosal ectropion by simple flap procedures. *Dis Colon Rectum* 1986;29:92.
2. Christensen MA, Pitsch RM, Cali RL, et al. "House" advancement pedicle flap for anal stenosis. *Dis Colon Rectum* 1992;35:201.
3. Corman ML, Veidenheimer MC, Coller JA. Anoplasty for anal stricture. *Surg Clin North Am* 1976;56:727.
4. Ferguson JA. Repair of "Whitehead deformity" of the anus. *Surg Gynecol Obstet* 1959;108:115.
5. Hudson AT. S-plasty repair of Whitehead deformity of the anus. *Dis Colon Rectum* 1967;10:57.
6. Kaplan HY, Freund H, Muggia-Sullam M, Wexler MR. Surgical correction of ectropion of the anal mucosa. *Surg Gynecol Obstet* 1982;154:83.
7. Nickell WB, Woodward ER. Advancement flaps for treatment of anal stricture. *Arch Surg* 1972;104:223.
8. Rosen L. Anoplasty. *Surg Clin North Am* 1988;68:1441.
9. Rosen L. V-Y advancement for anal ectropion. *Dis Colon Rectum* 1986;29:596.
10. Sarver JB. Plastic relief of anal stenosis. *Dis Colon Rectum* 1969;12:277.
11. Gingold BS, Arvanitis M. Y-V anoplasty for treatment of anal stricture. *Surg Gynecol Obstet* 1986;162:241.
12. Milson JW, Mazier WP. Classification and management of postsurgical anal stenosis. *Surg Gynecol Obstet* 1986;163:60.
13. Corman ML. *Colon and rectal surgery,* 2nd ed. Philadelphia: J.B. Lippincott, 1984;139–150.
14. Ferguson JA. Whitehead deformity of anus, S-plasty repair. *Dis Colon Rectum* 1979;22:286.
15. Pearl RK, Hooks VH, Abcarian H, et al. Island flap anoplasty for the treatment of anal stricture and mucosal ectropion. *Dis Colon Rectum* 1990;33:581.
16. Oh C, Zinberg J. Anoplasty for anal stricture. *Dis Colon Rectum* 1982;25:809.
17. Khubchandani IT. Mucosal advancement flap anoplasty. *Dis Colon Rectum* 1985;28:194.
18. Pidala MJ, Slezak FA, Porter JA. Island flap anoplasty for anal canal stenosis and mucosal ectropion. *Am Surg* 1994;60:194.
19. Pidala MJ, Slezak FA, Porter JA. Mucosal ectropion associated with complete rectal prolapse: treatment with combined Delorme procedure and island flap anoplasty. *Perspect Colon Rectal Surg* 1994;7:71.
20. Pidala MJ, Slezak FA, Porter JA. Island flap anoplasty. *Contemp Surg* 1995;47:11.

CHAPTER 443 ■ GLUTEUS MAXIMUS TRANSPOSITION FLAP FOR SPHINCTER RECONSTRUCTION

S. P. SEIDEL, K. E. GEORGESON, AND L. O. VASCONEZ

EDITORIAL COMMENT

The synergy of the gluteus maximus for anal sphincter control is superior to that of other muscles previously used, such as the gracilis. The internal sphincter, of course, is the most important sphincter to prevent incontinence but, in its absence, crossing the gluteus maximus and allowing contraction at will prevents soiling, even in children without an internal sphincter.

The gluteus maximus flap uses the lower third of the muscle bilaterally to reconstruct an innervated, voluntary, external sphincter. It is useful in cases of congenital, neurogenic, or traumatic incontinence, where direct sphincter repair is impossible or has failed.

INDICATIONS

Three components are necessary to maintain fecal continence: a reservoir (the rectum), intact sensation (including a sensate anal canal), and functioning internal and external sphincters. External sphincter reconstruction can be successful only when the other components are in place. A patient with a severely scarred and non-distensible rectum, or one that is insensate, will not benefit from reconstruction of the external sphincter. Preoperative evaluation should include such tests as anorectal manometry, barium enema, anorectal ultrasound, and video defecography, in order to optimize patient selection.

External sphincter incompetence can result from congenital anomalies such as imperforate anus, pelvic trauma, birth trauma, and surgery. Ideally, repair is aimed at reconstruction of the native external sphincter with a sphincteroplasty or related technique. However, when the sphincter is absent, hypoplastic, or damaged beyond repair, another form of correction must be utilized.

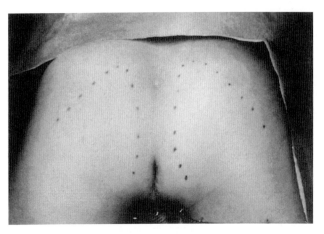

FIG. 1. Two mirror-image incisions are drawn over each buttock. Care is taken to be at least 2 cm from the anal canal.

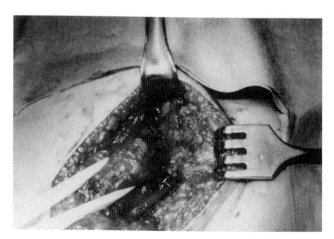

FIG. 3. Lower third of muscle isolated and encircled.

External sphincter reconstruction has traditionally relied on the transposition of surrounding musculature and encirclement of the anus to recreate a voluntary sphincter. The gracilis muscle sling has become the standard against which other repairs are measured (1). The gluteus maximus has potential advantages over the gracilis, which prompted its selection as a primary option for sphincter reconstruction.

ANATOMY

The paired gluteus maximus muscles are strong thigh extensors and lateral rotators of the hip. The muscle origin is from the superomedial ilium, posterolateral sacrum, coccyx, and sacrotuberous ligament; it insets on the femur and iliotibial tract. The blood supply is chiefly via the paired superior and inferior gluteal arteries, with contributions from branches of the medial and lateral circumflex vessels. The muscle is innervated by the inferior gluteal nerve, which originates from nerve roots of L-5, S-1, and S-2.

FLAP DESIGN AND DIMENSIONS

The inferior third of the paired gluteus maximus muscles can be readily harvested without detriment to gait or pelvic sta-

bility. The parallel fiber arrangement and large muscle mass lend themselves well to transposition and reconstruction of a sphincter with adequate bulk. Perhaps most important, the gluteus maximus normally serves as an accessory muscle of continence (2–4). After transposition, patients readily learn to contract their buttocks and bring the new sphincter into action; this is, in fact, a normal response to the urge to defecate.

OPERATIVE TECHNIQUE

The technique is actually a modification of a previously reported rectal sphincter construction using the origin of the gluteus maximus (2). Diverting colostomy is performed 2 to 3 weeks prior to sphincter reconstruction. The patient is given a Fleet enema or Dulcolax suppository on the evening prior to surgery. Intravenous ampicillin, gentamicin, and clindamycin are administered prior to making an incision. General endotracheal anesthesia is utilized, and the patient is placed in the prone, jackknife position.

Two mirror-image incisions are used (Figs. 1, 2). Access to the gluteus muscles is gained via bilateral incisions that parallel the caudal border of the muscle. They extend from the lateral sacral border to a point just inferior and lateral to the ischial tuberosity. The caudal portion of the gluteus maximus

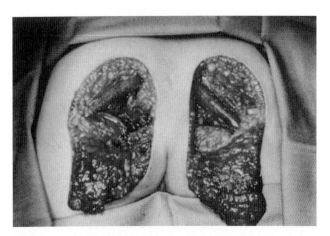

FIG. 2. Skin incised and inferior edge of gluteus maximus muscle exposed.

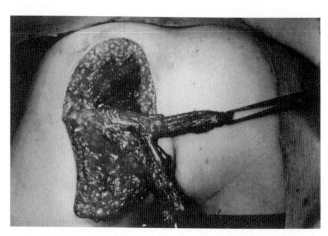

FIG. 4. Fascial attachments are divided and the muscle split longitudinally.

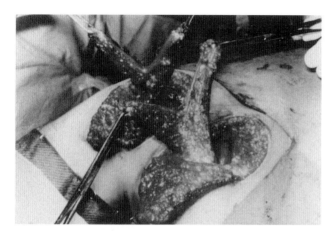

FIG. 5. Dissection completed and muscle ends split.

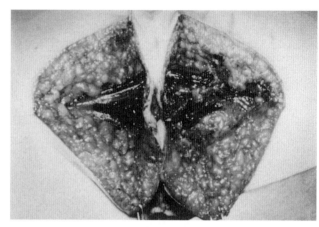

FIG. 7. Sling created by suturing opposing split muscles to each other about the rectum.

is exposed. The fibers are traced to their origin, and 4 cm of muscle are encircled and detached, along with a 6- to 10-mm rim of sacral and coccygeal fascia, from its origin (Fig. 3). The muscle is then reflected laterally. Frequently, fibrous attachments are identified, which must be divided to free the muscle sufficiently. Care must be taken to avoid injuring the neurovascular bundle, which lies just deep to the plane of dissection. The dissection is continued until the medial muscle edge will comfortably reach beyond the midline of the rectum (Figs. 4, 5).

The initial incisions are extended inferiorly in a curvilinear fashion lateral to the anus (Fig. 2). They must remain far enough outside the mucocutaneous junction to avoid scarring of the anal canal (at least 2 cm). A capacious tunnel is created superiorly and inferiorly around the rectum, connecting the two incisions. The dissected muscle is split lengthwise for 4 cm along the detached end and transposed (Figs. 6, 7). The superior portion is passed anteriorly, and the inferior portion posteriorly, around the rectum. The cut ends are opposed to each other with 2-0 PDS mattress sutures, incorporating any attached fascia to increase strength. A mirror-image procedure is performed on the contralateral side. This creates two, opposing, muscle slings that completely encircle the rectum (Fig. 7). The anal canal is also

effectively lengthened by 2 cm. Incisions are closed in the usual manner (Fig. 8).

Patients are given a high-fiber diet, as tolerated. Activity is ad libitum, with sitting prohibited for 14 days or until all incisions are well-healed. No attempts are made to delay a bowel movement. At 14 days, patients are instructed to begin "sphincter training." This consists of squeezing the buttocks, and thereby the neosphincter, with a digit placed in the anus, thus simulating the sensation of stool in the rectal vault. The scissoring action provided by contraction of the gluteus muscles effectively bars the passage of stool, additionally allowing for rectal distension and consequent sensation (3,4). With time, this response becomes nearly instinctive. Colostomy takedown is performed in a standard fashion after 3 months. No adjunctive tests or training are necessary.

CLINICAL RESULTS

Nine procedures have been completed to date; in seven cases, the colostomy has been taken down. All patients have the ability to generate good tone with gluteal contraction. Five of these patients have excellent results, with normal continence;

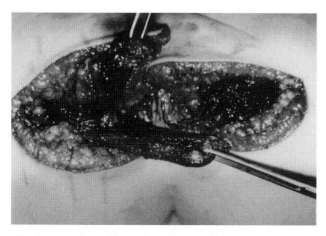

FIG. 6. Split muscle flap is transposed toward the rectum prior to creation of a sling.

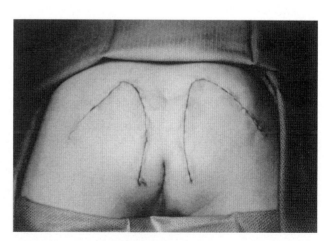

FIG. 8. Wound closed.

the other two have poor continence. We believe this is due to placement of the perianal incisions too close to the anal canal early in the series. This has led to scarring of the canal, preventing adequate sphincter contraction, despite a functional muscular sling. We are now carefully avoiding encroachment on the anal canal, by placing the incisions 2 cm from the mucosal border.

SUMMARY

The inferior gluteus maximus muscle, split to encircle the rectum, is the anal encirclement procedure that best restores voluntary extenal sphincter tone. It provides an excellent option for reconstruction of the external rectal sphincter, with little donor-site morbidity.

References

1. Pickrell KL, Broadbent TR, Masters FW, et al. Construction of a rectal sphincter and restoration of anal continence by transplanting the gracilis muscle. *Ann Surg* 1952;135:853.
2. Hentz VR. Construction of a rectal sphincter using the origin of the gluteus maximus muscle. *Plast Reconstr Surg* 1982;70:82.
3. Pearl RK, Prasad ML, Nelson RL, et al. Bilateral gluteus maximus transposition for anal incontinence. *Dis Colon Rectum* 1991;34:478.
4. Skef J, Radhakrishnana J, Reyes HM. Anorectal continence following sphincter reconstruction utilizing the gluteus maximus muscle: a case report. *J Ped Surg* 1983;18:779.

CHAPTER 444 ■ LIMBERG SKIN FLAPS

J. G. HOEHN

Even in the era of muscle and musculocutaneous flap reconstructions, the Limberg flap (1–6), because of its versatility of design and simplicity of surgical execution, continues to be my choice of treatment for small pressure ulcers (7).

INDICATIONS

There are four basic principles of pressure ulcer surgery that have been established in the last 40 years. They bear restatement:

1. Excision of the ulcer with the surrounding scar (removal of devitalized tissue and infection)
2. Ostectomy to remove the offending pressure point and the infected bone (removal of devitalized tissue and infection)
3. Muscle-flap transfer (obliteration of dead space, restoration of contour)
4. Reconstruction with flap transfer (replacement with like tissue, restoration of durable tissue)

Use of Limberg flaps for reconstruction satisfies principle 4 and permits achievement of principles 1 to 3 when each or all are required.

ANATOMY

The arterial supply of the Limberg flap arrives by means of the subdermal plexus. This random-pattern supply permits flap layout in any configuration (see Figs. 1 and 3A).

FLAP DESIGN AND DIMENSIONS

The geometric principles on which the flap is based must be understood. An equilateral parallelogram is geometrically termed a rhombus (Fig. 1). Rhomboid figures have several characteristics that lead to the conclusion that the minor angle should be 60 degrees for optimal Limberg flap transfers (3). Although 60 degrees is the angle that allows for exact satisfaction of the defect, skin elasticity permits variation in design, and surgical undermining will facilitate further adjustments in closure (3).

Knowledge of the patterns of skin elasticity and the position of the relaxed skin tension lines (RSTL) and their counterparts, the lines of maximum extensibility (LME), is paramount in planning Limberg flaps (6). Donor-site closure is facilitated by arranging the layout of the flap so that the donor-site scar coincides with the LME. This minimizes tension at the point of closure (Fig. 1, point cf, and see Fig. 2B).

When these two principles of flap design are understood, a variety of Limberg flaps can be planned for most defects (5) (Fig. 1). Excision of the defect is planned in a rhombic fashion, and the flap is then oriented so that the donor-site scar will fall in the LME (see Fig. 2A). Flap design is marked on the skin and followed throughout the operation. After the ulcer has been removed, the elasticity of the surrounding skin will produce an enlargement of the defect. The temptation to enlarge the flap size must be resisted. As wound closure is achieved, normal skin tension is restored (see Fig. 2B).

The inherent geometric design defines a length-width ratio of 1:1 (Fig. 1). This ratio relates to the adequacy of circulation in random flaps and establishes the safety factor of the flap. The high safety factor of Limberg flaps has been confirmed by their use in diverse sites under all conditions. The universal application and design potential of the Limberg flap should obviate any functional deficit.

The Dufourmentel flap (8) has proved a useful extension of the Limberg flap for irregular defects (2–4,6). Geometrically, the Dufourmentel flap is more complicated to design, but once planned, it is as technically easy to execute as the Limberg flap (Fig. 1).

Postoperative effects of muscle spasm are considered in flap planning to reduce tension on the repair. The RSTL and LME are assessed after final positioning, and the optimal location of the flap is noted. The rhombic excision is planned and oriented to be placed in the LME in the ultimate donor-site closure (see Figs. 2A, 3A).

OPERATIVE TECHNIQUE

Excision of the ulcer, intact when possible, includes skin margins, contaminated periulcer tissue, and the ulcer base (Fig. 2B). Osteophytes that are frequently a distinct part of the sacral pressure ulcer are removed with a broad chisel to restore a smooth surface (9–12).

Inspection of the defect for completeness of ulcer resection is pertinent at this time. Retention of "rind" will inevitably lead to delayed wound healing. As noted earlier, the size of the surgical defect may alarm the unfamiliar surgeon, but no change should be made in the original flap design.

The flap is elevated in the same plane as the excision and is transferred to the defect (Figs. 2B and 3B). If significant dead space exists, an adjacent muscle flap can be used to obliterate the dead space and offer additional soft tissue for padding.

Flap inset and closure are facilitated by prior closure of the donor site. Heavy retention sutures tied over gauze or cotton bolsters may aid in the closure of the donor site (Fig. 2B), but care must be taken to avoid strangulation of tissue.

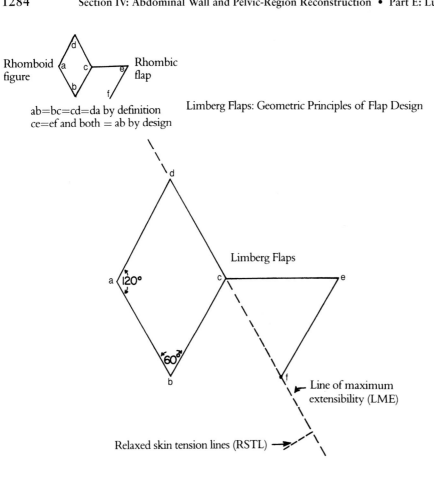

Rhomboid figure

Rhombic flap

ab=bc=cd=da by definition
ce=ef and both = ab by design

Limberg Flaps: Geometric Principles of Flap Design

Limberg Flaps

Line of maximum extensibility (LME)

Relaxed skin tension lines (RSTL) →

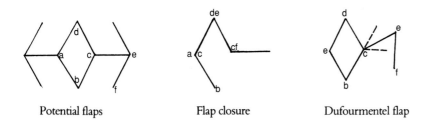

Potential flaps

Flap closure

Dufourmentel flap

FIG. 1. Basic geometric principles of Limberg flap design.

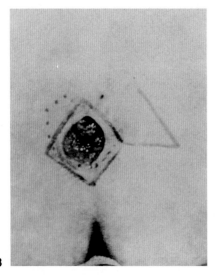
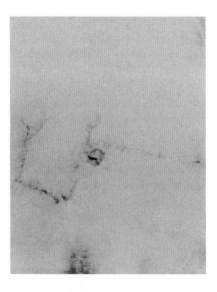

A,B

FIG. 2. A 44-year-old bedridden patient with multiple sclerosis required closure of a sacral pressure ulcer for hygienic reasons. The wound had been meticulously cared for at home and thus was small on presentation. **A:** Intraoperative photographs demonstrating the degree of undermining (*dotted line*), anticipated surgical resection designed in a rhomboid pattern, and Limberg flap design. Note location of rhomboid design and flap choice. Compare with Fig. 1. Three other Limberg flaps could be designed for this rhombus and an infinite number of rhombus figure designs could be planned, allowing maximum flexibility in design. **B:** Postoperative photograph at 7 days demonstrating flap closure. Note bolster stitches placed across point of maximum tension at apex of donor-site closure. (From Hoehn et al., ref. 7, with permission.)

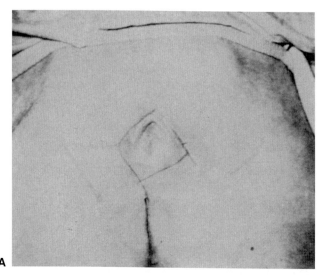
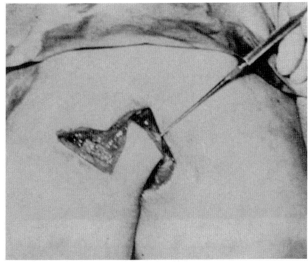

A

B

FIG. 3. A 24-year-old quadriplegic man of markedly asthenic habitus who presented with a recurrent sacral pressure ulcer. Fourteen months prior, a Limberg flap had been used to close a similar defect. The scar from the previous donor site and flap transfer can be seen on the right side of the wound. **A:** The old Limberg flap scars are on the right side. The rhombic excision is planned, and the new Limberg flap is designed on the contralateral side. **B:** The Limberg flap of uniform thickness is being rotated into position.

Although postoperative morbidity is minimal, the positional and nursing care requirements prolong the hospital stay. Hospital discharge is planned for 17 to 21 days.

CLINICAL RESULTS

In 20 years, 64 Limberg flaps were performed on 55 patients for reconstruction of small sacral decubitus ulcer defects. Review of 1- to 16-year follow-ups reveals that there were 14 recurrent sacral ulcers in the area of previous sacral ulcer repair by Limberg flaps. Two cases were reconstructed by transferring a contralateral Limberg flap (Fig. 3); the remainder required a larger flap. I do not think that ulcer recurrence and flap breakdown are related to flap design. Rather, various patient factors (spasticity, motivation, and/or job requirements) contribute to the recidivism rate (11,12).

SUMMARY

The Limberg flap and its variations can be satisfactorily used to close small sacral pressure ulcers.

References

1. Limberg AA. Design of local flaps. In: Gibson TA, ed. *Modern trends in plastic surgery.* London: Butterworth, 1966;38–61.
2. Lister GD, Gibson T. Closure of rhomboid skin defects: the flaps of Limberg and Dufourmentel. *Br J Plast Surg* 1972;25:300.
3. Koss N, Bullock JD. A mathematical analysis of the rhomboid flap. *Surg Gynecol Obstet* 1975;141:439.
4. Koss N. The mathematics of flaps. In: *Basic science in plastic surgery: an educational foundation symposium.* St. Louis: Mosby, 1979; 274–283.
5. Jervis W, Salyer KE, Busquets HA, Atkins RW. Further application of the Limberg and Dufourmental flaps. *Plast Reconstr Surg* 1974;54:335.
6. Borges AF. The rhombic flap. *Plast Reconstr Surg* 1981;67:458.
7. Hoehn JG, Elliott RA, Stayman JW. The use of Limberg flaps for repairing small decubitus ulcers. *Plast Reconstr Surg* 1977;60:548.
8. Dufourmentel C. La fermeture des pertes de substance cutanée limitées: le lambeau de rotation en L pour losange dit "LLL." *Ann Chir Plast* 1962;7:61.
9. Conway H, Griffith BH. Plastic surgical closure of decubitus ulcers in patients with paraplegia based on experience with 1000 cases. *Am J Surg* 1956;91:946.
10. Dansereau JG, Conway H. Closure of decubitus in paraplegics: report of 200 cases. *Plast Reconstr Surg* 1964;33:474.
11. Rogers J, Wilson LF. Preventing recurrent tissue breakdown after pressure sore closure. *Plast Reconstr Surg* 1975;56:419.
12. Constantian MB, ed. *Pressure ulcers: principles and techniques of management.* Boston: Little, Brown, 1980;173.

CHAPTER 445 ■ GLUTEAL ROTATION SKIN FLAP

B. H. GRIFFITH

Since the early days of pressure sore closure in 1945, the gluteal rotation flap has been the workhorse for the repair of ulcers in the sacral area (1). At first, closure was attempted by simple approximation of the edges of the wound, but the tension was too great and the procedure was usually unsuccessful. The rotation of adjacent skin and subcutaneous fat was a logical improvement in technique and has had a remarkably long and successful track record (2,3).

INDICATIONS

Coverage of the sacral area after excision of a sacral pressure ulcer is the chief use for this flap. However, it also can be used to close a sacral wound due to radiation injury, a meningomyelocele, and others.

ANATOMY

The blood supply of this random flap is derived from the superficial branch of the superior gluteal artery and from the inferior gluteal artery, which anastomose freely within the gluteus maximus and send perforating branches through the muscle to form a rich network in the subcutaneous fat and the overlying dermis.

FLAP DESIGN AND DIMENSIONS

The flap consists of the skin and subcutaneous fat of essentially the entire buttock. It is based inferiorly, i.e., over the distal edge of the gluteus maximus muscle (Figs. 1, 2). This ensures that the scar created by rotating the flap will not be in a position where it can be pressed on when the patient is sitting. If this rule is violated and the flap is based superiorly, i.e., over the upper buttock, the scar is made more vulnerable to the trauma of sitting, and recurrence of the ulcer is likely (Fig. 3).

The flap size obviously varies with the size of the patient and the width of the buttock, but it should extend from the edge of the defect over the sacrum to just medial to the posterior edge of the greater trochanter of the femur. The flap may therefore be 15 to 25 cm wide. If the length of the flap from base to distal edge does not exceed the width (a 1:1 ratio), there is no need for a delay; i.e., the flap may be raised and

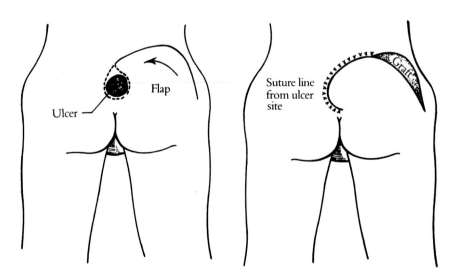

FIG. 1. Gluteal rotation skin flap. The flap extends from the edge of the defect to just medial to the posterior edge of the greater trochanter. A split-thickness skin graft is placed laterally over the gluteus muscle to take tension off the medial suture line. The flap crosses the midline 2 to 3 cm. The flap is based inferiorly to avoid a scar in an area subject to pressure from sitting. The length-to-width ratio is 1:1.

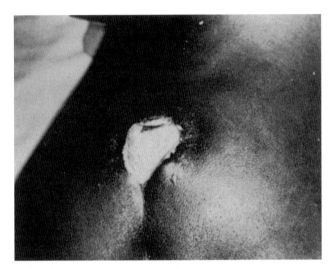
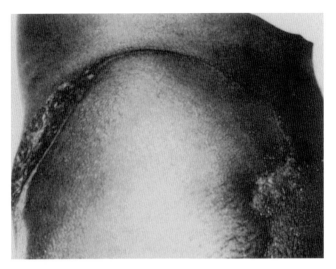

FIG. 2. Typical use of the gluteal rotation flap for closure of a sacral ulcer.

rotated in one stage. The pivot point is in the medial third of the base, and the arc of rotation is 25 to 40 degrees.

The flap should be as large as possible within the limits described above. The larger the flap, the more expandable it is, the farther away from the pressure of sitting its scar will be, and the more possible it will be to rotate it a second or even a third time should this be necessary. A small flap usually cannot be successfully rotated a second time because it is too narrow to reach and the old scar would be placed over an area of pressure.

OPERATIVE TECHNIQUE

The gluteus maximus and its fascia are *not* raised with the flap. However, turnover flaps of gluteal fascia should be used to cover the sacrum after the bone has been smoothed down and deprived of its bony prominences. It is usually necessary to place a skin graft over the muscle laterally to close part of the flap donor area in order to take tension off the important suture line over the sacrum (Fig. 1). Only when the buttock (and, therefore, the flap) is very wide and the flap is under no

tension when it is sutured into place can the skin graft be safely omitted (Fig. 4).

Rotation of the flap across the midline is usually possible for a distance of 2 to 3 cm. In the case of a large sacral defect that cannot be covered by one gluteal rotation flap, a second similar flap from the other buttock can be added (Fig. 5). When this is done, an inferior base should be used for the second flap for the same reasons that were given above for this design.

Postoperative hematoma is usually successfully prevented by the use of continuous suction by means of a catheter left in place under the flap for 2 full weeks (4–6). The patient is best kept prone on a well-padded Stryker frame or Circolectric bed for 1 to 2 days postoperatively and then turned prone to supine alternately every 2 hours for 2 weeks. Sutures are left in place for 2 weeks as well.

CLINICAL RESULTS

This is a very durable flap, providing that the underlying sacral prominences are smoothed down and pressure over the sacrum

A
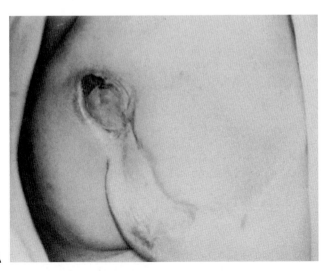
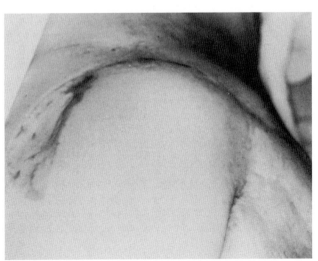
B

FIG. 3. A: Sacral ulcer unsuccessfully closed with a gluteal flap incorrectly based superiorly, with resultant loss of a portion of the flap and the scar in an area subject to trauma from sitting. (From Griffith et al., ref. 6, with permission.) B: Result after closure with a gluteal rotation flap as described.

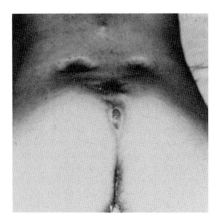
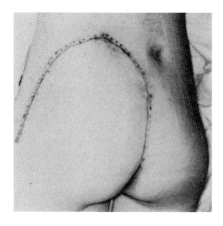

FIG. 4. Closure of a large sacral wound with a gluteal rotation flap in a patient with a wide pelvis. Skin graft not needed laterally.

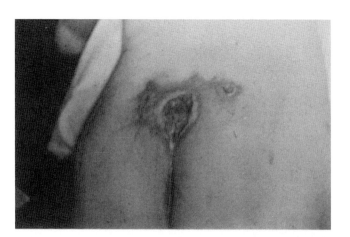
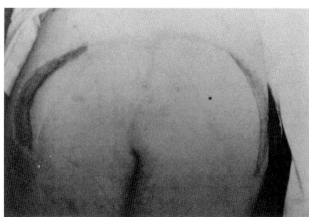

FIG. 5. Closure of an extremely large sacral ulcer with two gluteal rotation flaps. Note that both are based inferiorly to avoid a scar in the "sitting area." (From Griffith et al., ref. 6, with permission.)

is avoided in the future. Based on an experience with 1000 patients (2), the success rate was 95 percent, but there was an 11 percent recurrence rate of the ulcer in paraplegic patients who did not avoid later prolonged pressure over the sacral area.

Necrosis of even a small portion of the distal edge of the flap is extremely rare if the rules mentioned above are followed. Loss of the skin graft over the lateral muscle is an irritating, but rarely serious complication. There is no significant functional deficit.

SUMMARY

The inferiorly based gluteal rotation flap is still the standard and well-proven technique for repair of sacral defects.

References

1. Barker DEL Elkins CW, Poer DH. Methods of closure of decubitus ulcers in the paralyzed patient. *Ann Surg* 1946;123:523.
2. Conway H, Griffith BH. Plastic surgical closure of decubitus ulcers in patients with paraplegia: based on experience with 1000 cases. *Am J Surg* 1956;91:946.
3. Griffith BH, Schultz RC. The prevention and surgical treatment of recurrent decubitus ulcers in patients with paraplegia. *Plast Reconstr Surg* 1961; 27:248.
4. Griffith BH. Advances in the treatment of decubitus ulcers. *Surg North Am* 1963;43:245.
5. Griffith BH. Pressure sores. In: Grabb WC, Smith JW, eds. *Plastic surgery,* 3rd ed. Boston: Little, Brown, 1979.
6. Griffith BH, Lewis VL, Jr. Pressure Sores. In: Goldwyn RM, ed. *The unfavorable result in plastic surgery,* 2nd ed. Boston: Little, Brown, 1984; 1073–1084.

CHAPTER 446 ■ GLUTEUS MAXIMUS MUSCLE AND MUSCULOCUTANEOUS FLAPS

S. W. PARRY, E. C. ALMAGUER, AND L. O. VASCONEZ

Gluteus maximus muscle and musculocutaneous flaps (1–10) have provided more reliable coverage of the sacral area than techniques used in the past.

INDICATIONS

These flaps have several advantages over the random flaps previously employed:

1. Their excellent blood supply permits more versatility in flap design with a greater assurance of primary healing; this is especially useful in difficult secondary cases where random flaps are not available because of previous scarring.
2. The procedure, which is not technically difficult, is relatively bloodless because most of the dissection takes place in areolar tissue planes.
3. Since the continuity between the subcutaneous tissue and the muscle fascia is not disturbed, the natural resistance to shearing forces is preserved; the problem of nonadherence of the skin flap to the underlying structures is reduced.
4. These flaps also provide muscle padding in the pressure area.
5. The presence of well-vascularized muscle may promote healing in infected tissue (11).

The gluteus maximus muscle is not an expendable muscle. Loss of gluteus maximus function in an ambulatory patient results in significant hip instability. Therefore, only the superior or inferior half of the muscle may be used. In the paraplegic, the entire muscle may be employed for coverage (5).

ANATOMY

The gluteus maximus muscle is the most superficial of the gluteus muscle group. It is a thick, broad muscle originating from the posterior gluteal line of the ilium, as well as the lateral aspect of the sacrum and coccyx. The major portion of the muscle inserts into the iliotibial tract. The inferior deep portion inserts into the greater tuberosity of the femur between the vastus lateralis and the adductor magnus (5,7) (Fig. 1).

The gluteus maximus is a type III muscle with two dominant pedicles (10). The muscle is supplied by direct branches of the hypogastric artery—the superior and inferior gluteal arteries, each with an accompanying vein. These vessels arise separately from the hypogastric artery and exit the pelvis through the lateral border of the sacrum.

The superior gluteal artery, the larger of the two vessels, leaves the pelvis above the piriformis muscle, supplying the superior half of the gluteus maximus muscle. It then courses laterally to supply the gluteus medius and gluteus minimus muscles.

The inferior gluteal artery passes posterior to the piriformis muscle as it exits from the sciatic foramen adjacent to the sciatic nerve. The vessel supplies the inferior half of the gluteus maximus muscle and a portion of the posterior thigh (7). Thus the gluteus maximus muscle may be divided into superior and inferior halves, each with a distinct medially located vascular pedicle (Fig. 1). There are anastomotic channels between the superior and inferior gluteal arteries, but it is not known whether these are consistent.

The blood supply of the skin and subcutaneous tissue of the buttock is derived from numerous musculocutaneous

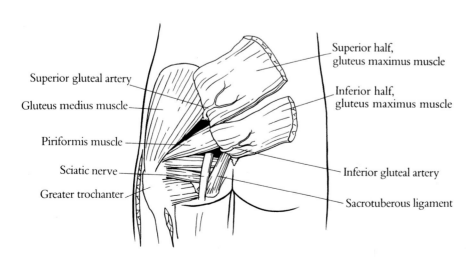

FIG. 1. Anatomy of the gluteus maximus muscle. It can be divided into halves based on either the superior or inferior gluteal arteries. (From Parry et al., ref. 9, with permission.)

Superior half, gluteus maximus muscle

Inferior half, gluteus maximus muscle

Inferior gluteal artery

Sacrotuberous ligament

Superior gluteal artery

Gluteus medius muscle

Piriformis muscle

Sciatic nerve

Greater trochanter

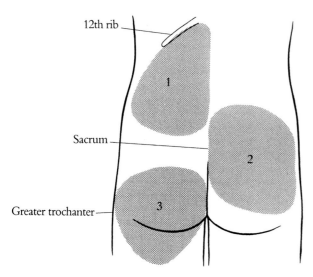

FIG. 2. Vascular territories of the lower back and gluteal region: (1) from the sacrospinalis muscle, (2) from the superior gluteal-supplied portion of the gluteus maximus muscle, and (3) from the inferior gluteal-supplied portion of the gluteus maximus muscle. (From Parry et al., ref. 9, with permission.)

perforators that exit on the superficial surface of the muscle. The skin over the lower buttock and the upper posterior thigh is nourished by branches of (1) the descending branch of the inferior gluteal artery, (2) the medial and lateral circumflex femoral arteries, and (3) the first perforating branch of the deep femoral artery (5). Specific vascular territories for the gluteal region have been described (6) (Fig. 2).

The gluteus maximus muscle functions as extensor and lateral rotator of the thigh. Additionally, it serves to raise the trunk from the stooping position by rotating the pelvis backward on the head of the femur (1). It is innervated by the inferior gluteal nerve (L5, S2), a pure motor nerve.

FLAP DESIGN AND DIMENSIONS

Rotation Flap

The gluteus maximus musculocutaneous rotation flap has proved to be quite reliable. It is based inferiorly and medially. Blood supply for sacral coverage is furnished by the superior gluteal artery. In designing the flap, the posterior

superior iliac spine and the greater trochanter are key anatomic landmarks (5). The superior gluteal artery exits from the pelvis approximately 5 cm inferior to the superior iliac spine and 5 cm lateral to the midline of the sacrum, on the deep surface of the gluteus maximus muscle (Fig. 3). The skin and subcutaneous portion of the flap may be designed as large as necessary to cover the sacral defect within the confines of the vascular territory (Fig. 4A). The flap may be designed to cross the midline without delay (4).

Muscle Transposition Flap

The muscle transposition flap or turnover flap is another reliable alternative for providing coverage for the sacrum. The entire gluteus muscle or one-half of it may be used. Again, the entire muscle should not be used in ambulatory patients.

The preferred incision for approaching this flap is the oblique incision across the buttock (Fig. 5B). A curvilinear incision over the iliac crest may be alternately employed for patients who have previously undergone gluteal rotation flaps (7) (Fig. 5C).

Island Musculocutaneous Flap

The gluteus maximus island musculocutaneous flap is another method of obtaining soft-tissue coverage of sacral defects (8–10). When employing this method, it is technically simpler to elevate the superior half of the gluteus maximus muscle and advance this to cover the sacral defect. In ambulatory patients, maintaining the inferior half of the gluteus maximus muscle intact preserves function and restores normal buttock contour (9,10).

When the sacral defect is less than 6 cm after debridement, a unilateral superior gluteal island musculocutaneous flap is usually adequate for closure (8,10). If the defect is larger, bilateral flaps may be necessary for coverage (9,10).

After the sacral prominence is excised and all the necrotic or chronically infected soft tissue is removed, the musculocutaneous island is outlined (Fig. 6A). It is advisable to design the skin island 3 to 4 cm larger than the defect to be covered to minimize tension.

OPERATIVE TECHNIQUES

Loss of tissue directly over the sacrum involves only subcutaneous tissue and skin. In the treatment of soft-tissue defects of

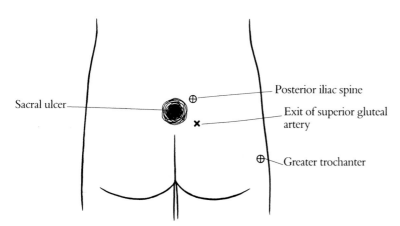

FIG. 3. Anatomic landmarks.

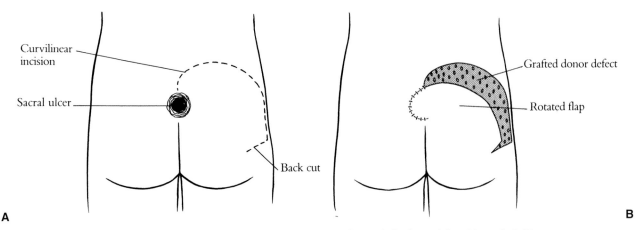

FIG. 4. A,B: Gluteus maximus musculocutaneous rotation flap with the donor defect skin-grafted. (From Parry et al., ref. 9, with permission.)

the sacrum, meticulous debridement of any devitalized tissue or granulation tissue must be performed. In addition, removal of exostoses, the bony prominence of the sacrum, and any infected sacral bone is mandatory. Coverage of the sacral soft-tissue defect may be obtained by employing the gluteus maximus musculocutaneous flap in several ways.

Rotation Flap

Once the flap is designed, the incision is made through the skin, subcutaneous tissues, and gluteus maximus muscle insertion.

The gluteus maximus muscle is incised along the inferior and lateral borders without undermining the subcutaneous tissues. The muscle is then elevated in the plane overlying the gluteus medius muscle.

At this point, the key structure in dissecting this anatomic region is the piriformis muscle. The superior gluteal artery and accompanying veins emerge from its superior edge about three fingerbreadths inferior to the iliac crest—a variable danger point (5). The piriformis muscle is identified, and elevation of the gluteus maximus muscle is continued in a superomedial direction. The superior gluteal artery with its accompanying vein is identified and preserved.

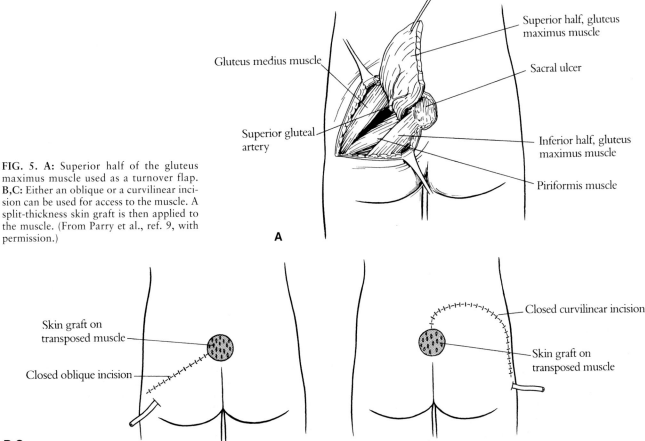

FIG. 5. A: Superior half of the gluteus maximus muscle used as a turnover flap. **B,C:** Either an oblique or a curvilinear incision can be used for access to the muscle. A split-thickness skin graft is then applied to the muscle. (From Parry et al., ref. 9, with permission.)

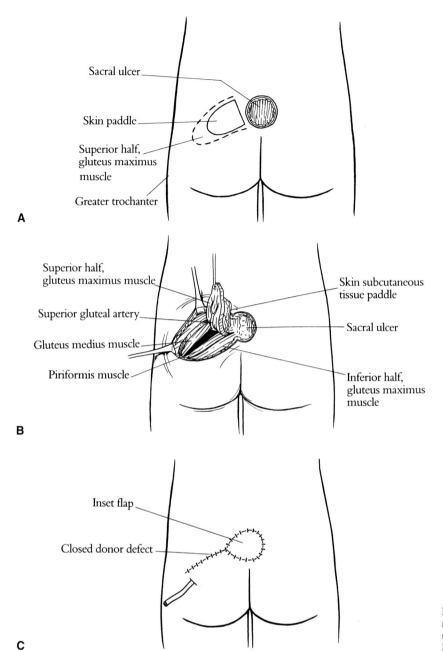

FIG. 6. A: Design of an island gluteus maximus musculocutaneous flap. B: The flap is based on the superior gluteal artery. C: The flap inset. (From Parry et al., ref. 9, with permission.)

Detachment of the gluteus maximus muscle from its origin is performed as widely as necessary (starting from its superior border) to allow the musculocutaneous flap to rotate properly (5).

For ambulatory patients, the entire gluteus maximus muscle should not be transected, for this may cause debilitating hip instability. For these patients, the inferior half of the muscle should remain intact. It may be necessary to backcut the flap, allowing the flap to rotate fully without tension, but caution must be exercised.

Once the flap is elevated, it is rotated over the sacral defect. Hemostasis is then achieved, and the gluteus maximus muscle fibers are sutured to the contralateral gluteus maximus muscle without tension. The subcutaneous tissue of the flap is inset into the sacral defect, and the skin is closed. Drains are placed within the donor defect, which may be grafted with split-thickness skin if necessary (Fig. 4B).

Muscle Transposition Flap

The gluteus maximus muscle is exposed by incising the skin and subcutaneous tissue flaps. The insertion of the muscle is detached from the greater trochanter and iliotibial tract. The dissection proceeds bluntly as the gluteus maximus is elevated off the underlying gluteus medius and reflected superiorly and medially (Fig. 5A).

The pivot point of the flap is the gluteal vessels when the whole muscle is transposed and the superior gluteal artery when the superior half of the gluteus maximus muscle is transferred (Fig. 5A). The flap is based superomedially and is turned over like the page of a book in a like direction, extending up to 5 cm past the midline. The transposed muscle is sutured to the base of the defect without tension. A split-thickness skin graft is then employed to cover the surface of the muscle. A drain is left to obliterate the dead space, and the incision is closed (1–3) (Fig. 5B and C).

Island Musculocutaneous Flap

The island of skin and subcutaneous tissue is incised down to the gluteus maximus fascia. Care should be taken not to undermine the island of skin and subcutaneous tissue from its attachment to the gluteus maximus muscle fascia. It is advisable to secure the subcutaneous tissue to the fascia temporarily. At this point, the skin and subcutaneous tissue surrounding the island flap are undermined, exposing the gluteus maximus muscle.

The superior half is detached from its insertion on the femur and iliotibial tract. The muscle with the island of skin and subcutaneous tissue is elevated in a superomedial direction, exposing the piriformis muscle. The superior gluteal artery and vein are exposed and preserved. Then the origin of the superior half of the gluteus muscle is detached, leaving the whole muscle and skin paddle attached only by the superior gluteal vessels (Fig. 6B).

The flap is advanced to cover the sacral defect. It also may be rotated in an inferomedial direction to cover ischial defects. The gluteus muscle origin is sutured to the contralateral border of the sacral defect, and the cutaneous island is inset. Care must be exercised to prevent tension on the vascular pedicle. The donor site is closed in V-to-Y advancement fashion, and drains are left in place (Fig. 6C).

Bilateral island musculocutaneous flaps may be employed when the sacral defect to be covered is larger than 6 cm. Once the flaps are dissected and advanced, the flaps are sutured to each other in the midline, recreating the intergluteal fold. The donor defects are again closed in a V-to-Y advancement fashion, and drains are left in place.

CLINICAL RESULTS

The muscle transposition flap is very durable, providing adequate muscle and subcutaneous tissue padding over the sacral defect. In ambulatory patients, this flap has shown long-term stability, as well as improved cosmetic appearance (9).

In using the muscle transposition flap, precautions to be taken while elevating the muscle are avoidance of damage to the gluteal vessels or sciatic nerve and prevention of hematoma or seroma by meticulous hemostasis. The complications of this flap are hematoma formation, skin-graft loss, loss of flap (full or partial), sciatic nerve damage, and wound infection. Fortunately, the incidence of flap loss is small, owing to the rich blood supply provided by the gluteal vessels. In Ger's experience (1), there were no instances of muscle necrosis, one instance of partial skin-graft loss, and one hematoma due to accidental early removal of the drain—a complication rate of 5.8 percent.

The possible complications of the island musculocutaneous flap are hemorrhage, hematoma formation, loss of the skin and subcutaneous tissue paddle, loss of the entire musculocutaneous flap, and wound infection. Virtually all these complications may be eliminated with meticulous and gentle technique and a thorough understanding of the anatomy involved.

SUMMARY

The gluteus maximus muscle can be used as a muscle or musculocutaneous flap for coverage of sacral defects.

References

1. Ger R. The surgical management of decubitus ulcers by muscle transposition. *Surgery* 1971;69:106.
2. Stallings JO, Delgado JP, Converse JM. Turnover island flap of gluteus maximus muscle for the repair of sacral decubitus ulcer. *Plast Reconstr Surg* 1974;54:52.
3. Mathes SJ, Vasconez LO, Jurkiewicz MJ. Extension and further applications of muscle flap transpositions. *Plast Reconstr Surg* 1977;60:6.
4. Vasconez LO, Schneider WJ, Jurkiewicz MJ. Pressure sores. *Curr Probl Surg* 1977;14:34.
5. Minami RT, Mills R, Pardoe R. Gluteus maximus myocutaneous flaps for repair of pressure sores. *Plast Reconstr Surg* 1977;60:242.
6. McCraw JB, Dibbell DG, Carraway JH. Clinical definition of independent and myocutaneous vascular territories. *Plast Reconstr Surg* 1977;60:341.
7. Mathes JM, Nahai F, eds. *Clinical atlas of muscle and musculocutaneous flaps.* St. Louis: Mosby, 1979;91–103.
8. Maruyama Y, Nakajima H, Wade M, et al. A gluteus maximus myocutaneous island flap for the repair of a sacral decubitus ulcer. *Br J Plast Surg* 1980;33:150.
9. Parry SW, Mathes SJ. Bilateral gluteus maximus myocutaneous advancement flaps: Sacral coverage for ambulatory patients. *Ann Plast Surg* 1980;8:443.
10. Mathes JM, Nahai F, eds. *Clinical applications for muscle and musculocutaneous flaps.* St. Louis: Mosby, 1982;426–432.
11. Chang N, Mathes SJ. Comparison of the effect of bacterial inoculation in musculocutaneous and random-pattern flaps. *Plast Reconstr Surg* 1982;70:1.

CHAPTER 447 ■ SLIDING GLUTEUS MAXIMUS FLAP

O. M. RAMIREZ AND J. N. POZNER

Variations of the gluteus maximus flap are useful for closure of lower trunk midline defects anywhere from the T12 level to the posterior perineum. The sliding type of operation allows this reconstruction to be performed while the structural integrity and function of the muscle unit are preserved (1–5).

INDICATIONS

This flap is useful for closure of defects due to radiation, pressure sores, trauma, chronic perineal wounds, osteomyelitis, and so on. Its main usefulness is in the nonparalyzed patient in whom functional preservation of the muscle is critical. This flap is contraindicated in patients in whom, because of the size or shape of the defect, the gluteal pedicles are close to the wound. Elevation of the flap in these patients will not allow closure of the defect. In this instance, a free muscle or musculocutaneous flap anastomosed to the gluteal vessels gives an excellent one-stage coverage. Despite the generally held belief, radiation has not been a contraindication for use of this flap. The relatively lateral position and deep location of the gluteal pedicles, in addition to the robust collateral circulation, have permitted complete survival of this flap in such instances.

ANATOMY

The gluteus maximus has the shape of a parallelogram. The pelvic border constitutes the fibers of origin from the ilium, sacrum, coccyx, sacrospinalis fascia, and sacrosciatic and sacrotuberous ligaments (3,6). The femoral border includes the osseous and fascial insertions of the muscle along the iliotibial tract and femur. The cephalic border corresponds to the gluteal aponeurosis. This aponeurosis is the common origin of the gluteus medius muscle as well. The caudal border corresponds to the gluteal fold.

The vascular territory of the gluteus maximus muscle extends from the T12 level down to the distal third of the posterior thigh. Laterally, this extends around the anterior superior iliac spine and from here to the lateral thigh, overlapping with the territory of the tensor fasciae latae flap. This muscle unit is probably the one with the largest vascular territory in the human body. The muscle has four vessels that enter its deep surface. The superior and inferior gluteal arteries with their venae comitantes enter the muscle about 5 cm from its fibers of origin on the pelvis. The medial circumflex and first perforating femoral arteries with their venae comitantes enter the muscle close to its femoral border. There are extensive intramuscular and subcutaneous anastomoses between the branches of these four vessels. In addition, there are anastomoses between the gluteal system and the lumbar perforators and between the femoral system (medial circumflex, first perforating) and other branches of the profunda femoris in the perifascial-subcutaneous plane of the skin of the corresponding territories. This explains the extension of the gluteal flap to the lumbar and thigh areas. Branches of the pudendal artery pierce the sacrotuberous ligament to enter the muscle. Some of them may be big enough (up to 2 mm in diameter) to cause confusion with the gluteal pedicles for the inexperienced surgeon.

The gluteus maximus muscle is innervated by the inferior gluteal nerve (L5,S1,S2) (3,6). This accompanies the inferior gluteal artery and vein. During flap elevation, this neurovascular pedicle should be preserved to allow preservation of function.

FLAP DESIGN AND DIMENSION

The flap shape and size will depend on the location and size of the defect. For defects up to 10 cm in diameter, no skin island or subcutaneous dissection is needed. This variation is called "sliding plication-gluteus maximus flap" (5). In this variation, the muscle and the skin are elevated en bloc and advanced to the midline (Figs. 1–3). For perineal defects, the lower fibers of origin of the muscle are detached and advanced to the depths of the cavity. The overlying skin is then closed independently in the midline. For sacral and sacrococcygeal defects, adjacent triangular skin islands overlying the corresponding muscles are made (Figs. 4–9). For large sacrolumbar defects, the triangular skin paddle overlying the sacral portion of the muscle is extended to the lumbar area on the superficial lumbar fascia (3).

OPERATIVE TECHNIQUE

Preoperatively a standard bowel prep including colon irrigation and antibiotics is administered. In addition, broad-spectrum antibiotics are administered at surgery and during the perioperative period.

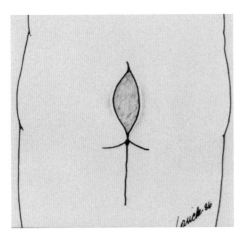

FIG. 1. Modified sliding gluteal plication.

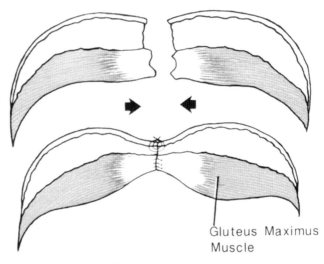

Gluteus Maximus Muscle

FIG. 3. Completed repair.

For the moderately sized defects, the initial approach should be the plication sliding type of operation. If a longer flap is needed and the decision to use a triangular skin island is made, the skin islands are incised first down to the muscle fibers. From there, a wide subcutaneous dissection is made away from the skin island. Both approaches then elevate the gluteus maximus along its periosteal origin on the sacrum and coccyx. Dissection is continued inferiorly to separate the ischiorectal fat from the muscle fibers. From there, dissection is continued to identify the sacrotuberous ligament. It is in this ligament that branches of the pudendal artery are found. This should be doubly ligated and divided. The fibers of the gluteus should be "shaved off" from this ligament. This ligament should not be transected; otherwise, the dissection becomes bloody and the anatomic landmarks are lost.

The inferior neurovascular bundle is identified next. This is located 1 cm superior to the sacrotuberous ligament and 5 cm from the lateral border of the sacrum. The superior gluteal artery and vein are located 3 cm above the inferior gluteal neurovascular pedicle. After both are identified and protected, the rest of the fibers of origin are detached. Separation of the gluteus maximus from the medius is another important step of the operation. However, this is done only if the size of the defect requires extensive mobilization of the gluteus maximus muscle. Both muscle boundaries are clearly identified close to the insertion of the gluteus maximus on the iliotibial tract, and separation is usually started there. Some of the fibers of insertion to the iliotibial tract are also detached if there is too

much lateral pull during flap advancement. Partial detachment usually does not affect the muscle function. At this point, usually the gluteus muscles are ready to be advanced and inset into the defect. Closure is done to its opposite member with figure-of-eight heavy Vicryl sutures. The donor defect is closed in a V-Y fashion, and enough subcutaneous dissection should be done to avoid lateral pulling of the muscle flap (Figs. 4–9).

Postoperative care is directed to avoid pressure and shearing forces on the gluteal flap. Our usual routine is for a 2-week

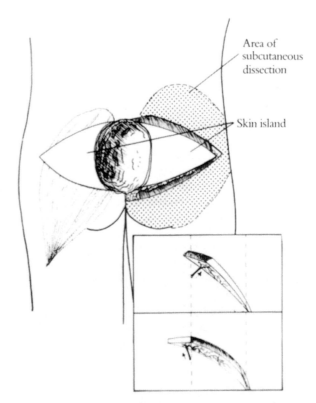

Area of subcutaneous dissection

Skin island

FIG. 4. Outline of the flap and extent of the subcutaneous dissection. Insert shows the orientation of the gluteal pedicles before and after flap advancement. (From Ramirez et al., ref. 1, with permission.)

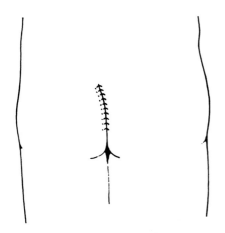

FIG. 2. Graphic depiction of the flap.

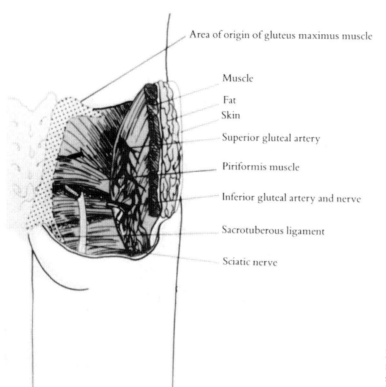

Area of origin of gluteus maximus muscle

Muscle

Fat

Skin

Superior gluteal artery

Piriformis muscle

Inferior gluteal artery and nerve

Sacrotuberous ligament

Sciatic nerve

FIG. 5. Relationship of the gluteal pedicles, piriformis muscle, sciatic nerve, and "gluteal lid." Observe the extensive muscle origin that needs to be detached. (From Ramirez et al., ref. 1, with permission.)

period of bed rest on a Clinatron bed followed by assisted ambulation with full activity by 6 weeks.

CLINICAL RESULTS

The senior author has used variations of the gluteus maximus flap to cover lower trunk midline defects in over 100 ambulatory patients. In the initial group of patients, functional evaluation was performed, including gait analysis, step climbing, and manual muscle strength. In a limited group of patients, electromyographic studies were also performed. These studies showed excellent preservation of muscle function (Figs. 10,11).

SUMMARY

The sliding gluteus maximus flap and its variations allow closure of small and truly massive lower trunk midline defects. This can be done with preservation of muscle function important in the ambulatory patient.

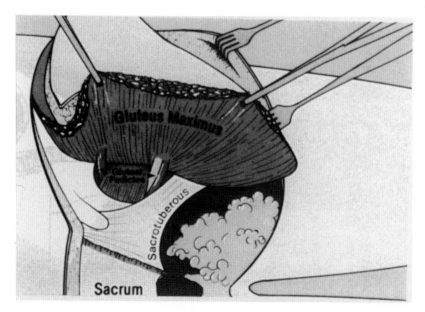

FIG. 6. Detachment of the muscle off the sacrotuberous ligament ischiorectal fat is key for its advancement. (From Ramirez et al., ref. 3, with permission.)

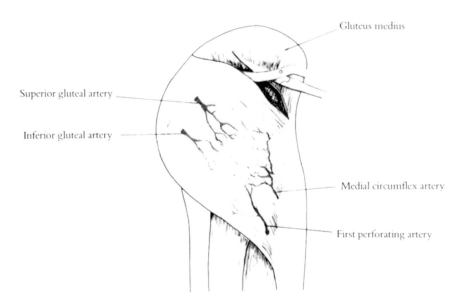

FIG. 7. The four vessels that supply the gluteus maximus muscle. Observe the orientation of the fibers of the gluteus medius. (From Ramirez et al., ref. 1, with permission.)

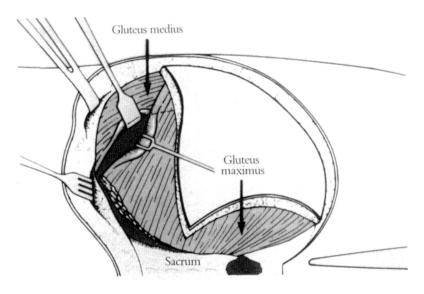

FIG. 8. Separation of the gluteus maximus off the medius is another important step of the operation. (From Ramirez et al., ref. 1, with permission.)

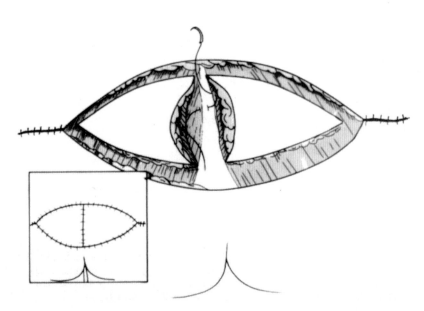

FIG. 9. The periosteal origin of the muscle is sutured to the opposite member. Closure of the donor defect in a V-Y fashion. (From Ramirez et al., ref. 1, with permission.)

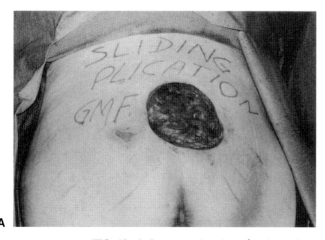

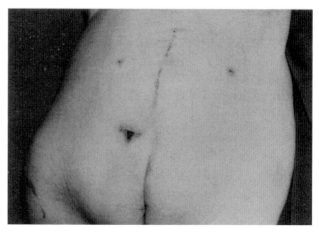

A   B

FIG. 10. A: Intraoperative view of patient prior to modified sliding gluteal plication. B: Postoperative view of patient following modified sliding gluteal plication.

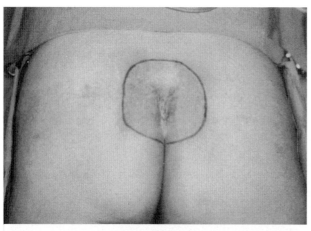

A,B

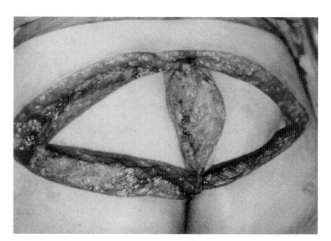

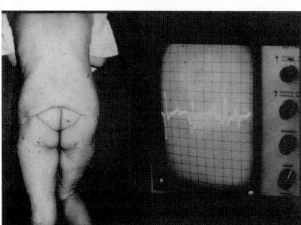

C

FIG. 11. A: Preoperative view of patient with large area of scarring from radiation necrosis. B: Intraoperative view showing triangular flaps incised and approximated in the midline. C: Postoperative view showing healed flaps. Electromyographic studies show intact neuromuscular function.

References

1. Ramirez OM, Orlando JC, Hurwitz DJ. The sliding gluteus maximus myocutaneous flap: its relevance in ambulatory patients. *Plast Reconstr Surg* 1984;74:68.
2. Ramirez OM, Hurwitz DJ, Futrell JW. The expansive gluteus maximus flap. *Plast Reconstr Surg* 1984;74:727.
3. Ramirez OM, Swartz WM, Futrell JW. The gluteus maximus muscle: experimental and clinical considerations relevant to reconstruction in ambulatory patients. *Br J Plast Surg* 1987;40:1.
4. Ramirez OM. The distal gluteus maximus advancement musculocutaneous flap for coverage of trochanteric pressure sores. *Ann Plast Surg* 1987; 18:295.
5. Ramirez OM. The sliding plication gluteus maximus musculocutaneous flap for reconstruction of sacrococcygeal wound. *Ann Plast Surg* 1990;24:223.
6. Williams PL, ed. *Gray's anatomy,* 38th ed. New York: Churchill Livingstone, 1995.

CHAPTER 448 ■ SLIDE-SWING SKIN AND MUSCULOCUTANEOUS FLAP

J. SCHRUDDE AND V. PETROVICI

The slide-swing skin and musculocutaneous flap is well suited for coverage of sacral defects (1–4).

INDICATIONS

None of the numerous other procedures offered over the years produces the advantages of the procedure described here (5–9). In recent publications, the use of various rotation flaps is frequently advocated (10–12); however, the rotation flap has some disadvantages. It can be used to close only relatively small bedsores. Extensive supplementary revisions are required when creating and mobilizing rotation flaps, causing additional scars; and scars, especially in paraplegics, offer little resistance to stress and can be the starting point for new bedsores.

The slide-swing flap (SSF) is used most often for covering large defects in the sacral region. Its application extends to chronic fistulas, unstable scars (Fig. 3), radiation ulcers (Fig. 4), pressure ulcers (Fig. 5), and various dysplasias, such as hairy nevi.

ANATOMY

Although the SSF is a random flap, the general direction of blood vessels should be considered in flap design. The anatomic particulars of the sacral region will influence the operative procedure, keeping in mind that the sacrum lies directly under the skin. The gluteal region provides great reserves of muscle and skin (see Figs. 4 and 5). The gluteus maximus muscle can be included with the flap to create a more robust musculocutaneous flap.

FLAP DESIGN AND DIMENSIONS (SEE CHAPTER 111)

The extent of the subsurface defect is explored by forceps, and the defect boundaries are drawn on the skin. After the extent of the defect has been determined, the flap can be planned.

In cases of an unfavorable ratio of length to width as in type II SSFs or in cases of very deep ulcers, portions of the gluteal muscle are included in the flap to ensure a better flap blood supply (Figs. 1, 2). If the defect is located in the upper region of the sacrum, inclusion of the lower portions of the latissimus dorsi in the flap will improve the results (see Fig. 5). Because mistakes in cutting the flap cannot be corrected, precise design and remeasurement of the flap are of great importance.

OPERATIVE TECHNIQUE

The incisions should be carried down to the muscle layer. Not only the ulcer proper but all scar tissue is excised. The excision should be carried out en bloc to avoid contact with infected surfaces.

The principles and technique of the slide-swing flap are discussed in more detail in Chapter 111. The donor site is closed before suturing the flap in place. Suction drainage, for about a week, is introduced to prevent any hematoma. With this method, two or three ulcers can be treated in one session.

All pressure on the flap must be avoided during the first few postoperative days. After the sutures are removed, 13 to 14 days postoperatively, the patient is permitted freedom of movement; however, sitting on the flap should not occur until after 5 to 6 weeks.

The same operative technique can be used in cases of chronic fistulas or radiation ulcers. Preoperative visualization of fistulas by contrast radiography is obligatory. In patients with radiation ulcers, preoperative radiographs are helpful in finding osteomyelitic bone.

CLINICAL RESULTS

Marginal or partial necrosis is the main complication. This is most likely to occur when the patient rests lying on his or her back and exerts pressure on the operated area. If granulation tissue or parts of a fistula have been left behind, recurrence of the fistula is most likely. Hematomas under the flap should be suctioned off at once. Healing by secondary intention is frequently observed in operated radiation ulcers, because radical excision cannot be achieved in all cases.

SUMMARY

The slide-swing skin or musculocutaneous flap can be effectively used for covering defects in the sacral region.

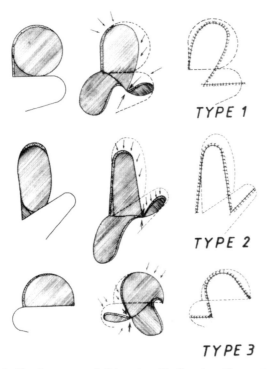

TYPE 1

TYPE 2

TYPE 3

FIG. 1. The three types of slide-swing skin flaps (see Chapter 102). (From Schrudde and Petrovici, ref. 4, with permission.)

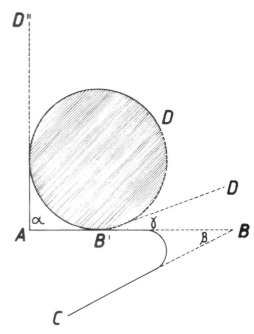

FIG. 2. Geometric principles of the slide-swing flap with exchange of asymmetrical triangles (see Chapter 111). (From Schrudde and Petrovici, ref. 4, with permission.)

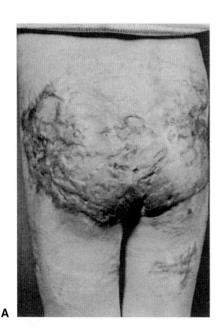

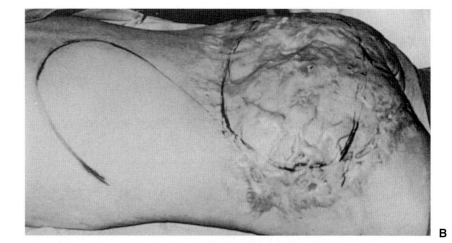

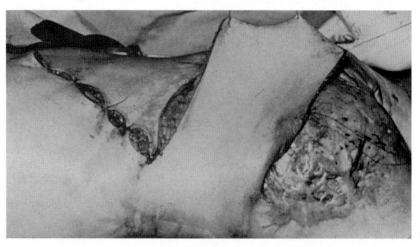

FIG. 3. **A:** Extensive burn scar area on buttocks of a 3-year-old child, causing a substantial functional deficit. **B:** A large type I slide-swing flap (SSF) from the back is planned. **C:** The flap has been cut and put into position to estimate how much of the scar area can be excised. *(Continued)*

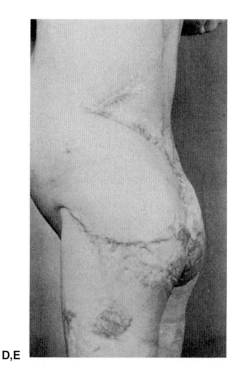
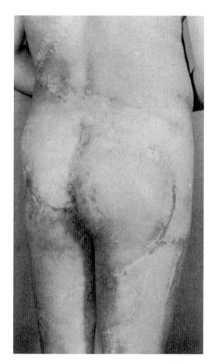

FIG. 3. *Continued* D: Result after 5 months. E: Final result after three more operations, including another SSF for coverage of right buttock.

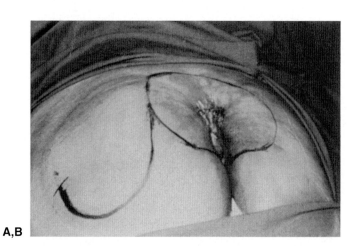
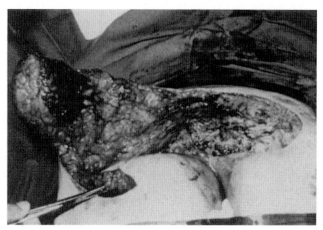

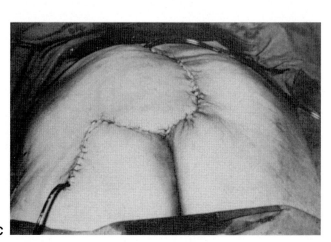

FIG. 4. A: Coverage of the sacrum with deep radiation damage. B: Portions of the gluteal musculature are included in this musculocutaneous flap. C: The flap inset and the donor site are closed primarily.

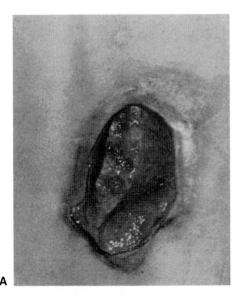

A

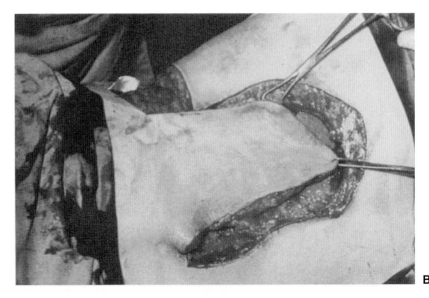

B

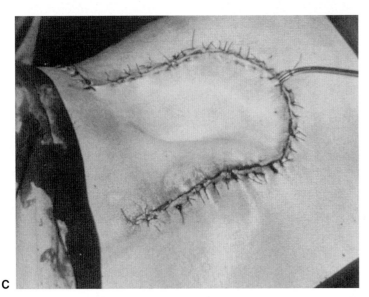

C

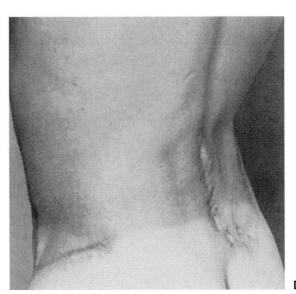

D

FIG. 5. **A:** Deep soft-tissue defect, 18 × 14 cm, due to pressure necrosis in lumbosacral region. **B:** Application of a slide-swing musculocutaneous flap, type I. The lower part of the latissimus dorsi muscle has been included in the flap. **C:** The flap inset and the donor site are closed primarily. **D:** Result 1 year.

References

1. Schrudde J. Deckung von Hautdefekten durch gestielte Lappenplastik. *Aesthet Med* 1963;12:166.
2. Wahle H, Schrudde J, Olivari N. Zur konservativen and operativen Behandlung von Druckgeschwueren bei Paraplegikem. *Z Neurolog Psych* 1971;39:653.
3. Olivari N, Schrudde J, Wahle H. The surgical treatment of bedsores in paraplegics. *Plast Reconstr Surg* 1972;50:477.
4. Schrudde J, Petrovici V. Unfallbedingte Spaetschaedigungen des Hautund Subkutangewebes. *Chir Geg* 1975;4:2.
5. Conway H, Griffith BH. Plastic surgery for closure of decubitus ulcers in patients with paraplegia: based on experience with 1000 cases. *Am J Surg* 1956;99:946.
6. Dansereau JG, Conway H. Closure of decubiti in paraplegics. *Plast Reconstr Surg* 1964;33:474.
7. Schmidt-Tintemann U. Die plastische Deckund des sacralen Dekubitus. *Langenbecks Arch Chir* 1965;309:117.
8. Zellner PR, Meinecke FW. Anzeigetechnik verschiedener plastischer Operationsverfahren bei Druckgeschwueren. *Chir Plast* 1966;2:115.
9. Griffith BH. Pressure Sores. In: Grabb WC, eds. *Plastic surgery.* Boston: Little, Brown, 3rd Ed., 1979;818.
10. Ger R, Levine SA. The management of decubitus ulcers by muscle transposition. *Plast Reconstr Surg* 1976;58:419.
11. Hurwitz DJ, Swartz WM, Mathes SJ. The gluteal thigh flap: a reliable sensate flap for the closure of buttock and perineal wounds. *Plast Reconstr Surg* 1981;68:521.
12. Scheflan M, Nahai F, Bostwick J. Gluteus maximus island musculocutaneous flap for closure of sacral and ischial ulcers. *Plast Reconstr Surg* 1981;68:533.

Online Chapter

CHAPTER 449. Thoracolumbar-Sacral Flap *J. H. Binns and S. C. Vyas*

www.encyclopediaofflaps.com

CHAPTER 450 ■ INTERCOSTAL NEUROVASCULAR ISLAND SKIN FLAP

R. K. DANIEL AND C. L. KERRIGAN

EDITORIAL COMMENT

This is a very innovative flap, particularly because it was hoped that it would provide sensibility to a paralyzed patient. The difficulty of the operative procedure and the variability of the sensibility results have decreased its use.

The intercostal island flap has many applications in torso reconstruction (1–5). It can provide a large skin area with a permanent blood supply to close defects secondary to radiation or tumor excision. With modifications, it can be used as a sensory skin flap for paraplegics or as a compound osteocutaneous flap for chest-wall reconstruction.

INDICATIONS

The clinical applications for torso reconstruction are virtually limitless, as any intercostal bundle on either side can be selected. Because the length is expandable, the flap can reach from the nape of the neck to the sacrum and sweep the torso like the hands of a clock, even reaching the contralateral chest. This flap is our first choice for children with multiple recurrent pressure sores overlying a prominent lumbar kyphosis.

ANATOMY

The anatomy of the intercostal flap is based on a thorough understanding of the course of an intercostal neurovascular bundle. For simplification, this course can be divided into four segments (see Fig. 1A, B). From the posterior midline to the anterior midline, the subdivisions consist of the vertebral, costal groove, intermuscular, and rectus segments. Throughout, the venous system parallels the arterial.

The *vertebral* segment extends from the aorta to the commencement of the costal groove of the rib and measures approximately 8 cm long. The segmental intercostal artery arises from the aorta and can be located in the middle of the interspace. As it continues distally, it approaches the cephalad rib to reach the beginning of the costal groove. The course of the intercostal nerve parallels the vessel and lies caudal to it. In the proximal portion of this segment, the artery gives rise to three branches: the dorsal branch, the nutrient branch to the rib, and the collateral branch that follows the main trunk but assumes a position adjacent to the caudal rib. This segment is not dissected in an island flap but is dissected for the transfer of a free intercostal flap. This

segment also does not contribute to the length of the flap, because the pivot point for rotation is the juncture of vertebral and costal groove segments.

The *costal groove* segment begins at the costal groove and extends to the level of insertion of the abdominal musculature and diaphragm onto the ribs. It measures approximately 12 cm long. Under protection of the costal groove, the neurovascular bundle assumes a course deep to the external and internal intercostal muscles but superficial to the innermost intercostal muscle and the parietal pleura. In this segment, the vessels give rise to numerous large musculocutaneous perforators at intervals of 1 to 3 cm. In the distal portion of the segment corresponding to the midaxillary line, vessels and nerves give off their lateral cutaneous branches that perforate the intercostal muscle to attain a subcutaneous position. This branch itself subsequently divides into posterior and anterior branches that travel in a subcutaneous course to supply and innervate the overlying cutaneous territory.

The *intermuscular* segment extends from the costal attachment of the abdominal musculature to the lateral border of the rectus muscle and is approximately 12 cm long. The neurovascular bundle travels in a plane between the internal oblique and the transversus abdominis muscle. The most confusing anatomy is at the transition point between the costal groove and intermuscular segments. At this level, the transversus abdominis and diaphragm are attached to the inner surface of the costal cartilages. The neurovascular bundle is located between this musculature and the costal cartilage.

The *rectus* segment corresponds to the width of the rectus muscle and averages 8 cm long. The neurovascular bundle courses deep to the rectus muscle, where it anastomoses with the epigastric vessels at the muscle midpoint. From this anastomosis arise perforators to supply the muscle and overlying skin.

FLAP DESIGN AND DIMENSIONS

The maximum dimensions of the cutaneous segment have not been determined. Experimental evidence suggests that one interspace can support a flap up to 8.6 interspaces wide; thus, flap size is limited by ease of donor-site closure. Our largest flap to date measures 18 × 12.5 cm. The location of the skin flap may be anywhere along the course of the intercostal neurovascular bundle. If located over the rectus segment, the blood supply will come from the deep vessels, the innervation will come from the main intercostal nerve, and the flap should be elevated in a submuscular plane. If the flap is located over the intermuscular or costal groove segment, the blood supply will come from the deep vessels, but innervation will come from the lateral cutaneous branch. Skin flaps that

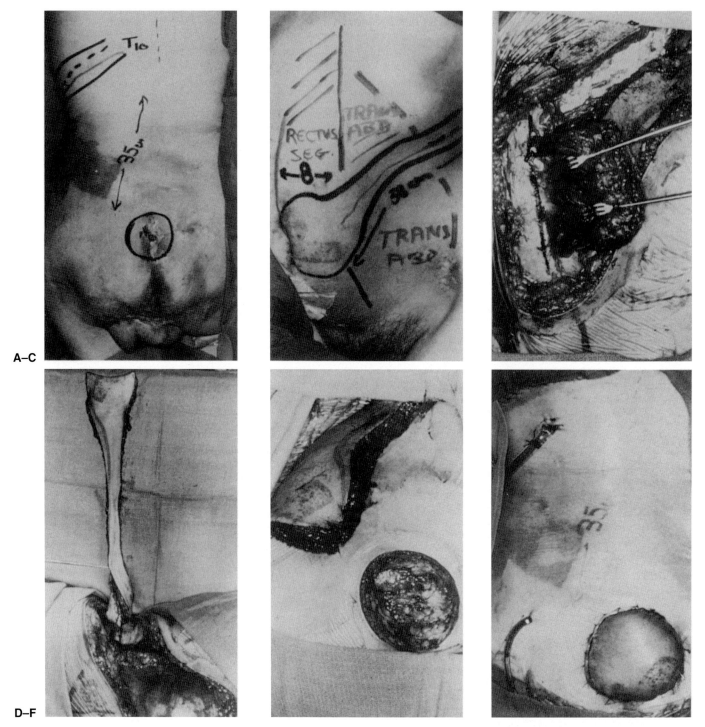

A–C

D–F

FIG. 1. Closure of a sacral ulcer in a paraplegic using an intercostal island flap. **A,B:** T10 neurovascular intercostal flap is outlined with the skin paddle overlying the rectus segment and abutting a previous midline incision. **C:** The lateral rectus segment is incorporated into the flap before the transversus abdominis. **D:** The flap completely isolated with the thorax opened but the peritoneum closed. **E:** The flap easily reaches the sacral defect. The skin overlying the pedicle is removed before passage through the tunnel. **F:** The flap in place following passage through the interconnecting tunnel.

cross the abdominal midline are dependent on somewhat sparse vascular connections and should not exceed the contralateral rectus segment.

The most dorsal pivot point of the island flap is the lateral border of the sacrospinatus muscles, corresponding to the posterior angle of the rib. The arc of rotation is 360 degrees, with an average radius of 38 cm. The flap may be rotated to the adjacent thorax, to the posterior aspect of the shoulder, to the ipsilateral and contralateral backs, to the posterior midline, and to the sacrum. The longest radius of this arc that we have used is 42 cm, from T9-10 interspace to the sacrum. It should be noted that superior rotation requires maximum resection of the rib above to avoid kinking the pedicle.

The approximate recipient-site requirements are determined, and the distance from this site to the pivot point of the flap is measured. The interspace to be used is chosen (usually T9 or T10), and the length of the pedicle along the interspace is drawn (see Fig. 1A, B). The cutaneous portion of the flap is then centered over the interspace at the appropriate distance from the pivot point. Sensory flaps are best designed with the patient's arm at the side so as not to distort the cutaneous interspace relationship.

OPERATIVE TECHNIQUE

Flap elevation is divided into three key steps: (1) isolation of the vascular pedicle, (2) elevation of the cutaneous paddle, and (3) fusion of the cutaneous paddle and its vascular pedicle (Fig. 1).

To isolate the vascular pedicle, an incision is made along the interspace to be used from the posterior pivot point to the dorsal outline of the flap. The incision is carried down to the fascia, and the skin is retracted superiorly and inferiorly to expose the ribs above and below the interspace. Scalpel incision is carried down to and through the rib periosteum on both ribs. A complete and careful subperiosteal dissection of the cephalad rib is carried out without damage to the intercostal vessels. The portion of the caudal rib adjacent to the selected interspace is similarly exposed. The cephalad rib is then excised as far dorsally as possible. The pleural cavity is entered next, and by sharp dissection, the entire length of the exposed interspace is divided from the interspace above and from the rib below.

To elevate the skin paddle, the incision around the skin flap is made down to the fascia. When the flap is located over the rectus segment, the greatest vascularity is ensured if the rectus muscle and the lateral third of its posterior sheath are elevated with it. The dissection is thus down to, but not through, the peritoneum. With the flap located over the intermuscular segment, the full thickness of abdominal musculature should be included to ensure preservation of the vascular network.

To join the cutaneous paddle to the proximal portion of its vascular pedicle, the deep surface of the flap is dissected free from the peritoneum until the diaphragm is encountered. The costal cartilage (if crossing over the path of the neurovascular bundle) is incised on both sides of the flap and may be left in place. The remaining soft tissues between the flap and the interspace then are divided.

Flap Insetting

A large subcutaneous tunnel is created from the pivot point of the flap to the recipient defect. This procedure is facilitated by the use of a tunneler (employed by vascular surgeons for femoral-popliteal bypasses). The flap is passed gently through the tunnel, being careful not to kink or twist the vascular pedicle. The flap is sutured in position, and the donor site is closed after placement of a chest tube in the pleural cavity.

CLINICAL RESULTS

In our series of 13 patients, we have used the flap to cover the following sites: (1) sacrum, 8; (2) chest wall, 2; and (3) axilla/shoulder, 3. The etiology of the defects included pressure ulceration, tumor excision, radiation, and infection. The youngest patient was aged 5 years, the oldest 63. The principal contraindications have been obesity and chronic pulmonary problems.

The reliability of the flap is excellent, and there has not been significant loss of any flap—a tribute to its durability. Sensation has been maintained in the island flaps, and, to date, pressure sores have not recurred in the sacral region. Our initial patient was seen 7 years postoperatively, and skin coverage was both stable and sensate.

The actual complications are relatively few: intraoperative damage of the neurovascular pedicle and postoperative compression of the pedicle. The former is prevented by a straight-through incision into the pleural cavity above and below the designated interspace rather than by attempting to tease the pedicle out without penetrating the pleura. Compression is best avoided by creating a broad interconnecting tunnel (8 cm minimum) and proximal resection of the rib, if it is transposed superiorly. Growth of a rib along the pedicle is inevitable if the periosteum is included, but it is of little consequence. As with any new surgical procedure, practice dissections in the anatomic laboratory will facilitate clinical execution.

SUMMARY

The intercostal island flap has multiple applications for torso reconstruction. It can be used to provide sensation to the sacral area in paraplegics, especially children.

References

1. Dibble DG. Use of a long island flap to bring sensation to the sacral area in young paraplegics. *Plast Reconstr Surg* 1974;54:220.
2. Daniel RK, Terzis JK, Cunningham DM. Sensory skin flaps for coverage of pressure sores in paraplegic patients: a preliminary report. *Plast Reconstr Surg* 1976;58:317.
3. Daniel RK, Kerrigan CL, Gard DA. The great potential of the intercostal flap for torso reconstruction. *Plast Reconstr Surg* 1978;61:653.
4. Kerrigan CL, Daniel RK. The intercostal flap: an anatomical and hemodynamic approach. *Ann Plast Surg* 1979;2:411.
5. Shively RE, Schafer ME, Kernahan DA. The spread of sensibility into previously anesthetic skin following intercostal flap transfer in a paraplegic. *Ann Plast Surg* 1980;5:396.
6. Little JW, Fontana DJ, McCulloch DT. The upper quadrant flap. *Plast Reconstr Surg* 1981;68:175.

CHAPTER 451 ■ UPPER QUADRANT ABDOMINAL MUSCULOCUTANEOUS RIB-SKIN FLAP

J. W. LITTLE, III

The intercostal neurovascular island skin flap (1–4), when sizable or extended toward the midline, is considered to require surgical delay (2–4) or double intercostal pedicles (3,5). The following expanded transpleural technique broadens and deepens the thoracic pedicle, the abdominal paddle, and the critical thoracoabdominal transition, thereby speeding elevation and enhancing the circulatory vigor of the flap (6).

The nomenclature emphasizes not the well-recognized intercostal nature of the thoracic pedicle, but the full-thickness nature of the abdominal paddle, representing, as it were, the virtual entire upper abdominal quadrant, with rectus muscle and deep epigastric systems included. Through the presence of these latter, impressive extensions of contralateral upper quadrant and ipsilateral lower-quadrant abdominal wall have been possible.

INDICATIONS

The execution of this flap, involving an open thoracoabdominal approach, must be considered an exceptional surgical undertaking and is not, therefore, indicated where surface flaps are available and will do as well. Beyond concerns for acute pulmonary complications and long-term abdominal support, operative morbidity includes 1 week of considerable postoperative pain. The special virtues of this flap, however, sensibility and remarkable vascularity through a long pedicle, easily justify its use in special circumstances.

In sensory reconstruction, of course, the pedicle must originate above the sensory level. Such is frequently possible when treating the dorsal defects of myelodysplastic children, in whom ulcers tend to overlie the spinal deformities and hence the sensory lesions themselves. It is less often possible in treating the conventional pressure sores of the acquired paraplegic. The highest pedicle that can cover the sacrum without insensible extension of its paddle is T8. Microsurgical anastomosis of the intercostal nerve to one above the level of sensory loss is a possible solution to this problem (3). The T11 pedicle with a modest inferior extension of the paddle can cover the ischial region and may be indicated for a troublesome ischial sore in a paraplegic with a sensory level fortuitously falling between T11 and L2-3. For levels below L2-3, which occur most commonly in myelodysplastic children, the sensory tensor fasciae latae flap carrying the lateral femoral cutaneous nerve remains the simpler and preferred source of innervated coverage.

In general reconstruction, the flap is most often indicated for large or difficult defects of the low trunk, where local solutions to sizable problems may be limited. Surely the clearest indication remains the complicated radiation defect of the lumbosacral or hip region, to which unsurpassed blood supply can be brought quickly from a remote area to ensure rapid per primam healing (see Fig. 3).

ANATOMY (3,4)

The thoracic course of the major neurovascular bundle is deep within the intercostal space, at points immediately applied to the parietal pleura; its abdominal course runs between the transversus abdominis and internal oblique abdominis muscles. Collateral vascular pathways also run within the musculature of the intercostal space. Innervation of the skin overlying the rectus muscle is by way of the main intercostal trunk, and that of the abdominal wall lateral to the muscle is through the lateral cutaneous branch that arises from the deep trunk in the midaxillary line and thereafter follows a subcutaneous course (Fig. 1).

Additional points are pertinent (6). The major neurovascular bundle, in passing from the intercostal space to the abdominal wall, runs deep to the chondral syncytium of the costal margin. The scanty transversus abdominis muscle arises from the inner surfaces of the cartilages of the lower six

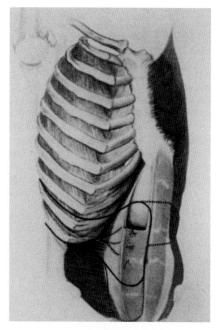

FIG. 1. Planned incisions. (From Little et al., ref. 6, with permission.)

ribs, in common with the diaphragm, at some distance within the costal margin. The deep intercostal vessels anastomose freely with the superior and inferior deep epigastric systems after perforating from beneath the lateral third of the posterior rectus sheath to reach the undersurface of the muscle. The perforating vessels of the anterior rectus sheath support an impressive circulation across the abdominal midline.

FLAP DESIGN AND DIMENSIONS

Extended skin paddles can exceed 25 × 25 cm and are considered limited only by the ability to restore the abdominal defect. Certainly, no flap has shown even marginal ischemia of any border at any time. The pivot point of this true island flap occurs at the intersection of the selected interspace with the lateral border of the sacrospinalis muscle, one hand's breadth off the spine. The arc of rotation of extended flaps is impressive. A T10 pedicle with extended paddle reaches the ipsilateral trochanter and ischium; a T9 pedicle with similar extension reaches the occiput (Fig. 2).

The ninth, tenth, or occasionally other intercostal space is selected as the pedicle for the flap, and spaces above and below are marked as superior and inferior margins. These relationships should be determined with the patient's arm at the side, so that the subcutaneous portion of the pedicle will not be displaced but will accurately overlie the desired interspace and thus carry the appropriate lateral cutaneous nerve. The abdominal paddle is drawn flush to the midline, centered at the umbilicus in the case of the T10 pedicle, somewhat higher for T9. Its size is limited only by the requirements of the defect. The pedicle marking then is blended to the abdominal paddle over the region of the costal margin.

OPERATIVE TECHNIQUE

Thoracic incisions are made to fascia and carried at this level to the rib of the selected interspace (the tenth, for a T10 pedicle) above and to its inferior neighbor (the eleventh) below, where they are deepened through muscle and periosteum onto rib (Fig. 3).

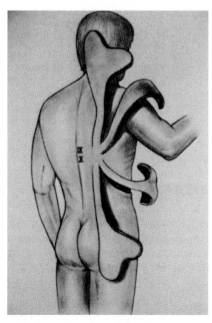

FIG. 2. Arcs of rotation.

Behind the posterior axillary line, it is neither necessary to include skin and subcutaneous tissue in the pedicle (the lateral cutaneous nerve does not become superficial until the midaxillary line) nor to divide the latissimus dorsi muscle, which instead may be retracted intact or used in some other way (as, for example, a reversed muscle flap (9)). The upper rib is removed subperiosteally from the sacrospinalis muscle to the costochondral junction, and the thorax is entered through the midportion of the periosteal bed over this extent. The superior border of the lower rib then is freed subperiosteally; without removing this rib, the superior aspect of its bed is similarly entered behind the rib.

Now that the pedicle has been completed by rapid, parallel full-thickness cuts into the thoracic cavity, attention is turned to the abdominal paddle. It is incised along the midline into the underlying rectus sheath and along the superior and inferior margins through both the anterior sheath and rectus muscle, dividing and ligating the deep epigastric vessels where encountered. The muscle is lifted bluntly from the underlying posterior sheath from medial to lateral until perforating vessels are encountered (usually at the junction of the middle and lateral thirds of the sheath). These vessels are necessary for survival of the undelayed flap across the midline and are spared by deepening the dissection through the posterior sheath onto the peritoneum just at their appearance.

The remainder of the abdominal dissection is rapidly performed at the level of the intact peritoneum, dividing skin, subcutaneous tissue, and abdominal wall musculature along the superior and inferior margins of the paddle until the costal margin is reached. Here the deep dissection of transversus muscle from peritoneum continues well beneath the costal margin onto the diaphragm. The elevated abdominal paddle is joined to the dissected thoracic pedicle. The cartilaginous portion of the upper rib is removed, and the upper incision is joined full-thickness. Below, the J-shaped portion of terminal cartilage crossing the interspace is divided flush with the lower incision and carried with the flap. This situation occurs regularly when the ninth interspace is used, including a portion of chondral tenth rib in the flap. It does not occur when the lower tenth interspace is used. The presence of the main neurovascular bundle deep to this cartilage and of the collateral systems superficial to it is considered to make its removal hazardous, jeopardizing the surviving length of ambitious flaps. Subsequent removal from the recipient site with the patient under local anesthesia remains a simple prospect, although no such removal has been necessary to date. Now the remaining soft-tissue attachments are divided, connecting paddle to pedicle and incorporating a small portion of diaphragm to ensure total inclusion of transversus abdominis muscle in this critical transition zone.

The initial design may incorporate paddle extensions across the midline to include the contralateral abdominal upper quadrant or inferiorly to include the ipsilateral lower quadrant (Fig. 1). When crossing the midline to include the former, the midline fusion is divided deeply at the level of the posterior rectus sheath. The contralateral anterior rectus sheath is included to carry the additional skin. When taking the lower abdominal wall, underlying rectus muscle is included, along with that portion of the lateral posterior sheath bearing perforating intercostal branches. Thus two thirds to three quarters of the abdominal wall can be transferred with ease and speed. The flap can be raised in less than 1 hour.

Of course, a considerable abdominal and thoracic wall defect remains in the wake of this elevation. The thoracic defect is closed in a straightforward manner by approximation of the remaining ribs with heavy intercostal sutures. It is usually necessary to remove an additional small part of cut proximal rib to ensure that intercostal closure does not compress

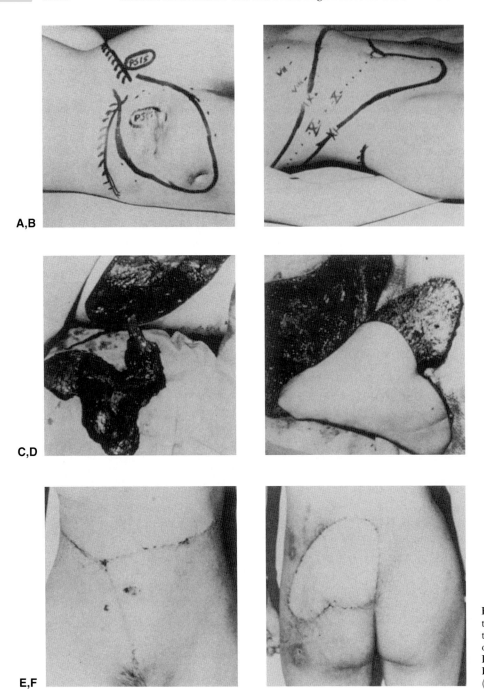

A,B

C,D

E,F

FIG. 3. A 19-year-old woman with radiation-treated sacroiliac sarcoma. **A:** Planned resection. **B:** Planned incisions. **C:** Extended paddle on T10 pedicle with part of secondary defect. **D:** Contralateral extension denuded for filler. **E, F:** Wounds healing without complication (From Little et al., ref. 6, with permission.)

the exiting pedicle. The diaphragm is reattached to the closed chest wall, but no effort is made to close the pleura, sealing the chest instead with a multiple overlapping soft-tissue closure. A chest tube is inserted.

The abdominal defect is more of a problem because support must be returned to that portion of abdominal wall between the residual posterior rectus sheath (medial two thirds) and the closed costal margin. This step is accomplished by splitting off flaps from the remaining abdominal musculature and fascia, including lower external oblique muscle and fascia and contralateral rectus sheath. Skin closure is accomplished directly after extensive undermining. The flap then is tunneled subcutaneously to the area of the wound, which is approached now that the chest and abdominal wounds have been closed. The skin of the pedicle is excised, conserving the subcutaneous component and its lateral cutaneous nerve.

Longitudinal traction on the pedicle does not appear to be detrimental, as the intact layer of parietal pleura prevents undue tension on the vessels themselves.

CLINICAL RESULTS

Of six flaps raised to or beyond the midline, all have survived entirely without signs of compromise. All healing was per primam, including three patients treated for extensive radiation defects. All flaps were sensate, four immediately and two after some delay. No defects have recurred over a 1- to 3-year follow-up.

There have been no complications in this series. All chest tubes were removed during the first week following an unremarkable pulmonary course in all patients.

Abdominal support has remained satisfactory in all patients. The segmental loss of rectus abdominis muscle has not been noticed. Vertical shortening of the hemithorax through rib resection and intercostal closure has produced no postural deformity.

SUMMARY

The upper quadrant abdominal musculocutaneous rib-skin flap is basically an extension of the intercostal neurovascular island flap. Although it involves a transpleural technique, it is a more robust flap that is technically less difficult to perform.

References

1. Dibbell DG. Use of a long island flap to bring sensation to the sacral area in young paraplegics: case report. *Plast Reconstr Surg* 1974;54:220.
2. Daniel RK, Terzis JK, Cunningham DM. Sensory skin flaps for coverage of pressure sores in paraplegic patients: a preliminary report. *Plast Reconstr Surg* 1976;58:317.
3. Daniel RK, Kerrigan CL, Gard DA. The great potential of the intercostal flap for torso reconstruction. *Plast Reconstr Surg* 1978;61:653.
4. Kerrigan CL, Daniel RK. The intercostal flap: anatomical and hemodynamic approach. *Ann Plast Surg* 1979;2:411.
5. Daniel RK. The upper quadrant flap (Discussion). *Plast Reconstr Surg* 1981;68:183.
6. Little JW, Fontana DJ, McCulloch DT. The upper quadrant flap. *Plast Reconstr Surg* 1981;68:175.

CHAPTER 452 ■ PARAVERTEBRAL OSTEOMUSCULAR FLAP

J. C. MUSTARDÉ

Most problems arising in the management of babies with spina bifida are due to damage to the spinal cord, occurring occasionally in later childhood, but most often during, after, and possibly before birth. It is obvious that the cord is more likely to be damaged in babies who are born with meningomyeloceles (Fig. 1), where the primitive neural tissue of the cord has remained untubed and where its surface is exposed, with failure of development also of the skin, muscle, bone, and neural coverings that are normally present along the spine.

INDICATIONS

Tubing, followed by dural covering of the neural plaque, presents little problem, but provision of adequate skin covering that will protect the spinal cord permanently is more difficult to achieve (Fig. 2A, B). Skin flaps in the dorsal region are not readily raised and moved without running into vascular problems, and they tend to leave scars close to the midline. Apart from this, skin flaps alone can offer little protection to the underlying cord in the event of blows to the lumbar region in later life.

FLAP DESIGN AND DIMENSIONS

A flap that is raised in the muscles of the paravertebral region and that includes the transverse processes of the bifid vertebrae will, on being turned over toward the midline (Fig. 2C, D) and firmly fixed to its opposite number by a line of sutures in the lumbodorsal fascia, produce a tunnel that will not only provide permanent protection for the underlying spinal cord but also will readily accept free skin grafts onto the muscle surface now exposed on the midline. This does away with the need for raising, and especially for undermining, dorsal skin flaps (1).

OPERATIVE TECHNIQUE

The neural plaque of the meningomyelocele should be tubed and closed with the dural covering. The osteomuscular flaps are developed by incising the paravertebral muscle mass and fracturing the transverse processes (Fig. 2). The lumbodorsal muscles are incised down to the tips of the lateral processes (Fig. 3A). Then the lumbodorsal muscle mass is grasped by Lane's tissue forceps and turned toward the midline, thus fracturing the lateral vertebral processes (Fig. 3B, C). The paravertebral osteomuscular flap therefore creates a protective bony canal for the spinal cord. The lumbodorsal muscle mass is included with the flap to carry the blood supply to the bone (Fig. 3D). Because the muscle is left exposed dorsally, it provides an excellent bed for skin grafts.

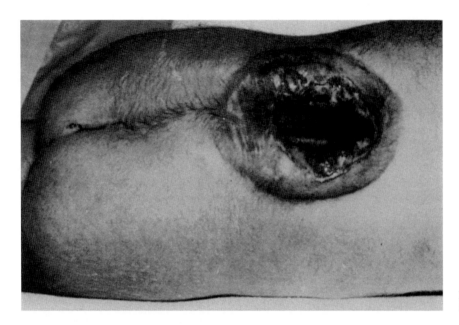

FIG. 1. Meningomyelocele in the newborn infant, showing exposed neural plaque.

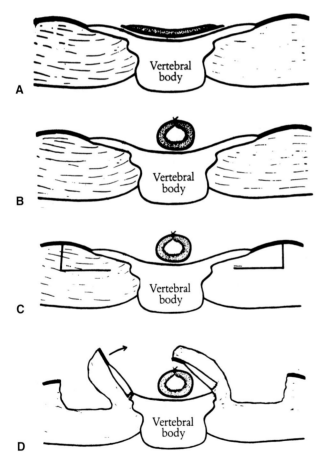

FIG. 2. Schematic representation of transverse section through a meningomyelocele. **A, B:** Tubing of the neural plaque with closure of dural covering. **C, D:** Development of the osteomuscular flaps by incising paravertebral muscle mass and fracturing the transverse processes. (From Mustardé, ref. 1, with permission.)

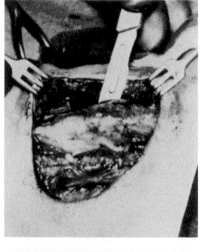
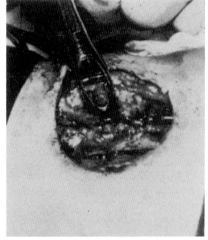

A,B

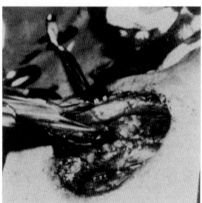
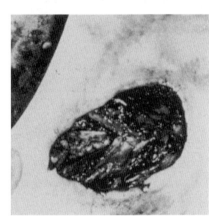
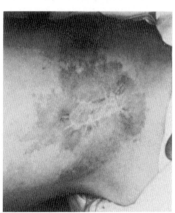

C–E

FIG. 3. Paravertebral osteomuscular flap used to construct a protective spinal canal. **A:** The cord has been tubed and the dural covering closed. The lumbodorsal muscles are being incised down to the tips of the lateral processes. **B, C:** The lumbodorsal muscle mass, grasped by Lane's tissue forceps and turned toward the midline, thus fracturing the lateral vertebrae processes. **D:** The osteomuscular flaps are being united from above down (the tubed cord is seen still exposed on the left), followed by union of the muscle layer superficially. **E:** Postoperative result showing well-healed skin graft over the reconstructed spine. Note development of widespread capillary nevus.

After the muscle layer is brought together in the midline, the skin of the back is closed as far as possible without any tension. The remaining defect is then skin-grafted (Fig. 3E).

CLINICAL RESULTS

An operation of this nature is obviously most effective if it can be carried out within 2 or 3 hours of birth, and in my experience, the procedure has led, if not to actual recovery of neurologic function, at least to diminution of the severity of neurologic problems in the developing child.

SUMMARY

The paravertebral osteomuscular flap can be used to close meningomyelocele defects. It provides a protective bony canal for the newly closed neural plaque. At the same time, the muscular bed permits the skin defect to be grafted.

Reference

1. Mustardé JC. *Plastic surgery in infancy and childhood*, 2nd ed. Edinburgh: Churchill-Livingstone, 1979; Chap. 26.

CHAPTER 453 ■ TRANSVERSE LUMBOSACRAL BACK FLAP

H. L. HILL, JR.

The transverse lumbosacral back flap (TLBF) (1) is presented as a reasonable alternative procedure in the coverage of medium to large soft-tissue defects of the lower lumbar spine, sacrum, and upper coccygeal areas. It applies particularly to the treatment of sacral pressure sores.

INDICATIONS

Advantages of this flap include the following: (1) it is a quick and easy procedure, (2) the flap elevation itself is relatively bloodless, (3) the donor defect is in a non-weight-bearing area, (4) muscle is not sacrificed (possibly of importance in the ambulatory patient), and (5) surgical options are preserved in cases of recurrence. (The flap itself may be reelevated and inset in some cases of recurrence.)

The primary disadvantages of the TLBF are relative and should be considered when determining the surgical options. First, the TBLF is composed of skin (albeit thick) and subcutaneous tissue, consequently lacking the bulky padding afforded by alternative musculocutaneous flaps. Second, the vascularity of the flap tip (i.e., the portion covering the defect) is empirically less dependable than that of a musculocutaneous flap. Finally, the donor defect is large, cannot usually be closed primarily, and, in the occasional patient, may prove of cosmetic concern.

Candidates for flap coverage of sacral defects are usually those in whom rehabilitation can be anticipated. Occasionally, though, it can be justified to improve hygiene and facilitate nursing care in an otherwise chronically nonrehabilitatable person.

ANATOMY

The blood supply to the skin and subcutaneous region between the lower ribs and posterior iliac crest is largely segmental. It appears that the primary vascular supply is from posterior perforating arteries of the lower intercostal vessels through the latissimus dorsi muscle and lumbar arteries through the lumbar triangle. Additional contributors include musculocutaneous perforators from the gluteus maximus muscle inferiorly and inconsistent paraspinous perforators in the midline and sacrospinalis area (1) (Fig. 1A,B).

Closer dissection of the lumbar perforators, especially L3, exposes a medially directed branch, "axially" providing blood supply to the skin near the midline (2). In the human, transaortic injection of fluorescein in a lumbar artery intraoperatively fluoresces significantly across the midline (Fig. 2A,B). The midline need not be considered a relatively avascular barrier to flap design (3–5). Specifically in regard to the transverse lumbosacral back flap, when the lumbar perforators are preserved, a portion of the flap is probably axial with a random extension across the midline.

FLAP DESIGN AND DIMENSIONS

The TLBF is designed so that its vascular pedicle is preserved along the lateral aspect of the paraspinous muscles on either side (Fig. 3A). It is extended across the midline several centimeters lateral to the contralateral perforators, which are usually identified and located. The limit of the lateral extent of this flap is unclear, although it is routinely safe 2 to 3 cm lateral to the opposite paraspinous border. There has been at least one instance in which marginal necrosis occurred with this length, but routinely, such flaps do well. (One early patient had a significant flap loss which, in retrospect, was obviously due to elevation past the vascular pedicle.) It might be recommended that fluorescein determinations of flap viability be carried out at the appropriate time in questionable flaps.

Flap width should be such that most of the lower lumbar skin is included. This prevents the secondary defect from extending over the pressure-bearing area of the sacrum.

OPERATIVE TECHNIQUE

The involved tissue is excised, and limited removal of the underlying bone is performed (Fig. 4A). The flap is usually elevated from the tip to the base, resorting to blunt dissection as the pedicles are approached, identified, and preserved. To enhance rotation, the flap may be backcut for 2 to 3 cm (probably more, because theoretically it may survive as an island). On backcutting, the vascular pedicles obviously must be included in the flap.

Following flap rotation and inset, one or two large suction drains are used. The wound is closed in two layers. The donor defect is covered with a meshed split-thickness skin graft.

Postoperative care usually includes removal of drains at 3 to 5 days and avoidance of weight-bearing on the flap for about 2 weeks.

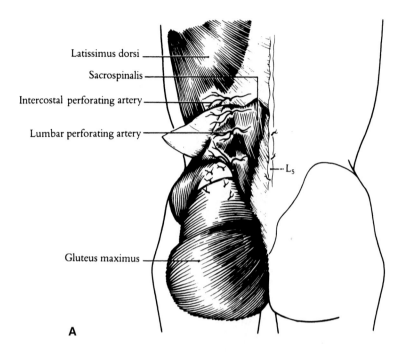

Latissimus dorsi

Sacrospinalis

Intercostal perforating artery

Lumbar perforating artery

L5

Gluteus maximus

A

Cross Section

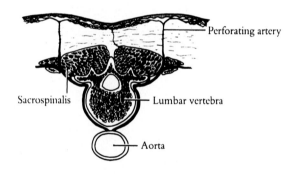

Perforating artery

Sacrospinalis

Lumbar vertebra

Aorta

Subdermal Plexus Across Midline

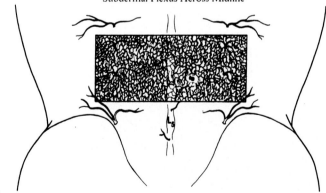

B

FIG. 1. **A:** Vascular supply of the lumbosacral skin. **B:** The existence of a vascular supply across the midline has been confirmed by experimental, cadaver, and clinical investigations. (From Hill et al., ref. 1, with permission.)

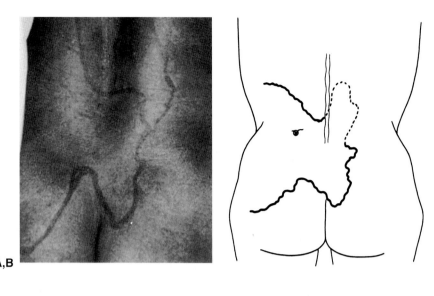

FIG. 2. A,B: Area of fluorescence outlined on the lumbosacral area of a patient injected transabdominally in a lumbar artery while undergoing abdominal aneurysmectomy. (From Hill et al., ref. 1, with permission.)

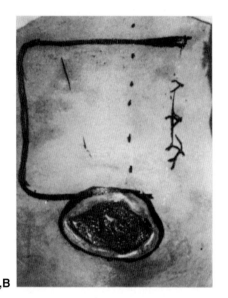
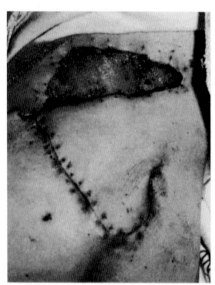

FIG. 3. A: Paraplegic with pressure sore (flap outlined). B: Two weeks postoperatively. (From Hill et al., ref. 1, with permission.)

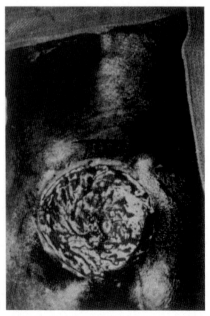
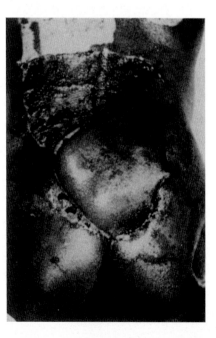

FIG. 4. A: Large sacral pressure sore following debridement. B: Three weeks postoperatively. (From Hill et al., ref. 1, with permission.)

CLINICAL RESULTS

Complications directly relating to surgery have been gratifyingly few, despite contamination of the initial wound and the relative debilitation of the patients. Partial flap loss is unusual.

SUMMARY

Approximately one fourth of all pressure sores are sacral, particularly in paralyzed or bed-ridden patients. Recurrence is all too frequent. The TLBF is a reliable surgical alternative in these usually sick and debilitated patients.

References

1. Hill HL, Brown RG, Jurkiewicz MJ. The transverse lumbosacral back flap. *Plast Reconstr Surg* 1978;62:177.
2. Daniel RK. The anatomy and hemodynamics of the cutaneous circulation and their influence on skin flap design. In: Grabb WC, Myers MB, eds. *Skin flaps.* Boston: Little, Brown, 1975;111–131.
3. Baroudi R, Pinotti JA, Edwald MK. A transverse thoracic abdominal skin flap for closure after radical mastectomy. *Plast Reconstr Surg* 1978; 61:547.
4. Hartrampf CR, Scheflan M, Black PW. Breast reconstruction following total mastectomy with a transverse abdominal island flap: anatomic and clinical observations. *Plast Reconstr Surg* 1982;69:216.
5. Davies D, Adendorff D. A large rotational flap raised across the midline to close lumbosacral defects. *Br J Plast Surg* 1977;30:1663.

CHAPTER 454 ■ BILATERAL LATISSIMUS DORSI MUSCULOCUTANEOUS ADVANCEMENT FLAPS FOR CLOSURE OF MENINGOMYELOCELE DEFECTS

J. B. MCGRAW AND J. O. PENIX

> ### EDITORIAL COMMENT
>
> The reader is advised to refer also to Chapters 416 and 419 for alternative methods of closure.

One of every 800 infants is born with spina bifida cystica. The disease includes a number of conditions in which epithelium-lined sacs filled with cerebrospinal fluid (CSF) are in free communication with the spinal subarachnoid space; there is usually associated maldevelopment of the spinal cord, some paralysis of the lower limbs and sphincter, and a variable sensory deficit.

Obtaining good coverage of the meninges is a lifesaving measure that prevents major complications and preserves maximum function. The main challenge presented by the spina bifida defect is to repair the dura adequately and to create a durable surface cover without functional loss and without excessive traumatization of very small, newborn infants.

INDICATIONS

Eighty-five percent of patients with spina bifida cystica have a myelomeningocele, with protrusion of the meningeal membranes through a defect in the vertebral column and with nerve elements found within the sac. These patients almost always have an associated motor and sensory deficit of the lower limbs, rectum, and bladder.

Fourteen percent of spina bifida cystica patients have a meningocele with no nerve elements in the sac and no associated paralysis. Rarer forms of the disease are syringomyelocele and myelocele, expressed as dilatations of the central canal of the cord and an incomplete closure of the neural groove.

All forms of the disease can be associated with other congenital anomalies, including hydrocephalus, clubfoot, dislocation of the hip, absent ribs, exstrophy of the bladder, prolapse of the uterus, Klippel-Feil deformity, congenital heart disease, and umbilical hernias. Previous options for closure included primary repair, skin grafts, or more complex repairs using rotation skin flaps or the "reversed" latissimus dorsi muscle flap.

Primary repair is rarely possible and is associated with a high incidence of wound dehiscence. Skin grafting of the meninges is frequently complicated by poor graft take, early or late breakdown of the graft, the associated meningitis, and death. Rotation flaps can provide durable coverage but at the expense of significant blood loss, an extensive and lengthy procedure, and large donor-site skin grafts. The "reversed" latissimus dorsi muscle flap offers a tedious dissection and unpredictable variability of the vascular pedicles; it also compromises latissimus dorsi muscular function, which is important to these paraplegic patients in transfer activities.

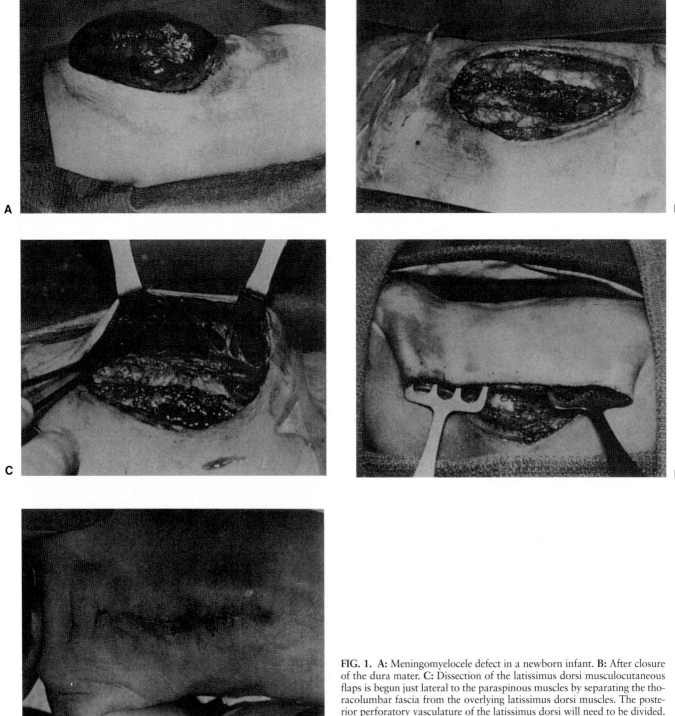

FIG. 1. A: Meningomyelocele defect in a newborn infant. **B:** After closure of the dura mater. **C:** Dissection of the latissimus dorsi musculocutaneous flaps is begun just lateral to the paraspinous muscles by separating the thoracolumbar fascia from the overlying latissimus dorsi muscles. The posterior perforatory vasculature of the latissimus dorsi will need to be divided. **D:** The latissimus dorsi musculocutaneous flap is advanced to the midline. **E:** Final result. Note that the dog-ears are setting well.

FLAP DESIGN AND DIMENSIONS

Excellent soft-tissue coverage can be obtained by using bilateral latissimus dorsi musculocutaneous advancement flaps (1); CSF shunts can be employed within 5 days of initial surgery; and discharge within 2 weeks can be reasonably expected. When a myelomeningocele defect occurs in the lower sacral area, bilateral latissimus dorsi advancement flaps are insufficient to provide total muscular coverage of the meninges. Advancement flaps of external oblique muscle or turnover flaps of gluteus maximus muscle then can be used to supplement the latissimus dorsi in these patients (2).

For cervical and high thoracic defects, bilateral trapezius musculocutaneous flaps can be advanced in much the same way as latissimus dorsi units. The muscles are exposed through a midline thoracic incision and are elevated from the paraspinous and rhomboid muscles. The lower margins of the origins are then divided, and the units can easily be advanced into the midline.

OPERATIVE PROCEDURE

The goals of the neurosurgical part of the procedure are straightforward. Neural elements are freed from cutaneous elements, a subarachnoid space is developed, and a watertight dural closure is obtained. The CSF is drained through an incision in the epidermal-arachnoid junction. Then, using sharp dissection, a circumferential incision of the dura is completed, and the epidermal-arachnoid membrane is excised flush with the neural plaque, taking care to remove all epidermal tissue from the plaque.

At this point, an anatomic arachnoid surface is created by folding the neural plaque inward, along the axis of the spine, and closing it with 4-0 chromic catgut. The dura mater is dissected laterally to the dura-dermis fusion line, or the "junctional zone."

After the dura is circumferentially separated from the dermis, it is elevated away from the underlying lumbosacral fascia, dysplastic paraspinal muscles, and posterior bony elements. It is closed in the axis of the spine using a running suture of 4-0 chromic reinforced with a layer of running 4-0 Prolene. If a significant kyphosis that will complicate or jeopardize the flap closure is present, it should be partially removed.

Dissection of the bilateral latissimus dorsi musculocutaneous flaps is begun just lateral to the paraspinous muscles by separating the thoracolumbar fascia from the overlying latissimus dorsi muscles. The plane between the paraspinous muscular fascia and the posterior edge of the latissimus dorsi muscle is often ill defined in the area of the deformity, but it can be identified superiorly in the region of the trapezius muscle. The separation between the latissimus dorsi and external oblique muscles is identified, and a submuscular plane of dissection is developed between the two muscles.

Care should be taken to avoid dissecting beneath the external oblique muscle, because a peritoneal perforation can result. The posterior perforating vasculature of the latissimus dorsi muscle is divided when encountered approximately 6 cm lateral to the midline.

Separating the origin of the latissimus dorsi muscle from the iliac crest will give additional exposure of the anterior muscle. The dissection then can be continued on the deep surface of the latissimus dorsi muscle until the anterior margin of the muscle is encountered and completely released from its fascial attachments to the skin and chest wall.

Once this dissection is completed bilaterally, the two musculocutaneous units will advance to the midline for closure. Closure should be carried out in three layers: muscle, fascia, and skin. The midline closure of the latissimus dorsi muscle is carried out with 3-0 Vicryl rather than a less substantial suture. The deep fascia and subcutaneous layers are closed with 4-0 Vicryl (Fig. 1).

CLINICAL RESULTS

The usual operative time for harvesting bilateral latissimus dorsi musculocutaneous advancement flaps is 1 hour or less, with an average blood loss of only 30 to 35 ml. These flaps are unmatched in reliability, and the dissection is straightforward. Although there is some controversy regarding the timing of the coverage, in our experience, the best results are obtained when medical and surgical interventions are carried out within the first 24 hours of life. Because of the age and size of these patients, anesthesia, monitoring, and core body temperature maintenance are essential to the success of the procedure.

In our unit, this operative procedure has been performed 147 times without a mortality. This is a significant improvement over an observed mortality of 3% to 7% with skin grafts and random skin flaps.

SUMMARY

Local musculocutaneous advancement flaps offer a safe, simple, and effective closure of myelomeningocele defects in the newborn infant. These procedures have proven to be lifesaving, decreasing mortality and morbidity without adding any long-term disability.

References

1. McCraw JB, Penix JD, Baker JW. Repair of major defects of the chest wall and spine with the latissimus dorsi myocutaneous flap. *Plast Reconstr Surg* 1978;62:197.
2. Ramirez DM, Ramasastry SS, Granick MS, et al. A new surgical approach to closure of large lumbosacral meningomyelocele defects. *Plast Reconstr Surg* 1987;80:799.

CHAPTER 455 ■ BILATERAL INTERCONNECTED LATISSIMUS DORSI–GLUTEUS MAXIMUS MUSCULOCUTANEOUS FLAPS FOR CLOSURE OF LARGE LUMBOSACRAL MENINGOMYELOCELE DEFECTS

S. S. RAMASASTRY AND O. M. RAMIREZ

EDITORIAL COMMENT

The extension of the latissimus dorsi into the gluteus is more reliable than if one were to extend it laterally. Consequently, this is a useful extension for the closure of very large and low meningomyeloceles.

To overcome the problems of significant flap complications, increased operating time, and blood loss, the en bloc advancement of bilateral interconnected latissimus dorsi and gluteus maximus musculocutaneous units without lateral relaxing incisions and back cuts can achieve primary closure of large lumbosacral meningomyelocele defects (1).

INDICATIONS

Primary wound healing can be achieved in most small thoracolumbar and lumbosacral meningomyelocele defects with wide undermining of the wound edges and direct closure of the wound. (In a series of 130 patients (2), it was discovered that only 25% required more elaborate closure techniques.)

Large meningomyelocele defects can be difficult to repair, however, and are associated with problems of wound breakdown and infection (3). We recommend a technique of closure for defects 5 cm or greater in width, where wide undermining of the skin only is fraught with significant wound complications. The procedure has been used instead of previously described methods such as advancement flaps, bipedicle flaps, rotation flaps, the paraspinous musculoosseous Mustardé technique (4) (see Chapter 452), and the latissimus dorsi musculocutaneous flap described by McCraw et al. (5) (see Chapter 454).

This technique is preferable to earlier ones for the following reasons: (1) no relaxing incisions or backcuts are used; (2) no skin grafts are needed; (3) the blood supply of the intervening skin between the latissimus dorsi and gluteus maximus muscles is more reliable; (4) the inclusion of the gluteus maximus muscle as a musculocutaneous unit provides significant superomedial advancement, facilitating closure of large defects in the low thoracolumbar and lumbosacral areas without tension; and (5) transfer of the gluteus maximus muscle should not cause any functional deficit. In addition, this composite muscle flap provides good soft-tissue padding over the neural repair.

The only contraindication is the decision by the neurosurgeon not to intervene surgically in a child with severe neurologic deficit (one patient in our series of 18 patients) or multiple severe congenital anomalies.

ANATOMY

The anatomic details of the latissimus dorsi and gluteus maximus muscles and their relevance to reconstructive surgery have been well described (6–8) (Fig. 1). The basis for our technique, using latissimus dorsi-gluteus maximus musculocutaneous flaps as a single unit, derives from injection studies of the gluteal arterial system in 20 adult and 2 neonatal cadavers. A rich anastomotic network exists between the vasculature of the skin overlying the gluteus maximus and the latissimus dorsi muscles (7). Adequate skin circulation of the lumbar area skin between the latissimus dorsi and gluteus maximus musculocutaneous territories is maintained if dissection of both these muscles is done in continuity, even if paraspinous perforators are sacrificed (Fig. 2).

OPERATIVE TECHNIQUE

During the initial neurosurgical closure of the dural defect, undermining of the skin should be avoided (Fig. 3). Following the dural repair, flap elevation is begun by incising the thoracolumbar fascia over the paraspinous muscles and carrying the dissection under the latissimus dorsi to its free border laterally. The perforating vessels are cauterized and divided in the process.

The entire latissimus dorsi then is based on the thoracodorsal vessels, which should be preserved. The latissimus dorsi muscle is then freed from its attachments to the external oblique and serratus posterior muscles by sharp dissection. The gluteus maximus muscle is detached from the iliac

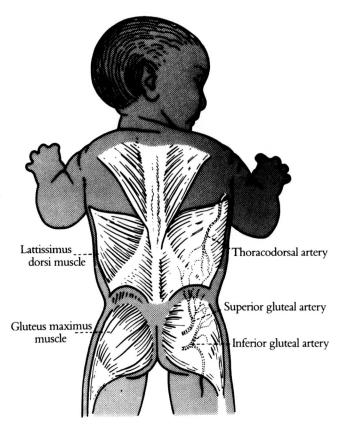

FIG. 1. The latissimus dorsi and gluteus maximus muscles shown with the major vascular pedicles: the thoracodorsal artery and the superior and inferior gluteal arteries. (The paravertebral and perforating vessels are not shown.)

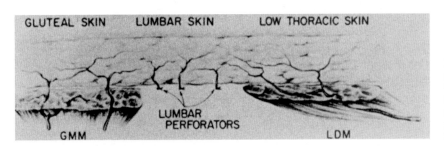

FIG. 2. Cross-sectional illustration showing the rich anastomoses between the latissimus dorsi vessels and the superior gluteal vessels supplying the lumbar skin, maintained by submuscular dissection without skin undermining. GMM, gluteus maximus muscle; LDM, latissimus dorsi muscle.

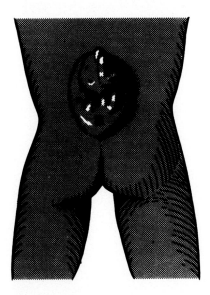

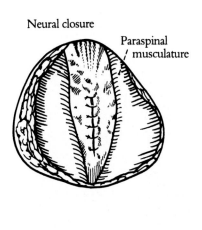

FIG. 3. Preoperative appearance of a meningomyelocele lesion and the neural closure (schematic).

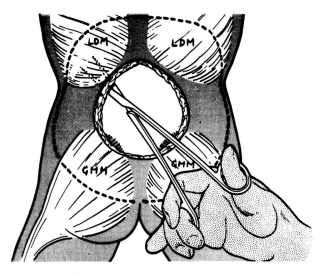

FIG. 4. The submuscular dissection of the latissimus dorsi and gluteus maximus musculocutaneous units bilaterally. Dotted line indicates the area of undermining at the submuscular level beneath the latissimus dorsi (*LDM*) and gluteus maximus muscles (*GMM*).

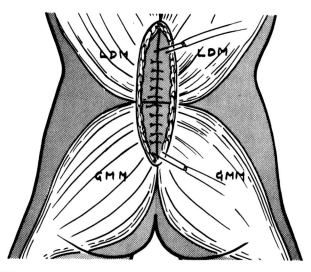

FIG. 5. Schematic illustration showing the approximation of the latissimus dorsi (*LDM*) and gluteus maximus (*GMM*) musculocutaneous units in the midline (seen through a cutaneous window for clarity). No back cuts are made in the skin.

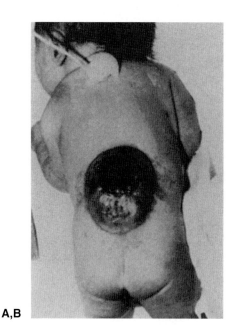
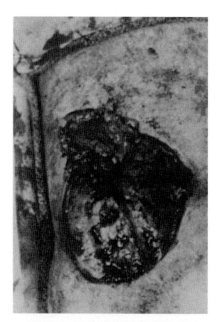

A,B

FIG. 6. A: A 14-hour-old full-term infant was referred with a 10 × 8-cm lumbosacral meningomyelocele. The child had flaccid paralysis of both lower extremities and no anal wink. **B:** The exposed neural plate was dissected free, and the dura was repaired, obtaining a watertight closure. The kyphos was resected, and a small portion of abnormal skin around the myelorachischisis was excised. The technique as described was used to obtain a three-layer closure of the soft-tissue defect in a stepwise fashion. **C:** Mobilization of bilateral compound musculocutaneous flaps. **D:** Appearance of the repair at the end of the operation. The child's postoperative course was complicated by upper respiratory infection that delayed placement of the ventriculoperitoneal shunt. The back wound healed uneventfully, and the child was discharged on postoperative day 21. **E:** Appearance of the repair at 6 months.

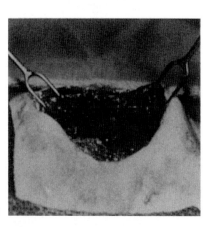
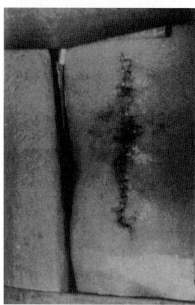
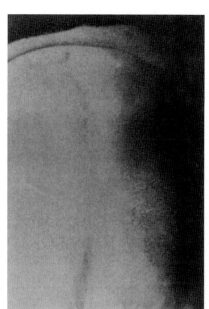

C–E

crest and sacrum, and the dissection is carried into the plane between the gluteus maximus and medius. Care should be taken to preserve the gluteal vessels (Fig. 4).

The quadratus lumborum muscle is often poorly developed in the infant, and retroperitoneal structures, including the ureter, must be safeguarded. No lateral relaxing incisions or backcuts are made. The submuscular dissection of the flap is carried all the way to the posterior or midaxillary line, as needed (Fig. 5). The flaps meet in the midline with minimal tension and can be approximated in three layers (Fig. 6).

CLINICAL RESULTS

This technique has been used in the last 3 years in 18 thoracolumbar and lumbosacral defects that could not be repaired by direct primary closure. Primary reconstruction was carried out in the 18 patients immediately following neurosurgical management of the meningomyelocele. Blood loss was less than 20 ml in all patients, and blood transfusion was not necessary.

All reconstructions were completed in one stage, with no complications. Good healing was noted at 14 months' mean follow-up, and there has been no deterioration of neurologic function. There was one death following correction of Fallot's tetralogy in the late postoperative period. No flap was lost, and no wound infections or disruptions were noted.

Potential disadvantages associated with dissection of such an extensive nature are significant blood loss and prolonged operating time. The use of electrocautery and meticulous dissection with attention to hemostasis have eliminated significant blood loss and the need for blood transfusion in all our patients.

SUMMARY

A new method for reconstruction of large thoracolumbar and lumbosacral meningomyelocele defects involves the medial advancement of latissimus dorsi and gluteus maximus musculocutaneous units and reapproximation in the midline. This permits primary closure of the defect in three layers. The flaps are based on the thoracodorsal and superior gluteal vessels and the intervening thoracolumbar fascia. They provide tension-free, durable, and viable soft-tissue coverage over the dural repair. The flaps do not alter the nerve supply of the muscles and merely redefine the muscle origins.

References

1. Ramirez OM, Ramasastry SS, Granick MS, et al. A new surgical approach to closure of large lumbosacral meningomyelocele defects. *Plast Reconstr Surg* 1987;80:799.
2. Patterson, TJ, Till K. The use of rotation flaps following excision of lumbar myelomeningoceles: an aid to closure of large defects. *Br J Surg* 1959;46:606.
3. Luce EA, Walsh J. Wound closure of the meningomyelocele defect. *Plast Reconstr Surg* 1985;75:389.
4. Mustardé JC. Meningomyelocele: the problem of skin cover. *Br J Surg* 1969;53:36.
5. McCraw JB, Fenix JO, Baker JW. Repair of major defects of the chest wall and spine with the latissimus dorsi myocutaneous flap. *Plast Reconstr Surg* 1978;62:197.
6. Mathes SJ, Nahai F. *Clinical atlas of muscle and musculocutaneous flaps.* St. Louis: Mosby, 1979;91–103, 369–391.
7. Mathes SJ, Nahai F. *Clinical applications for muscle and musculocutaneous flaps.* St. Louis: Mosby, 1982;5, 7–9, 13, 20, 24, 66–69, 114–115, 317, 352–360, 460–465, 470–471.
8. Ramirez OM, Swartz WM, Futrell JW. The gluteus maximus muscle: experimental and clinical considerations relevant to reconstruction in ambulatory patients. *Plast Surg Forum* 1984;7:27.

CHAPTER 456 ■ THIGH TRANSPOSITION SKIN FLAP

B. H. GRIFFITH

For closure of small pressure sores in the ischial area, excision of the ulcer, the bursa, and the entire ischium and primary closure with approximation of the local muscles, subcutaneous tissues and skin, plus postoperative wound suction, may be satisfactory. If the ischial defect is large, however, simple approximation is inadequate (1). The deep hole must be filled, and this is best done with muscle (1–5). The biceps femoris sometimes augmented with the semitendinosus or semimembranosus, has generally proven to be the best muscle. Exposure of these thigh muscles necessitates a large wound. The thigh transposition flap evolved to solve the problems of exposure and coverage (3–5).

INDICATIONS

The principal use for this flap is the closure of an ischial pressure sore (Fig. 2). It is also useful for the closure of ulcers between the ischial area and the trochanter (Fig. 3).

ANATOMY

The blood supply for this random flap is from the inferior gluteal artery and anastomoses between it and the posterior branch of the obturator and the medial circumflex femoral arteries by means of perforators that come through the adductor magnus and gracilis muscles.

FLAP DESIGN AND DIMENSIONS

This is a large flap consisting of skin and the underlying fibroadipose tissue of most of the posterior thigh (Fig. 1). Its upper edge is at and lateral to the ischial defect. Its base is on the posteromedial thigh, its distal free edge along a line running longitudinally down the thigh from a point just medial to the posterior edge of the greater trochanter. It extends distally on the thigh to a few centimeters above the popliteal fold.

The width of the pedicle, that is the transverse dimension of the flap, is usually about twice the length from base to free margin. Depending on the size of the patient, it may measure 20 × 10 cm to 30 × 15 cm (see Fig. 1).

Basing the flaps on the lateral edge of the thigh not only provides a less abundant blood supply but also makes the superomedial edge of the flap very difficult to suture along the gluteal fold. A separation of the wound often results if this is done (4,5).

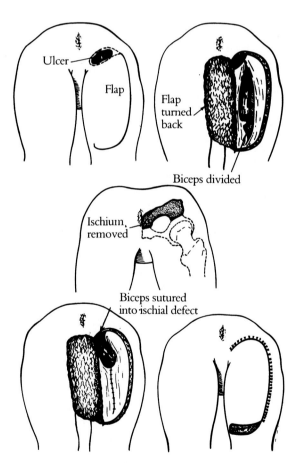

FIG. 1. Schematic drawing of thigh transposition skin flap used for closure of an ischial pressure sore. The flap is wide, large, and based on the posteromedial edge of the thigh. Its elevation affords excellent access to the muscle used to obturate the large hole made by total ischiectomy. A split-thickness skin graft is used distally on the thigh to avoid tension on the upper wound edge. (From Griffith, ref. 5, with permission.)

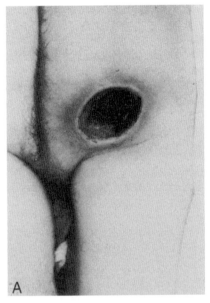
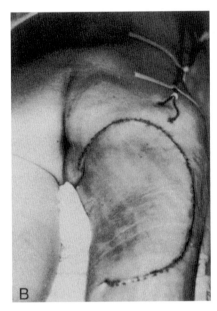
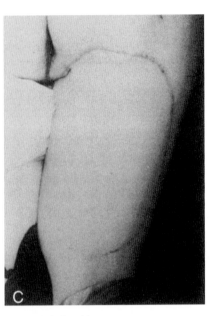

FIG. 2. A: Large right ischial pressure sore. B: Thigh transposition flap 1 week postoperatively with Hemovac drains in place. C: Final result.

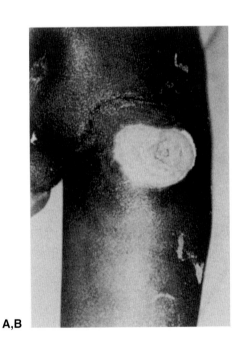
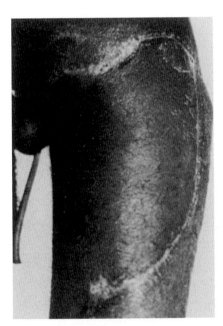

A,B

FIG. 3. A: Large ulcer between the ischial area and the trochanter. It occurred following ischiectomy, biceps flap, and thigh transposition flap. B: Repair using the thigh flap a second time.

OPERATIVE TECHNIQUE

The flap is raised off the fascia covering the hamstrings. After the ischiectomy has been completed and the muscle flap has been turned into the defect, the skin flap is advanced laterally (superiorly) and sutured in place with a double-layer closure. A split-thickness skin graft is usually needed to cover the distal flap donor site to avoid tension on the proximal suture line (see Fig. 1).

CLINICAL RESULTS

The reported 97% success rate (4) has been maintained; however, I have seen late recurrences of ischial ulcers in paraplegic patients who have been sitting up in their wheelchairs for extended periods. On occasion, the very large size of the flap has permitted its use a second time.

Flexor muscle spasms must be relieved in paraplegics before this flap can be used safely. Otherwise, the wound may be violently torn apart by the spasms. The use of continuous wound suction for 2 weeks postoperatively has virtually eliminated the problems of postoperative hematoma and secondary sinus formation that I used to see when I depended unrealistically on "pressure dressing" postoperatively. The patient is kept on a Stryker frame or Circolectric bed and turned, front to back, alternately every 2 hours for 2 weeks postoperatively to prevent flexion of the hips and to facilitate general care. Infection is kept to a minimum by antibiotics. Necrosis of these flaps has been a negligible problem, even though they are elevated and advanced without a preliminary delay.

There is no deficit from the use of this flap. The accompanying muscle flap(s) presumably could be troublesome in patients with intact spinal cords but are not troublesome in paraplegics, for whom the flap is usually employed.

SUMMARY

The thigh transposition flap gives good exposure for transfer of the biceps muscle into an ischial defect as well as supplying good, stable cover.

References

1. Blocksma R, Kostrubala JG, Greeley PW. The surgical repair of decubitus ulcers in paraplegics: further observations. *Plast Reconstr Surg* 1949;4:123.
2. Bors E, Comarr AE. Ischial decubitus ulcer. *Surgery* 1948;24:680.
3. Gelb J. Plastic surgical closure of decubitus ulcers in paraplegics as a result of civilian injuries. *Plast Reconstr Surg* 1952;9:525.
4. Conway HC, Griffith BH. Plastic surgical closure of decubitus ulcers in patients with paraplegia: based on experience with 1000 cases. *Am J Surg* 1956;91:946.
5. Griffith BH. Pressure sores. In: Grabb WC, Smith JW, eds. *Plastic surgery* 3rd ed. Boston: Little, Brown, 1979; Chapter 50; 818.

CHAPTER 457 ■ SCROTAL FLAP

I. KAPLAN AND M. BEN-BASSAT

EDITORIAL COMMENT

The scrotum will cover small adjacent defects, particularly if they are traumatic; however, for recurrent pressure sores, the success rate is much lower and the procedure is of only temporary value.

Experience in the treatment of ischial pressure sores in paraplegics has led to the frustration of repeated breakdown of scars and flaps despite excision of the ischial tuberosity. In a small series of patients, the use of rotation flaps from the scrotum provided very gratifying results (1–3).

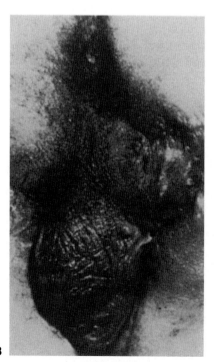 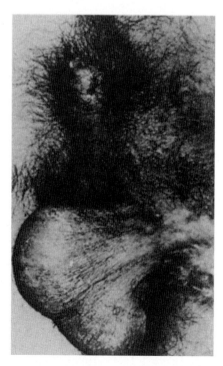

FIG. 1. A: Scrotal flap used to repair an ischial ulcer that had repeatedly broken down after several attempts at repair with other rotation flaps. Note that in this patient the ischial tuberosity was not resected. **B:** The result 5 years later. (From Kaplan, ref. 1, with permission.)

A,B

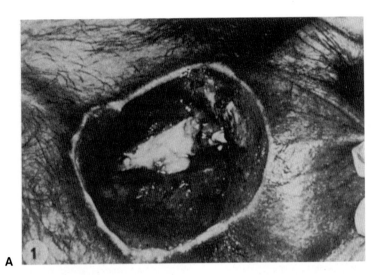

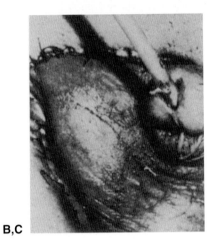
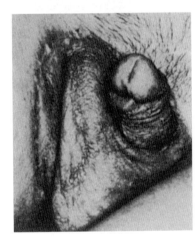

A

B,C

FIG. 2. **A:** A 24-year-old man who had been injured in a car accident 5 years before with damage to the spinal cord at the D7-8 level. He had a deep ulcer measuring 10 × 12 cm in the right groin. In addition, he had multiple smaller ulcers all around the pelvis and over the sacral area, the left and right trochanteric areas, and both ischial areas. Following correction of his anemia and hypoalbuminemia, the ulcer was debrided. It became apparent that the ulcer was extremely large. Laterally, the cavity abutted on the femoral vessels, and distally, it reached almost to the adductor canal. The pubic ramus was involved, the cavity extending behind the penile shaft. An adductor muscle flap was rotated from its proximal insertion to cover the femoral vessels. Following this procedure, a large medial cavity remained that we judged could not be adequately covered with a skin flap alone. **B:** A rotation flap of the scrotum was used, bringing the right testicle into the defect to fill the dead space. Suction drainage was continued for a week. A large amount of sterile fluid, probably lymph, was discharged by means of the drain, but after the drain removal, the discharge ceased. **C:** Healed result at 14 days. The patient can now undergo closure of his other sores. (From Taube et al., ref. 3, with permission.)

INDICATIONS

The advantages of the scrotum as cover for these defects are numerous. The scrotum in paraplegics is usually large and pendulous, and there is almost no limit to the amount of tissue available, as half or even more of the scrotum can be used, with closure of the donor site presenting no problem (Fig. 1).

ANATOMY

Because of the presence of the dartos muscle, the scrotum provides a highly vascular and thick covering ideal for a weight-bearing area. Existing anatomic relationships make the scrotum an excellent choice.

CLINICAL RESULTS

The etiology of these groin ulcers is not quite understood. We surmise that prolonged pressure of a urine bottle over the anesthetic region is largely contributory.

SUMMARY

The versatility of the scrotal flap is now established through its use in sores of the ischium, pubis, and inguinal area. In one patient, the testicle also was used as a space filler (Fig. 2).

References

1. Kaplan I. The scrotal flap in ischial decubitus ulcer. *Br J Plast Surg* 1972;25:22.
2. Kaplan I. The scrotal flap repair for ischial decubitus ulcers: a follow-up. *Br J Plast Surg* 1976;29:34.
3. Taube E, Labandter H, Kaplan I. Decubitus ulcer in the groin: repair using a testiculoscrotal flap. *Br J Plast Surg* 1977;30:86.

CHAPTER 458 ■ GLUTEUS MAXIMUS MUSCULOCUTANEOUS FLAP

R. L. MILLS

The gluteus maximus musculocutaneous flap has found its place in the surgery of spinal cord-injured patients (1) (Fig. 2), in whom functional loss from use of the muscle is not a consideration.

INDICATIONS

The gluteus maximus muscle is important to posture and gait in normal patients. Clinical or experimental evidence is not available to indicate how much of a normally functioning gluteus maximus might be sacrificed without adverse effect. Rather than using a normal muscle, an alternate repair should be sought.

For the ischial area, which is critical to weight bearing, there seems no indication for use of the gluteus maximus muscle alone, although this has been done. The muscle also has been used for repair of the trochanter and sacrum with a skin-grafted surface.

ANATOMY

See Chapter 466.

FLAP DESIGN AND DIMENSIONS

The surface design is a simple rotation flap with excess muscle taken to fill space in the wound (see Fig. 1). The incisions are planned so that the flap is as large as possible and will not encroach on pressure points. Ischial repairs do not require use of skin that does not directly overlie the muscle, except perhaps inferiorly. An island flap can be designed for ischial repairs, if necessary, to meet the requirements of the case (2,3).

OPERATIVE TECHNIQUE

For ischial repairs, the muscle is elevated from its inferior border, which usually appears as part of the wall of a soft-tissue defect over the prominence of the ischial tuberosity. The muscle is elevated by dissecting in the areolar plane (although often somewhat scarred) deep to the muscle and superficial to the sciatic nerve. The blood supply is protected by being closely attached to the deep surface of the muscle, except near the piriformis muscle margin, where it emerges from the pelvis.

The incision is made through skin and subcutaneous tissue to the muscle fascia, which is quite thin. The dissection then bares the muscle surface for several centimeters distal to the skin incision (Fig. 1). The muscle is transected at a point where a mass adequate to fill the deep portions of the wound has been included. In the lateral part of the wound, it may be necessary to backcut parallel to the muscle fibers to achieve adequate mobility.

The tip of the flap is drawn into place by suturing the excess muscle into the depths of the wound. If the flap is suitably designed, the flap donor site can nearly always be closed without a skin graft. The long side of the surface wound is often shortened by excision of a Burow's triangle, but it is sometimes appropriate to lengthen the short side by a backcut.

CLINICAL RESULTS

Adequacy of blood supply has not, in my experience, been a problem, even in the presence of scars in the skin and subcutaneous tissue. Complications such as wound hematoma,

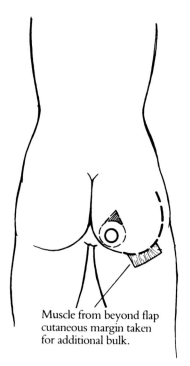

Muscle from beyond flap cutaneous margin taken for additional bulk.

FIG. 1. Excess muscle is taken beyond the cutaneous incision (for anatomy, see Chapter 466).

1326

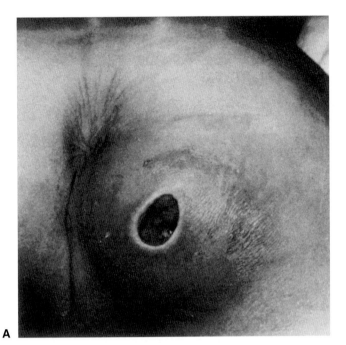
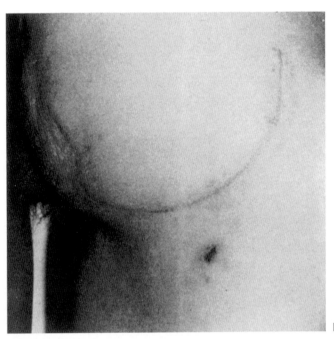

A

B

FIG. 2. **A:** Ischial pressure sore. **B:** Following repair.

seroma, or infection have related to the nature of the wound rather than to the nature of the flap.

SUMMARY

The gluteus maximus musculocutaneous flap can be reliably used for ischial ulcer repair.

References

1. Minami RT, Mills RL, Pardoe R. Gluteus maximus myocutaneous flaps for repair of pressure sores. *Plast Reconstr Surg* 1977;60:242.
2. Mathes SJ, Nahai F, eds. *Clinical atlas of muscle and musculocutaneous flaps.* St. Louis: Mosby, 1979;91–103.
3. Mathes SJ, Nahai F, eds. *Clinical applications for muscle and musculocutaneous flaps.* St. Louis: Mosby, 1982;434–437.

CHAPTER 459 ■ GRACILIS MUSCLE AND MUSCULOCUTANEOUS FLAPS

F. R. HECKLER

The gracilis muscle and musculocutaneous flaps are ideal for covering ischial pressure sores (1,2). For a complete discussion of indications, anatomy, flap design and dimensions, and operative technique, see Chapter 421.

INDICATIONS

The ischium lies well within the reach of standard-sized musculocutaneous flaps. Caution is advised in the use of these flaps in paraplegics with severe muscle atrophy because failure of the skin portion of such flaps has been a problem. No such problem has been encountered in paralyzed patients who have retained reasonably normal muscle bulk.

OPERATIVE TECHNIQUE

The operative procedure is performed with the patient in the lithotomy or prone position, depending on which gives the

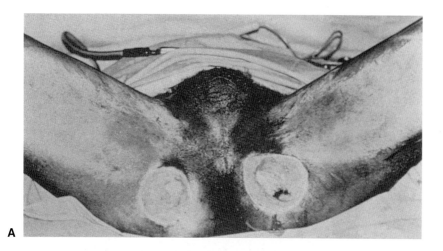

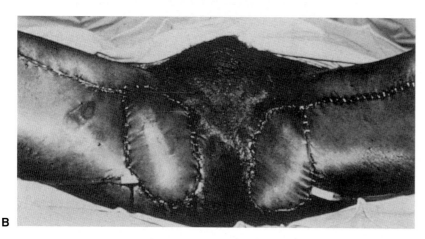

FIG. 1. A: Large bilateral ischial pressure sores in a paraplegic patient. B: After wide excision and removal of the bony prominences, bilateral gracilis musculocutaneous flaps were used to close the defects. (Courtesy of Philip Antypas, M.D.)

best access to the recipient site. The ulcer and inciting bony prominence are removed, and the flap is transferred and sutured into place over suction drains (3,4) (Fig. 1).

CLINICAL RESULTS

Improper location of the skin-paddle design and subsequent partial separation of the skin and muscle components of the musculocutaneous unit are, in my opinion, the most common causes of failure in the use of this flap. In my series of 53 patients with various perineal problems, none of the flaps failed. This success rate is particularly gratifying because the gracilis musculocutaneous flap seems to have gained some notoriety for relative lack of reliability.

SUMMARY

The gracilis muscle and musculocutaneous flap can be reliably used for coverage of ischial defects.

References

1. Mathes SJ, Nahai, F, eds. *Clinical atlas of muscle and musculocutaneous flaps.* St. Louis: Mosby, 1979;13–31.
2. Mathes SJ, Nahai, F, eds. *Clinical applications for muscle and musculocutaneous flaps.* St. Louis: Mosby, 1982;438–439.
3. Labandter HB. The gracilis muscle flap and musculocutaneous flap in the repair of perineal and ischial defects. *Br J Plast Surg* 1980;33:95.
4. Wingate GF, Friedland, JA. Repair of ischial pressure ulcers with gracilis myocutaneous island flaps. *Plast Reconstr Surg* 1978;62:245.

CHAPTER 460 ■ BICEPS FEMORIS FLAPS

G. R. TOBIN

EDITORIAL COMMENT

With use of this flap as a V-Y advancement, one must be assured that the flap sits comfortably without any tension in the area of the defect with the hip flexed. Failure to confirm this will create a significant incidence of dehiscence in patients having this procedure.

The biceps femoris muscle long head provides the basis for several reliable flaps for ischial pressure ulcer reconstruction. These flaps include musculocutaneous advancement, hamstring V-Y, and turnover muscle flaps (1–3) (see Figs. 1–4). Among these and alternative ischial flaps described in this encyclopedia, the author's first choice is the biceps femoris musculocutaneous advancement flap (3) (see Figs. 1,2, and 4).

The biceps femoris musculocutaneous unit (4,5), when used clinically as a transposition flap, resulted in significant tissue loss, and the flap fell into disrepute (5,6). These tissue losses occurred because transposition requires division of distal major vascular pedicles to this segmentally supplied muscle. The advancement modification described preserves all neurovascular pedicles and results in reliable flap survival (3).

INDICATIONS

The advantages of this flap are as follows: (1) it easily covers large ischial defects; (2) it is highly reliable; (3) a maximum number of reconstructive options are preserved for recurrent ischial ulcers, and use of the flap does not preclude subsequent use of alternative flaps, in contrast to most other ischial flaps; and (4) it transfers both muscle and skin over the ischium, providing greater bulk that protects the membranous urethra and better balances the pelvis in sitting (3,7). The muscle component provides greater reliability in contaminated wounds, presumably because of better vascular perfusion of muscle (8).

ANATOMY

The biceps femoris long head originates on the ischial tuberosity and inserts principally on the fibular head. The flap vascular supply is from segmental vascular pedicles from profundus femoris vessels, which are accompanied along an obliquely caudal course by branches of the sciatic nerve (9). Most of these pedicles enter the muscle belly in its distal half (the anatomic basis for better survival of advancement flaps compared with transposition flaps) (3).

The overlying thigh skin derives its vascular supply from biceps femoris musculocutaneous perforators (3–5). It receives secondary vascular supplies from axial branches of the inferior gluteal artery (when preserved), the dermal-subdermal plexus of a medial or lateral cutaneous pedicle (when preserved), and musculocutaneous perforators from the semitendinosus and semimembranosus muscles (when preserved) (3,10–12). Flap innervation is from sciatic nerve motor branches to the biceps femoris and hamstring muscles and from the posterior cutaneous nerve of the thigh (9).

Hamstring muscles are prime knee flexors, and they function in normal gait to decelerate leg swing immediately before heel strike, thus contributing to forward momentum of the thigh and upper body (13). In paraplegics, however, the hamstring muscles are usually either useless or spastic. Accordingly, their division and transfer leave no functional loss and may relieve knee flexion spasticity or contracture (3). Therefore, when voluntary knee flexion is present, as in patients with normal innervation or partial spinal cord lesions, I transfer only the biceps femoris long head with the flap. In complete spinal cord lesions, I include the semitendinosus and semimembranosus muscles (3).

FLAP DESIGN AND DIMENSIONS

This flap consists of the biceps femoris long head and its overlying musculocutaneous territory, the posterior thigh skin (Fig. 1). The flap is advanced cephalad into the ischial defect on both its neurovascular pedicles and a wide medial or lateral cutaneous pedicle (3). Also, the flap may be reelevated and readvanced (14). Subsequently, the cutaneous and muscle components can be independently, sequentially used (1,10,15) (Fig. 2).

The flap extends vertically from the gluteal to the popliteal creases and transversely from the gracilis muscle to the fascia lata. Thus it comprises one third of thigh circumference at all levels and provides the largest described skin paddle for ischial ulcer reconstruction (approximately 45 × 20 cm). Deeply, it includes the long head of the biceps femoris muscle. In addition, it also may include semitendinosus and semimembranosus muscles if these units are not required to preserve voluntary knee flexion (3,11).

The flap pivots on the entrances of its vascular pedicles into the posterior thigh. It may be advanced cephalad 10 cm without division of any neurovascular pedicle. To date, I have found this maneuver sufficient to cover all ischial ulcers.

Because of its musculocutaneous vascular supply, the cutaneous portion of this flap may be elevated as an island (3,11) (Fig. 3); however, I prefer to preserve a wide medial or lateral cutaneous pedicle. A medial cutaneous pedicle is chosen when a tensor fasciae latae flap has been or may be needed for trochanteric ulcers (see Fig. 1). Alternatively, a lateral cutaneous pedicle that carries the sensory nerves may be designed (Fig. 4).

OPERATIVE TECHNIQUE

Procedures to relieve hip flexor spasm either precede flap transfer or are done simultaneously (8). The ulcer is excised en

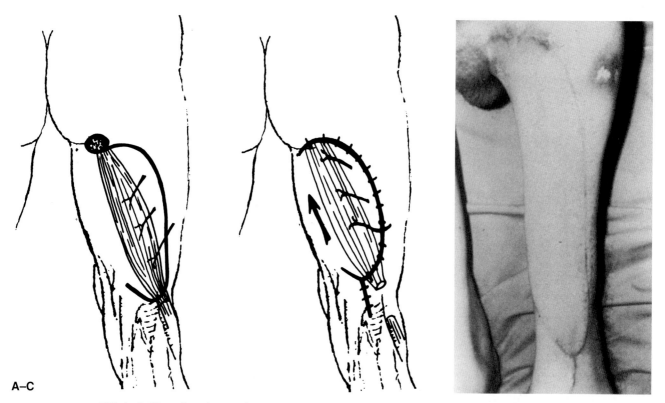

A–C

FIG. 1. A: Biceps femoris musculocutaneous advancement flap with a medial cutaneous pedicle. **B:** Flap inset after cephalad advancement, reorientation of vascular pedicles, transection of tendons, and V-Y closure of donor defect. **C:** Biceps femoris musculocutaneous advancement flap closure of ischial pressure ulcer. (From Tobin et al., ref. 3, with permission.)

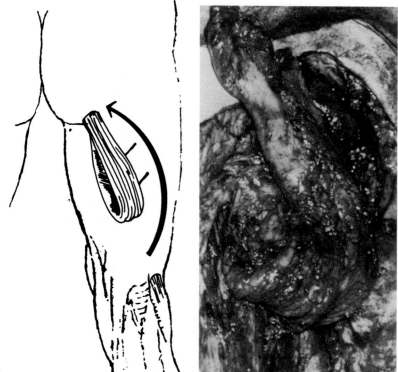

A,B

FIG. 2. A: Biceps femoris turnover muscle flap closure of ischial pressure ulcer. **B:** Combined hamstring muscle flap turned over to close an ischial ulcer. Skingraft application and successful closure followed.

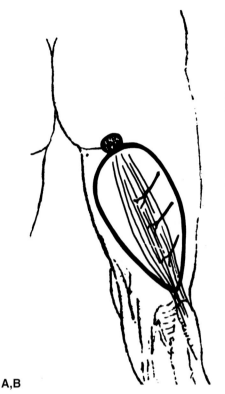
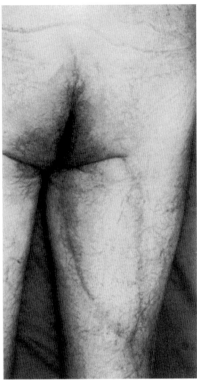

A,B

FIG. 3. A: Alternative island cutaneous design of biceps femoris musculocutaneous advancement flap. B: Island biceps femoris musculocutaneous advancement flap closure of ischial ulcer. (From Tobin et al., ref. 3, with permission.)

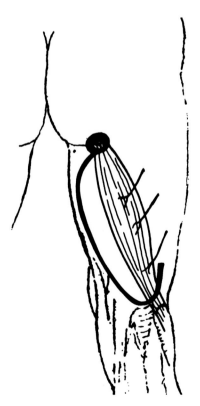

FIG. 4. Alternative cutaneous design of biceps femoris musculocutaneous advancement flap. Lateral cutaneous pedicle preserved.

bloc (16). The ischial tuberosity is excised, and the ischium is contoured to broaden the pressure point. Total and subtotal ischiectomies are avoided (7). Specific systemic perioperative prophylactic antibiotics are given.

The flap cutaneous margins are incised and elevated deep to the underlying fascia. Cutaneous sensory nerves that lie lateral to the ischial tuberosity are preserved if they are functional. At the muscle-component borders, the dissection enters the plane deep to the muscles, and neurovascular pedicles are identified and mobilized.

Laterally, the sciatic nerve is the guiding landmark to the deep dissection. The biceps femoris long head is included in the flap by surgical separation from the short head. Medially, the semitendinosus and semimembranosus muscles are included in the flap unless they are needed to preserve voluntary knee flexion (3,11). The flap muscles are transected at origin and insertion tendon junctions. After mobilization, the flap is advanced into the ischial defect and its neurovascular pedicles are redirected cephalad (see Fig. 1). First, the proximal half of the flap is inset without tension; then the distal flap and cutaneous donor defect are closed by V-Y technique (17). Skin grafts may be used for the donor defect, but I have not needed them to date.

CLINICAL RESULTS

I have had experience with more than 20 clinical flaps. Clinical experience with biceps femoris musculocutaneous advancement flaps has been excellent; there have been no partial or complete losses to date (3). This success rate presumably results from preservation of distal segmental vascular pedicles, as reports of transposition flaps describe a high partial failure rate (5,6).

SUMMARY

Biceps femoris musculocutaneous advancement flaps provide a large posterior thigh skin paddle carried on underlying muscle mass. This flap has proven most reliable and versatile for reconstruction of ischial ulcers.

References

1. Gelb J. Plastic surgical closure of decubitus ulcers in paraplegics as a result of civilian injuries. *Plast Reconstr Surg* 1952;9:525.
2. Pappas C, Goldich G, Cundy K, Wong W. Skin flaps vs. muscle flaps: coping with infection in the presence of a foreign body. *Plast Surg Forum* 1980;3:133.
3. Tobin GR, Pompi-Sanders B, Man D, Weiner LJ. The biceps femoris myocutaneous advancement flap: a useful modification for ischial pressure ulcer reconstruction. *Ann Plast Surg* 1981;6:396.
4. McCraw JB, Dibbell DG. Experimental definition of independent myocutaneous vascular territories. *Plast Reconstr Surg* 1977;60:212.
5. McCraw JB, Dibbell DG, Carraway JH. Clinical definition of independent and myocutaneous vascular territories. *Plast Reconstr Surg* 1977;60:341.
6. McCraw JB. Closure of defects of the lower extremity by myocutaneous flaps. In: Converse JM, ed. *Reconstruction plastic surgery,* 2nd ed. Philadelphia: Saunders, 1977;3560–3566.
7. Comarr AE, Bors E. Perineal urethral diverticulum: complications of removal of ischium. *JAMA* 1958;168:2000.
8. Michaelis L, ed. *Orthopedic surgery of the limbs in paraplegia.* Berlin: Springer-Verlag, 1965;8012.
9. Brash JC, ed. *Neurovascular hila of limb muscles.* Edinburgh: Livingstone, 1965;54, 55.
10. Conway H, Griffith BH. Plastic surgery for closure of decubitus ulcers in patients with paraplegia. *Am J Surg* 1956;91:946.
11. Hurteau JE, Bostwick J, Nahai F, Hester R, Jurkiewicz MJ. V-Y advancement of hamstring musculocutaneous flap for coverage of ischial pressure sores. *Plast Reconstr Surg* 1981;68:539.
12. Hurwitz DS, Swartz WM, Mathes SJ. The gluteal thigh flap: a reliable sensate flap for the closure of buttock and perineal wounds. *Plast Reconstr Surg* 1981;68:521.
13. Simon SR, Mann RA, Hagy JL, Larsen U. Role of the posterior calf muscles in normal gait. *J Bone Joint Surg* 1978;60A:465.
14. Tobin GR, Gordon JA, Smith BA, Schusterman MS. Preserving motor function by splitting muscle and myocutaneous pedicles. *Plast Surg Forum* 1980;3:160.
15. Baker DC, Barton FE, Converse TM. A combined biceps and semitendinosus muscle flap in the repair of ischial sores. *Br J Plast Surg* 1978;31:26.
16. Guttman L. The treatment and rehabilitation of patients with injuries of the spinal cord. In: MacNalty AS, Cope Z, eds. *British history of World War II surgery.* London: His Majesty's Stationery Office, 1953;486–496.
17. Campbell RM, Delgado JP. The pressure sore. In: Converse JM, ed. *Reconstructive plastic surgery.* Philadelphia: Saunders, 1977;3787.

CHAPTER 461. Limberg Skin Flaps *J.G. Hoehn*
www.encyclopediaofflaps.com

CHAPTER 462 ■ THIGH TRANSPOSITION AND ROTATION SKIN FLAPS

M. B. CONSTANTIAN

EDITORIAL COMMENT

It is now well known that including the underlying fascia corresponding to the tensor fasciae latae territory will increase the vascularity and safety of this flap.

Defects over the greater trochanter can present some unique problems. If caused by pressure, trochanteric ulcers may reach sizable proportions and may communicate with a pyarthrosis in the hip or with nearby sacral or ischial ulcers. Because of proximity to the hip joint and its powerful muscle groups, the trochanteric ulcer cannot be easily managed without good control of muscle spasticity. Flexion contractures that prohibit joint movement or positioning must be corrected before ulcer closure. Finally, because balance and positioning depend on the function and anatomy of the hips, bony excision or disarticulation must be planned intelligently and with forethought. Management by a number of surgical specialists may be necessary in some circumstances.

INDICATIONS

Because of the common association of bursal and joint abnormalities, trochanteric defects, especially pressure ulcers, can have a surprisingly benign appearance for all the trouble they can cause. Gentle probing of a wound that does not respond to conservative care may reveal a long sinus, heterotopic calcifications, or communication with the hip joint or a nearby bursa. Such abnormalities can be investigated by sinography and plain radiographs.

Drainage of loculated pus must be carried out prior to ulcer closure. Treatment of an involved hip joint should be part of the preoperative plan. Unexpected bony manipulation at surgery is a sign of inadequate diagnosis of the deformity.

If the cephalad extension of the ulcer does not communicate with the hip joint, the problem is one of readying the wound for closure. If the ulcer communicates with the hip joint, it has been my experience that conservative measures have not succeeded in controlling the pyarthrosis; the ultimate solution has virtually always involved resection of the head and neck of the femur. Protracted attempts at conservative treatment of the joint infection may lead to osteomyelitis of the acetabulum or ilium, a much more profound problem for which there is no good surgical answer. Patients who develop this degree of bony involvement usually require proximal disarticulation of the femur, saucerization of the acetabulum and ilium, revision or resection of the ischium, and closure with a large, anteriorly based thigh flap (1).

ANATOMY

A number of bursae are found near the greater trochanter (Fig. 1) and may be involved in a nearby pressure ulcer or traumatic defect. A large, frequently multiloculated bursa separates the greater trochanter from the gluteus maximus; a second bursa is located between the gluteus medius and gluteus minimus muscles; a third bursa appears between the tendons of the gluteus maximus and vastus lateralis muscles. This is a random flap supplied by branches of the lateral femoral circumflex artery and a superficial circumflex iliac artery.

FLAP DESIGN AND DIMENSIONS

A variety of skin and musculocutaneous flaps will reach the trochanteric area. If the defect is a pressure ulcer, however, the surgeon is wise to select a flap that is large and thus can be advanced a second or third time to close a secondary (recurrent) ulcer. A superiorly based transposition or rotation skin flap fills these requirements well (2–6) (Fig. 2).

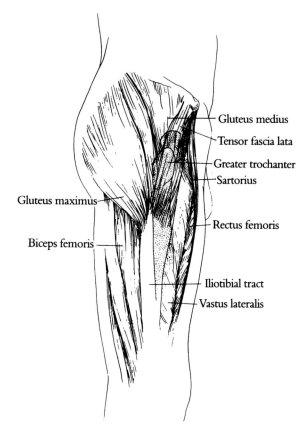

FIG. 1. Surgical anatomy of the trochanteric area. Stippled areas represent the major bursae.

A superiorly based skin flap can be outlined and raised at the level of the deep fascia (Fig. 3). The flap is usually designed with a width of approximately 8 to 10 cm and a length of 20 to 25 cm, and it can be raised without delay if constructed properly.

The only limitation to the use of such a flap concerns closure of the counter defect, which may require split-thickness skin grafting if the primary defect is posterior to the trochanter. The more posterior the primary defect, the larger the flap must be to close it. Frequently, the soft tissues posterior to the ulcer can be advanced several centimeters anteriorly to meet the margin of the flap. When the trochanteric ulcer is anterior to the greater trochanter, the flap is planned in the same location but should be curved anteriorly around the ulcer. The width of the flap is determined, of course, by the size of the defect.

Generally, the anterior border of the flap runs along the anterior border of the tensor fasciae latae muscle. The general outline of the flap is in a quartercircle shape, which facilitates closure of the secondary defect. The narrower the flap, the wider the arc of rotation but the harder it is to close the secondary defect. The wider the flap, the shorter the arc of rotation but the easier it is to close the secondary defect.

OPERATIVE TECHNIQUE

The patient should lie supine on the operating table with a sandbag or rolled sheet inserted beneath the ipsilateral buttock to elevate the trochanteric area. A superiorly based skin flap then can be outlined and raised at the level of the deep fascia (see Fig. 3).

When a portion of the greater trochanter presents in the wound, some bony debridement or modification will be neces-

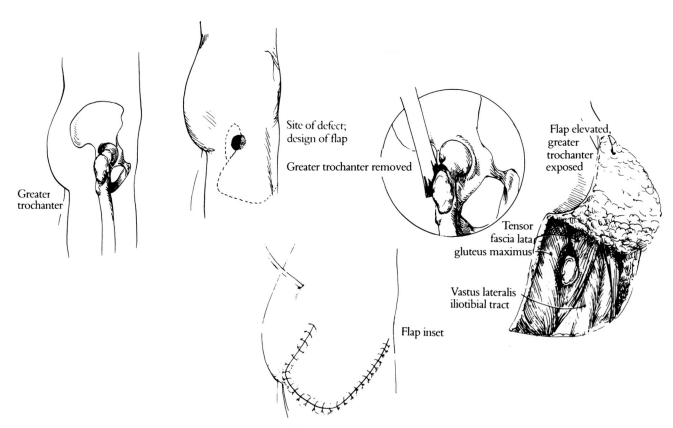

FIG. 2. Closure of trochanteric defect with superiorly based transposition flap.

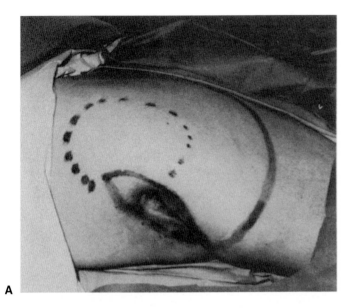
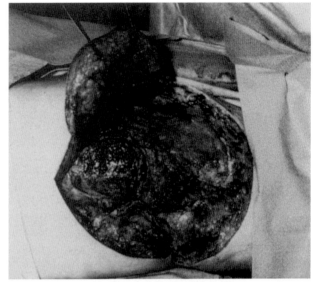
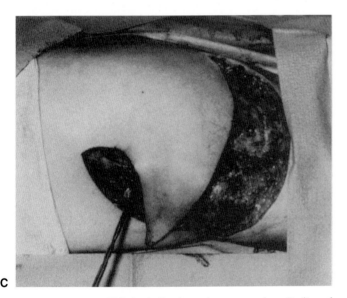
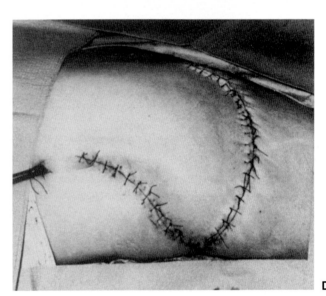

FIG. 3. A: Trochanteric pressure ulcer. Outline of excision and proposed flap. Dotted line indicates size of cavity into which ulcer leads. **B:** Flap elevated, cavity lining excised, trochanter leveled. **C:** Transfer of flap. **D:** Closure.

sary. Even in the case of a trochanteric pressure ulcer, it is not always necessary to excise the entire greater trochanter. In fact, removal of the trochanter is contraindicated in nonparaplegics, because proper insertion of the gluteus medius is critical to maintenance of a normal gait. In either case, the greater trochanter and any other bony projections are merely leveled to provide a smooth surface that will not protrude through whatever soft tissues are brought to cover them.

The secondary defect usually can be closed primarily if the flap is well designed, but it may be covered with a split-thickness skin graft if necessary. Drainage by means of a large siliconized suction catheter is advisable. One special point of postoperative care is that the patient should not lie on the contralateral hip because in this position the operated side tends to flex automatically, placing tension on the wound closure. In the case of paraplegics or quadriplegics, the patient should be repositioned every 2 to 3 hours, if feasible, alternating between prone and semiprone positions.

A variation in this flap is the inclusion or addition of the tensor fasciae latae muscle, which, although thin, has a predictable, proximal, dominant vascular supply. The tensor fasciae latae is routinely uncovered during elevation of the superiorly based skin flap and thus may be added under direct vision as a separate muscle flap or raised with the overlying skin as a musculocutaneous flap. If properly done, the donor site may still often be closed primarily (6).

CLINICAL RESULTS

In a recent review of 50 superiorly based rotation flaps of this design (6), 72% had no complications and 18% had hematoma, defined as any amount of blood requiring at least one aspiration. Wound separation (10%), partial flap loss (8%), and infection (4%) were less common. Although the superiorly based transposition flap is generally reliable and well vascularized, the rate of complications in this particular review indicates the relatively high incidence of wound complications in cord-injured patients with chronic open wounds.

SUMMARY

The superiorly based thigh transposition flap can be used in conjunction with treatment of underlying pyarthrosis or sinuses, to cover trochanteric pressure ulcers.

References

1. Constantian MB, Jackson HS. The complex problem. In: Constantian MB, ed. *Pressure ulcers: principles and techniques of management.* Boston: Little, Brown, 1980.
2. Barker DE. Surgical treatment of decubitus ulcers. *JAMA* 1945;129:160.
3. Conway H, Kraissl CJ, Clifford RH, et al. Plastic surgical closure of decubitus ulcers in patients with paraplegia. *Surg Gynecol Obstet* 1947;85:321.
4. Kostrubala JG, Greeley PW. The problem of decubitus ulcers in paraplegics. *Plast Reconstr Surg* 1947;2:403.
5. Blocksma R, Kostrubala JG, Greeley PW. Surgical management of decubitus ulcer in paraplegics: further observations. *Plast Reconstr Surg* 1949;4:123.
6. Constantian MB, Jackson HS. The trochanteric ulcer. In: Constantian MB, ed. *Pressure ulcers: principles and techniques of management.* Boston: Little, Brown, 1980.

CHAPTER 463 ■ THIGH BIPEDICLE ADVANCEMENT SKIN FLAP

B. H. GRIFFITH

> ### EDITORIAL COMMENT
>
> This bipedicle random flap may, in some instances, be the only solution to the problem. However, first choice would be a flap with a more secure circulation such as a musculocutaneous or a fasciocutaneous flap.

Pressure sores in the region of the greater trochanter of the femur were closed for some years by means of rotation skin flaps (1,2); however, frequent problems with partial necrosis led to the use of a more reliable means of closure. A bipedicle flap advanced laterally from the anterolateral thigh has proven extremely useful for the repair of defects in this area (3,4).

INDICATIONS

This flap is uniquely suited to the closure of an oval or round trochanteric wound (see Fig. 2).

ANATOMY

The blood supply of the thigh bipedicle advancement flap is derived mainly from the superficial circumflex iliac branch of the femoral artery and the lateral circumflex femoral branch of the profunda femoris artery. They anastomose with each other and with branches of the deep circumflex iliac artery and send perforating branches through the tensor fasciae latae, sartorius, and rectus femoris muscles to provide a rich network of vessels in the subcutaneous tissue and skin. Because the flap is elevated off the underlying muscle fascia, the circulation depends on the dermal-subdermal plexus fed from both pedicles.

FLAP DESIGN AND DIMENSIONS

The flap consists of skin and the underlying fibroadipose tissue and is basically longitudinally oriented. Its lateral edge is adjacent to the trochanteric defect, and its medial edge lies just lateral to the anterior superior iliac spine proximally and to the femoral triangle on the anterior thigh distally. Its size varies with the size of the patient and the size of the defect to be closed from 10 × 20 cm to 15 × 30 cm. A 2:1 ratio of length to width should not be exceeded (Fig. 1).

When the trochanteric wound is especially large, the proximal pedicle may be somewhat narrower than the distal pedicle because the distance between the edge of the trochanteric wound and the anterior superior iliac spine may be short. However, the proximal pedicle should be kept lateral to the iliac spine to avoid having to put a skin graft directly over the bone.

OPERATIVE TECHNIQUE

The flap is elevated off the underlying muscle fascia and shifted laterally to cover the trochanteric defect. When used to repair a trochanteric pressure sore, the underlying greater trochanter should, of course, be resected along with the ulcer, bursa, and any soft-tissue calcifications that may be present (Fig. 1). The stump of the trochanter should be completely covered with a rotation flap of tensor fasciae latae or turnover flaps of fascia lata or muscle fascia before the bipedicle flap is advanced into the wound.

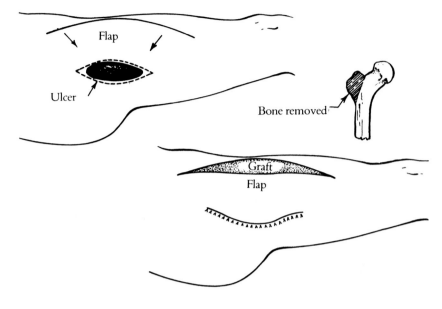

FIG. 1. Thigh bipedicle advancement skin flap for closure of trochanteric pressure sore. The medial edge of the flap is really farther anterior than can be shown in this two-dimensional diagram. Note the split-thickness skin graft placed on the anterior thigh to relieve tension on the lateral suture line. Note also the resection of the trochanter and a little of the lateral cortex of the femur below it to avoid a new pressure point. (From Griffith, ref. 3, with permission.)

A–C

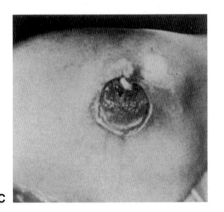
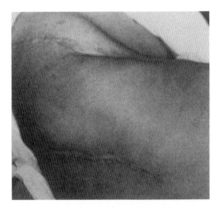
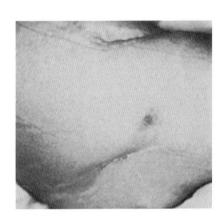

FIG. 2. A: Large right trochanteric ulcer with exposed bursa and bone. **B:** After bipedicle advancement flap with split-thickness skin graft to close the flap donor area. **C:** Same area 10 years later.

This flap is particularly useful when the trochanteric ulcer is very large and has caused a separation of the subcutaneous tissue from the underlying tensor fasciae latae muscle, thus making a musculocutaneous flap impossible. A delay has never been necessary. A split-thickness skin graft must be placed on the anterior thigh to cover the flap donor site to avoid tension on the important lateral suture line (see Fig. 2).

CLINICAL RESULTS

The success rate of this flap in my hands has been in excess of 95% both in the short term (2 weeks) and in the long run (follow-up of 4 to 25 years). The blood supply by means of the two pedicles is so rich that I have not had a problem with circulation in the flap.

Continuous wound suction for 2 weeks postoperatively has kept the hematoma rate to under 10%. Sutures are left in for 2 weeks, and the patient is turned prone to supine alternately on a Stryker frame every 2 hours for 2 weeks before flexion of the hip is permitted. There has been no functional deficit.

SUMMARY

A bipedicle skin flap is a reliable method of closing trochanteric defects.

References

1. Conway H, Griffith BH. Plastic surgical closure of decubitus ulcers in patients with paraplegia: based on experience with 1000 cases. *Am J Surg* 1956;91:946.
2. Griffith BH, Schultz RC. The prevention and surgical treatment of recurrent decubitus ulcers in patients with paraplegia. *Plast Reconstr Surg* 1961; 27:248.
3. Griffith BH. Pressure sores. In: Grabb WC, Smith JW, eds. *Plastic surgery,* 3rd ed. Boston: Little, Brown, 1979; Chap. 50;818.
4. Griffith BH, Lewis VL Jr. Pressure sores. In: Goldwyn RM, ed. *The unfavorable result in plastic surgery,* 2nd ed. Boston: Little, Brown, 1984; Chap. 52;1073–1084

CHAPTER 464 ■ GLUTEAL THIGH FLAP FOR RECONSTRUCTION OF LATERAL THIGH DEFECTS

J. BUNKIS, R. L. WALTON, AND D. J. HURWITZ

The gluteal thigh flap provides an excellent source of sensate tissue for defects of the proximal lateral thigh, particularly those overlying the greater trochanter (1,2). This flap has advantages in ambulatory patients in that it allows repair of proximal lateral lower extremity defects without sacrifice of major lower limb muscle units.

INDICATIONS

The gluteal thigh flap can be used to cover most defects over the proximal lateral thigh. The most common indication for its use in this region is trochanteric pressure sores and exposed total hip prostheses (see Fig. 3). It also can be used to reconstruct the lateral thigh or to cover the femur following tumor extirpation for sarcomas or following localized trauma to the proximal lateral thigh.

This flap is particularly useful in the nonparaplegic patient because it provides a flap with excellent sensibility without sacrificing important motor units. We have used both peninsular and island designs of this flap for coverage of trochanteric defects.

ANATOMY

See Chap. 420 (Fig. 1).

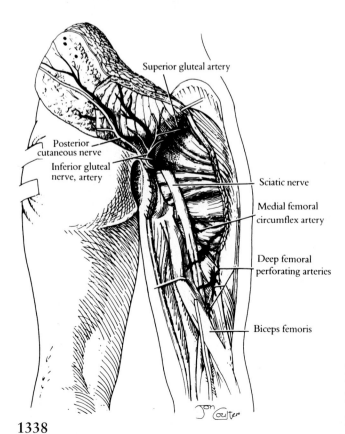

Superior gluteal artery

Posterior cutaneous nerve

Inferior gluteal nerve, artery

Sciatic nerve

Medial femoral circumflex artery

Deep femoral perforating arteries

Biceps femoris

FIG. 1. Flap anatomy. The gluteal thigh flap includes the skin, subcutaneous tissue, and femoral fascia of the posterior thigh region. Note the relationship of the posterior cutaneous nerve to the descending branch of the inferior gluteal artery. (From Hurwitz et al., ref. 1, with permission.)

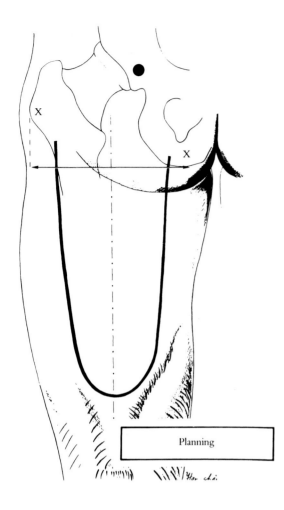

Planning

FIG. 2. Flap design. The central axis of the flap (halfway between the greater trochanter and the ischial tuberosity) overlies the extrapelvic course of the inferior gluteal artery. The entire posterior aspect of the thigh can be incorporated into the flap. (From Hurwitz et al., ref. 1, with permission.)

FLAP DESIGN AND DIMENSIONS

See Chap. 420 (Figs. 2 and 3B).

OPERATIVE TECHNIQUE

See Chap. 420 (Fig. 3).

CLINICAL RESULTS

To date, we have employed the gluteal thigh flap for coverage of 11 lateral thigh defects. One patient dehisced a wound over a trochanter secondary to an underlying hematoma. Another developed dysesthesia in an island flap transferred to close a trochanteric defect, presumably as a result of tethering of the nerve during a tight closure. Other than decreased sensibility

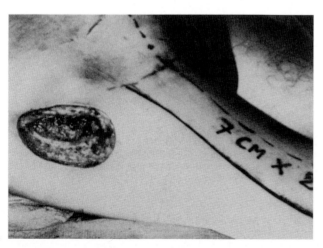
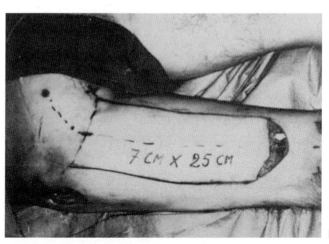

A   **B**

FIG. 3. A: Left trochanteric pressure sore has been excised with the patient in the prone position. **B:** Gluteal thigh flap design. Distal incision has been carried through the femoral fascia, and the distal neurovascular pedicle has been identified (*arrow*). *(Continued)*

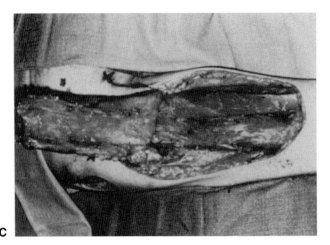

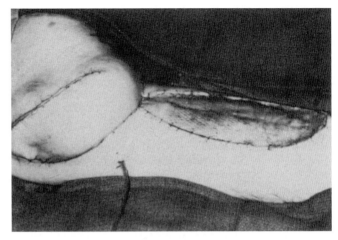

C

D

FIG. 3. *Continued.* **C:** Flap has been elevated to the inferior border of the gluteus maximus muscle. More proximal dissection can increase flap length, but care must be taken to avoid placing incisions over the ischial tuberosity, as to do so may predispose the patient to pressure sores in this area. **D:** The interposing skin bridge has been divided and the peninsular flap inset into the trochanteric defect. A split-thickness skin graft was employed to avoid a tight closure in this thin male patient.

in the donor area and occasional temporary tightness in the thigh (resulting from donor-site closure), no functional deficits were encountered.

The gluteal thigh flap has proven quite reliable if designed and elevated with care. All the complications encountered thus far were avoidable and not the result of intrinsic pitfalls in flap anatomy or design.

SUMMARY

The inferior gluteal thigh flap can be used to close trochanteric pressure ulcers and is especially useful in nonparaplegic patients.

References

1. Hurwitz DJ, Swartz WM, Mathes SJ. The gluteal thigh flap: a reliable sensate flap for the closure of buttocks and perineal wounds. *Plast Reconstr Surg* 1981;68:521.
2. Walton RL. The inferior gluteal thigh flap. In: Mathes SJ, Nahai F, eds. *Clinical applications for muscle and musculocutaneous flaps.* St. Louis: Mosby, 1981.

CHAPTER 465 ■ TOTAL THIGH FLAP

G. S. GEORGIADE

> ### EDITORIAL COMMENT
>
> This is a useful procedure that was more common in the past. Currently, better management and/or prevention of pressure sores have decreased its use.

The total thigh flap has been successfully applied to manage difficult recurrent pressure sores for more than 30 years (1–5).

This flap is particularly useful in paraplegic patients with large, multiple, recurrent ulcers or for large trochanteric ulcers associated with pyarthrosis of the hip joint and widespread osteomyelitis of the femur and pelvis.

INDICATIONS

With the development of versatile regional musculocutaneous flaps, the application of the total thigh flap is currently limited to the patient with ulceration around the hip, sacral, or ischial

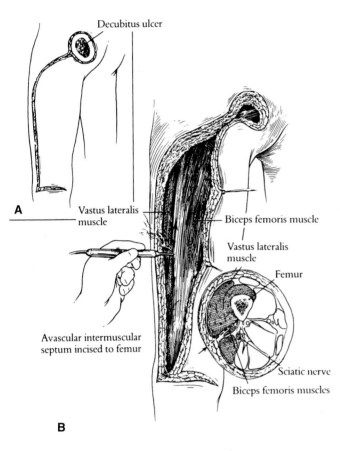

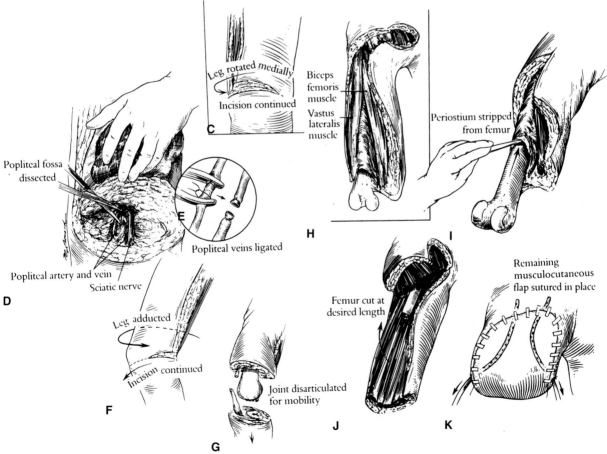

FIG. 1. Diagrammatic representation of the steps in the operative procedure.

regions who does not have available musculocutaneous flaps or whose ulcer is so massive that no regional flap is of sufficient dimensions to resurface the defect.

The total thigh flap will provide a significant amount of tissue for closure of large defects in the trochanteric region. The flap may be extended below the knee to cover combined defects in the ischial, trochanteric, and sacral regions. The flap should be designed so that the thigh muscles can be maximally used. If recurrent ulceration develops in the same region, the femur may be further shortened and the flap advanced superiorly for coverage. The thigh flap is a relatively safe procedure, is not technically difficult, and is reliable when executed properly.

OPERATIVE TECHNIQUE

Patients undergoing this procedure should be monitored with extreme care because of vasomotor instability. Substantial blood loss should be anticipated, and transfusion should be initiated at the onset of surgery.

The incision is marked on the midlateral aspect of the femur and extends from the trochanteric region to the level of the knee. The incision is begun superiorly and is extended inferiorly along the femur and then circumferentially around the knee just above the patella or below the patella if a longer flap is required (Fig. 1A). The popliteal vessels are identified in the popliteal fossa and are ligated. After the tibial and peroneal nerves are ligated and divided, the dissection is carried along the lateral intermuscular septum, located along the lateral border of the long head of the biceps muscle, and is extended superiorly. The incision along the lateral muscular septum is relatively avascular and provides a cleavage plane between the biceps femoris muscle and the vastus lateralis muscle. The quadriceps and hamstring muscles are divided, and the dissection is extended subperiosteally, completely freeing the femur from the muscle mass of the thigh (Fig. 1B). By remaining in close proximity to the femur, the superficial femoral artery, the essential blood supply to the thigh flap, is avoided (Fig. 1C–K). In patients not requiring resection of the femoral head, acetabulum, or pelvis for control of osteomyelitis, a segment of femur 8 to 12 cm below the greater trochanter is preserved to provide adequate stability and balance when the patient is in the sitting position.

If disarticulation is necessary, the subperiosteal dissection is extended to the level of the greater trochanter. The gluteus maximus muscle is retracted superiorly, and the external rotator muscles are divided, exposing the hip joint. The disarticulation is accomplished at the joint level after incising the joint capsule, retracting the femoral head laterally, and then ligating and transecting the ligamentum teres. At the subperiosteal level, the dissection is extended by releasing all the muscular attachments to the femur. The entire femur and the portion of the lower extremity to be discarded are now detached from the thigh flap (Fig. 1H–J).

The dissection as described is altered when there is extensive osteomyelitis or pyarthrosis of the hip joint. Extensive resection of the affected bone, including the acetabulum and ischium, is often necessary as part of the dissection.

The distal end of the flap is then rotated into the defect, and the deeper layers are sutured, progressively approximating the flap to the underlying musculature in multiple layers. Two suction drains are inserted into the depths of the wound for a period of 4 to 6 days.

CLINICAL RESULTS

The most common postoperative problem is hematoma, especially in patients requiring extensive resection of the pelvis. Postoperative infection is also common and is probably due to fecal contamination of the wound. Sinus tracts are frequent in patients with pyarthrosis and osteomyelitis of the hip joint. Partial wound separation is also common, and secondary wound closure may be necessary. Recurrent urinary tract infections, hydronephrosis, and acute pyelonephritis are constant possibilities during the postoperative period.

SUMMARY

The thigh flap is useful when regional musculocutaneous flaps are not available for the management of extensive tissue necrosis in the paraplegic patient.

References

1. Georgiade N, Pickrell K, Maguire C. Total thigh flaps for extensive decubitus ulcers. *Plast Reconstr Surg* 1956;17:220.
2. Berkas EM, Chesler MD, Sako Y. Multiple decubitus ulcer treatment by hip disarticulation and soft-tissue flaps from the lower limbs. *Plast Reconstr Surg* 1961;27:618.
3. Spira M, Hardy SB. Our experience with high thigh amputations in paraplegics. *Plast Reconstr Surg* 1963;31:344.
4. Steiger R, Curtiss P. The use of a total thigh flap procedure for chronic infection of the hip joint. *J Bone Joint Surg* 1968;50:1429.
5. Royer J, Pickrell K, Georgiade N, et al. Total thigh flaps for extensive decubitus ulcers: a 16-year review of 41 total thigh flaps. *Plast Reconstr Surg* 1969;44:109.

CHAPTER 466 ■ GLUTEUS MAXIMUS MUSCLE AND MUSCULOCUTANEOUS FLAPS

R. L. MILLS

The gluteus maximus muscle flap is used to repair defects centered over the trochanter, such as typical pressure sores, although use of the gluteus musculocutaneous flap is limited because of other more suitable repairs.

ANATOMY

The gluteus maximus muscle arises from the posterior part of the ilium, the posterior surface of the lower sacrum, and the side of the coccyx. It passes downward and laterally to insert into the iliotibial band and the gluteal tuberosity of the femur. Its blood supply is from the superior and inferior gluteal arteries that emerge from the pelvis through the greater sciatic foramen above and below the piriformis muscle (Fig. 1). Both arteries arborize on the inferior surface of the muscle before penetrating to supply the muscle and overlying skin. The superior gluteal artery passes beyond the gluteus maximus to supply the gluteus medius and minimus muscles. The inferior gluteal artery extends beyond the muscle to supply much of the posterior thigh skin.

Use of the muscle or a musculocutaneous flap designed to repair trochanteric defects takes advantage of a rich blood supply from the inferior gluteal artery and the vascular contri-bution to the area from the medial and lateral femoral circumflex and first perforating arteries (the cruciate anastomosis of Henry) (1). In a defect centered over the trochanter (such as a typical pressure sore), a portion of the gluteus muscle passes beyond (distal and posterior to) the defect with its blood supply intact.

FLAP DESIGN AND DIMENSIONS

That portion of the gluteus that passes beyond the defect with its blood supply intact and with or without its overlying skin can be rotated laterally and cephalad to cover the trochanter. The surface design can be circular as a rotation flap (Fig. 2) or rectangular if a skin graft is anticipated. A distally based muscle flap of the inferior half of the gluteus muscle can be turned over to cover trochanteric defects (2).

OPERATIVE TECHNIQUE

The dissection usually begins from within the defect where the margin of the muscle can be seen after excision of the tissue lining the defect (3). The insertion of the muscle is carefully

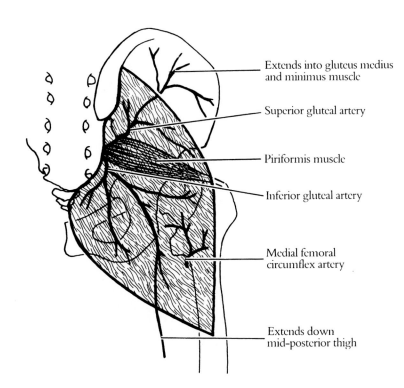

Extends into gluteus medius and minimus muscle

Superior gluteal artery

Piriformis muscle

Inferior gluteal artery

Medial femoral circumflex artery

Extends down mid-posterior thigh

FIG. 1. Vascular supply of gluteus muscle.

1343

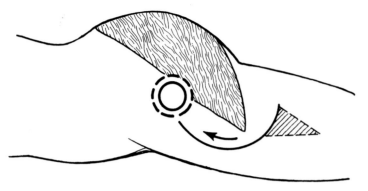

FIG. 2. Rotation flap design.

freed from the femur. The perforating vessels will be found just behind the insertion in fatty tissue. Some of these may be divided, if necessary, to gain additional mobility of the flap. A distally based muscle flap depends on the cruciate anastomosis, since the inferior gluteal artery must be divided proximally in the reflection of the flap. The muscle is covered with a skin graft to complete the repair.

CLINICAL RESULTS

Experience with this variant of the gluteus musculocutaneous flap is limited because of other suitable repairs.

SUMMARY

The gluteus muscle and musculocutaneous flap can be used for coverage of trochanteric pressure sores. It can be based proximally on the inferior gluteal blood supply or distally on the cruciate anastomosis.

References

1. Henry AK, ed. *Extensile exposure*, 2nd ed. Edinburgh: Churchill-Livingstone, 1970.
2. Becker H. The distally based gluteus maximus muscle flap. *Plast Reconstr Surg* 1979;63:653.
3. Minami RT, Mills RL, Pardoe R. Gluteus maximus myocutaneous flaps for repair of pressure sores. *Plast Reconstr Surg* 1977;60:242.

CHAPTER 467 ■ VASTUS LATERALIS MUSCLE FLAP

R. L. MILLS

The vastus lateralis is not suitable for musculocutaneous flaps. Its most common use has been in muscle flaps for trochanteric pressure-sore repairs in patients with spinal cord injuries (see Fig. 2). It is available for defects of whatever cause in the middle and upper thigh and hip region that need to be filled with vascular tissue, where a subsequent skin graft as cover would be satisfactory (1).

ANATOMY

The vastus lateralis muscle arises from a broad aponeurosis that is attached to the intertrochanteric line, to the anterior and inferior borders of the greater trochanter, to the lateral lip of the gluteal tuberosity, and to the upper half of the linea aspera. It inserts through a flat tendon into the lateral border of the patella, blending with the quadriceps femoris tendon.

The blood supply is from the lateral femoral circumflex vessels that enter the medial edge of the muscle approximately a

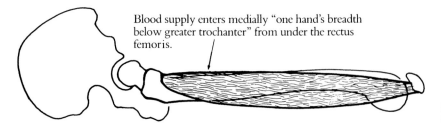

Blood supply enters medially "one hand's breadth below greater trochanter" from under the rectus femoris.

FIG. 1. Vastus lateralis muscle with location of vascular pedicle.

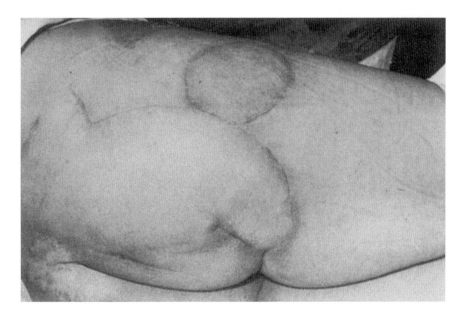

FIG. 2. Trochanteric defect repaired with vastus lateralis muscle flap with skin graft.

hand's breadth below the greater trochanter (Fig. 1). The overlying skin is part of the tensor fasciae latae vascular territory.

OPERATIVE TECHNIQUE

The medial border of the muscle is exposed through a longitudinal incision along a line between the anterior superior iliac spine and the lateral border of the patella. The muscle is beneath the fascia lata, which is incised along the same line. The vastus is then separated from the rectus femoris, taking care to avoid the neurovascular bundle. If necessary, the origin also may be divided if it facilitates placing the muscle into the defect to be repaired. The superficial surface of the muscle is most suitable for accepting a skin graft (Fig. 2). The muscle is sutured to the margins of the defect and covered with a skin graft of intermediate thickness.

CLINICAL RESULTS

With use of the vastus lateralis muscle flap, complications are unusual. The use of a normal muscle does not seriously affect use of the leg because the other parts of the quadriceps continue to act as strong knee extensors. An occasional skin graft has failed and required secondary replacement. Vascularity of the muscle is dependable. Some atrophy of the muscle can be expected, and there is a difference of opinion as to the implications of this problem with regard to durability of repair. Many of these repairs have stood up well over many years in paraplegic patients.

SUMMARY

The vastus lateralis muscle flap can be used to cover trochanteric pressure sores. The muscle must be covered with a split-thickness skin graft, as this flap does not have an associated cutaneous territory.

References

1. Mathes SJ, Nahai F, eds. *Clinical applications for muscle and musculocutaneous flaps.* St. Louis: Mosby, 1982;482–483.

CHAPTER 468 ■ TENSOR FASCIAE LATAE MUSCULOCUTANEOUS FLAP

T. R. STEVENSON AND F. NAHAI

A pressure sore centered at and involving the greater trochanter is amenable to closure with a tensor fasciae latae musculocutaneous flap (1–3). Skin flaps alone often do not provide stable coverage of this sore.

ANATOMY

The tensor fasciae latae (TFL) is a short, flat muscle of the lateral thigh 12 to 15 cm long. It is invested by two layers of the iliotibial tract that is continuous with the fascia lata. The muscle serves as an accessory flexor and medial rotator of the thigh.

The anterior aspect of the outer lip of the iliac crest, the lateral surface of the anterior superior iliac spine, and the deep surface of the fascia lata give origin to the TPL. At its origin, the TFL lies between the gluteus medius and sartorius muscles, superficial to the vastus lateralis and lateral to the origin of the sartorius. The muscle blends with and inserts into the fascia lata in the middle third of the thigh.

The TFL is nourished by a single major vessel that is predictable in location: the transverse branch of the lateral femoral circumflex artery (Fig. 1). The branch usually arises from the deep femoral artery, although it may originate from the common femoral artery. It emerges from beneath the rectus femoris muscle, anterior to the vastus lateralis. The artery enters the muscle on its deep (medial) surface 6 to 8 cm from the anterior superior iliac spine. The vessel is 2 to 3 mm in diameter at its origin. Venous drainage is accomplished by venae comitantes measuring 1.8 to 2.5 mm in diameter and closely associated with the major artery.

On entering the TFL, the artery branches into vessels that run parallel to the muscle fibers and send perforators to the skin. A descending artery continues beyond the muscle to supply skin of the anterolateral midthigh and part of the lower thigh. Skin overlying the muscle is supplied by numerous musculocutaneous perforators. Axial musculocutaneous perforators extend a considerable distance beyond the muscle, increasing the TFL skin territory.

The motor nerve to the TFL is an inferior branch of the superior gluteal nerve (L4 and L5). It emerges between the gluteus maximus and gluteus medius muscles and pierces the deep surface of the muscle.

The skin territory of the TFL is supplied by two sensory nerves. The lateral cutaneous branch of the twelfth thoracic nerve exits between the internal and external oblique muscles in the anterior axillary line. It descends across the iliac crest approximately 6 cm behind the anterior superior iliac spine. This nerve supplies skin over the iliac crest and upper portion of the TFL. The lateral cutaneous nerve of the thigh is a branch of the second and third lumbar nerves. It enters the thigh below the inguinal ligament, passes 1 to 2 cm medial to the anterior superior iliac spine, and runs in a plane on the surface of the sartorius. It provides sensibility to the skin of the anterolateral thigh.

FLAP DESIGN AND DIMENSIONS

The TFL musculocutaneous flap commands a skin territory of up to 600 cm^2 (15 ×14 cm), representing a skin area three times as large as the surface of the muscle. A line 10 to 15 cm long drawn on the skin over the iliac crest, beginning at the anterior superior iliac spine and passing posteriorly, marks the origin of the TFL muscle. The skin territory extends at least 2 cm above this line. The lower border of the skin territory is 8 cm above the lateral femoral condyle. A line drawn from the greater trochanter distally to the head of the fibula marks the

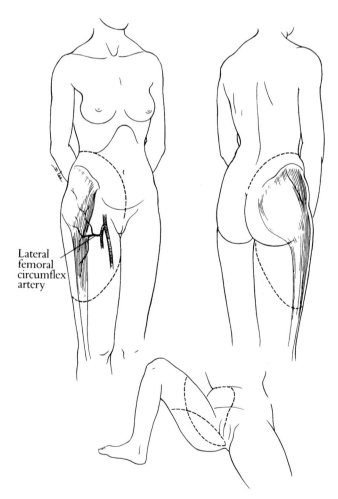

Lateral femoral circumflex artery

FIG. 1. Fascial anatomy and potential areas of coverage of the tensor fasciae latae musculocutaneous flap.

1346

posterior margin of the skin territory. Anteriorly, the skin island can be carried to a line overlying the midportion of the rectus femoris muscle. The skin, muscle, and underlying fascia are elevated as a unit based on the dominant vascular pedicle. The pedicle determines the point of rotation and is located 6 to 8 cm below the anterior superior iliac spine.

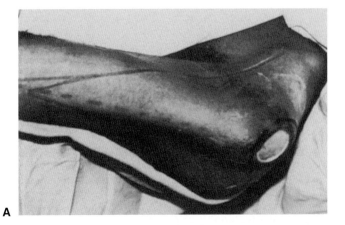

A

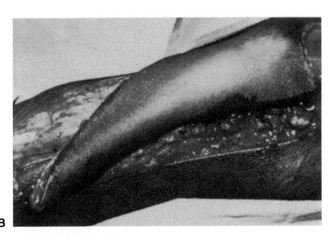

B

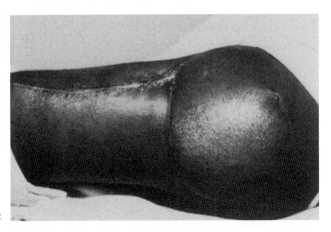

C

FIG. 2. **A:** Outline of tensor fasciae latae musculocutaneous flap. **B:** Elevation and beginning rotation of tensor fasciae latae musculocutaneous flap. **C:** Healed tensor fasciae latae musculocutaneous flap seen 3 months postoperatively.

OPERATIVE TECHNIQUE

The ulcer and its bursa are excised. The prominence of the greater trochanter is removed with an osteotome. A TFL flap is outlined (Fig. 2), raised, and rotated posteriorly over the defect (Fig. 2B). The donor site is closed primarily, or a split-thickness skin graft is applied. The patient is allowed to bear weight on the flap 3 weeks postoperatively (Fig. 2C).

The first step in raising the TFL flap is outlining the desired skin island. An incision is made through the skin, subcutaneous tissues, and fascia lata at the distal skin border. Temporary sutures are placed between the dermis and the fascia lata to prevent dislodging the skin. The anterior and posterior skin borders are incised distal to proximal through the fascia lata. The dissection is carried from the distal end of the flap proximally in a plane deep to the fascia lata overlying the vastus lateralis. If the unit is to be used as a rotation flap to cover the greater trochanter, the vascular pedicle need not be identified. The tissues are dissected proximally until enough is raised for rotation into the defect.

If an island flap is planned, the vascular pedicle must be identified. The plane deep to the fascia lata and TFL is followed proximally until the vessels are seen entering the TFL 6 to 8 cm below the anterior superior iliac spine. Just before it enters the TFL, the lateral femoral circumflex artery gives off a superior branch to the gluteus minimus muscle. This branch may be divided. Once the pedicle is identified, the skin incisions are completed and the origin of the TFL muscle is dissected free of the iliac crest. The TFL muscle is also released from its attachments to the gluteus minimus muscle. The donor site of the TFL musculocutaneous flap is closed primarily or, if too large for direct closure, covered with a split-thickness skin graft.

CLINICAL RESULTS

Complications have occurred with the use of this procedure. Infection in the operative site is treated by drainage and systemic antibiotics. Necrosis of the distal portion of the flap may result if the skin-island length exceeds the design limits. If bleeding of the dermis is sluggish at the time of operation, fluorescein is given and ultraviolet light is used to assess skin circulation. Any areas that do not fluoresce are excised.

Use of the TFL muscle in a flap results in little functional deficit. The muscle is a minor accessory flexor and medial rotator of the thigh, and its loss is well tolerated.

SUMMARY

The TFL flap will reliably cover an excised trochanteric pressure sore. A recurrence of the sore can be anticipated if prolonged and excessive pressure is applied to the site.

References

1. Hill H, Nahai F, Vasconez L. The tensor fascia lata musculocutaneous free flap. *Plast Reconstr Surg* 1978;61:517.
2. Nahai F, Silverton J, Hill H, Vasconez L. The tensor fascia lata musculocutaneous flap. *Ann Plast Surg* 1978;1:372.
3. Nahai F, Hill H, Hester TR. Experiences with the tensor fascia lata flap. *Plast Reconstr Surg* 1979;63:788.

CHAPTER 469 ■ PROXIMAL TFL (GLUTEUS MEDIUS-TENSOR FASCIAE LATAE) MUSCULOCUTANEOUS FLAP

J. W. LITTLE, III AND J. R. LYONS

The proximal TFL flap is recommended for the repair of uncomplicated defects around the trochanter. It is based on the forgotten proximal portions of the tensor fasciae latae muscle and its neighboring gluteus medius muscle, providing closure through the principle of rotation advancement.

It uses an area previously unused in the musculocutaneous repair of pressure sores, an area that remains unavailable to other pressure-sore sites. It transfers a bulky muscle pad of gluteus medius to the exact ostectomy site and presents a secondary defect that is readily closed from a remote and unscarred secondary area. Its use spares other flaps of the region and retains in reserve such major reconstructive units as the traditional tensor fasciae latae musculocutaneous (1–5) and vastus lateralis (6,7) muscle flaps for future needs.

INDICATIONS

We consider it our flap of choice for closure of uncomplicated primary and secondary defects of the trochanter (see Fig. 3). In this role it surpasses the thin, conventional TFL flap by bringing in a considerable muscle pad where desired and by rarely, if ever, requiring a skin graft. We continue to use the conventional TFL flap where tandem defects exist over the ischium or sacrum. We prefer the vastus lateralis system to obliterate a complex dead space, especially where the hip joint has been involved.

ANATOMY

The narrow tensor fasciae latae muscle arises from a short segment of the outer lip of the iliac crest immediately behind the anterior superior iliac spine. It descends vertically some distance before inserting into the tough iliotibial tract of the lateral thigh. Immediately deep and posterior arises the broad gluteus medius, whose origin occupies essentially the entire sweep of the outer crest as well as the posterior half of the external iliac wing below the crest. Finally, deep to both arises the gluteus minimus from the anterior half of the remaining iliac wing to insert, with the medius, into the superior aspect of the greater trochanter of the femur (Fig. 1).

The blood supply of the tensor fasciae latae muscle and fascia is well described (3,4). The lateral circumflex femoral artery of the profunda femoral system gives off a major ascending branch that terminates as the dominant pedicle to the tensor fasciae latae muscle, passing between the rectus femoris and vastus lateralis muscles to reach the tensor some 8 cm below the anterior superior iliac spine. Immediately before entering the muscle, the artery divides into descending, trans- verse, and ascending branches. The descending branch supplies an impressive territory, including the distal fascia lata and lateral integument of the thigh. The transverse branch, which immediately gives off a small branch to the gluteus minimus, nurtures the main belly of the muscle, and the ascending branch feeds the upper muscle and a segment of iliac crest. The blood supply of the gluteus medius is by way of the deep branch of the superior gluteal artery of the internal iliac system. Both the tensor fasciae latae and the gluteus medius muscles are innervated by the superior gluteal nerve.

Apparent inconsistencies arise when considering the anatomy of the tensor fasciae latae muscle, causing confusion in its classification (4). We prefer to think of this strange little mongrel as sharing anatomic traits, functions, and vascular supplies with both the lateral group of femoral muscles acting at the hip (glutei) and the anterior group of femoral muscles acting at the knee (sartorius, quadriceps). We consider the tensor as squarely occupying that common vascular territory joining the internal and external iliac systems as they anastomose about the hip. Seen this way, both the superior and inferior rami of the deep branch of the superior gluteal artery anastomose freely with the terminal ascending branch of the lateral circumflex femoral artery through the region of the tensor and minor gluteus muscles. Certainly, when separating the tensor along its posterior border from the gluteus medius, rich vascular connections must be divided. It is this generous collateral flow around the hip, we contend, that allows inclusion of a major portion of gluteus medius muscle as a true nutritive musculocutaneous extension of the anteriorly supplied tensor fasciae latae muscle in the flap to be described.

FLAP DESIGN AND DIMENSIONS

The flap can measure from 15 cm or more in width to 20 cm in length, with its base falling along a line joining the greater trochanter to the estimated pedicle of the TFL some 8 cm below the anterior superior iliac spine. This latter determination also represents the pivot point of the flap, which can be shifted laterally by backcutting (through skin and fat only) along the base toward the trochanter. The arc of rotation includes the entire hip and trochanteric region anterior to the gluteus maximus muscle.

After appropriate preparation of the wound and ostectomy of the trochanter, the flap is outlined (Fig. 2). Beginning at the posterior superior margin of the defect, a rotation arc is inscribed, rising to the height of the iliac crest and dropping back inferior to its anterior superior iliac spine to end near the estimated location of the pedicle of the tensor fasciae latae some 8 cm below.

1348

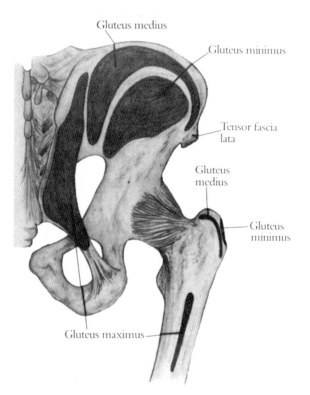

FIG. 1. Bony origins and insertions of TFL and gluteus muscles. (From Little and Lyons, ref. 5, with permission.)

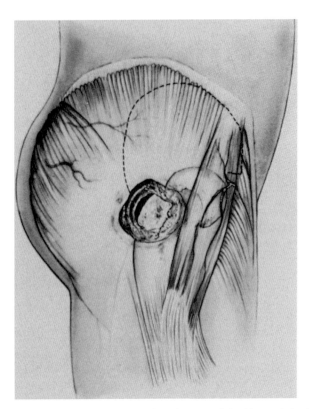

FIG. 2. Planned incision. (From Little and Lyons, ref. 5, with permission.)

This flap has not been performed on an ambulatory patient. Whereas the tensor itself remains expendable, the gluteus medius is quite important to normal gait. As a potent thigh abductor, it pulls the pelvis toward the trochanter of the weight-bearing leg, preventing pelvic collapse on the unsupported side while that leg is raised. As a medial rotator, it then swings the pelvis forward as the step is executed. Although the gluteus minimus remains to continue these functions, total loss of the gluteus medius component would likely create a Trendelenburg gait. For this reason, the conventional TFL flap is preferred in the ambulatory patient.

OPERATIVE TECHNIQUE

The incision is made through skin, fat, and dense gluteal aponeurosis onto muscle. Beginning anteriorly, the narrow tensor fasciae latae is divided from the crest. A finger is now introduced around the anterior border of gluteus medius, between its thin muscle sheet and the underlying deeply situated gluteus minimus. This sheet is progressively divided until its thicker portion is reached over the posterior wing. Usually, the division of medius can now swing inferiorly toward the defect. When the defect is large or posteriorly located, however, greater portions of posterior deeper medius are included, up to but not beyond the overlapping free edge of gluteus maximus. Anteriorly, a distinct plane exists between the gluteus medius muscle fibers and underlying dense fascia of the gluteus minimus. Posteriorly, the gluteus medius itself must be cut across. It is here that multiple significant branches of the superior gluteal artery are routinely divided on their way to anastomosis with the lateral circumflex femoral system.

No muscles are divided beyond the anterior border of the tensor. Subcutaneous dissection proceeds with care as the level of the anterior pedicle is approached, although the vessels themselves are not sought. The lateral femoral cutaneous nerve, if encountered, is spared for later possible reinnervation. Rotation is now attempted and occasionally must be aided by backcutting through skin and subcutaneous tissue alone. With rotation complete, layered closure is performed over multiple drains.

The secondary defect resulting from this rotation transposition is a crescent-shaped area of exposed gluteus minimus fascia anteriorly and a cut surface of gluteus medius muscle posteriorly. Rapid undermining (to the umbilicus, if necessary) and direct advancement of the skin of the lower abdominal quadrant across the iliac crest achieve closure. If the dense fascia over the crest has been lifted with the abdominal flap, this is advanced and secured to the exposed fascia of the gluteus minimus with heavy sutures near the margin of the rotated flap, allowing tension-free closure of skin and fat. Should a skin graft be required to close a portion of the defect after advancement (an unlikely occurrence), it would lie protected in the concavity between crest and trochanter.

Because the vascular pedicle has not been disturbed, the entire traditional tensor fasciae latae musculocutaneous flap remains available for later requirements, as do virtually all useful axial flaps of the region that have been described.

CLINICAL RESULTS

This flap has been used in eight paraplegic patients over the past 2 years (Fig. 3), with all flaps surviving entirely and healing per primam. There have been no recurrences to date. Moreover, there have been no wound or other complications in this small series.

SUMMARY

The proximal TFL flap, which includes a portion of the gluteus medius muscle, is used to close uncomplicated defects

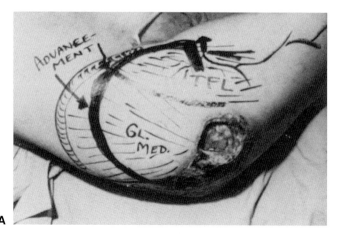
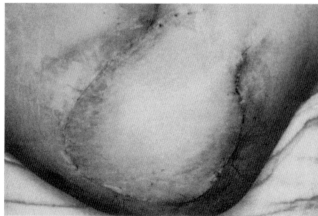

A   B

FIG. 3. A 43-year-old woman with multiple sclerosis. **A:** Primary trochanteric sore with posterior extension showing the flap design and the proposed secondary defect that will be closed by abdominal advancement. **B:** Early postoperative result. (From Little and Lyons, ref. 5, with permission.)

around the greater trochanter. Its use does not preclude later use of the standard TFL flap for the same area if necessary.

References

1. Nahai F, Silverton JS, Hill HK, Vasconez LO. The tensor fascia lata musculocutaneous flap. *Ann Plast Surg* 1978;1:372.
2. Nahai F, Hill HL, Hester TR. Experiences with the tensor fascia lata flap. *Plast Reconstr Surg* 1979;63:788.
3. Mathes SJ, Nahai F, eds. *Clinical atlas of muscle and musculocutaneous flaps.* St. Louis: Mosby, 1979;63–85.
4. Nahai F. The tensor fascia lata flap. *Clin Plast Surg* 1980;7:51.
5. Little JW III, Lyons JR. The gluteus medius–tensor fasciae latae flap. *Plast Reconstr Surg* 1983;71:366.
6. Mathes SJ, Vasconez LO, Jurkiewicz MJ. Extensions and further applications of muscle flap transposition. *Plast Reconstr Surg* 1977;60:6.
7. Minami RT, Hentz VR, Vistnes LM. Use of vastus lateralis muscle flap for repair of trochanteric pressure sores. *Plast Reconstr Surg* 1977;60:364.

CHAPTER 470 ■ UPPER TRANSVERSE RECTUS ABDOMINIS FLAP: THE FLAG FLAP

R. DE LA PLAZA

EDITORIAL COMMENT

This is an excellent flap, with the donor site often hidden in the submammary area and with a long arc of rotation, since it is based on the deep inferior epigastric vessels. The flap can easily reach the region of the trochanter or as low as the distal third of the thigh.

This flap is a reverse of the lower transverse rectus abdominis (TRAM) flap (1–4). The rectus muscle represents a flagpole, and the skin of the upper abdomen, a flag, q.e.d., "flag flap."

INDICATIONS

The flap is most useful for coverage of large defects in the superior abdomen, the flanks, hips, trochanteric area, and above-the-knee amputation stumps. It can also be utilized for the anterior, internal, and lateral aspects of the thighs, almost down to the knee and the perineal region (Fig. 1E).

ANATOMY

The blood supply of the flap is ensured by the inferior epigastric artery, a branch of the external iliac, which has a caliber of 2 to 3 mm. The inferior epigastric vessel enters the distal third

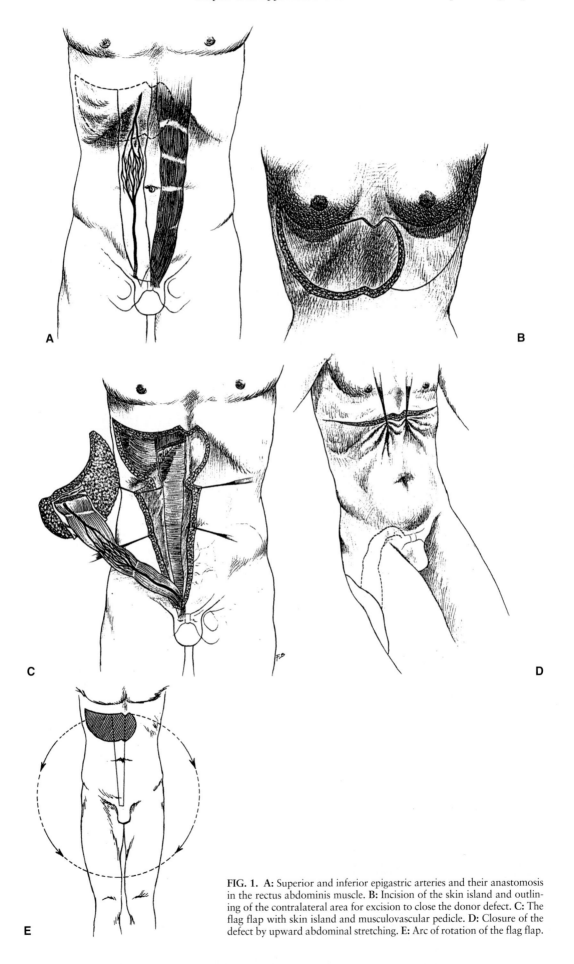

FIG. 1. A: Superior and inferior epigastric arteries and their anastomosis in the rectus abdominis muscle. **B:** Incision of the skin island and outlining of the contralateral area for excision to close the donor defect. **C:** The flag flap with skin island and musculovascular pedicle. **D:** Closure of the defect by upward abdominal stretching. **E:** Arc of rotation of the flag flap.

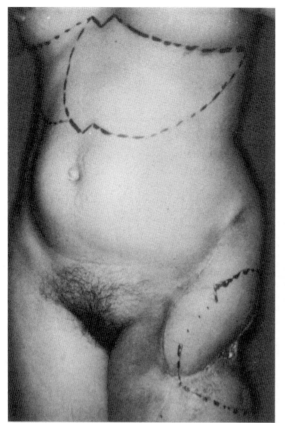

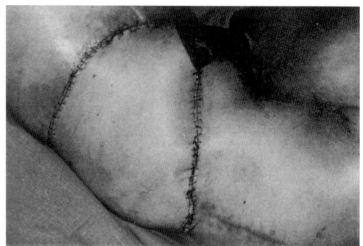

A,B

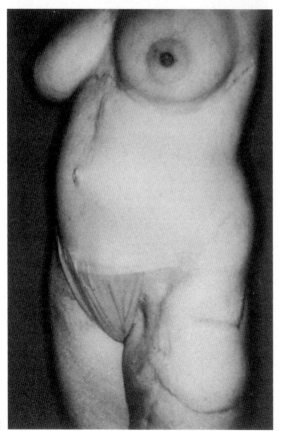

C

FIG. 2. A 30-year-old female with a large tissue defect after excision of a liposarcoma on the upper lateral aspect of the thigh and subsequent radiotherapy and radionecrosis. **A:** Preoperative outline of flag flap and area to be covered on the thigh. **B:** The flap sutured in position, leaving part of the muscle pedicle exteriorized. This was covered by a mesh skin graft. In this case, the pedicle was not completely covered, because of the intense radiation damage to the skin in Scarpa's triangle. The donor area was closed primarily, as in a reverse dermolipectomy. **C:** Appearance 1 month after division of the pedicle and adaptation of the skin edges.

of the rectus abdominis muscle on its posterior surface, where it is easily seen as it courses superiorly in a cephalic direction. Just above the umbilicus, the artery anastomoses in what appears to be a wide network of vessels with similar branches from the superior epigastric. This epigastric arcade is known to send perforating vessels segmentally and penetrates the anterior rectus sheath to supply the overlying skin (Fig. 1B). There are also connections between the epigastric arcade and the segmental intercostal vessels. Most of them are divided as the flap is freed for transfer.

The inclusion of a portion of the anterior rectus sheath throughout the extent of the muscle seems to be important, in light of recent studies of the anastomotic network at the level of the fascia. The flap procedure could be carried out using only a portion of the rectus muscle; we have done this in some cases, but only up to the umbilicus. Above the umbilicus, the division of the muscle would enter the zone of anastomosis of both arterial systems, making hemostasis more difficult and damaging flap irrigation. Nevertheless, the most caudal part of the muscle can be left in place, up to where it penetrates the arteriovenous pedicle. Given the great musculocutaneous mass of the flap, great care must be taken not to produce extreme traction on the pedicle, which could lead to its rupture, avulsion, or elongation, with subsequent stenosis.

FLAP DESIGN AND DIMENSIONS

The flap consists of an island of skin outlined and elevated from the upper abdomen, and extending to the submammary fold in females (Fig. 1A). Laterally, the island can safely extend to the anterior axillary line on the ipsilateral side of the rectus muscle chosen and to the lateral edge of the contralateral rectus. Skin flaps of 25 to 30 cm long by 12 to 20 cm wide can be taken, depending on the amount of abdominal laxity that will allow primary closure. The cutaneous island can be amplified with a caudal extension in the middle zone, providing more skin and modifying the form of the island, thus allowing a better adaptation to certain types of defects.

It is helpful to mark out a symmetrical area to the opposite anterior axillary line, keeping in mind that a good portion of that skin will be discarded. Theoretically, all the skin marked from one to the other axillary line could be utilized in its entirety by taking both rectus muscles; however, this alternative would be very rare and we have had no experience with it. Utilization of the two halves, with their corresponding muscles, might occasionally be indicated, particularly in the reconstruction of very extensive defects in the perineal region.

OPERATIVE TECHNIQUE

An incision is made at the lower edge of the flap, continuing to the opposite anterior axillary line. Dissection of the skin of the lower abdomen follows. This can be done bluntly to some extent, but attention must be paid to the segmental perforators that need to be divided between ligature clips, rather than by electrocautery. If necessary, the umbilicus is transected and taken with the abdominal flap, or circumscribed and later exteriorized at the proper level, as in a reverse abdominal dermolipectomy. Incision of the remaining edges of the flap is carried out.

Flap elevation begins on the contralateral side and continues up to the midline linea alba. The skin flap on the side of the carrier muscle is elevated to the lateral edge of the rectus muscle. At this point, the superior end of the incision is made down to the costal margin and includes the anterior rectus sheath and the muscle insertion. The linea alba is preserved,

and the anterior rectus sheath is divided longitudinally on the ipsilateral side of the midline, in a rectangular shape up to the lateral edge of the muscle. The underlying muscle is freed from the posterior sheath by blunt and sharp dissection.

The abdominal flap is elevated, exposing the anterior rectus sheath, a portion of which (approximately 3 to 4 cm wide) is included along the line of the perforating vessels. The underlying rectus muscle is lifted, completely freeing its medial and lateral attachments. The segmental intercostal vessels are divided between ligatures, as far as necessary. The superior portion of the rectus muscle and sheath is completely divided, with suture ligation of the upper epigastric vessels. The flap is now free and ready to be transferred to the surgical defect (Fig. 1C).

In cases in which defects are situated above the inguinal folds, the pedicle will remain inside the abdominal wall. When this limit is passed, the flap and pedicle will be exteriorized through an incision in the inferior region of the abdomen or in the actual inguinal fold. Care must be taken not to section the inferior superficial abdominal vessels (the superficial epigastric artery, external pudendal artery, and superficial circumflex iliac artery). Protecting these vessels is necessary, to provide a blood supply to the upper abdominal skin, thus preventing ischemia and necrosis. Burying the pedicle in the subcutaneous tissue under the skin of the thigh or hip may also cause flap ischemia, due to compression. As an alternative, the pedicle may be covered with a mesh skin graft taken from the contralateral cutaneous area that was discarded.

Although there is no significant potential for the development of a hernia in the upper abdomen, as the posterior rectus sheath is intact, Marlex mesh or a dermal graft taken from the discarded cutaneous area can be used to avoid epigastric softening or bulging. The mesh or dermal graft is inserted into the gap from the costal margin along the medial and lateral remnants of the anterior rectus sheath, down to the inferior border. We have never had a problem below the semicircular line. Most of the time, the muscle turns at that level and maintains the integrity of this segment of the abdominal wall. The upper abdominal skin has previously been undermined, and it is relatively simple to close the wound primarily by a reverse type of abdominal lipectomy (Fig. 1D). Suction drainage is placed on both sides of the abdomen.

The patient is encouraged to ambulate during days 3 to 4 postoperatively, although the flap is closely observed for venous congestion.

CLINICAL RESULTS

Partial or total flap necrosis is improbable; vascularization of the flag flap is excellent, and substantially better than that of the TRAM flap because: (a) the deep inferior epigastric artery has a caliber two or three times that of the upper artery; and (b) the flow of blood through an arterial system of larger caliber to another of lesser caliber causes an increase in the pressure and speed of blood circulation (5), and thus better flap perfusion. The opposite is true for the TRAM flap.

The possibility of hernia development is minimal as the posterior rectus aponeurotic sheath is preserved, and the anterior sheath is not resected below the semicircular line. Other complications, such as hematoma and infection, are similar in incidence to those of other procedures in this area (Fig. 2).

SUMMARY

The upper transverse rectus abdominis flap, with its wide arc of rotation, has numerous applications over a wide area and is provided with more secure vascularization than the TRAM flap.

References

1. DeFranzo AJ, Nesmith RL. Reconstruction of large soft tissue defects of the lower torso with rectus abdominis musculocutaneous flaps. *Eur J Plast Surg* 1990;13:26.
2. De la Plaza R, Arroyo JM, Vasconez LO. Upper transverse rectus abdominis flap: the flag flap. *Ann Plast Surg* 1984;12:410.
3. Drever JM. The epigastric island flap. *Plast Reconstr Surg* 1977;59:343.
4. Rodrigo Cucalon M, Vinue J, Esarte J, et al. Reconstruction de los grandes defectos de la pared abdominal con colgajos miocutaneo. *Cir Plast Ibero-Latinamer* 1987;13:111.
5. Bernoulli D. *Hydrodinamyca*, 1738. Bernoulli's equation is easy to find in modern texts on hydrodynamic physics.

CHAPTER 471 ■ INFERIORLY-BASED RECTUS MUSCLE FLAP IN FLANK WOUND COVERAGE

B. M. GREENBERG

The rectus muscle flap lends itself to either superior or inferior transfer on the superior epigastric or inferior epigastric vascular system, respectively (1).

INDICATIONS

The inferior rectus myocutaneous flap is indicated for coverage of ipsilateral defects within the lower abdominal wall, groin, hip, and flank. Closure of large wounds in the lower back and flank in ambulatory patients has been problematic (2,3). Local muscle transfers, such as superior and inferior gluteal flaps, risk the loss of hip extension and may limit ambulation (4). Substantial soft-tissue coverage to fill large volumetric defects is often required (5).

The rectus muscle is easily mobilized and tunneled to a flank defect, thus restoring contour without undue bulk. The muscle and skin component maintains a robust blood supply, because the flap can be based on the dominant inferior epigastric system in an axial pattern. The rectus island flap is well-suited for posterolateral flank defects and has also been used for perineal reconstruction (6), closure of difficult wounds of the upper thigh (7), and wounds of the posterior superior iliac spine (8).

ANATOMY

Skin perfusion is maximal periumbilically, based on 1- to 2-mm perforators. The flap-skin island should not be dissected past the midline, but may be planned within 2 to 3 cm lateral to the palpable edge of the rectus muscle. Inferiorly, it is advisable to maintain the inferior edge of the flap above the inguinal ligament.

FLAP DESIGN AND DIMENSIONS AND OPERATIVE TECHNIQUE

The inferiorly-based rectus island flap is hardy, and its excellent arc of rotation makes it a viable option when planning the closure of a complex open wound of the pelvis, perineum, or flank. The flap can be utilized without its accompanying skin paddle, if the added bulk of fatty tissue is a detriment to transfer or would result in an unacceptable cosmetic outcome. In the case of muscle requirements alone, a skin graft can be applied following transfer. The use of a liberal subcutaneous tunnel may shorten the distance of transfer. Additionally, isolating the inferior system will facilitate coverage by lengthening the flap and increasing the arc of rotation.

The size of the defect in three dimensions, following any needed debridement, should be measured prior to flap design. A decision to incorporate a skin island as part of the dissection will depend on the nature and depth of the defect, the adiposity of the patient, and aesthetic considerations.

The rectus muscle should be harvested in its entire width, to incorporate the maximal number of perforating vessels. (Denervation atrophy has been shown to result in a nonworking muscle, in any case.) The flap is raised, identifying and preserving the inferior epigastric pedicle. Careful attention to bipolar coagulation of the muscle, both proximally and distally, should be paid, to obviate against later recipient-site hematoma. Small branch vessels should be tied with fine silk, when adjacent to the proximal pedicle, to prevent injury. Identification and ligation of the superior epigastric artery is necessary, after determining the length of muscle required.

A tunnel, passing over the lateral aspect of the inguinal ligament, may facilitate inset into flank wounds.

The donor site is usually reconstructed with Marlex mesh, which is sutured into position with 0-Tevdek under moderate tension, after releasing the lateral portion of the external oblique muscle. Generally, suction drains are used in both donor and recipient sites.

SUMMARY

The hardiness of the rectus island flap is well-suited for posteriolateral flank defects. Flap robustness and an excellent arc of rotation make it a viable option when planning the closure of a complex open wound of the pelvis, perineum, or flank.

References

1. Bentivegna PE, Greenberg BM. Use of an inferiorly based rectus muscle flap in flank wound coverage. *Ann Plast Surg* 1992;22:261.
2. Hill L, Brown RG, Jurkiewicz MJ. The transverse lumbosacral back flap. *Plast Reconstr Surg* 1978;62:177.
3. McGraw JB, Arnold PG, eds. *Atlas of muscle and musculocutaneous flaps.* Norfolk, VA: Hampton Press, 1986;265–295.
4. Ger R, Levine SA. The management of decubitus ulcers by muscle transposition. *Plast Reconstr Surg* 58:419, 428.
5. Taylor GE, Corlett R, Boyd JB. The extended deep inferior epigastric flap: a clinical technique. *Plast Reconstr Surg* 1983;72:751.
6. Tobin GR, Day TG. Vaginal and pelvic reconstruction with distally based rectus abdominis myocutaneous flaps. *Plast Reconstr Surg* 1988;81:62.
7. Gottlieb ME, Chandrosekhar B, Terz JJ, et al. Clinical applications of the extended deep inferior epigastric flap. *Plast Reconstr Surg* 1986;78:782.
8. Lineaweaver WC, Buncke GM, Bentivegna PE, Buncke HJ. Subtransversalis passage of a rectus abdominis island flap for treatment of osteomyelitis of the posterior superior iliac spine. *Ann Plast Surg* 1989;22:539.

 CHAPTER 472. Open-Jump Skin Flap from Abdomen to Thigh *S.C. Morgan*
www.encyclopediaofflaps.com

CHAPTER 473 ■ FREE MICROVASCULAR POSTEROLATERAL THIGH FLAPS

T. R. HEINZ AND L. O. VASCONEZ

EDITORIAL COMMENT

This is a dependable flap that can be harvested relatively easily. The quality of the skin is reasonably thin.

The free lateral thigh flap offers the possibility of harvesting a very large (up to 20 × 30 cm) pliable, thin, and generally hairless fasciocutaneous free flap for practically any type of requirement.

INDICATIONS

This flap has the advantage of incorporation in a chimeric fashion with the iliac bone, vastus lateralis, tensor fasciae latae muscles, or TRAM-flap territories, for very extensive combined defects. The term "lateral thigh flap" is misleading, since two flaps based in the lateral thigh territory have been described based on quite different arterial systems. A cutaneous posterolateral thigh flap, based on the third perforator of the profunda femoris artery (1), will be described first. A second flap, which can be called the anterolateral thigh flap, is based on the cutaneous branch of the descending branch of the lateral circumflex femoral system (1–6) and is described in Chap. 522. Either of these flaps may be innervated, typically with a branch of the lateral or posterior femoral cutaneous nerve.

ANATOMY

The posterior thigh flap is based on a branch of the profunda femoris artery, which gives off four perforating arteries that supply the muscles and skin of the posterolateral aspect of the thigh. The third cutaneous perforator is generally the largest, usually approximately 1.0 to 2.0 mm in diameter. It traverses the space between the iliotibial tract and the biceps femoris muscle, giving muscular branches to each, and emerges from that space immediately distal to the adductor brevis. This branch pierces the origin of the vastus lateralis muscle along the linea aspera, about half the distance from the greater trochanteric to the lateral femoral condyle.

The artery continues on to give a muscular branch to the biceps femoris muscle and is approximately 2 mm in diameter at this point. It then traverses the muscle fibers of the short head of the biceps femoris to become a cutaneous branch of about 1.0 to 1.5 mm in diameter (Fig. 1).

Posterolateral Thigh Flap

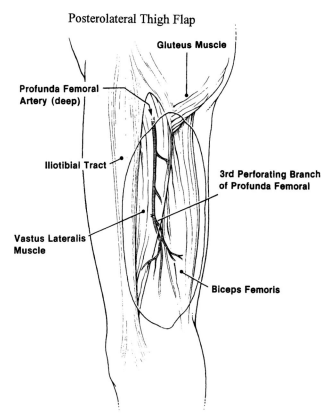

FIG. 1. Vascular anatomy and usual flap orientation of the posterolateral thigh flap. Note that vastus lateralis may be harvested.

The artery is accompanied by a vena comitans, usually of good caliber and quality. The length of the vascular pedicle that can be used is about 5 cm.

The nerve supply to this portion of the thigh is derived from the posterior and lateral femoral cutaneous nerves, and one or both may be used, as needed, according to the design of the flap.

FLAP DESIGN AND DIMENSIONS

The vascular pedicle can be located by the Doppler flowmeter and marked (Fig. 1). These vessels should be large and are easily identified. Since the pedicle emerges between the iliotibial tract and the biceps femoris, these may be identified with the patient in the supine position, the knee slightly flexed, and the hip internally rotated.

With the pedicle approximately half the distance from the greater trochanter to the lateral epicondyle of the femur, an oval flap of up to 20 × 30 cm may be outlined in this area. The flap is typically incised superiorly and subfascial dissection is used, with care toward the center of the flap at the

point of fascial penetration of the pedicle vessels. The deeper fascia is incised at this point, and careful dissection is used to expose the vascular pedicle fully. A portion of the intermuscular septum on both sides of the vascular bundle should be taken with this structure.

OPERATIVE TECHNIQUE

The patient is placed in the lateral decubitus position for exposure of the lateral and posterior thigh. The pedicle is located with the Doppler flowmeter at one-half the distance from the greater trochanter to the lateral femoral epicondyle, along the line of the posterior border of the iliotibial tract. The lateral femoral cutaneous nerve of the thigh in the anterior portion of this flap territory emerges from behind the inguinal ligament near the anterior superior iliac spine and descends inferolaterally to innervate the anterior portion of this thigh skin territory.

The posterior femoral cutaneous nerve of the thigh emerges just below the gluteal fold at one-half the distance from the ischium to the trochanter. It then descends almost longitudinally caudally, to provide sensation to the posterior thigh. These points may be marked and the skin flap raised from superior centrally in the subfascial plane. As one approaches the pedicle, care is taken to avoid injury, as the deep fascial layer is penetrated for better definition of the pedicle itself. With this under control, the remainder of the flap may be safely raised quite rapidly, to include the iliotibial tract fibers. Muscular branches will be ligated as the deeper dissection of the pedicle proceeds. Splitting the linea aspera is also helpful to allow identification of the accompanying vein.

The donor site may be closed directly to up to 15 cm in width or skin-grafted, as required.

SUMMARY

The posterolateral thigh free flap is quite useful. It is relatively easy to harvest, has a long pedicle and vessels of good diameter, can be frequently closed primarily, and may be harvested with the patient supine.

References

1. Song Y, Chen G, Song Y. The free thigh flap: a new free flap concept based on the septocutaneous artery. *Br J Plast Surg* 1984;37:149.
2. Baek SM. Two new cutaneous free flaps: the medial and lateral thigh flaps. *Plast Reconstr Surg* 1983;71:354.
3. Kajiyama K, Kawashima T. Experience with anterolateral thigh flaps. *Jpn J Plast Reconstr Surg* 1986;29:398.
4. Koshima I, Eudoh T, Uchida A, et al. Clinical experience with free anterolateral thigh flaps. *J Jpn Soc Plast Reconstr Surg* 1986;6:260.
5. Xu D-C, Zhang S-Z, King J-M, et al. Applied anatomy of the anterolateral femoral flap. *Plast Reconstr Surg* 1988;82:305.
6. Koshima I, Fukudo H, Utonomiya R, Soeda S. The anterolateral thigh flap: variation in vascular pedicles. *Br J Plast Surg* 1989;42:260.

LOWER EXTREMITY RECONSTRUCTION

CHAPTER 474. Slide-Swing Skin Flap *J. Schrudde and V. Petrovici*

www.encyclopediaofflaps.com

CHAPTER 475. Bipedicle Crural Skin Flap *S. W. Hartwell, Jr.*

www.encyclopediaofflaps.com

CHAPTER 476 ■ ISLAND FLAP IN RECONSTRUCTIVE SURGERY OF THE LEGS

F. C. BEHAN

EDITORIAL COMMENT

The design versatility of fasciocutaneous flaps, particularly in the lower extremity, is due to our knowledge of the blood supply through the septocutaneous vessels. As long as the surgeon maintains one septocutaneous perforator vessel, he or she could outline a flap either proximally or distally based or as a turnover flap, or as the authors demonstrate, in an elegant way, with what they call the "keystone flap."

The keystone-design perforator island flap (KDPIF), used to reconstruct soft-tissue defects and to avoid complex reconstruction, is described.

INDICATIONS

The principle of island-flap repair has a long history (1–5). The KDPIF is a curvilinear trapezoidal flap. It is essentially two V-Y end-to-side flaps (see Fig. 3). The curvilinear shape of the flap fits well into various body contours. This chapter describes the use of an island flap that is effective in many areas of the body, provides effective skin coverage, and achieves excellent aesthetic results.

ANATOMY

The KDPIF is designed within the dermatomal segments or precincts (Fig. 1) and straddles the longitudinal running structures (6,7) [e.g., the cutaneous nerves and superficial veins (8)], which are incorporated in the flap. Aligning the flaps along the cutaneous nerve supply, when possible, incorporates the perforators that accompany the peripheral nerves (8,9). These are in addition to the subcutaneous, fascial, and muscular perforators that support the viability of the flap (10). Blunt dissection allows the retention of the majority of venous communications (8). Doppler localization techniques have not been used preoperatively or intraoperatively.

FLAP DESIGN AND DIMENSIONS

The vascular basis of this keystone flap is essentially that of a fasciocutaneous perforator and has been well described by us and others (1–5). Hence, we use the terminology *keystone design perforator island flap*. It is really an extension of the angiotome principle, designed as an island based on axial

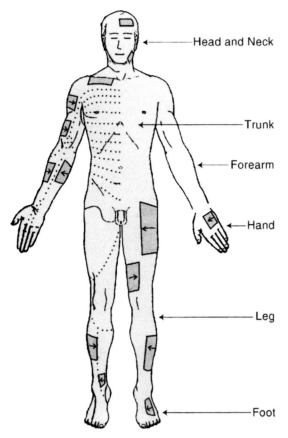

FIG. 1. Keystone design perforator island flaps designed along the dermatomal segments. The longitudinal axis of the flap sits along the dermatomal segment and superimposes on septocutaneous, musculocutaneous and fasciocutaneous perforator vessels that ensure the viability of the flap.

perforators from the underlying structures. However, to design a flap the same width as the primary defect immediately adjacent to it, which has essentially the same mobility characteristics, and to expect this not only to close that defect but also to permit direct closure of its own larger secondary defect, seems empirically daring. What is it about the design that enables this to occur when the rules of length-breadth ratio seem to be overruled? It was S. H. Milton in 1971, remarking on the experimental studies on island flaps, who said, "an island is safer than a peninsula."

The flap has certain characteristics of a bipedicled flap (6,7), yet this keystone flap is really two V-Y flaps side by side, but facing in opposite directions. In a conventional bipedicled design, the secondary defect is usually larger than the primary and is not closeable without grafting. By converting this bipedicled flap into an island with V-Y advancement at each end, the longitudinal tension in the flap is released, thus creating laxity and redundancy in its midportion, which can then be moved farther in a horizontal direction toward the defect. Closure of the V-Y defects at each end narrows the whole defect complex, so that the flap does not have to move so far horizontally. Similarly, the secondary defect on the opposite side of the flap is reduced by this maneuver. Wide, blunt dissection preserving the neurovascular structures, and teasing of the surrounding tissue, facilitate centripetal movement inward circumferentially around the flap. Although considerable tension exists peripherally, the central portion of the flap does not move excessively, relative to its underlying vertical perforators. These are consequently not subjected to the same tension.

Flap Subtypes

- Type I: standard flap design and closure are suitable for defects up to 2 cm in width over most areas of the body.
- Type IIA: division of deep fascia. For larger areas of reconstruction located over the muscular compartments, the deep fascia over the muscular compartment is divided along the outer curvature of the flap, to permit further mobilization of the keystone flap.
- Type IIB: with split-thickness skin graft to secondary defect. Where excess tension exists, the secondary defect may be skin grafted (e.g., where tissue has limited elastic stretch on the lower third of the lower limb and the lower third of the forearm). This retains the advantage, however, of allowing the flap to cover vital structures while the graft allows wound healing.
- Type III: double-keystone flaps. For considerably larger defects (5 to 10 cm), a double-keystone design can be carried out, to exploit maximal laxity of the surrounding tissues. This is suitable for large defects in the calf or sacral regions.
- Type IV: rotational keystone flap. Occasionally, to facilitate rotation across joint contractures or compound fractures with exposed bone, the keystone flap is raised with undermining up to 50% of the flap subfascially. The undermined fasciocutaneous part of the flap, which could be either proximally or distally based, can then be transposed across large joint contractures of the elbow and knee, or can be used to cover the exposed bone in compound fractures. Perforator support is derived from the attached part of the flap.

OPERATIVE TECHNIQUE

The lesion should be excised in an elliptical manner, with its axis parallel to the line of the cutaneous nerves, veins, known vascular perforators, or a combination of these. In the upper and lower limbs, this location is generally longitudinally placed (Fig. 1). The side of the defect that has the greater laxity is chosen for the flap site. In the lower leg, where these flaps are particularly well suited, the flap is best sited posterior to the defect, so that the increasing laxity of skin over the posterior compartment can be exploited to close the secondary defect (e.g., upper, middle, and lower calf areas in the lower limb).

In the upper limb, these techniques are well applied to the biceps and triceps areas of the upper arm, and the proximal flexor and extensor areas of the forearm. An incision at 90 degrees at either end of the defect meets the curvilinear line of the flap markout. This curvature or keystone shape is then mobilized. The width of the flap equals the width of the defect (Fig. 2). Its length is governed by the size of the elliptical excision.

Once the excisional defect is created after the removal of a lesion, the KDPIF has a ratio of 1:1 for the width of the defect to the width of the flap. The length of the flap is determined by the size of the excisional defect. A right angle is formed at the limits of the excision to create the keystone design (Fig. 2A and B).

Blunt dissection allows mobilization of the surrounding tissue while advancing the flap to facilitate wound approximation (Fig. 3A). Careful teasing of the circumferential tissue is performed without any flap undermining, so as to preserve the integrity of the perforators. Where possible, all subcutaneous longitudinal venous and neural structures that support the flap should also be retained within the limits of the surgical

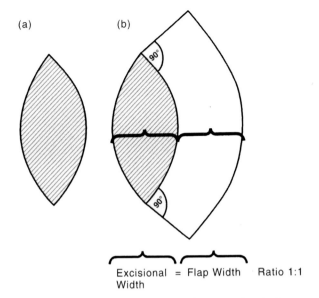

(a)   (b)

Excisional = Flap Width   Ratio 1:1
Width

FIG. 2. A: Mitotic lesion or traumatic defect excised with clearance; **B:** Keystone design perforator island flap. The trapezoid-shaped flap is contoured along the side of the excisional defect with 90-degree angle at the limits of the island flap.

procedure. Any inadvertent trauma to the venous drainage system is repaired. The deep fascia is left intact for smaller lesions up to 2 cm (type I keystone). Where increased mobilization is required, the lateral deep fascial margin is released, particularly in the areas of the calf, thigh, forearm, and upper arm (type II keystone).

The first step in wound closure is direct apposition of the defect with interrupted single-layer nylon sutures (Fig. 4C). Depending on the size of the defect, that may be two, three, or four stay sutures in this single-layer-closure technique. Then the V-Y advancement of each end of the flap in the longitudinal axis is completed (Fig. 3B). This creates redundancy and laxity in the flap tissue at the right-angle points of the flap, which are excised. This also serves to narrow the whole defect. Wound closure of the relaxed keystone flap can now be completed, using a hemming suture advanced in the horizontal axis into the original defect and sutured. Further undermining and release allow even distribution of tension, and facilitate circumferential wound closure. A continuous, everting, horizontal mattress suture also helps to distribute tension evenly around the flap margins.

To close the V-Y points initially may reduce tension. However, our technique of direct closure of the midpoint helps to determine the need for a graft, if undue tension is present. Stay sutures must be left intact for 14 to 17 days, to prevent wound dehiscence.

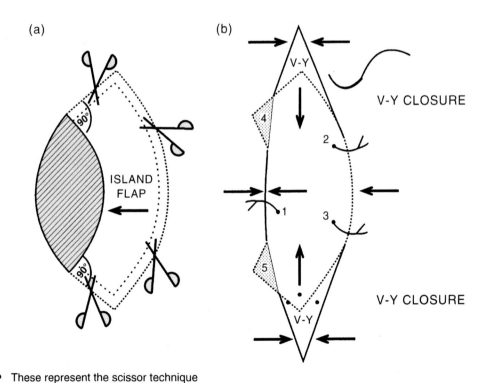

These represent the scissor technique
used for the Blunt Dissection

FIG. 3. A: Blunt-dissection mobilization around the limits of the flap. *Note:* No dissection is done beneath the island flap to preserve the integrity of the perforators, while retaining, if possible, all longitudinal venous and neural structures that support the flap. The deep fascia is divided along the outer curvilinear line in types IIA, IIB, III and IV, in which the undue tension exists. No deep fascia is divided beneath the flap canopy, the site of the random perforator. **B:** The keystone island flap in position. Interrupted sutures (*1–3*) bring the flap into alignment, creating lines of tension. Closure of the double V-Y apposition points at the limits of the flap creates a relative redundancy in the central portion of the flap and relaxes the horizontal tension. The *shaded areas* (*4* and *5*) are redundant and are excised. The wound closure is completed with the Hemming suture.

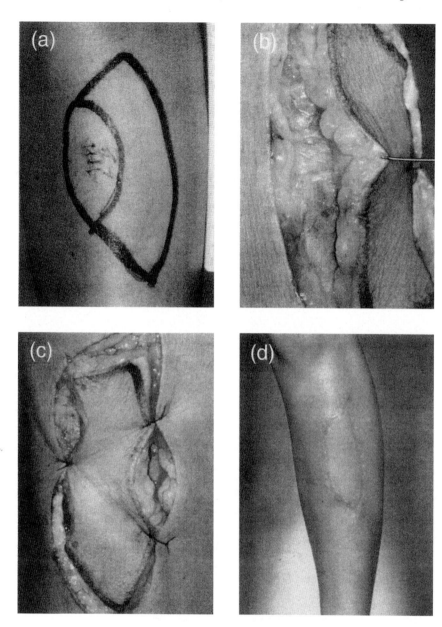

FIG. 4. A–D: The use of a type IIA keystone flap to reconstruct a 5- × 2.6-cm soft tissue defect on the lower leg after a wide local excision for a level II malignant melanoma.

CLINICAL RESULTS

Since 1995, we have performed more than 300 keystone-design flaps, with only one case of partial flap necrosis. Superficial flap necrosis occurred in the leg of a 78-year-old diabetic patient. Thus the flap-survival rate in this whole series has been 99.6%. The procedure has been associated with excellent healing, minimal postoperative pain, minimal postoperative edema, and superior aesthetics.

When initially islanded, flaps appear hyperemic, perhaps because of denervation or vessel vasodilatation. It is conjectured that this is a sympathetic response, and a sympathectomy is being performed to the small vessels via the blunt dissection. We have observed striking vascular changes in these island flaps. This may make them intrinsically more robust than skin-based flaps, which rely on horizontal blood flow and are more subject to tensional forces (4,5,8,10). The red-dot sign at a suture point is where arterial blood oozes on the surface of the flap, which is not seen around the perimeter of the insert. The vascular flare is seen consistently in those KDPIFs that have a myocutaneous base for the perforators.

To facilitate closure of the secondary defect, the flap should be sited along the side of the excision margin that has the greater tissue laxity. This may not be significantly different at either side, but it is the tissue beyond the flap itself that must ultimately move to close the defect. It is this progressive movement outward into looser territory that enables direct closure of the secondary defect. In the lower limb, for instance, tissue is mobile over the medial, and especially over the posterior, compartment. Here, the calf and thigh muscles themselves can move with the overlying skin, compared with the tighter fascial or periosteal beds of the anterolateral aspect, which allows very little direct advancement of overlying skin.

The perforating skin vessels of the lax muscle compartment are also longer and more stretchable than the short tighter vessel of the anterior region. In this sense, the design is somewhat akin to the principle of the bibbed flap, in which the first flap closes the main defect, and the smaller second flap (because it is now taken from laxer tissues) is able to close the secondary defect. In this case, however, the second flap is direct advancement.

Postoperative pain is negligible, and narcotics are rarely needed. When healing is complete, the surrounding nerve supply usually returns to normal, although some patients do complain of mild dysesthesia, particularly in the large flaps in the front of the thigh. Somewhat surprisingly, postoperative pin-cushion–type flap edema has been minimal, despite the islanded flap design. No doubt the underlying perforator support plays a role, as well as the relatively large size of the flaps.

SUMMARY

The reliability of this island flap design is possibly due to the fact that the circulation is based on vertically orientated perforators and dispenses with the subdermal plexus. This could explain why lines of transverse tension across the flap, so commonly seen on direct suturing, validate that perfusion is reliable to the limits of the flap, because the island design is supported by such vessels. The ability to close relatively large defects totally with flap tissue from the immediate vicinity maximizes the aesthetic appearance, compared with grafts or distant flaps, which have poor color match, poor contour, and secondary deformity. The nature of the curvilinear design of

the keystone flap fits well into body contour dimensions (i.e., straight lines stand out; curves fit into the creases).

References

1. Behan FC, Wilson I. The principle of the angiotome, a system of linked axial pattern flaps. In: *Transactions of the 6th International Congress of Plastic and Reconstructive Surgery*. Paris: Masson, 1975.
2. Littler JW. Neurovascular pedicle transfer of tissue in reconstructive surgery of the hand. *J Bone Joint Surg* 1956;38A:917.
3. Behan FC, Cavallo AV, Terrill P. Ring avulsion injuries managed with homodigital and heterodigital venous island conduit (VIC) flaps. *Br J Plast Surg* 1998;23B:465.
4. Behan FC, Terrill PJ, Breidahi A, et al. Island flaps including the Bezier type in the treatment of malignant melanoma. *Aust N Z J Surg* 1995;65:870.
5. Behan FC. The fasciocutaneous island flap: an extension of the angiotome concept. *Aust N Z J Surg* 1992;62:874.
6. Onizuka T, Akagawa T, Kondo S, et al. The length: breadth ratio of skin flaps on the trunk: two new long narrow flaps. *Br J Plast Surg* 1975;28:123.
7. Schwabegger A, Ninkovic M, Wechselberger G, Anderl H. The bipedicled flap on the lower leg, a valuable old method? Its indications and limitations in 12 cases. *Scand J Plast Reconstr Surg Hand Surg* 1996;30:87.
8. Shalaby HA, Saad MA. The venous island flap: is it purely venous? *Br J Plast Surg* 1993;46:285.
9. Nakajima H, Imanishi N, Fukuzumi S, et al. Accompanying arteries of the cutaneous veins and cutaneous nerves in the extremities: anatomical study and a concept of the venoadipofascial and/or neuroadipofascial pedicled fasciocutaneous flap. *Plast Reconstr Surg* 1998;102:779.
10. Braverman IM. The cutaneous microcirculation. *J Invest Dermatol Symp Proc* 2000;5:3.

CHAPTER 477 ■ SLIDING TRANSPOSITION SKIN FLAP

S. H. HARRISON AND M. N. SAAD

The use of local flaps in the leg has long been known to be hazardous (1–4), partly because of the limited collateral circulation in that area but also due to faulty design. A basic but neglected factor that has been responsible for the large percentage of failed flaps in the leg is the convexity of its surface.

INDICATIONS

The lateral movement of a standard transposition flap across the convex surface of the leg results in transverse tension across the pedicle and embarrassment of its blood supply (5). The bipedicle or "strap" flap is similarly at risk (Fig. 1A). The transverse excursion of both pedicles across the convex surface results in tension, thus depriving the central part of the flap of its blood supply, causing necrosis at the very site where skin cover is required. Use of

the sliding transposition flap in the leg obviates transverse tension by insetting the distal oblique edge of the flap into the contralateral side of the defect (Fig. 1B), thus draping the long axis of the flap loosely across the convex surface (6).

FLAP DESIGN AND DIMENSIONS

A suitable donor site is selected medial or lateral to the defect (Fig. 2A). From the lower end of the defect, an oblique line is drawn, this being the distal edge of the flap. Its length should be equal to the contralateral side of the defect. From the end of this line, the lateral edge of the flap is drawn proximally toward its base. The width of the base of the flap should be adequate to sustain the circulation of the flap, bearing in mind that excess width will limit mobility. A length-to-width ratio of 3:2, in our experience, has been more than adequate.

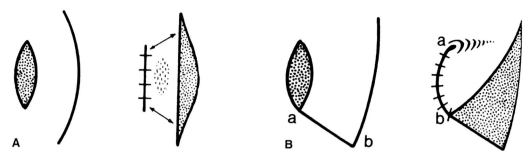

FIG. 1. A: The standard bipedicle flap frequently fails because the midportion of the flap, which is already under considerable tension, must reach over the convex surface of the leg. B: Note, however, that the long axis of the sliding transposition flap drapes easily over the convex surface of the leg. (From Harrison and Saad, ref. 6, with permission.)

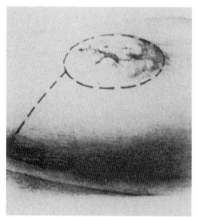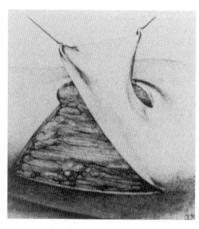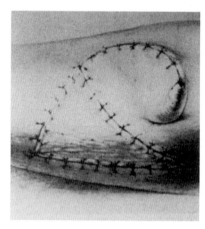

A–C

FIG. 2. A: A leg defect with the sliding transposition flap outlined. B: The flap easily reaches the defect without tension. Because the anatomy of the blood supply to the fascia and skin of the leg has been recently clarified, the fascia is now included with the flap. (This illustration depicts the older method of including just skin and subcutaneous tissue.) C: The donor site is covered with a split-thickness skin graft. (From Harrison and Saad, ref. 6, with permission.)

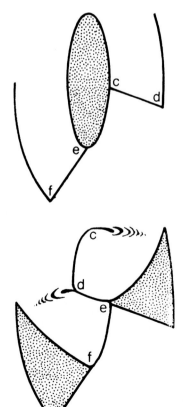

FIG. 3. A larger defect can be closed with two sliding transposition flaps. Note that both are proximally based. (From Harrison and Saad, ref. 6, with permission.)

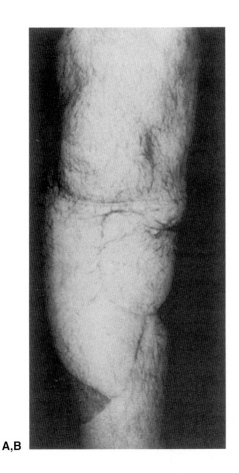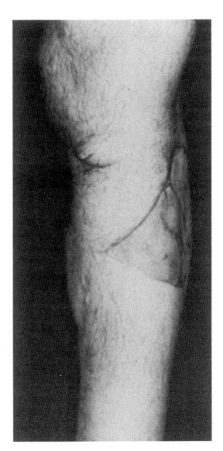

A,B

FIG. 4. An upper tibial defect has been covered with two sliding transposition skin flaps. Split-thickness skin grafts have been applied to the donor defects. (From Harrison and Saad, ref. 6, with permission.)

OPERATIVE TECHNIQUE

In our earlier patients, the flaps were raised superficial to the deep fascia, but more recently, we have included the deep fascia in our flaps (7) (see Chap. 481). After raising the flap (Fig. 2B), the recipient site is prepared and the flap is inset so that its long lateral edge is sutured to the contralateral side of the defect (Fig. 2C). The flap donor site is grafted. For larger defects, two flaps can be used (Figs. 3 and 4), both being proximally based. The degree of excursion of the flap results in an obvious dog-ear, which usually regresses with time.

CLINICAL RESULTS

In the first 13 patients reviewed in 1969, none of the flaps using this technique was lost in part or in whole, and the principle for establishing full-thickness skin cover using this method can be accepted as one available in selected patients.

SUMMARY

The sliding transposition flap is a reliable method of covering defects of the leg in selected patients.

References

1. Crawford BS. The repair of defects of the lower limbs using a local flap. *Br J Plast Surg* 1957;10:32.
2. Harrison, SH. Fractures of the tibia complicated by skin loss. *Br J Plast Surg* 1968;21:262.
3. Connelly JR. Reconstructive procedures of the lower extremity. In: Grabb WC, Smith JW, eds. *Plastic surgery.* Boston: Little, Brown, 1968;784.
4. Saad MN. The problems of traumatic skin loss of the lower limbs, especially when associated with skeletal injury. *Br J Surg* 1970;57:604.
5. Patterson TJS. The effects of tension on the survival of skin flaps. In: *Transactions of the fifth international congress of plastic and reconstructive surgery.* Melbourne, Australia: Butterworth, 1971;807.
6. Harrison SH, Saad MN. The sliding transposition flap: its application to leg defects. *Br J Plast Surg* 1977;30:54.
7. Pontén B. The fasciocutaneous flap: its use in soft-tissue defects of the lower leg. *Br J Plast Surg* 1981;34:215.

CHAPTER 478 ■ SAPHENOUS VENOUS FLAP

R. L. THATTE, M. S. WAGH, AND M. R. THATTE

The saphenous venous flap is useful for covering defects on both the anterior and posterior surfaces of the leg, including the popliteal fossa and knee joint.

INDICATIONS

This flap has been used most frequently for compound fractures of the tibia in emergency procedures, or for the same type of defect at a later stage after fixation of fractures has been achieved. It also has been used for dense adherent scars over the tibia, as a prelude to secondary bone surgery, or to hasten union in tardy healing of fractures. When swung to the posterior surface of the leg (Figs. 2 and 3) and also to the popliteal fossa, it has been used to fill defects created by release of post-traumatic or post-burn contractures (Figs. 4 and 5). In addition, it has been found to be extremely useful in coverage of the knee joint (Figs. 6–8).

ANATOMY

The saphenous venous flap (1) is a unipedicled type-1 venous flap (2) based on the saphenous vein in the upper two-thirds of the leg. The long saphenous vein ascends for 2.5 cm anterior to the medial malleolus of the tibia and then crosses medial to the tibia, lying about 1 to 2 cm medial to the medial border of the bone, until it reaches the medial condyle of the tibia (Fig. 1). It then courses on the medial surface of the thigh, ultimately draining into the femoral vein. A vertical rectangular territory on either side of the vein is available for the flap.

Earlier reports of unipedicled venous flaps (3–5) postulated a to-and-fro flow pattern in the vein, seemingly supported by experimental and mathematical models. This explanation of venous flow has been contradicted more recently (6). The survival of unipedicled type-1 venous flaps has now been attributed to either the perivenous or perineural capillary network.

FLAP DESIGN AND DIMENSIONS

The flap consists of a rectangular fasciocutaneous island, longer at the vertical axis along the vein, and shorter in the transverse dimension across the vein (Fig. 1). It can be based only on a patent, long, saphenous vein. It is preferable not to use this flap when adherent, deep scars are seen in the area of the surface markings of the vein. Vein patency can be gauged

by tying a tourniquet in the lower third of the thigh. If the vein is not visible during this maneuver, palpation can assist in demonstrating a turgid, full vein. In the event of difficulties with both these techniques, a small incision at the proposed base of the flap and dissection through the deeper layers of the

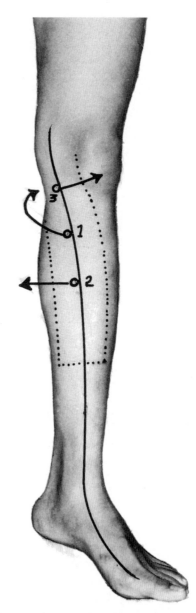

FIG. 1. Schematic diagram showing anatomy and design of the saphenous venous flap. A unipedicle flap can be raised based proximally at location 1 or 2. Dotted area shows the largest flap possible. (From Thatte and Thatte, ref. 1, with permission.)

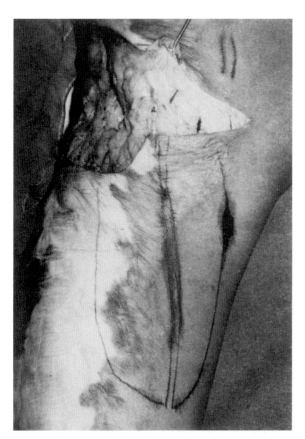

FIG. 2. Defect in popliteal fossa and flap design inferior to defect for postero-superior rotation. (From Thatte and Thatte, ref. 1, with permission.)

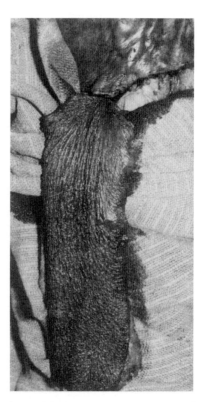

FIG. 4. Flap designed for burn contracture in the middle third of the leg. (From Thatte and Thatte, ref. 1, with permission.)

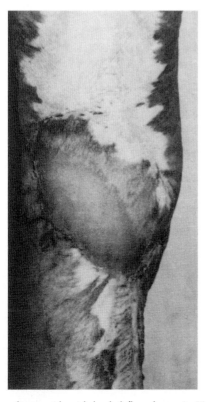

FIG. 3. Late photograph with healed flap shown in Fig. 2. (From Thatte and Thatte, ref. 1, with permission.)

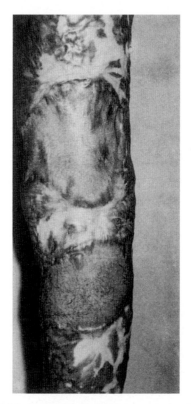

FIG. 5. Healed flap. Upper defect has been grafted and lower defect has been covered by the flap. (From Thatte and Thatte, ref. 1, with permission.)

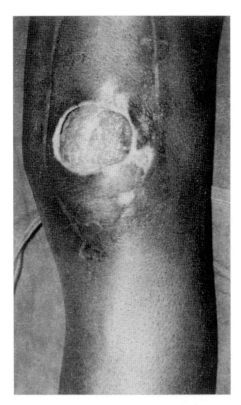

FIG. 6. Defect over anterior aspect of the knee. (From Thatte and Thatte, ref. 1, with permission.)

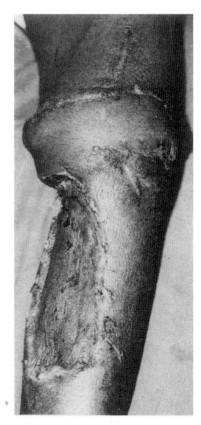

FIG. 8. Healed flap. (From Thatte and Thatte, ref. 1, with permission.)

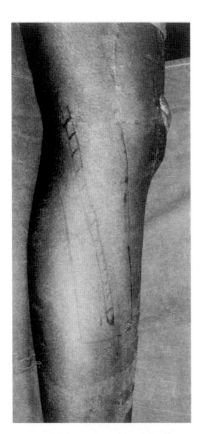

FIG. 7. Flap design to cover defect. (From Thatte and Thatte, ref. 1, with permission.)

subcutaneous fat will demonstrate vein patency. The saphenous venous flap island can be designed as a 1: 3 proportioned rectangle, the vein remaining in the middle along the length of the fasciocutaneous island.

The base of the flap in our series has never been below the midpoint of the leg, and the lowermost limit of the flap has never extended into the lower third of the leg. The medial extension of the flap usually stops around the area of the subcutaneous portion of the tibia, which is approximately 3 to 5 cm from the long saphenous vein in the upper two-thirds of the leg. An equal breadth is available on the posteromedial surface of the leg.

Total flap dimensions of 8 cm in width and 24 cm in length are therefore available in the upper two-thirds of the leg to cover defects by medial, superior, lateral, or posterior transfer of the saphenous venous island. The base of the island consists of only the long saphenous vein, with its adventitia and surrounding areolar tissue. This narrow base allows for flap mobility in an arc from 0 to 170 degrees. The flap is an island, and therefore seals and covers the defect on all sides.

OPERATIVE TECHNIQUE

The dissection is performed under tourniquet. The skin is incised down to and including the deep fascia in the vertical dimension on either side of the saphenous vein after a small incision has confirmed the patency and exact location of the vein at the flap base. A fasciocutaneous rectangle is then completed by making a transverse incision at the lower end and extending the exploratory incision at the upper end. Only the saphenous vein with its intact adventitia and surrounding areolar tissue is preserved at both ends.

After tourniquet release and achievement of hemostasis, heparin 100 U/kg is given subcutaneously and, after a further check of hemostasis, the vein at the lower end is clamped, ligated, and cut. The flap is transposed to the defect, and a split-thickness skin graft is applied to the donor site from which the flap was raised.

CLINICAL RESULTS

Seven of eight flaps in our series were successful, with five surviving completely without complication. One flap that was entirely lost was utilized in an elderly hypertensive patient who developed a large hematoma underneath the flap, due to a clotted suction drain. In this case, the saphenous vein had been teased off its fatty envelope over a length of about 3 cm, which may have contributed to thrombosis. The patient had received intraoperative heparin intravenously.

Two flaps had marginal distal loss, one also following a hematoma under the flap. This patient also had received intraoperative intravenous heparin, leading to excessive oozing. The defect resulting from flap loss required a small skin graft, but the flap fulfilled its original purpose of coverage.

The other marginal loss in one corner of the flap was anticipated, because the vein entered the distal (caudal) end of the flap eccentrically. The contralateral part of the distal end was probably not perfused by the venous network. Again, this flap also fulfilled its purpose in coverage of the defect.

SUMMARY

The saphenous venous flap can be raised at any level along the saphenous vein in the upper half of the leg. It provides a versatile technique for extensive scarring following extremity burns or trauma and is an improvement over previously used methods.

References

1. Thatte RL, Thatte MR. The saphenous venous flap. Br J Plast Surg 1989; 42: 399.
2. Thatte MR, Thatte RL. Venous flaps. Plast Reconstr Surg 1993; 91: 747.
3. Thatte RL, Thatte MR. The cephalic venous flap. Br J Plast Surg 1987; 40: 16.
4. Thatte MR, Kamdar NB, Khakkar DV, et al. Static and dynamic computerized radioactive tracer studies, vital dye staining, and theoretical methematical calculations to ascertain the mode of survival of single cephalad channel venous island flaps. Br J Plast Surg 1989; 42: 405.
5. Thatte MR, Healy C, McGrouther DA. Laser Doppler and microvascular pulsed Doppler studies of the physiology of venous flaps. Eur J Plast Surg 1993; 16:134.
6. Smith RJ, Fukuta K, Wheatley M, Jackson IT. Role of perivenous areolar tissue and recipient bed in the viability of venous flaps in the rabbit ear model. Br J Plast Surg 1994; 147:10.

CHAPTER 479 ■ LATERAL GENICULAR ARTERY FLAP

A. HAYASHI AND Y. MARUYAMA

EDITORIAL COMMENT

This is a useful and reliable flap for this location.

The lateral genicular artery flap allows single-stage reconstruction of soft-tissue defects around the knee. Because of its thinness, it also provides for an excellent result in contour at the recipient site.

INDICATIONS

For reconstruction of soft-tissue defects around the knee, the goals are to preserve function and to restore knee contour. Among possible solutions to these problems are the lateral and medial genicular artery flaps, and the posterior popliteal thigh flap. All these flaps are distally-based cutaneous and fasciocutaneous flaps harvested from the lower thigh (1–3). The lateral genicular artery flap is indicated for soft-tissue defects of the distal third of the thigh, the knee, the popliteal fossa, and the proximal third of the lower leg, with the exception of the medial aspects of these regions.

The flap has the following advantages. It allows single-stage reconstruction, as well as providing excellent results at the recipient site. A donor site less than 10 cm in width can be closed primarily in most instances, and no functional or sensory loss occurs in the lower extremity. The flap is certainly an effective alternative to previously reported muscle, musculocutaneous, and fasciocutaneous flaps (4–6). Since the posterior popliteal thigh flap and the medial genicular artery flap are also fasciocutaneous flaps based on the septocutaneous perforators around the knee, they share the same advantages as the lateral genicular artery flap. The choice among these flaps depends on the location of the defect and tissue availability at the donor site.

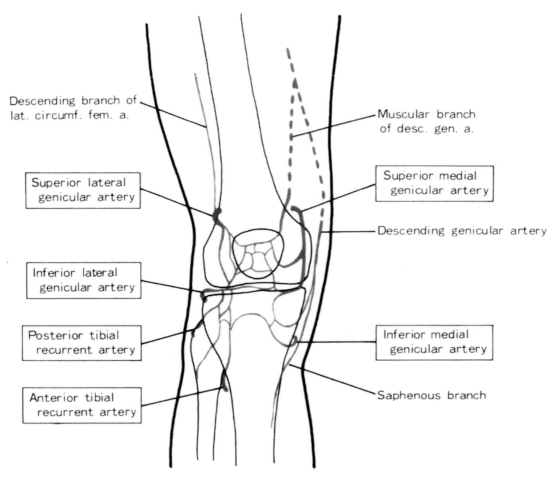

FIG. 1. Vascular anatomy of the anterior aspect of the knee showing cutaneous perforators and their communication.

ANATOMY (FIG. 1)

The superior lateral genicular artery (SLGA) usually originates from the popliteal artery. It courses superolaterally, giving off branches to the vastus lateralis, biceps femoris, and the knee joint. After traveling in the intermuscular space between the vastus lateralis and the short head of the biceps femoris, the SLGA penetrates the deep fascia (or iliotibial tract) just proximal to the lateral condyle of the femur. The point at which the cutaneous perforator of the SLGA penetrates the deep fascia is about 5 cm from the plane of the knee joint.

The cutaneous perforator of the SLGA terminates in small cutaneous branches that follow a radial pattern. These branches anastomose freely with the rete patellae, the lateral perforator of the profunda femoris artery, the musculocutaneous perforators from the popliteal artery, and the musculocutaneous or septocutaneous perforators (or both) from the descending branch of the lateral circumflex femoral artery (Fig. 1). Among these anastomoses, the communication between the SLGA and the lateral perforators of the profunda femoris artery are predominant; this arterial communication is well-developed in the mid-layer of the subcutaneous adipose tissue (1).

FLAP DESIGN AND DIMENSIONS

The skin island is designed on the lateral aspect of the lower thigh. The distal end of the flap must cover the skin over the lateral condyle of the femur, to include the emergence of the cutaneous perforator of the SLGA. The proximal end of

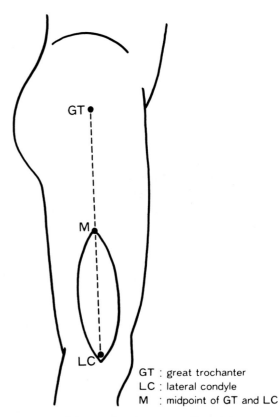

GT : great trochanter
LC : lateral condyle
M : midpoint of GT and LC

FIG. 2. Design of the lateral genicular artery flap in relation to surface landmarks.

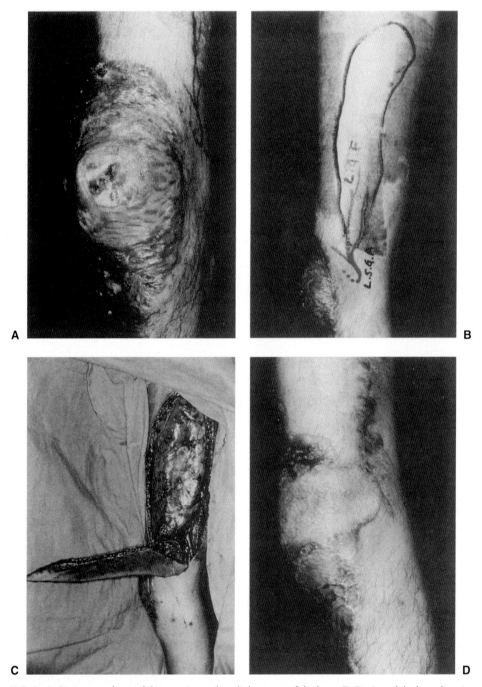

FIG. 3. **A:** Recurrent ulcers of the anterior and medial aspects of the knee. **B:** Design of the lateral genicular artery flap. **C:** Island flap was elevated, and donor site was closed primarily. **D:** Postoperative view showing complete survival of the flap and good recontouring of the knee. (From Hayashi and Maruyama, ref. 1, with permission.)

the flap can be safely extended to the mid-point between the greater trochanter and the lateral condyle of the femur (Fig. 2).

OPERATIVE TECHNIQUE

The incision is begun from the proximal apex of the flap, and the plane of dissection is maintained on the loose areolar layer over the deep fascia. Distal to the point 10 cm above the knee joint, the dissection should be carried down to the iliotibial tract for the safe dissection of the intermuscular septum between the vastus lateralis and the short head of the biceps

femoris. After division, the vascular pedicle can be identified just above the lateral condyle of the femur.

This island lateral genicular artery flap is then elevated and transferred to the defect. The flap arc of rotation reaches the distal third of the thigh, knee, and popliteal fossa, and the proximal third of the lower leg, with the exception of the medial aspects of these regions (Fig. 3).

CLINICAL RESULTS

Defects around the knee have been well-recontoured because of the thinness of the flap. However, when the patient cannot accept the donor-site scarring on the lateral aspect of the thigh, the posterior popliteal thigh flap might be a better alternative.

SUMMARY

The lateral genicular artery flap is useful for reconstruction of soft-tissue defects around the knee. The flap is thin, provides excellent results in knee contour, and produces no functional or sensory loss in the lower extremity.

References

1. Hayashi A, Maruyama Y. The lateral genicular artery flap. *Ann Plast Surg* 1990;24:310.
2. Hayashi A, Maruyama Y. The medial genicular artery flap. *Ann Plast Surg* 1990;25:174.
3. Maruyama Y, Iwahira Y. Popliteo-posterior thigh fasciocutaneous island flap for closure around the knee. *Br J Plast Surg* 1990;42:140.
4. Feldmann JJ, Cohen BE, May JW. The medial gastrocnemius myocutaneous flap. *Plast Reconstr Surg* 1978;61:531.
5. Swartz WM, Ramasastry SS, McGill JR, et al. Distally based vastus lateralis muscle flap for coverage of wounds about the knee. *Plast Reconstr Surg* 1987;80:255.
6. Acland RD, Godina MSM, Eder E, et al. The saphenous neurovascular free flap. *Plast Reconstr Surg* 1981;67:763.

CHAPTER 480 ■ THREE ANTEROMEDIAL FASCIOCUTANEOUS LEG ISLAND FLAPS

A. A. KHASHABA AND M. M. EL-SAADI

> **EDITORIAL COMMENT**
>
> The versatility of the flap is increased, as the flap can be converted into an island with preservation of its vascular pedicle.

These three fasciocutaneous island flaps (upper, middle, and lower) are based on three segments of the anteromedial aspect of the leg. Depending on the location of the nearest flap pedicle and the size of the defect, they can be used for reconstruction over almost any site in the lower two-thirds of the leg.

INDICATIONS

The upper and middle flaps are indicated mainly for coverage of bony and soft-tissue defects of the upper and middle thirds of the anterolateral aspect of the leg. The use of the lowest flap, perhaps the most important of the three, includes the difficult areas of the medial and lateral malleolus, the back of the calcaneum, and the Achilles tendon (1–6).

ANATOMY (7–9)

The medial septocutaneous vessels originate from the posterior tibial vessels and are enclosed in the deep transverse fascial septum of the leg, i.e., the septum that separates the soleus and gastrocnemius from the deep muscular compartment of the posterior leg. The upper and middle septocutaneous vessels supplying the upper and middle flaps pierce the fascia after passing through the tibial origin of the soleus just behind the medial border of the tibia. The lower septocutaneous vessels supplying the lower flap pierce the fascia, after passing between the flexor digitorum longus and soleus muscles and the Achilles tendon.

The three segments along the medial side of the leg where their feeding vessels are most frequently identified lie between 9–12 cm, 17–19 cm, and 22–24 cm, respectively, from the tip of the medial malleolus (Fig. 1). The external diameter of these vessels varies from 0.5 to 1.5 mm, those with larger diameter being found at the middle third of the leg.

FLAP DESIGN AND DIMENSIONS

The flaps are designed in accordance with the size of the defect and the site of the nearest pedicle (upper, middle, or lower). Generally speaking, the skin of the entire calf area can be raised on any of the three pedicles, but it is always safer not to transgress the midline posteriorly by more than 2 cm.

OPERATIVE TECHNIQUE

Raising the flap begins from its posterior edge in a subfascial plane. The pedicles will appear just before the medial border of the tibia is reached. After identifying and dissecting the pedicle, the flap is raised from all its edges. The greater saphenous vein will often be encountered at the anterior edge of the flap, and an effort should always be made to preserve it. The flap is then transferred to cover the defect, and a split-thickness skin graft is utilized at the donor site (Figs. 2–4).

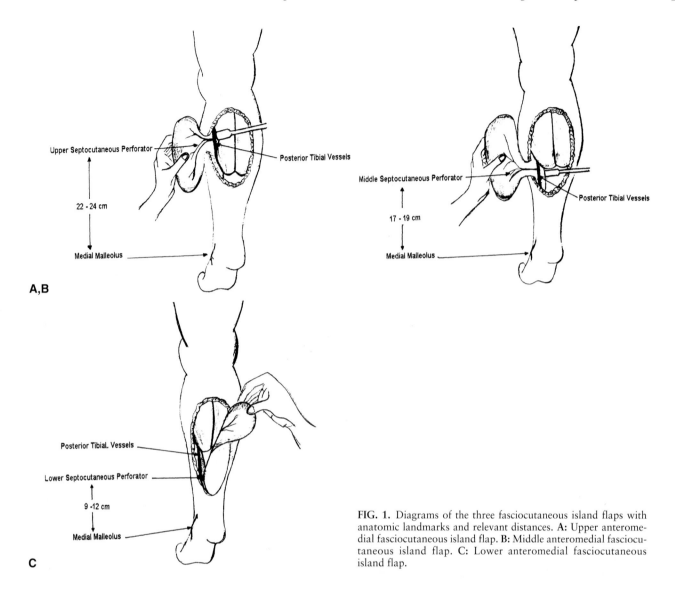

FIG. 1. Diagrams of the three fasciocutaneous island flaps with anatomic landmarks and relevant distances. A: Upper anteromedial fasciocutaneous island flap. B: Middle anteromedial fasciocutaneous island flap. C: Lower anteromedial fasciocutaneous island flap.

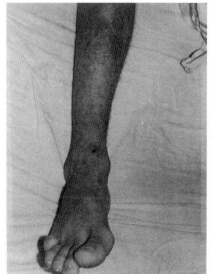
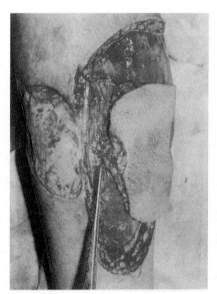
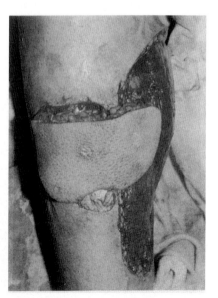

FIG. 2. A: Chronic leg ulcer of 2 years' duration over the shin of the tibia. B: The defect and a flap based on the uppermost segment (forceps point to pedicle). C: The flap rotated 90 degrees to cover the defect. *(Continued)*

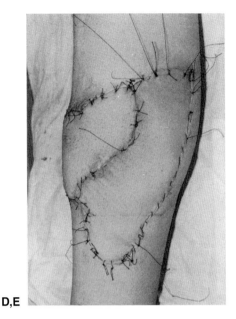

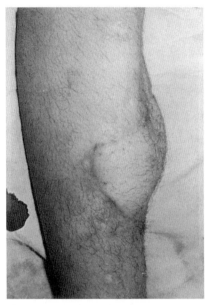

D,E

FIG. 2. *Continued.* D: Flap inset and sutured, and donor site skin grafted. E: Late postoperative view at 2 months. (From El-Saadi and Khashaba, ref. 1, with permission.)

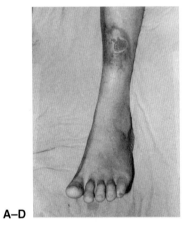
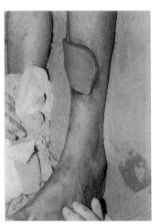
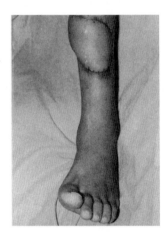
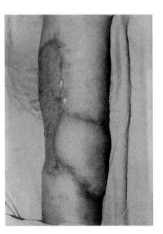

A–D

FIG. 3. A: Chronic post-traumatic leg ulcer of 3 years' duration. B: Flap based on the middle segment covering the defect. C: Early postoperative view. D: Late postoperative view of flap donor site. (From El-Saadi and Khashaba, ref. 1, with permission.)

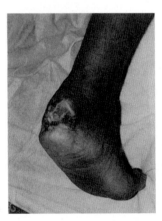
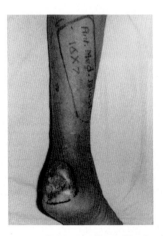
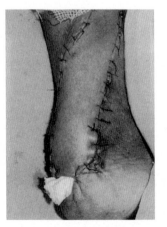
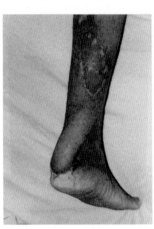

A–D

FIG. 4. A: Chronic post-traumatic ulcer of back of the calcaneum of 12 years' duration. B: Extent of excision and flap design based on the lower segment. C: Immediate postoperative view. D: Flap and donor site 2 months postoperatively. (From El-Saadi and Khashaba and ref. 1, with permission.)

CLINICAL RESULTS

In a series of eight flaps utilized for patients with chronic leg ulcers, all flaps survived completely; healing was uneventful without even minimal necrosis. The medial septocutaneous vessels are constant and are situated at relatively fixed points. Each vessel can support a reliable island flap. All three flaps have the following advantages. The flaps are thin, reliable, and easy to elevate. Based on the three segments described, coverage can be provided for almost any site in the lower two-thirds of the leg. The arc of rotation is extensive, and the flaps can fit the defect exactly and comfortably, with no axial tension or kinking. The operating time and donor-site morbidity are kept to a minimum, and the patient remains conveniently supine during the operation.

SUMMARY

The three anteromedial fasciocutaneous island flaps, based on the medial septocutaneous vessels of the leg, can be used for coverage in almost any site in the lower two-thirds of the leg.

References

1. El-Saadi MM, Khashaba AA. Three anteromedial fasciocutaneous leg island flaps for covering defects of the lower two-thirds of the leg. *Br J Plast Surg* 1990;43:536.
2. Moscona AR, Govrin-Yehudain J, Hirschowitz B. The island fasciocutaneous flap: A new type of flap for defects of the knee. *Br J Plast Surg* 1985;38:512.
3. Pontén B. The fasciocutaneous flap: its use in soft tissue defects of the lower leg. *Br J Plast Surg* 1981;34:215.
4. Thatte RL. One stage random-pattern de-epithelialised "turn-over" flaps in the leg. *Br J Plast Surg* 1982;35:287.
5. Tom S, Namiki Y, Hayashi Y. Anterolateral leg island flap. *Br J Plast Surg* 1987;40:236.
6. Walton RL, Bunkis J. The posterior calf fasciocutaneous free flap. *Plast Reconstr Surg* 1984;74:76.
7. Amarante J, Costa H, Soares R. A new distally based fasciocutaneous flap of the leg. *Br J Plast Surg* 1986;39:338.
8. Carriquiry C, Costa MA, Vasconez LO. An anatomic study of the septocutaneous vessels of the leg. *Plast Reconstr Surg* 1985;76:354.
9. Donski PK, Fogdestam I. Distally based fasciocutaneous flap from the sural region: a preliminary report. *Scand J Plast Reconstr Surg* 1983; 17:191.

CHAPTER 481 ■ FASCIOCUTANEOUS FLAP

B. PONTÉN

It is generally assumed that arterial blood supply to the fascia, subcutaneous fat, and skin is highly dependent on perforating vessels from the underlying muscle. Successful musculocutaneous flaps, free flaps, and many anatomic studies demonstrate the validity of this assumption; however, experience and practical observations have also furnished proof of another type of arterial circulatory system.

The sliding of muscles needs the loose connective tissue underneath the fascia and must not be hampered by more vessels than are absolutely necessary. Distally, the tendons give off no vessels whatsoever. It is also well known that after making an incision in a compartment, blunt dissection between the muscle and fascia can be performed without any bleeding worth mentioning. In addition, a large muscle can be rotated as a flap from its original position without any circulatory problems in the remaining overlying fascia, fat, and skin. A crush injury or a compartment syndrome can more or less destroy a muscle through ischemia, but the circulatory system to the superficial structures will still function. A high-tension electric current through an extremity can severely reduce or eliminate the circulation in a muscle but still leave the skin intact.

These observations, plus many years of experience in treating skin defects below the knee, with or without complications, made me realize that skin, fat, and fascia derive nutrition from the proximal vessels and have an important circulatory system of their own. Thus arose the idea of including the fascia in cross-leg flaps and in local flaps of the leg and foot (1).

ANATOMY

The arterial circulation of the fascia and the layers superficial to the fascia are usually scantily described in anatomy textbooks. The topography of the main arteries is always well described, but the less conspicuous superficial arteries are seldom shown, and few have names. The increasing use of free flaps, muscle, and musculocutaneous flaps has necessitated detailed studies of the vessels from the muscle as well as of

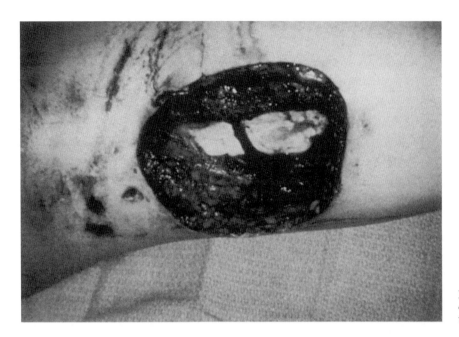

FIG. 1. A 45-year-old man with an avulsion of skin exposing the proximal third of the left tibia.

those giving rise to the fascial plexus. Recently, investigators stimulated by the successful use of fasciocutaneous flaps have verified in postmortem studies that the fascial plexus is much more extensive than had been assumed earlier.

The anatomic arrangements of the circulation in the skin of the leg and probably also in that of the arm, follow the same principles. There are long arteries following the axis of the extremity proximally under the fascia, eventually penetrating and creating a plexus in and on the fascia. The vessels are clearly visible from underneath when the fascia is lifted from the muscle. Some fairly large axial long vessels run parallel to the superficial nerves: the saphenous nerve, the sural nerves, and several long branches of cutaneous nerves in the leg and foot.

There are also shorter musculocutaneous arteries penetrating the fascia and forming a plexus, and they seem to adopt the same pattern; that is, they run close to the fascia before penetrating.

On the medial side of the tibia, the main axial vessel is the saphenous artery. There are also proximal vessels from the inferior genicular artery; further distally, constant branches from the posterior tibial artery form a longitudinal plexus on the superficial surface of the deep fascia.

On the lateral side, vessels from the anterior tibial artery pierce the anterior part of the fascia. Four or five branches have been found at the anterior border of the lateral compartment; together with lateroposterior branches from the peroneal artery, they form a longitudinal plexus of fascia covering the lateral compartment of the leg.

Each one of the three arteries of the leg gives off segmented branches that perforate the fascia of the leg and arborize on top of the fascia and form connections with the superior and inferior branch. These are the septocutaneous vessels. If one includes at least one septocutaneous perforator, it is possible to outline and elevate safely and reliably fasciocutaneous flaps, proximally or distally based (2,3).

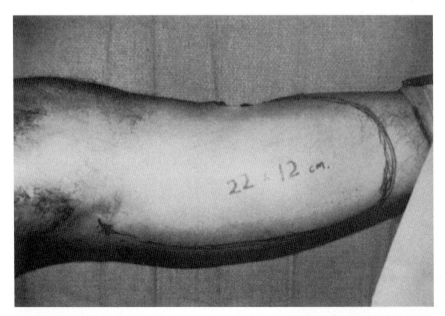

FIG. 2. A fasciocutaneous flap outlined over the medial head of the gastrocnemius muscle. Note the dimensions: 22 × 12 cm.

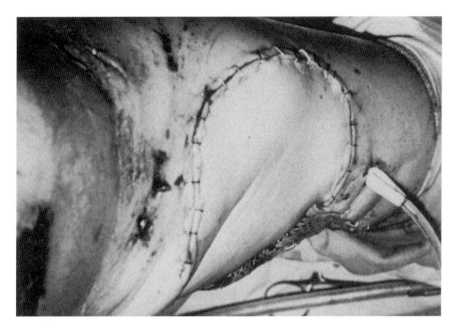

FIG. 3. A flap transposed to cover the entire defect without any tension.

On the middle part of the posterior side, there are usually two or three longitudinal vessels deriving their blood supply from a branch of the popliteal artery. Flaps from the posterior side are very useful because they can be made quite broad and long. The dorsum of the foot also can be used, at least on the proximal part, the distal border sited where the tendon sheaths begin.

FLAP DESIGN AND DIMENSIONS

The arc of rotation of the fasciocutaneous flap is often quite extensive, and it is therefore important to plan the position of the patient on the table in advance. The surgeon may have to begin with the patient face down, and it may be necessary to turn the patient during the operation when rotating the flap.

After marking the outline of the defect, the best fasciocutaneous flap for the particular patient should be planned and marked. Because it is easy to rotate these long flaps, I prefer to use longitudinal incisions along the axis of the leg. The basic rules are the same as when planning other flaps: It is essential to avoid tension. I prefer to have a long and broad flap that falls into place without being under tension (Figs. 1–5).

OPERATIVE TECHNIQUE

Before beginning the incision, one should remember not to touch or disturb the circulation between the fascia and skin. This implies that the incision should go through skin, fat, and fascia. Hooks always should be used in the fascia, and not in the skin, when handling the flap. If hooks are placed in the skin in an attempt to lift a long and heavy flap, it is easy to destroy at least part of the delicate tissue between the fat and the fascia.

The incision should be started in an area where the fascia is easily identified and where there normally is an adequate space between fascia and muscle. From this incision, a finger through the opening in the fascia can lift it from the muscle underneath by blunt dissection. This maneuver is usually easy to perform, but in certain areas there is a septum between the muscle compartments underneath the flap. In such cases, it is advisable to undermine from both sides, after which the

septum should be carefully cut after transecting the distal part. The flap will be loose and freely mobile.

Utmost attention should be paid to preserving a segment of septum continuous with the base of the flap because often a

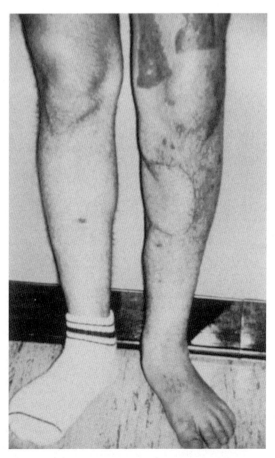

FIG. 4. A healed flap 3 months postoperatively. Patient is walking normally.

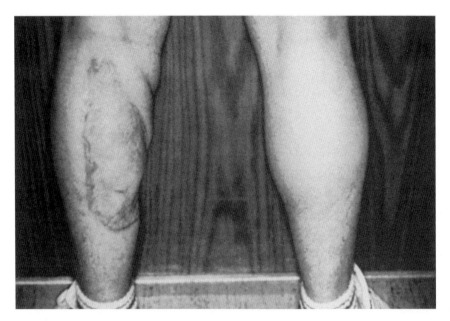

FIG. 5. A secondary defect that was mesh-grafted immediately.

septocutaneous vessel is included there and it may be essential for flap survival.

It is well known that the fascia is rather tough, which might hamper flap rotation. To lengthen the flap and facilitate rotation, a backcut in the fascia (not in the skin or fat) is useful. Even a small backcut can give an extra centimeter that might be necessary in order to have an absolutely relaxed flap lying over the defect. It is self-evident that cutting the vessels that can be seen in the fascia should be avoided.

The rotation can be quite extensive, and a longitudinal incision flap border can end up in a horizontal position. Flap stability and good flap circulation make delay procedures unnecessary. All my flaps have been raised and rotated in one stage.

Bleeding from the borders of the incision usually does not create any problems, and diffuse bleeding from the loose connective tissue separating the fascia and muscle is generally insignificant. The area to be covered should, of course, be surrounded by normal skin or at least skin with good circulation, but this is not mandatory.

The edges of the area to be covered are undermined, and the rotated fascia is sutured underneath the skin. As a rule, I do not have any bandage on the flap itself, except perhaps a few tapes, especially in cases where there is risk for bleeding under the flap. In a few cases, I have used suction for 24 hours. The secondary defect can be covered immediately with a split-thickness skin graft, but it also can be left uncovered.

Flap transposition almost inevitably results in a "pig's ear," but this irregularity soon reduces considerably by itself, and, if necessary, it is very easy to remove the little extra piece of skin later.

Because many of the vessels follow the cutaneous sensory nerves, the patient will lose sensation in an area peripheral to the defect after flap transfer. This should be regarded as an insignificant sequela, considering the effective solution of the main problem.

CLINICAL RESULTS

Previous authors have observed that circulation in a flap is better if the fascia is included. The technique has been used when covering pretibial skin defects with delayed bipedicle flaps and as part of a delay procedure. It has been noted that the deltopectoral flap can be extended and has better circulation if the fascia is included. The same observations have been made in cross-leg flap surgery (Fig. 4).

The fasciocutaneous flap is reliable (1,3), and it can take rotation and kinking to a surprisingly high degree. Delay procedures are needless and it is, of course, possible to make two flaps in the same stage (Fig. 5).

The good circulation of the flap will make it especially useful when working with complicated cases (fractures, nerve and vessel injuries, cut tendons, for example). The flap can be used after tumor excision, in any kind of soft tissue defect after a trauma with or without fractures, in cases where osteosynthetic material is exposed, in combination with bone grafting, in chronic osteomyelitis, in pressure sores, and even in postthrombotic ulcers. There are only minor postoperative problems, even with the elderly patient, because patients do not need any extra fixation and can be in a wheelchair the next day provided the leg is kept in a horizontal position. The operative procedure is simple and short, the flap is safe and stable, and the technique should always be considered when one is faced with the problem of covering a soft-tissue defect on the lower leg.

References

1. Pontén B. The fasciocutaneous flap: its use in soft tissue defects of the lower leg. *Br J Plast Surg* 1981;34:215.
2. Carriquiry C, Costa MA, Vasconez LO. An anatomic study of the septocutaneous vessels of the leg. *Plast Reconstr Surg* 1985;76:354.
3. Tolhurst DE, Haeseker B. Fasciocutaneous flaps in the axillary region. *Br J Plast Surg* 1982;35:430.

CHAPTER 482 ■ ANTERIOR TIBIAL FLAP

J. F. R. ROCHA AND A. GILBERT

The anterior tibial artery supplies a great part of the antero-lateral surface of the lower leg. It participates equally in the vascularization of the foot and anterior compartment without being an indispensable element. Consequently, proximally and distally based island tibial flaps can be created to cover losses of substance of the lower leg and the calcaneal region.

ANATOMY

The flap is supplied by terminal branches of the superficial peroneal nerve satellite artery (SPA) that come from the superior and inferior peroneus lateralis arteries. These two muscular branches of the anterior tibial artery also participate in the cutaneous vascular supply by means of perforating twigs directly to the skin (Fig. 1) (1–4).

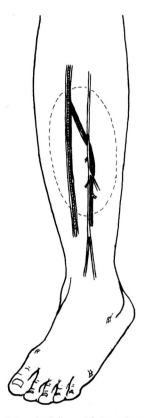

FIG. 1. Anatomy of the tibial flap with its axis over one of the peroneus lateralis arteries.

Superior Peroneus Lateralis Artery (SPLA)

This vessel branches off from the anterior tibial at variable levels. We measured it at an average of 25.6 cm from the lateral malleolus, with extremes of 20 cm in a 33-cm female lower leg to 32 cm in a 41-cm male lower leg (4).

As it runs over the interosseous membrane and the anterior surface of the fibula, the SPLA crosses the extensor digitorum longus before reaching the space between the peroneus lateralis and the anterior peroneal septum. The SPLA always gives some branches to the peroneus longus at this level. The caliber varies greatly from 1.2 to 2.5 mm (average, 1.63 mm), and its length ranges from 6 to 12 cm (average, 7.1 cm).

Inferior Peroneus Lateralis Artery (IPLA)

This vessel is found in 70% of cases. It branches off from he anterior tibial artery at an average of 17.2 cm from the lateral malleolus, with extremes of 12 cm in a 33-cm female lower leg to 20 cm in a 40-cm male lower leg. It has a shorter course than the SPLA, although with similar anatomic references. It gives some branches to the peroneus brevis before becoming an entirely cutaneous artery. The caliber varies from 1 to 2 mm (average, 1.4 mm), and its length ranges from 3.6 to 7.5 cm (average, 5 cm).

Superficial Peroneal Nerve Satellite Artery (SPNA)

This vessel provides vascularization to the nerve and the skin all along its descending path at the anterolateral surface of the lower leg (Fig. 2). It comes from the SPLA in 30% of the cases, from the IPLA in 40%, and from both the SPLA and IPLA in 30% of the cases.

The first cutaneous branch, at an average of 20 cm from the lateral malleolus, perforates the superficial aponeurotic sheet directly. It supplies all the anterolateral middle third and part of the upper third of the leg. The SPNA runs along the entire subcutaneous path of the superficial peroneal nerve at the lower leg. A second cutaneous branch that supplies part of the anterolateral middle and lower thirds of the leg is normally seen branching off the SPNA right after the perforating point of the superficial peroneal nerve. We measured this point at an average of 13.5 cm from the lateral malleolus, with extremes from 9 to 17 cm. The third group of cutaneous branches is identified along their subcutaneous descending path where the superficial peroneal nerve gives some sensory branches to the anterior lower third of the leg.

In general, the SPNA ends by anastomosing with the dorsalis pedis artery (55% of cases), the peroneal artery (35%), or the lateral malleolar artery (5%). In 5% of cases, there were no anastomoses evident. The caliber of the SPNA is, on average, 0.9 mm, with extremes from 0.6 to 1.5 mm.

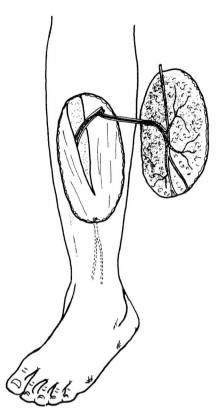

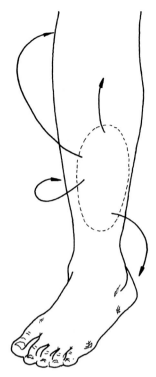

FIG. 3. The tibial flap can cover losses of substance at several sites in the lower leg.

FIG. 2. A split of the anterolateral superficial aponeurosis along the anterior peroneal septum allows identification of interseptal cutaneous branches of the anterior tibial artery. Note the superficial peroneal nerve attached to the flap and followed by its satellite artery.

is performed, whether preserving the SPN or not, and the flap is entirely liberated from the donor site according to the accurate position of the cutaneous branches and to the size of the flap (see Fig. 3).

FLAP DESIGN AND DIMENSIONS

The largest flap we have raised measured 20 cm long and 8 cm wide. The anterior and posterior tibial arteries must be clinically examined before surgery to ensure the feasibility of the flap. The outline of the skin flap is drawn inside the anterolateral middle and lower thirds of the leg. It is limited anteriorly by the tibial crest and posteriorly by the external border of the lateral gastrocnemius (Fig. 3).

OPERATIVE TECHNIQUE

The anterior peroneal septum is most easily approached with the patient lying supine and the lower leg kept in a mild internal rotation. We start raising the flap anteriorly by blunt dissection between the subcutaneous tissue and the aponeurotic sheet of the leg. The cutaneous branches of the SPNA can be easily seen along the anterior peroneal septum. An ascending splitting of the superficial fascia is carried out, starting from the aponeurotic perforating point of the superficial peroneal nerve. Then the lateral peroneal muscles are separated from the anterior peroneal septum. The SPNA and the superficial peroneal nerve are easily dissected proximally toward the vascular trunk. When an entire dissection of the pedicle is required, detachment of the extensor digitorum longus and extensor hallucis longus from the fibula and interosseous membrane allows exposure of the anterior tibial bundle.

An average of five twigs to the peroneus longus and brevis must be ligated between the first cutaneous branch and the trunk.

If an innervated skin transfer is desirable, the superficial peroneal nerve must be included in the flap. The distal incision

Island Tibial Flap

Generally, skin coverage of the anterior tibial tubercle, the anterior and lateral surfaces of the knee joint, and the upper third of the leg does not require the distal ligature of the anterior tibial vessels. The SPLA gives the flap a long arc of rotation. If the loss is more extensive or in patients with a shorter pedicle, the distal portion of the anterior tibial artery may need to be transected.

When inner surfaces are to be covered, the flap is raised more proximally and is tunneled between the anterior compartment and the tibia. It must pass behind the anterior tibial bundle to avoid any damage to the vascular and motor branches of the anterior muscles.

Reverse Tibial Flap

The feasibility of retrograde blood flow into the anterior tibial artery and venae comitantes permits this flap to be used for lower third, malleolar, or calcaneal skin cover (Fig. 4). The blood supply is provided by the plantar perforating branch of the dorsalis pedis artery that joins together both anterior and posterior tibial systems.

The two venae comitantes drain the flap to the greater and lesser saphenous veins by means of anastomoses with the dorsalis pedis venous arch. Venous drainage sometimes is impaired by the countless valves, thus requiring microsuture between one of the venae comitantes at its proximal end and a vein close to the recipient site.

If an innervated skin transfer is recommended, the reverse tibial flap must be raised, including part of the lower third, where cutaneous branches of the superficial peroneal nerve

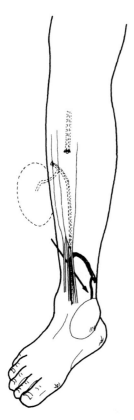

FIG. 4. When inner areas of the lower leg are to be covered, the flap must be tunneled under the anterior muscles or tendons for a looser turndown of the anterior tibial artery and the cutaneous pedicle.

are present. The nerve can be sutured to a sensory branch of the posterior tibial nerve or just interposed by a nerve graft. It is equally possible to reconstruct the posterior tibial nerve in which scar tissue is present by means of the superficial peroneal nerve vascularized by the tibial flap.

CLINICAL RESULTS

Finally, the donor site is covered by a split-thickness skin graft over the superficial aponeurosis of the lower leg. The unpleasant aspect of the donor site does not seem very significant when balanced against the multiple advantages of this flap.

SUMMARY

The anterior tibial flap can be used as an island flap to cover defects about the lower knee or as a reversed tibial flap for ankle and heel defects.

References

1. Dubreui C. *Variations des artères du membre inférieure.* Paris: Masson, 1933.
2. Salmon M. *Les artères de muscles, des membres et du tronc.* Paris: Masson, 1933.
3. Haerstch P. The blood supply to the skin of the leg: a post mortem investigation. *Br J Plast Surg* 1981;34:470.
4. Rocha JF, Izquierdo MP, Gilbert A, Hureau J. Les branches cutanées de l'artère tibiale antérieure. Biomédicale de St. Pères: Service d'orthopédie et chirurgie réparatrice de l'enfant. Communication to the Société Anatomique de Paris, October, 1984.

CHAPTER 483. Cross-Leg Skin Flap *A. M. Morris*

www.encyclopediaofflaps.com

CHAPTER 484 ■ SARTORIUS MUSCLE AND MUSCULOCUTANEOUS FLAP

M. ORTICOCHEA

EDITORIAL COMMENT

This innovative use of skin and muscle brought on a wave of enthusiasm and study for the musculocutaneous flap. All plastic surgeons are in debt to Dr. Orticochea for introducing and clarifying the principles of the musculocutaneous flap.

During the nineteenth and twentieth centuries, many surgeons described musculocutaneous flaps that were used for different purposes, for example, reconstruction of the palate (1), filling of facial losses (2), and penis reconstruction (3). I believe that two patients with different problems—a penis reconstruction and raw surfaces of a lower extremity—were responsible for my 1972 article, in which I conceived of the musculocutaneous flap as a substitute for delaying cutaneous flaps (3–6).

INDICATIONS

The rich irrigation of the superior pedicle of the sartorius, together with its great length, provides great versatility for

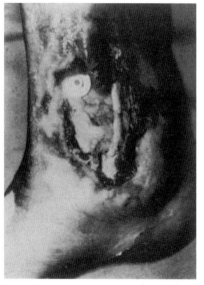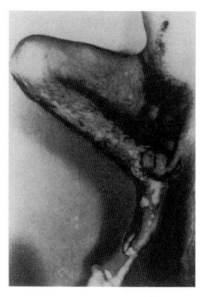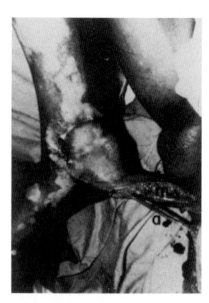

A–C

FIG. 1. **A:** Defect of the medial malleolus. **B:** Sartorius flap sutured to the defect. **C:** At the time of division of the flap, both the muscle (m) and the third arterial pedicle (a) (arising from the superficial artery) can be seen. (From Orticochea, ref. 5, with permission.)

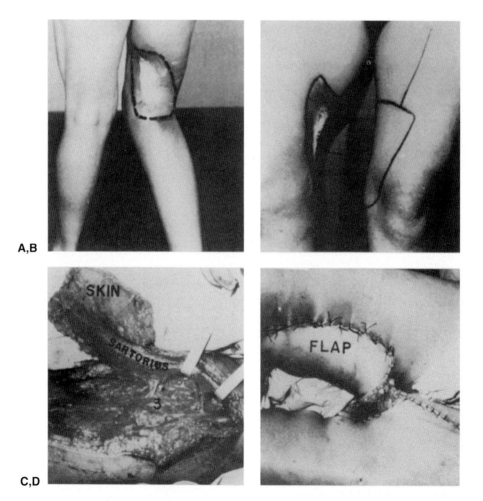

A,B

C,D

FIG. 2. **A:** Defect just medial and superior to the knee. **B:** Defect outlined and flap designed. The proximal border of the skin flap lies at the level of the vascular pedicle. The distal border may extend beyond the insertion of the muscle if required. **C:** Flap elevated. Note the sartorius muscle and skin paddle. The two vascular pedicles to the sartorius muscle from the profunda femoris are displayed. The proximal end of the sartorius is also divided. **D:** Flap sutured to the defect. The flap may be rotated through 90 degrees without occluding the vessels. *(Continued.)*

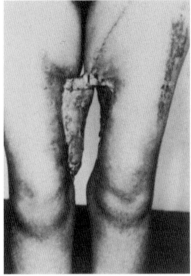
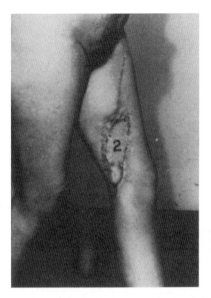
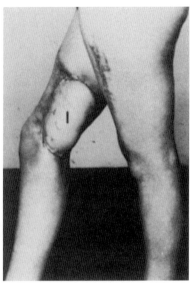

E–G

FIG. 2. *(Continued.)* **E:** Four weeks later, the flap is ready to be divided. **F:** Donor site skin-grafted. **G:** Final result. (From Orticochea, ref. 5, with permission.)

transfer of skin to the lower abdominal wall, external genitalia, perineum, and opposite thigh.

ANATOMY

The sartorius muscle goes through the anterior aspect of the thigh, from superior to inferior and from lateral to medial, extending from the anterior superior iliac spine to the medial aspect of the upper end of the tibia. The sartorius has a segmental vascular supply but receives its proximal and principal vascular pedicle from the profunda femoris vessels. This superior proximal pedicle is several centimeters long, giving great mobility to musculocutaneous flaps of the sartorius muscle. At the level of Hunter's canal, the inferior pedicle of the sartorius is formed by small vessels that are branches of the femoral vessels.

OPERATIVE TECHNIQUE

The greater saphenous vein, owing to its easy dissection, must be included in the superior proximal pedicle of the sartorius muscle. Two additional points are stressed. The proximal edge of the cutaneous part of the flap should overlie the vascular pedicles to the muscle. In other words, the area supplied by the vascular pedicles is distal to their site of entry into the

muscle. Second, the skin is attached to the muscle by a layer of superficial fascia. The small perforating blood vessels pass through this layer and may easily be damaged if any shearing stress is imparted to the skin during the operation. When the muscle is divided, therefore, the ends should be sutured with catgut to the overlying fat (Figs. 1 and 2).

SUMMARY

The sartorius muscle can be used with or without the overlying skin for coverage of various leg defects.

References

1. Bakamjian V. A technique for primary reconstruction of the palate after radical maxillectomy for cancer. *Plast Reconstr Surg* 1963;31:103.
2. Owens N. A compound neck pedicle designed for the repair of massive facial defects: formation, development and application. *Plast Reconstr Surg* 1955;15:369.
3. Orticochea M. A new method of total reconstruction of the penis. *Br J Plast Surg* 1972;25:106.
4. Orticochea M. The musculocutaneous flap method: an immediate and heroic substitute for the method of delay. *Br J Plast Surg* 1972;25:106.
5. Orticochea M. Immediate (undelayed) musculocutaneous island cross-leg flaps. *Br J Plast Surg* 1978;31:205.
6. Orticochea M. The musculocutaneous flap: personal history. *Plast Reconstr Surg* 1981;67:258.

CHAPTER 485 ■ GASTROCNEMIUS MUSCLE AND MUSCULOCUTANEOUS FLAPS

B. E. COHEN AND M. E. CIARAVINO

Use of the gastrocnemius as either a muscle or musculocutaneous flap has proven to be highly effective in the management of knee and upper leg wounds. The constant dominant proximal vascular pedicle that runs down the length of the muscle makes this one of the most reliable flaps in the body. The muscle can be raised easily, quickly, and safely if attention is paid to the relevant technical and anatomic details. It is generally unnecessary to operate in the vicinity of its high vascular pedicle, thereby decreasing the possibility of inadvertent damage to the flap's blood supply. Transposition of the gastrocnemius results in little or no functional deficit, providing that the soleus and the other head of the gastrocnemius are left intact and functioning. If necessary, subsequent bony procedures can be carried out by elevating the healed flap with the assurance of a good vascular supply.

INDICATIONS

Because of their separate anatomic characteristics and locations within the leg, the two muscle heads are not completely interchangeable. Since the medial head is larger, longer, and more optimally positioned along the tibial border, it is used much more often for coverage of defects in the leg and knee.

As a muscle flap, the medial head can cover wounds of the knee and upper third of the tibia. Because of its smaller size and the intervening muscles of the anterior and lateral compartments, the lateral head has a smaller reach. It can be applied to upper lateral leg and knee wounds of somewhat lesser dimensions.

As a musculocutaneous flap, the medial gastrocnemius range of coverage is expanded to include the lower thigh, knee, and upper two-thirds of the tibia. The lateral gastrocnemius musculocutaneous flap can cover defects of the lower thigh, lateral knee, and upper third of the tibia.

Although a longer and broader flap can be created by elevating the gastrocnemius as a musculocutaneous flap, the major disadvantage is the obligatory skin graft on the flap donor site and the resultant deformity of the leg contour. Because of the lessened donor deformity, as well as its greater ability to fill three-dimensional defects, the gastrocnemius muscle alone is generally preferred.

ANATOMY

The gastrocnemius is the most superficial muscle within the posterior compartment of the leg (Fig. 1) (1–3). It is comprised of two heads that arise separately from the lower femur, the femoral condyles, and the posterior knee capsule. The anterior edge of the medial head lies along the medial border of the tibia, while that of the lateral head is separated from the tibia

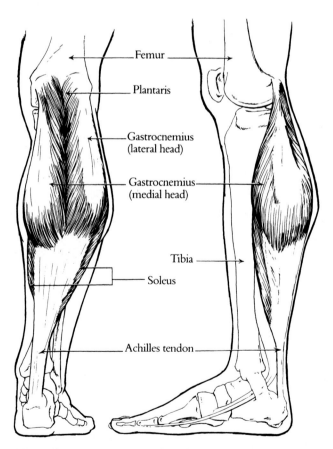

FIG. 1. The gastrocnemius muscle and its neighboring structures are depicted in posterior and medial views of the leg. Its tendon joins with that of the soleus to form the Achilles tendon.

1384

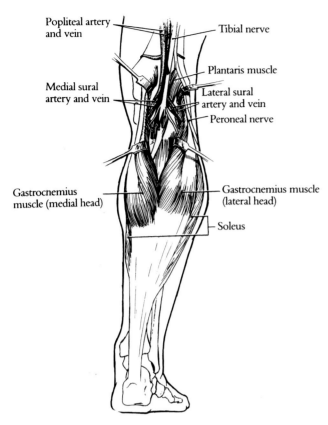

FIG. 2. The medial and lateral heads are retracted to show their neurovascular supply by the sural vessels and branches of the tibial nerve. The plantaris and soleus muscles lie immediately deep to the gastrocnemius.

by the muscles of the anterior and lateral compartments. Posteriorly, the muscle bellies converge in the midline of the calf, intermingling and running together inferiorly. The tendon of the gastrocnemius joins with that of the soleus to form the Achilles tendon. These muscles act in concert to plantar flex the foot. Because it crosses the knee, the gastrocnemius contributes to the flexion of that joint.

The medial and lateral sural arteries provide independent blood supply to the two muscle heads (Fig. 2). These vessels arise from the popliteal artery above the level of the knee joint (4). Each courses a few centimeters with its venae comitantes before entering the anterior aspect of the proximal muscle belly with the innervating branches of the tibial nerve. The vessels then pass down the longitudinal axis of the muscle bellies. This vascular arrangement is constant and effectively constitutes the sole supply of the muscle (Mathes and Nahai Type 1) (2), making it ideally suited for use as a flap. The independent neurovascular supply of the two muscle bellies allows them to be used as separate muscle and musculocutaneous flaps.

FLAP DESIGN AND DIMENSIONS (FIGS. 3 AND 4)

Muscle Flap

The position of the muscle in the leg can readily be determined by inspection and palpation in most instances. One entire muscle belly or the other is chosen, depending on the clinical situation (1–3).

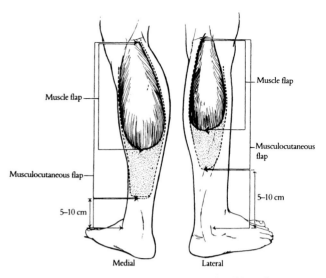

FIG. 3. The potential dimensions of the medial and lateral gastrocnemius muscle (solid line) and musculocutaneous (dashed line) flaps are shown. The medial flap is larger and can be made longer than the lateral one.

Musculocutaneous Flap

The medial head can support a skin flap that extends in width from the medial border of the tibia to the posterior midline of the calf. The point of rotation is the midline popliteal fossa, near the origin of the muscle and its blood supply. The level of the defect determines the length of the flap. This always includes the skin overlying the muscle and often a "random" extension of skin and subcutaneous tissue distal to the muscle. This extension is quite safely included with the flap when its length-to-width ratio is 1:1 or less. Generally, this reaches to a point approximately 10 cm above the malleolus. The age of the patient, the state of the

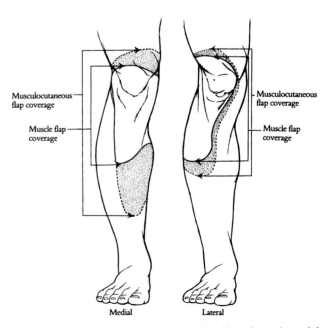

FIG. 4. The areas of coverage of the medial and lateral muscles (solid line) and musculocutaneous (dashed line) flaps are shown.

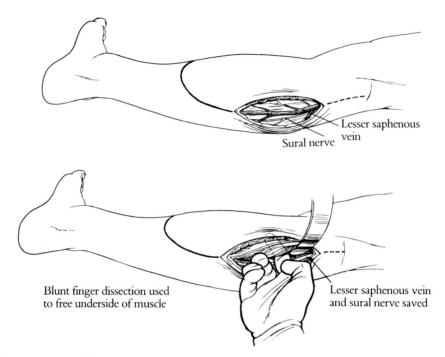

Lesser saphenous vein

Sural nerve

Blunt finger dissection used to free underside of muscle

Lesser saphenous vein and sural nerve saved

FIG. 5. Posterior midline approach with lesser saphenous vein and sural nerve landmarks. Once the fascia is incised, blunt dissection is used to develop the submuscular plane.

peripheral vascular circulation, and the degree of trauma to the leg will determine the safety of extending the flap past this point. If unsure, a delay of this distal portion should be done prior to the flap transfer.

The lateral gastrocnemius supports a flap of smaller dimensions. Its width extends from the posterior midline to a point over the lateral muscle compartment. In addition to the skin over the muscle, some skin distal to the muscle may be carried with the flap. The same constraints for the distal extension of the medial head apply here. Generally speaking, it is safe to extend this flap to within 10 to 15 cm of the lateral malleolus (Figs. 3 and 4).

OPERATIVE TECHNIQUE

Medial Gastrocnemius Muscle Flap

The posterior dissection is generally done first through a posterior midline incision or a longitudinal incision between the midline and the defect (Figs. 5 and 6). The posterior anatomy is clear and unlikely to have been damaged or obscured by the anterior trauma. The sural nerve and lesser saphenous vein are two key landmarks which are seen superficial to the muscle bellies and preserved. These structures

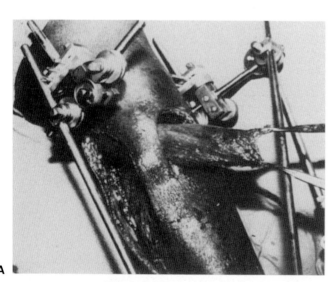

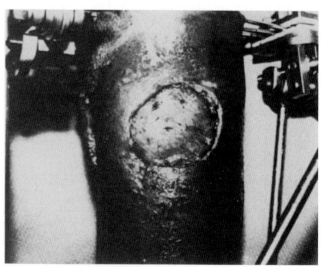

FIG. 6. A 34-year-old man with a large left upper leg defect **A:** Muscle flap elevated through separate longitudinal incision. Muscle passed through tunnel to defect. **B:** Muscle sutured in place and ready for skin graft. (Courtesy of Dr. David Buchanan).

are in the midline and help to locate the natural cleavage between the two upper muscle bellies, a distinction not so easily made more distally. The muscle fascia is split, and the junction of the two heads is incised. Gentle blunt finger dissection is used to seek the plane between the gastrocnemius and the underlying soleus muscle and plantaris tendon. The loose avascular areolar tissue can be progressively swept through with the finger down to the tendinous junction of the muscle with the soleus. The superficial dissection is then performed, and the muscle is transected distally with a cuff of tendon attached for use in fixation to the wound edge. Anteriorly, incisions extend the defect superiorly and inferiorly as needed for adequate exposure. The tunnel through which the muscle is passed should be of adequate size so as not to constrict the blood supply of the flap. The superficial surface of the muscle may remain so or be rotated to lie deeply, depending on how it best transfers. Drains are left in the muscle bed and the muscle is skin grafted.

Medial Gastrocnemius Musculocutaneous Flap

The midline posterior incision is made in the upper calf, and after identifying the sural nerve and lesser saphenous vein, the deep dissection is done as described above for the muscle flap. The remainder of the peripheral skin incision is then made, and the compound muscle and skin flap is elevated (Fig. 7). The peritenon over the exposed soleus fascia and Achilles tendon should be carefully preserved in this dissection to provide a suitable bed for application of skin grafts. The greater saphenous vein is generally, although not necessarily, transected during elevation of the distal portion of the flap. In dissecting the distal skin and subcutaneous portion of the flap toward the muscle, the tendinous contribution to the Achilles tendon is encountered and incised, thus converting the subcutaneous plane at this point to the previously dissected submuscular one. Backcuts of the proximal skin and subcutaneous tissue may be made as needed to allow for

easier rotation to the defect. A suction drain is generally placed beneath the flap. The flap is then sewn into the periphery of the prepared wound. Split-thickness skin grafts are applied to the flap donor site and are held in place with a tie-over dressing.

Lateral Gastrocnemius Muscle and Musculocutaneous Flaps

Techniques and approaches outlined for the medial side are generally applicable here. Again, the lesser saphenous vein and sural nerve are used as landmarks and should be preserved. In dissecting superiorly, one must be aware not to injure the peroneal nerve, which crosses from medial to lateral over the upper portion of the muscle belly (Fig. 8).

FLAP MODIFICATIONS

Local Coverage

Transposition Flap

In most instances, the muscle or musculocutaneous flap will be used as described above, as a transposition flap to cover a local defect (1–14). Various techniques for improving wound coverage and aesthetics have been described. Making the flap into an island by detaching the origin of the muscle head will result in extra reach for either flap. However, the proximity of the origin to the vascular supply adds a degree of complexity and risk to this latter maneuver. Additional length and improved contour may also be achieved by incising the muscle fascia. The appearance of the gastrocnemius musculocutaneous flap may be improved by placing the skin paddle over the distal edge of the muscle and limiting its dimensions to that required by the defect. These modifications help to minimize the contour deformity and may obviate the need for skin grafting (15).

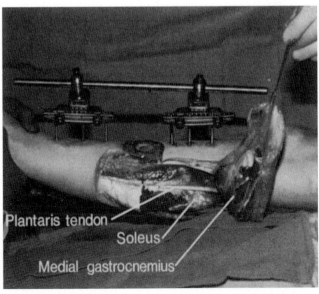
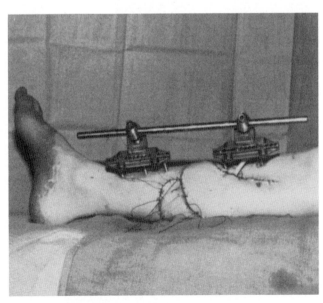

A   B

Plantaris tendon
Soleus
Medial gastrocnemius

FIG. 7. A 27-year-old man with an exposed fracture of the right midtibia 4 months after injury. A: The defect has been debrided and the musculocutaneous flap elevated and reflected with landmarks noted. B: Transposed flap with skin graft applied to donor site (posterior grafts not visible).

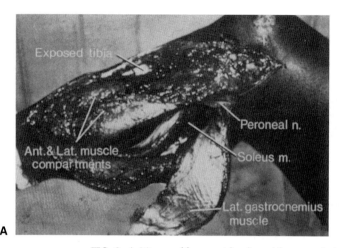

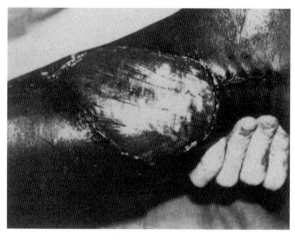

A

B

FIG. 8. A 20-year-old man with a lateral leg wound. **A:** Lateral gastrocnemius dissected prior to transposition to exposed tibial defect. **B:** Muscle flap transposed to defect and sutured into place. (Courtesy of Dr. David Buchanan.)

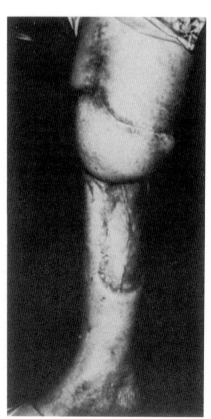

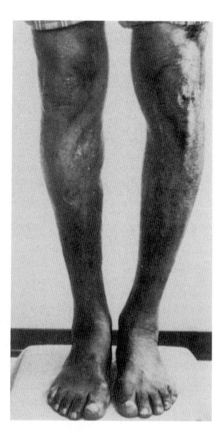

A,B

FIG. 9. The gastrocnemius musculocutaneous flap produces a considerable cosmetic deformity when used to cover a knee defect (**A**) compared to a midtibial defect (**B**).

Advancement Flap

By undermining in the submuscular plane, with or without opening the posterior midline, enough advancement of the musculocutaneous unit may be achieved to cover certain upper tibial defects (16).

Posterior Flap in Below-Knee Amputation

Both heads are left in the posterior skin flap, which is then turned up for closure as a musculocutaneous flap (17).

Fasciocutaneous Flap

In this modification, the skin, subcutaneous tissue, and muscle fascia are elevated as a flap, while the muscle is left in situ (18,19). This is further described in Chapter 481.

Distant Coverage

Cross-Leg Flap (12–14)

Generally, the medial head is chosen and used as a musculocutaneous flap for this purpose. The flap may not be as well oriented as a random cross-leg flap and must usually undergo some torsion to reach the defect in the opposite leg or foot. This is compensated for by the long and reliably robust flap that can be elevated without a preliminary delay procedure. External bony fixation devices may be used to hold the flap donor leg in a fixed position relative to the recipient leg while healing. Most authors have recommended that this well-perfused flap be divided in stages in order to stimulate neovascularization adequate to nourish the transposed tissue—a clinical concept supported by experimental evidence (20). However, the inherent disadvantages of prolonged immobilization and the need for staged procedures make cross-leg flaps primarily useful as a salvage operation.

Free Flap

Although either head is anatomically suited, there is no obvious situation in which the flap would be chosen over the many other available sites.

CLINICAL RESULTS

The gastrocnemius flap has provided reliable local soft-tissue coverage for traumatic defects, reconstruction following tumor resection, and the salvage of exposed knee prostheses. In cases where the muscle alone is employed, there is relatively little contour deformity, although a skin graft must be placed anteriorly over the muscle flap. The gastrocnemius musculocutaneous flap, in contrast, produces a considerable contour deformity. This latter effect is most obvious when the musculocutaneous flap is used for a high defect in an obese patient. In this instance, a rather large amount of tissue is added to the pretibial or knee area and a simultaneous loss of posterior bulk occurs (Fig. 9A). This deformity is least obvious when the musculocutaneous flap is used in a thin patient for a middle or low tibial defect (Fig. 9B).

SUMMARY

The medial and lateral gastrocnemius muscle flaps and, to a lesser extent, the gastrocnemius musculocutaneous flaps are effective flaps to use when confronted with an upper leg or knee defect.

References

1. McCraw JB, Dibbell DG, Carraway JH. Clinical definition of independent myocutaneous vascular territories. *Plast Reconstr Surg* 1977;60:341.
2. Mathes S, Nahai F, eds. *Clinical atlas of muscle and musculocutaneous flaps.* St. Louis: Mosby, 1979.
3. Mathes S, Nahai F, eds. *Clinical applications for muscle and musculocutaneous flaps.* St. Louis: Mosby, 1982.
4. Whitney T, Heckler F, White M. Gastrocnemius muscle transposition to the femur: how high can you go? *Ann Plast Surg* 1995;34:415.
5. Robertson IM, Barron JS. A method of treatment of chronic infective osteitis. *J Bone Joint Surg* 1946;28B:19.
6. Barford B, Pers M. Gastrocnemius plasty for primary closure of compound injuries of the knee. *J Bone Joint Surg* 1970;52B:124.
7. Ger R. The technique of muscle transposition in the operative treatment of traumatic and ulcerative lesions of the leg. *J Trauma* 1971;11:502.
8. Pers M, Pedgyesi S. Pedicle muscle flaps and their applications in the surgery of repair. *Br J Plast Surg* 1973;26:313.
9. Mathes SJ, McCraw JB, Vasconez LO. Muscle transposition flaps for coverage of lower extremity defects. *Surg Clin North Am* 1974;54:1337.
10. Vasconez LO, Bostwick J III, McCraw JB. Coverage of exposed bone by muscle transposition and skin grafting. *Plast Reconstr Surg* 1974;53:526.
11. Feldman JJ, Cohen BE, May JW. The medial gastrocnemius myocutaneous flap. *Plast Reconstr Surg* 1978;61:531.
12. McCraw JB, Fishman JH, Sharzer, LA. The versatile gastrocnemius myocutaneous flap. *Plast Reconstr Surg* 1978;62:15.
13. Furnas DW, Anzel SH. Two consecutive repairs of the lower limb with a single gastrocnemius musculocutaneous cross-leg flap. *Plast Reconstr Surg* 1980;66:137.
14. Dibbell DG, Edstrom LE. The gastrocnemius myocutaneous flap. *Clin Plast Surg* 1980;7:45.
15. Kroll J, Marcadis A. Aesthetic considerations of the medical gastrocnemius myocutaneous flap. *Plast and Reconstr Surg* 1987;79:67.
16. Riley WB Jr, Garren S, Ramey SJ. Variations in gastrocnemius and solus flap surgery (Abstract). *Plast Surg Forum* 1981;4:128.
17. Dellon AL, Morgan RF. Myodermal flap closure of below the knee amputation. *Surg Gynecol Obstet* 1981;153:383.
18. Ponten B. The fasciocutaneous flap: its use in soft-tissue defects of the lower leg. *Br J Plast Surg* 1981;34:215.
19. Reeder RC. The medial gastrocnemius skin-fascia flap (Abstract). *Plast Surg Forum* 1981;4:185.
20. Cohen BE. Beneficial effect of staged division of pedicle in experimental axial-pattern flaps. *Plast Reconstr Surg* 1979;64:366.

CHAPTER 486 ■ VASTUS MEDIALIS MUSCULOCUTANEOUS AND MUSCULOCUTANEOUS-TENDINOUS FLAPS FOR KNEE RECONSTRUCTION

G. R. TOBIN

The vastus medialis musculocutaneous flap is most useful for reconstruction of defects of the knee and distal thigh. This flap is designed as a medially based advancement flap, with V-Y cutaneous donor-defect closure (1,2) (see Fig. 2). An especially valuable option of this flap is its ability to carry vascularized quadriceps femoris tendon segments for patellar or distal quadriceps femoris tendon reconstruction. Thus, the flap may be designed as a musculocutaneous-tendinous composite flap (1,2) (see Fig. 3).

INDICATIONS

Vastus medialis musculocutaneous flaps are used for defects of the anterior or medial knee joint and distal thigh. The vastus medialis musculocutaneous tendinous composite flap is used to reconstruct segmental defects of the distal quadriceps femoris or patellar tendons (1,2) (see Figs. 3 and 5). If skin overlying the muscle is missing, the muscle only can be used to cover the anterior knee (3). A vastus medialis musculotendinous flap can be designed if knee skin cover is not needed (2).

ANATOMY

The vastus medialis muscle lies medial to the other components of the quadriceps femoris muscles and ventral to the thigh adductor muscles. Its long origin on the linea aspera femoris extends from the intertrochanteric line to the medial supracondylar line; its insertion is on the quadriceps femoris tendon and medial border of the patella.

The vastus medialis vascular supply usually consists of three to six segmentally arranged vascular pedicles from the superficial femoral vessels that enter the vascular hila along the medial side of the muscle (1,2,4) (Fig. 1).

Musculocutaneous perforators from the vastus medialis supply a large musculocutaneous territory centered over the muscle and extending beyond the muscle borders. This musculocutaneous territory is a large triangle with a wide base at the knee level anteriorly and an apex in the proximal medial thigh. In the midthigh, this musculocutaneous territory lies between the rectus femoris and gracilis musculocutaneous territories. In the distal thigh, this musculocutaneous territory occupies nearly half of the thigh circumference and covers the anterior and medial thigh.

The anatomic basis for the vastus medialis musculocutaneous-tendinous composite flap is a vascular supply from the

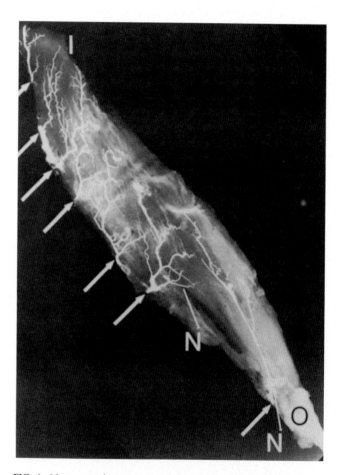

FIG. 1. Neurovascular anatomy of the vastus medialis muscle shown on specimen angiogram. Segmental vascular pedicles (arrows) from superficial femoral vessels enter medial muscle border. Pins show hila of motor nerves. Muscle origin (O) and insertion (I) are indicated.

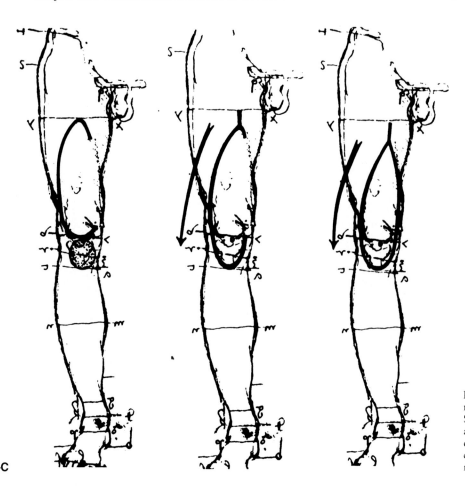

A–C

FIG. 2. The vastus medialis musculocutaneous flap. **A:** Cutaneous paddle design. Stippled area indicates knee defect. **B:** Flap advancement covers knee defect. V-Y donor defect closure. **C:** Flap designed as cutaneous island. (Modified from Mathe, ref. 5.)

vastus medialis muscle to the quadriceps femoris tendon along the course of the muscle-tendon junction. A series of vessels from muscle to tendon is found in the peritenon. This allows the medial half of the distal quadriceps femoris tendon to be transferred with the muscle as a vascularized tendon segment for distal patellar or quadriceps femoris tendon reconstruction (see Figs. 3 and 5).

Motor supply to the vastus medialis is two muscular branches of the femoral nerve that follow the plane of the vascular pedicle (see Fig. 1). The major motor branch enters a neural hilum on the ventral medial surface of the muscle near the muscle midpoint. A second motor branch enters a neurovascular hilum on the most proximal part of the muscle (1,2,4). Sensory nerves to the cutaneous paddle of the flap are

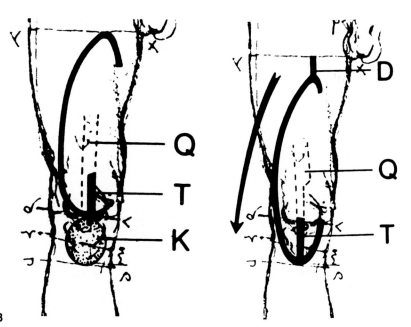

A,B

FIG. 3. The vastus medialis musculocutaneous-tendinous composite flap. **A:** Distal quadriceps femoris tendon (Q) is split to create vascularized tendon segment (T) to bridge knee defect (K). **B:** Vascularized tendon segment (T) is advanced with flap and interposed between quadriceps femoris tendon (Q) and insertion point. V-Y closure of donor defect (D). (Modified from Mathe, ref. 5.)

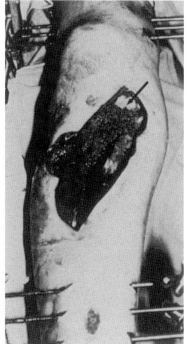
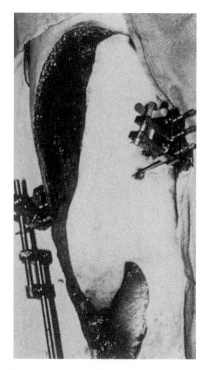
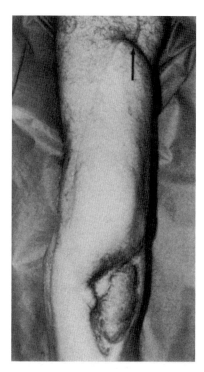

A–C

FIG. 4. Flap designed with medial cutaneous pedicle for cover of exposed knee joint and proximal tibia. A: Skin loss exposes knee cartilage (arrow) and tibial fracture. B: Composite flap with medial cutaneous base advanced. Tibial coverage supplemented by gastrocnemius muscle flap. C: Anterior view of extended leg showing successful postoperative result. V-Y closure of cutaneous donor defect (arrow). Note the large size of this flap.

branches of the medial cutaneous and intermediate cutaneous nerves of the thigh.

FLAP DESIGN AND DIMENSIONS

Vastus medialis musculocutaneous or musculocutaneous-tendinous flaps are designed as medially based advancement flaps with V-Y cutaneous donor-defect closure (Figs. 2 and 3). The vastus medialis musculocutaneous flap is the largest flap available from the distal thigh. The cutaneous paddle can be made as wide as half the distal thigh circumference. Flap length is the distal three fourths of the thigh (see Figs. 2, 4, and 5). The flap base is the segmental vascular pedicles from the superficial femoral vessels along the muscle origin medially (see Fig. 1). The arc of transfer of this advancement flap is 12 cm, which is sufficient to advance the flap from the upper patellar border to the tibial tubercle.

OPERATIVE TECHNIQUE

Skin paddles are incised as shown in Fig. 2. Although this flap has been successfully transferred as a cutaneous island, it is recommended that a medial cutaneous pedicle be maintained to preserve cutaneous sensory nerves and subcutaneous venous drainage (Figs. 2A, B, and Fig. 3).

After the cutaneous component of the flap is incised, the vastus medialis muscle is raised in continuity with the skin paddle by a dissection of the plane deep to the muscle. This dissection proceeds from the quadriceps femoris tendon toward the muscle origin. If a musculocutaneous-tendinous composite flap is required, the quadriceps femoris tendon is split along its midline to create a sufficiently long tendon segment in continuity with the muscle to bridge the tendon defect

(see Figs. 3 and 5). The muscle origin on the proximal femur may be transected to allow greater flap mobilization for large knee defects. If a vascularized quadriceps femoris tendon segment is transferred, the distal end of the tendon is sutured to the tibial tubercle or patellar tendon stump and the proximal border of the tendon is sutured to the lateral half of the split quadriceps femoris tendon that had been left in situ (see Figs. 3 and 5). The cutaneous donor defect in the proximal thigh is managed by V-Y closure (see Figs. 2 and 3).

Closed suction drainage is routinely used. Prolonged knee immobilization is used when tendon reconstruction is done.

CLINICAL RESULTS

This flap is highly reliable. Complete flap survival has been the result in all patients to date.

This flap is designed to avoid the functional deficit that would result from loss of this prime knee extensor. Motor innervation is retained, and muscle insertion is restored. When the musculocutaneous flap is used, the muscle is reinserted into the quadriceps femoris tendon and patella distally. When a musculocutaneous-tendinous flap is used, the tendon is reinserted into the patellar tendon stump or tibial tubercle. Thus, function is always preserved (see Figs. 3 and 5).

SUMMARY

Vastus medialis musculocutaneous flaps are highly reliable, are ideally located for reconstruction of knee and distal thigh defects, and cause no functional deficits. Moreover, they can be designed as composite musculocutaneous-tendinous flaps that carry vascularized quadriceps femoris tendon segments for patellar tendon reconstruction.

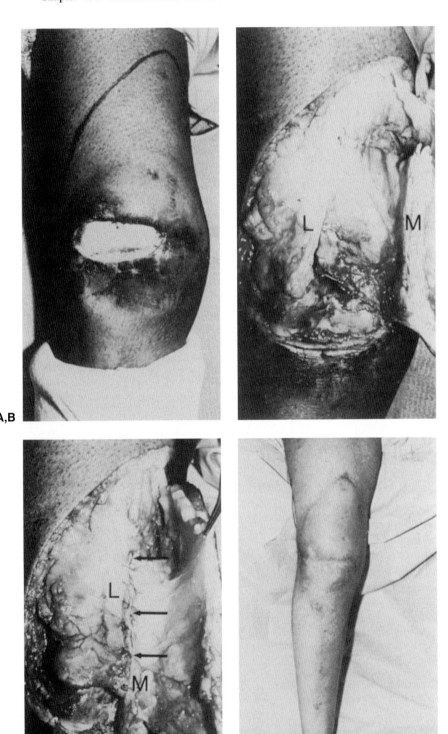

FIG. 5. Composite transfer of vascularized quadriceps femoris tendon segment. **A:** Medially based flap outlined above exposed knee joint with missing patella and patellar tendon. **B:** Distal quadriceps femoris tendon split. Medial half of tendon (*M*) transferred on flap. Lateral half (*L*) left in situ. **C:** Inset of vascularized medial tendon segment (*M*). Distal suture (*white arrow*) is made end-to-end to patellar tendon stump. Proximally, the edge of the tendon is sutured (*black arrow*) side-to-side to the distal quadriceps femoris tendon (*L*). **D:** Extended leg showing postoperative result with defect closed and knee extension restored.

References

1. Tobin GR. The vastus medialis musculocutaneous flap: a comparison with other regional flaps for complex knee defects. *Plast Surg Forum* 1982;5:223.
2. Tobin GR. Unpublished data.
3. Arnold PG, Prunes-Carrilo F. Vastus medialis muscle flap for functional closure of the exposed knee joint. *Plast Reconstr Surg* 1981;68:69.
4. Brash JC. *Neurovascular hila of limb muscles.* Edinburgh: Livingstone, 1955;68–70.
5. Mathe J. *Leonardo daVinci: anatomical drawings.* Fribourg: Production Liber SA, 1978.

CHAPTER 487 ■ SOLEUS FLAPS

G. R. TOBIN

The soleus muscle provides several reliable flaps that are frequently first choices for repair of defects between the knee and ankle.

INDICATIONS

These flaps are used to cover defects in the middle third (soleus and hemisoleus muscle) and distal third (soleus musculocutaneous and reverse medial hemisoleus muscle) of the leg that cannot be covered with skin grafts and are not so massive as to require large free or cross leg flaps. These defects include exposed bone or open fractures of the long bones or malleoli, exposed internal fixation devices, exposed vessels or vascular grafts, exposed tendocalcaneus or other tendons, and surgically excised osteomyelitis, stasis ulcers, and unstable scars (1–12). Compared with skin or fasciocutaneous flaps, soleus muscle flaps are more effective for contaminated or ischemic defects, presumably because of better vascular perfusion of muscle (13).

ANATOMY

The value and versatility of soleus-based flaps result from the following anatomic features: (1) The soleus is the largest, longest muscle beyond the knee. (2) It extends distally on the leg. (3) Its bipennate morphology and dual neurovascular supply permit vertical splitting of the two soleus bellies into lateral or medial hemisoleus muscle flaps (14) (Fig. 1). (4) Both muscle bellies carry overlying musculocutaneous and extended fasciocutaneous territories that permit design of wide, distally extended musculocutaneous flaps for distal leg and ankle defects (15) (Figs. 2–4). (5) Distal segmental vascular pedicles permit reversal of soleus segments on this distal vascular supply for distal leg and ankle defects (16–18) (Fig. 5).

The soleus lies immediately deep to the gastrocnemius and plantaris musculotendinous units in the posterior leg compartment. It has a bipennate morphology. It originates on the proximal third of both tibia and fibula, and it tapers to insert on the tendocalcaneus just above the ankle.

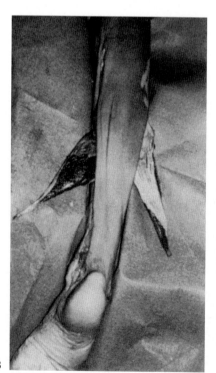
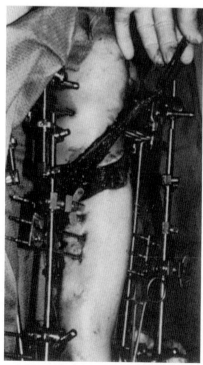

FIG. 1. **A:** Medial and lateral hemisoleus flaps raised simultaneously in a cadaver leg. **B:** Medial hemisoleus muscle flap raised for early cover of open midtibial fracture. Flap inset, successful skin-graft application, and fracture union resulted. (From Tobin, ref. 19, with permission.)

A,B

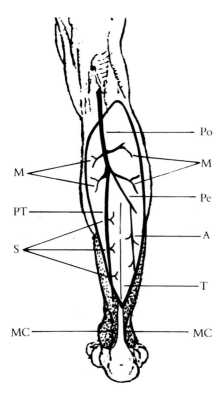

FIG. 2. Vascular anatomy of soleus flaps. Po, popliteal artery; PT, posterior tibial artery; Pe, peroneal artery; M, major vascular pedicles to proximal soleus; S, segmental posterior tibial vascular pedicles to soleus medial belly; A, longitudinal, intramuscular pedicles to lateral soleus belly; T, tendinous midline raphe separating medial and lateral soleus bellies; MC (*stippled area*), extended fasciocutaneous territories of soleus musculocutaneous flaps. (From Tobin, ref. 19, with permission.)

The soleus vascular supply is from popliteal, posterior tibial, and peroneal vascular pedicles to the proximal muscle, peroneal pedicles to the distal lateral belly, and segmental posterior tibial pedicles to the distal medial belly (see Fig. 2) [the basis for reversed soleus and reversed medial hemisoleus flaps (19)] (see Fig. 5).

Cutaneous perforators from each distal soleus belly supply overlying musculocutaneous and extended fasciocutaneous territories that extend from the posterior midline to the anterior borders of the posterior compartment and reach distally to the malleoli (15) (see Figs. 2–4). These perforators provide medial and lateral musculocutaneous flaps that extend well beyond their underlying hemisoleus muscles to cover the most distal leg and ankle (15). Both medial and lateral soleus bellies are independently innervated by branches of the medial popliteal and posterior tibial nerves (20).

FLAP DESIGN AND DIMENSIONS

The soleus provides the largest, longest regional flaps for the distal two thirds of the lower leg. Soleus muscle dimensions taper from the proximal third of the leg, where the soleus constitutes approximately 45% of leg circumference, to its narrow insertion. At the tibial midpoint, the soleus constitutes approximately 35% of leg circumference (21). Compared with soleus muscle flaps, hemisoleus muscle flaps are slightly longer when transposed and about half as wide (14).

The arc of rotation for fully mobilized, proximally based soleus and hemisoleus muscle flaps is the distance from the pivot point to insertion. The pivot point is at the junction of the proximal and middle thirds of the leg (the origin of major vascular pedicles to the proximal muscle) (19) (see Fig. 2). The muscle insertion is on the tendocalcaneus 6.0 ± 1.7 cm (X ± SD) above the calcaneus (21).

Soleus musculocutaneous flaps have the same pivot point as their muscle components, but their arcs of rotation are substantially longer when distally extending skin peninsulas are carried. Undelayed flaps extend a short distance beyond the malleoli; delayed flaps extend well beyond the malleoli (15) (see Figs. 2–4). Soleus musculocutaneous flaps also provide substantially wider flaps than their component hemisoleus muscles. Their skin peninsulas may extend from the ipsilateral border of the tendocalcaneus to the ipsilateral margin of the posterior compartment (the tibia or fibula) (15) (see Figs. 2–4). In the distal leg, medial soleus musculocutaneous flaps comprise one third of leg circumference, and lateral soleus musculocutaneous flaps comprise one fourth of leg circumference (15) (see Fig. 3).

Reversed medial hemisoleus and soleus muscle flaps have a pivot point that is the proximal of the two most distal posterior tibial vascular pedicles. This pedicle is usually located 7

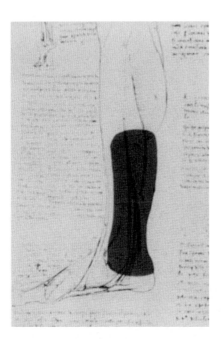

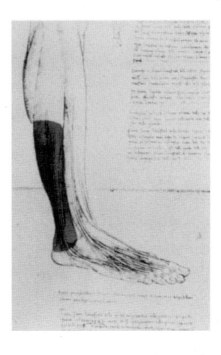

FIG. 3. Medial soleus musculocutaneous territory (left) and lateral soleus musculocutaneous territory (right). Soleus musculocutaneous flaps are designed within these boundaries. (Modified from O'Malley, ref. 26, with permission.)

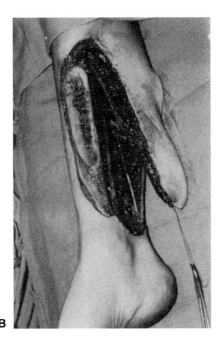
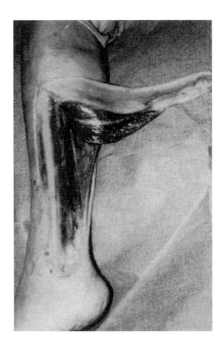

A,B

FIG. 4. A: Undelayed medial soleus musculocutaneous flap carried by medial hemisoleus muscle and raised to the malleolus. Complete flap survival and successful cover of resected unstable scar and tibial osteomyelitis resulted. B: Lateral soleus musculocutaneous flap carried by lateral hemisoleus muscle and raised beyond the malleolus. Note the anteriorly and distally extending fasciocutaneous components of this extended flap.

cm proximal to the malleolar flair (16) (see Fig. 5). Reversed soleus flaps reliably carry only the distal one half to two thirds of the muscle (16,17). Reversed transfer of the lateral hemisoleus muscle is questionable, as I find no major distal segmental peroneal pedicles to the lateral belly and no major vascular connections from posterior tibial pedicles crossing the distal muscle midline (19) (see Fig. 2).

The entire soleus muscle can be reversed by an alternative technique in which the posterior tibial vessels are divided at their popliteal origin and the posterior tibial vessels and attached soleus are reversed together (22); however, this technique involves major alteration of the extremity blood supply.

These flap dimensions permit coverage of leg middle-third defects with soleus and hemisoleus muscle flaps and coverage of leg distal two thirds and ankle defects with soleus musculocutaneous and reversed muscle flaps (14–18).

OPERATIVE TECHNIQUE

Soleus flaps are usually approached through either medial or lateral midline incisions placed over the respective borders of the leg posterior compartment (Figs. 5 and 6). Major subcutaneous nerves and veins, such as saphenous and sural trunks, are preserved when possible. The calf muscles are exposed by

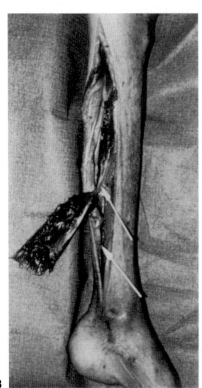
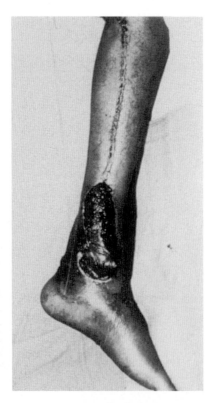

A,B

FIG. 5. A: Reversed medial hemisoleus muscle flap based on the two most distal posterior tibial vascular pedicles (located by *arrows*). B: Reversed medial hemisoleus muscle flap covering exposed malleolar fracture and internal fixation hardware. Successful skin-graft application and wound closure resulted. (From Tobin, ref. 19, with permission.)

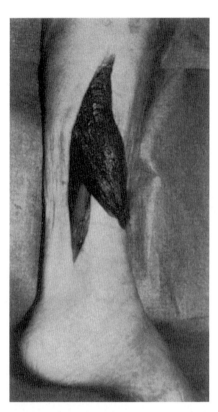

FIG. 6. Soleus muscle flap transposed through a medial midline incision. Transposition through lateral incision permits similar coverage of lateral leg midthird defects.

opening the posterior compartment deep fascia. In the leg midsection, well-defined planes usually separate the soleus from overlying gastrocnemius tendon and underlying vessels and deep muscles. If not present, the plane between soleus and gastrocnemius tendons must be surgically created. The plantaris tendon transverses the superficial plane. Vascular pedicles from the posterior tibial and peroneal vessels cross the deep plane.

At this stage of dissection, the muscle may be designed into proximally based soleus, hemisoleus, or reversed flaps. Proximally based soleus flaps require sharp separation of the overlying tendocalcaneus and division of tethering distal segmental vascular pedicles. Lateral or medial hemisoleus flaps are fashioned by separating the belly to be transferred from the belly left in situ by dissection along a midline raphe that separates them distally (14,19) (see Fig. 2). Reversed medial hemisoleus and soleus flaps are created by transversely dividing the muscle proximally and reversing the distal segment on the two most distal posterior tibial vascular pedicles (16) (see Fig. 5). Only one half to two thirds of the muscle can be reliably reversed (16,17).

Soleus musculocutaneous flaps are approached by means of incisions along a border of the skin peninsula (see Figs. 2–4). Usually, this is the posterior border that overlies the tendocalcaneus ipsilateral edge. The skin peninsula is raised deep to the underlying fascia, and the underlying hemisoleus belly is raised in continuity with the skin peninsula. The muscle border epimysium is sutured to overlying fascia to protect musculocutaneous perforators from shearing. Skin grafts are immediately applied to muscle flap and musculocutaneous flap donor sites.

CLINICAL RESULTS

The anatomy and experiences described in this chapter are derived from my studies of more than 100 cadaver legs and 50

clinical flaps. Proximally based soleus, hemisoleus, and soleus musculocutaneous flaps are exceptionally hearty and highly reliable. These flaps may fail if their proximal vascular pedicles or the major vascular supply of the limb are compromised by trauma or arteriosclerosis obliterans (23). Soleus musculocutaneous flaps may fail distally if the skin peninsula is extended too far or if small skin vessels are diseased (15).

Reversed soleus flaps have reported failure rates greater than 21% (16,17). Accordingly, reversed soleus flaps usually are reserved for secondary salvage procedures (16,17). This failure rate may be reduced by transferring only the distal half of the muscle on two distal vascular pedicles and by using only the medial hemisoleus belly (16,19).

Although the soleus is the prime ankle plantar flexor, functional deficit following transfer is lessened by both surgical maneuvers and synergistic muscle strengthening and alteration of gait (14,24,25). When hemisoleus flaps are used, the contralateral muscle belly remains in situ to preserve soleus function (14,25). Strengthening of gastrocnemius and deep calf muscle compensates for loss of soleus power. In ambulation, calf muscles serve to oppose dorsiflexion and to stabilize the ankle during ipsilateral weight bearing, thus allowing greater forward lean and stride length (24). Soleus deficit not relieved by synergistic calf-muscle strengthening is compensated for by lessening of forward lean, earlier contralateral heel strike, and shorter stride (24).

SUMMARY

The size, location, and anatomy of the soleus muscle allow several useful, reliable soleus-based flaps for cover of distal leg and ankle defects.

References

1. Stark WJ. The use of pedicled muscle flaps in the surgical treatment of chronic osteomyelitis resulting from compound fractures. *J Bone Joint Surg* 1946;28B:343.
2. Ger R. The operative treatment of the advanced stasis ulcer: a preliminary communication. *Am J Surg* 1966;11:659.
3. Ger R. The management of pretibial skin loss. *Surgery* 1968;63:757.
4. Ger R. Operative treatment of the advanced stasis ulcer using muscle transposition: a follow-up study. *Am J Surg* 1970;120:376.
5. Ger R. The technique of muscle transposition in the operative treatment of traumatic and ulcerative lesions of the leg. *J Trauma* 1971;11:502.
6. Ger R. Surgical management of ulcerative lesions of the leg. *Curr Prob Surg* 1972;3:1.
7. Pers M, Medgyesi S. Pedicle muscle flaps and their applications in the surgery of repair. *Br J Plast Surg* 1973;26:313.
8. Vasconez LO, Bostwick J, McCraw J. Coverage of exposed bone by muscle transposition and skin grafting. *Plast Reconstr Surg* 1974;53:525.
9. Mathes SJ, Vasconez LO, Jurkiewicz MJ. Extensions and further applications of muscle flap transposition. *Plast Reconstr Surg* 1977;60:6.
10. Ger R. The management of stasis ulcers of the leg where the tendocalcaneus is exposed. *Plast Reconstr Surg* 1977;60:337.
11. Ger R. Closure of defects of the lower extremity by muscle flaps. In: Converse JM, ed., *Reconstructive plastic surgery*, 2d ed. Philadelphia: Saunders, 1977;3549–3560.
12. Byrd HS, Cierny G III, Tebbetts JB. The management of open tibial fractures with associated soft-tissue loss: external pin fixation with early flap coverage. *Plast Reconstr Surg* 1981;68:73.
13. Pappas C, Goldich G, Cundy K, Wong W. Skin flaps vs. muscle flaps: coping with infection in the presence of a foreign body. *Plast Surg Forum* 1980;3:133.
14. Tobin GR, Moberg AW, Adcock R, Gemberling RM. Hemisoleus flaps. *Plast Surg Forum* 1981;4:126.
15. Tobin GR, Moberg AW, Pompi-Sanders B, Bundrick L Jr. Soleus musculocutaneous flaps. Unpublished data.
16. McGee WP, Gilbert DA, McInnis WD. Extended muscle and musculocutaneous flaps, *Clin Plast Surg* 1980;7:63.
17. McCraw JB. Selection of alternative local flaps in the leg and foot. *Clin Plast Surg* 1979;6:227.
18. Townsend PLG. An inferiorly based soleus muscle flap. *Br J Plast Surg* 1978;31:210.

19. Tobin GR. Hemisoleus and reversed hemisoleus flaps. *Plast Reconstr Surg* 1985;76:87.
20. Brash IC. *Neurovascular hila of limb muscles.* Edinburgh: Livingstone, 1965;88–89.
21. Tobin GR. Unpublished data, 1980.
22. Guyuron B, Dinner MI, Dowden RV, Labandter HP. Muscle flaps and the vascular detour principle: the soleus. *Ann Plast Surg* 1982;8:132.
23. Riley WB Jr, Cotlar SW, Long JK. The injury-compromised gastrocnemius musculocutaneous flap: lessons and limits. *Plast Surg Forum* 1980;3:136.
24. Simon SR, Mann RA, Hagy JL, Larsen L.J. Role of the posterior calf muscles in normal gait. *J Bone Joint Surg* 1978;60A:465.
25. Tobin GR, Gordon JA, Smith BS, Schusterman MA. Preserving motor function by splitting muscle and myocutaneous pedicles. *Plast Surg Forum* 1980;3:160.
26. O'Malley CD, Saunders JB, De CM, eds. *Leonardo da Vinci on the Human Body.* New York: Henry Schuman, 1952.

CHAPTER 488 ■ TIBIALIS ANTERIOR MUSCLE FLAP

M. PERS, S. MEDGYESI, AND B. KIRKBY

EDITORIAL COMMENT
(Chaps. 488, 489)

The use of transposition muscle flaps in the lower extremity continues to be very valuable. It is particularly so for coverage of defects of the proximal and middle thirds of the leg. As one approaches the distal third of the leg, particularly the foot and the ankle, microvascular surgery is most indicated.

To cover defects exposing the upper third of the tibial shaft (1–8), a medial or lateral gastrocnemius musculocutaneous flap should be the first choice; however, if the defect is located at a somewhat lower level, between the upper and middle third (see Fig. 1), and if the belly of the tibialis anterior muscle is already exposed in the defect, it may be a tempting alternative to mobilize this powerful muscle (6–8).

ANATOMY

The muscle has its bony origin from the lateral tibial condyle above to about halfway down the lateral side of the tibia. Blood is supplied from the tibialis anterior artery by several branches entering the muscle from behind. The vessels lie deeply on the interosseous membrane between the tibialis anterior and the extensors. The segmental supply means that the muscle may be transected safely at any level as long as the main vessels are intact. The cutaneous territory of this muscle is generally not useful for transfer because the donor defect may leave the anterior tibial artery and the deep peroneal nerve exposed.

FLAP DESIGN AND DIMENSIONS

The origin and the close relationship to the tibial shaft indicate that the muscle needs to be transferred only a very short

distance to cover a fracture line or an exposed orthopedic screw in a defect located laterally between the upper and middle thirds of the tibial shaft (Figs. 1 and 2).

The tibialis anterior muscle has an important normal function, however. Foot dorsiflexion and inversion will be impaired if the tendon is completely cut and the function of the tibialis anterior muscle is not taken over by other muscles (e.g., the extensor hallucis longus or extensor digitorum longus), although they have similar innervation from the deep peroneal nerve and are situated in the same anterolateral compartment as the tibialis anterior muscle. When it has been decided to mobilize the tibialis anterior muscle, one should therefore use only part of it, preserving the tendon to preserve dorsiflexion and inversion of the foot.

OPERATIVE TECHNIQUE

In transposing the tibialis anterior muscle, it may be feasible to chisel off the sharp anterior border of the tibia. The muscle then is detached from its bony origin and freed from the interosseous membrane as far as necessary for easy transfer (see Fig. 2B).

CLINICAL RESULTS

This muscle flap has been used to cover exposed bone following compound fracture in four patients. No necrosis has occurred; however, in one patient, it became necessary to amputate the leg: an older woman suffering from anterior-sclerosis in whom the additional operative trauma further impaired the blood supply to the fracture area and foot. This was a typical case of overestimation of the possible use of muscle flaps. Splitting the muscle has not resulted in any hematomas.

SUMMARY

The tibialis anterior muscle can be used to cover defects at the junction of the upper and middle thirds of the tibia. Only a

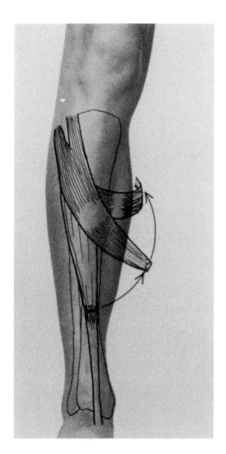

FIG. 1. Transposition of the superficial part of the tibialis anterior muscle. Diagram shows arc of rotation.

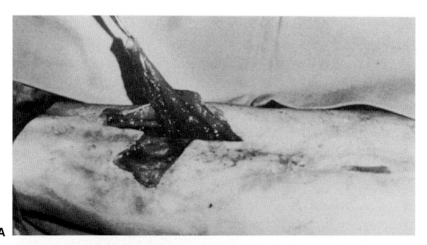

A

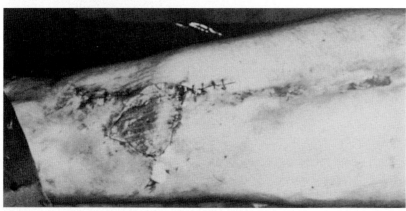

B

FIG. 2. A: Superficial part of tibialis anterior muscle mobilized. **B:** The muscle flap transferred to defect and covered with split-thickness skin graft.

portion of muscle should be used because a significant functional deficit will result from use of the complete muscle.

References

1. Ger R. The technique of muscle transposition in the operative treatment of traumatic and ulcerative lesions of the leg. *J Trauma* 1971;11:502.
2. Pers M, Medgyesi S. Pedicle muscle flaps and their applications in the surgery of repair. *Br J Plast Surg* 1973;26:313.
3. Mathes SJ, McCraw JB, Vasconez LO. Muscle transposition flaps for coverage of lower extremity defects. *Surg Clin North Am* 1974;54:1337.
4. McHugh M, Prindiville JB. Muscle flaps in the repair of skin defects over the exposed tibia. *Br J Plast Surg* 1975;28:205.
5. Pers M. Muscle flaps in reconstructive surgery. In: Barron JN, Saad MN, eds. *Operative plastic and reconstructive surgery,* Vol. 1. London: Churchill-Livingstone, 1981;115–135.
6. Robbins TH. Use of fasciomuscle flaps to repair defects in the lower leg. *Plast Reconstr Surg* 1976;57:460.
7. Mathes SJ, Nahai F, eds. *Clinical atlas of muscle and musculocutaneous flaps.* St. Louis: Mosby, 1979;133–261.
8. Mathes SJ, Nahai F, eds. *Clinical applications for muscle and musculocutaneous flaps.* St. Louis: Mosby, 1982;565, 577.

CHAPTER 489 ■ FLEXOR DIGITORUM LONGUS MUSCLE FLAP

M. PERS, S. MEDGYESI, AND B. KIRKBY

The muscle may be transferred as a supplement in combination with the medial constituents of the soleus or one of the peroneal muscles to defects in the distal third of the lower leg (1–3).

INDICATIONS

The flexor digitorum longus muscle has several qualities that make it useful for a soft-tissue reconstruction over the middle or distal part of the tibia (Fig. 1). First, the muscle fibers extend very far distally, nearly to the ankle joint. Second, its function, which is flexion of the distal phalanx of the lateral toes, is insignificant when intact flexor digitorum brevis muscle preserves the more important function of flexion in the proximal phalanges. With its close relationship to the medial aspect of the tibia, the flexor digitorum longus flap occasionally may prove useful as a filling material in bony cavities or fistulas in the middle third of the lower leg.

ANATOMY

The muscle is located in the medial compartment of the lower leg (Fig. 1). Its proximal part is felt just under the skin along the medial border of the tibial shaft. The muscle is only about 3 cm wide and rather thin. It has a distal location just in front of the medial part of the soleus muscle. The muscle has an extensive origin from the posteromedial surface of the tibial shaft, from just distal to the soleal line to within a hand's breadth from the tip of the medial malleolus (see Fig. 2).

The posterior tibial artery gives off four to five branches to the muscle. Proximally, the artery is located deeply behind the muscle, but more distally the vessels become superficial to follow the tendon on its way behind the medial malleolus to the plantar aspect of the foot.

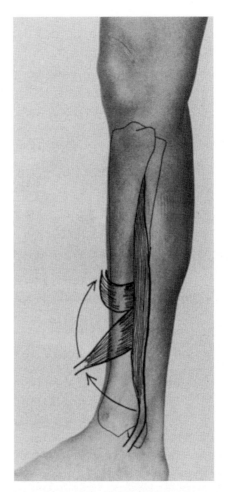

FIG. 1. Transposition of flexor digitorum longus muscle. Diagram shows arc of rotation.

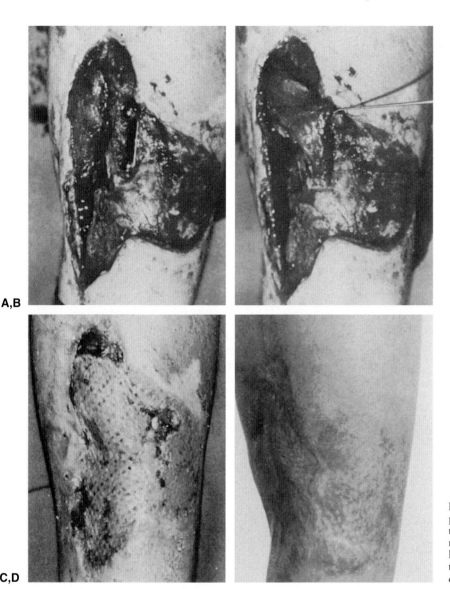

A,B

C,D

FIG. 2. **A:** Defect following skin necrosis. Metal plate exposed on the medial surface of the fractured tibia. **B:** The flexor digitorum muscle is mobilized from the medial compartment of the lower leg. **C:** Primary "take" of a meshed split-thickness skin graft on the transposed muscle flap covering the metal plate. **D:** Final result.

OPERATIVE TECHNIQUE

The flexor digitorum longus is approached through an incision close to the medial border of the tibia, followed by sharp dissection close to the medial aspect of the tibial shaft. When the tendon is cut distally, the tibialis posterior vessels should be carefully avoided, but one or two branches to the distal part of the mobilized muscle have to be severed (Fig. 2).

CLINICAL RESULTS

We have had four opportunities to use this muscle. In one patient, the muscle necrosed, presumably from pressure on the pedicle from the sharp anterior tibial edge. In the other patients, no necrosis occurred, and the primarily applied split-thickness skin grafts all "took" well.

SUMMARY

The flexor digitorum longus muscle flap can be used alone for small defects but is usually combined with either the soleus or peroneal muscles to close lower-third leg defects.

References

1. Pers M, Medgyesi S. Pedicle muscle flaps and their applications in the surgery of repair. *Br J Plast Surg* 1973;26:313.
2. Pers M. Muscle flaps in reconstructive surgery. In: Barron JN, Saad MN, eds. *Operative plastic and reconstructive surgery,* Vol. 1. London: Churchill-Livingstone, 1981;115–135.
3. Mathes SJ, Nahai F, eds. *Clinical applications for muscle and musculocutaneous flaps.* St. Louis: Mosby, 1982;563.

CHAPTER 490 ■ COMBINED EXTENSOR DIGITORUM LONGUS AND PERONEUS LONGUS MUSCULOCUTANEOUS FLAP

R. J. BLOCH, L. M. CORDERO,* AND J. M. PSILLAKIS

EDITORIAL COMMENT

The skin, fascia, and underlying two muscles probably work as independent territories. The limiting factor, then, is to what extent the fasciocutaneous flap will survive and also at what point the peroneus muscle becomes tendinous and able to provide useful transfer. As the distal third of the leg is approached, coverage becomes more tenuous and risky.

The loss of substance of the lower third of the tibia is a challenging reconstructive problem.

INDICATIONS

We studied and used the extensor digitorum longus (EDL) and peroneus longus (PL) in a single stage because they are capable of maintaining the viability of the skin covering and of providing muscular tissue to an area with a poor blood supply (1).

The two muscles were used in conjunction for the following reasons. The EDL provides greater volume and width, vascularizing the soft tissue to be transferred, and the PL supplies distally placed muscle fibers next to the lateral malleolus. The technique has been used for exposed fractures and osteomyelitis of the lower third of the tibia.

ANATOMY

Peroneus Longus

The PL is the widest of the two muscles of the posterior group on the lateral surface of the leg (see Fig. 4). It lies superficially to the peroneus brevis and the EDL (Fig. 1). It arises from the head and upper two thirds of the lateral surface of the fibula. This muscle inserts in the lateral side of the base of the first metatarsal and the medial cuneiform bone by means of a tendon passing through the sulcus behind the lateral malleolus. Innervation is supplied by the superficial peroneal nerve that enters the deep surface of the muscle at its origin. This muscle everts and plantar flexes the foot.

Dissections on 50 cadavers showed that the blood supply (Fig. 2) is provided by the peroneal artery (PeA) in 4% of the cases, by the anterior tibial artery (ATA) in 32%, and by

branches from both in 64%. Therefore, the anterior tibial artery provides pedicles for the muscle in 96% of all cases.

We observed that the vascular distribution of the PL differs from that found by others (2,3). The PeA was the sole nutrient only in 4% of the cases dissected by us. Our dissections revealed that the pedicles are composed of branches from two arteries: the ATA and the PeA. These originate separately from the popliteal artery; however, it should be pointed out that the anterior tibial artery irrigates practically all the nutrient pedicles.

Extensor Digitorum Longus

The EDL is found in the anterior compartment of the leg (Figs. 1, 3, and 4). It arises from the lateral condyle of the tibia, the upper three fourths of the medial surface of the fibula, and the anterior surface of the interosseous membrane. Together with the extensor digitorum brevis and the expansions of the interosseous and lumbrical muscles, it inserts in the proximal and distal phalanges of the four lesser toes. The function of the EDL is to extend the toes and dorsiflex the foot in synergy with the other muscles. Innervation is provided by the deep peroneal nerve.

The EDL is supplied segmentally by multiple branches that pass laterally from the ATA. Laboratory dissections of 18

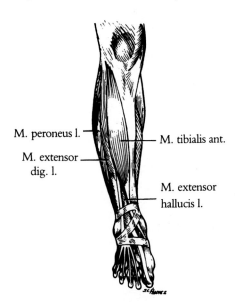

FIG. 1. The anatomy of the extensor digitorum longus and peroneus longus muscles and their relationship to other structures.

* Deceased.

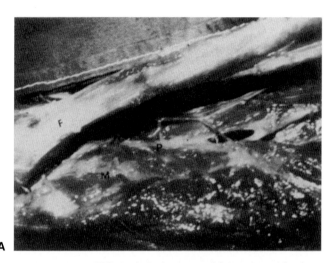
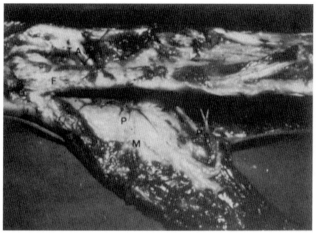

FIG. 2. A, B: Anatomy of the peroneous longus. Note the pedicles of the PeA and anterior tibial artery (ATA). *F*, fibula; *M*, muscle; *P*, pedicle of the ATA; *Pe*, pedicle of the PeA.

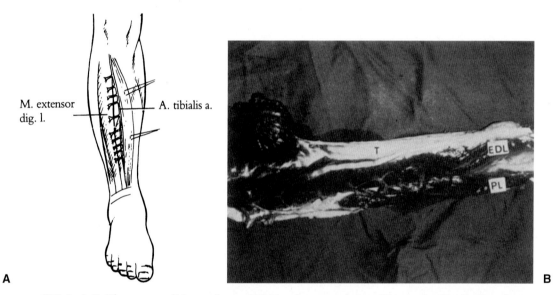

M. extensor dig. l.

A. tibialis a.

FIG. 3. A, B: The extensor digitorum longus *(EDL)* and peroneus longus *(PL)* muscles. Distribution of the nutrient pedicles. *T*, tibia; *p*, nutrient pedicles.

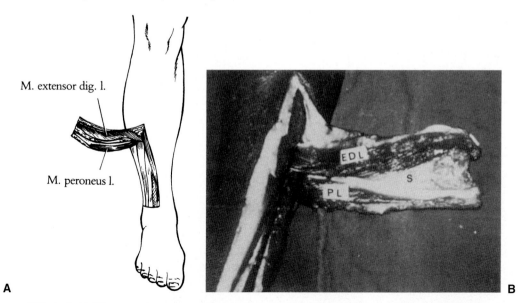

M. extensor dig. l.

M. peroneus l.

FIG. 4. A, B: The musculocutaneous flap made up of the extensor digitorum longus and peroneus longus. *S*, skin.

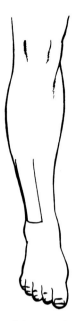

FIG. 5. Design of the musculocutaneous flap.

cadavers demonstrated that the muscle has eight pedicles in 50% of cases, nine pedicles in 5.5%, 10 pedicles in 22%, 11 pedicles in 5.5%, and 12 pedicles in 17%. All were derived from the ATA. The most proximal pedicle originates at an average distance of 4.68 cm from the head of the fibula, the most distal at 33.33 cm. It should be pointed out that the muscle has three or four main superior pedicles with a diameter of 0.75 to 1.0 mm. They leave the ATA directly, penetrating the superoposterior portion of the muscle belly. Vessels from the ATA penetrate the medioinferior aspect of the muscle belly after traversing through the extensor hallucis longus. At this point, the average diameter is 0.5 mm.

With respect to the distance of the pedicle from the reference point, we found the first pedicle at a distance of 4.68 cm. This finding agrees with the findings of others (4), who reported an average distance of 5 cm. Another important finding was that there are vessels with a wider lumen on the proximal side of the muscle, which enables the raising of a musculocutaneous flap with a proximal pedicle of four or five perforators. The use of a muscle flap based on the inferior pedicles has been reported (4).

Regarding the EDL, in all the cases studied, the single nutrient artery was the ATA, which furnishes a variable number of branches or pedicles (8 to 12). These findings differ from those of others (3), who reported 6 to 8 pedicles. Eight pedicles were found in only 50% of the cases we dissected.

Statistical analysis enabled us to conclude (1) that the origin of the arterial pedicles is from the ATA and PeA; (2) that the branches from the ATA are more proximal to the intercondyle line in relation to the branches from the PeA; (3) that the branches originating from the ATA are shorter compared with those from the PeA; and (4) that the external diameters of the branches from the ATA are not significantly different in cases with a single pedicle from those with two pedicles, one from the ATA and the other from the PeA.

FLAP DESIGN AND DIMENSIONS

The flap is outlined 2 cm from the external malleolus (Fig. 5), an average of 7 cm wide. The midline of the flap should descend vertically over the lateral malleolus. Two other lines are drawn on the anterolateral and posteromedial surfaces of the leg.

OPERATIVE TECHNIQUE

The incision is extended down until the tendon of the extensor digitorum is located at the level of the inferior extensor retinaculum, between the tendons of the extensor hallucis longus and peroneus brevis muscles. The dissection proceeds, and the four or five distal pedicles of the EDL are divided. The tendons are divided and the flap elevated to the lower-third tibial level (Fig. 6). The same technique is followed with the tendon of the PL behind the external malleolus.

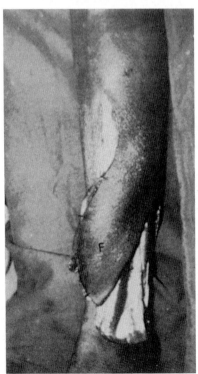

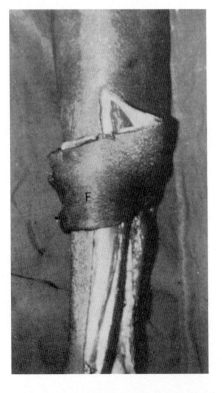

A,B

FIG. 6. A, B: Elevation and rotation of the musculocutaneous flap (F).

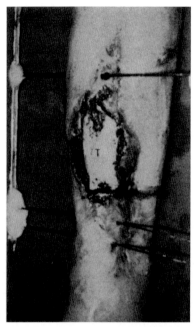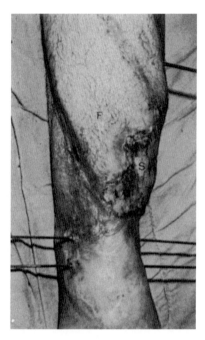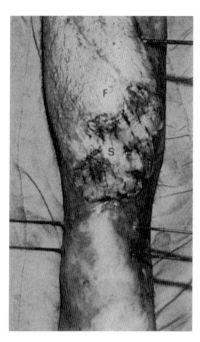

A–C

FIG. 7. **A:** Patient with a compound fracture and exposed tibia showing the focus of the fracture distally. **B, C:** Late result with integration of the musculocutaneous flap and a skin graft over the peroneus longus. *T*, tibia; *F*, musculocutaneous flap; *S*, skin graft.

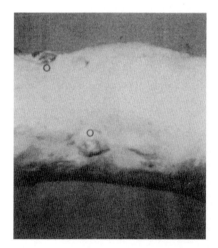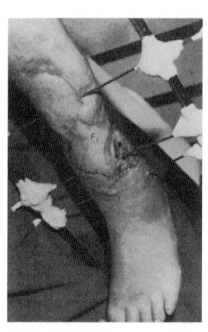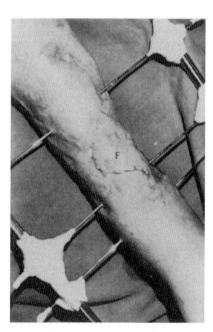

A–C

FIG. 8. **A:** Patient with chronic osteomyelitis and bone sequestrum. *O*, focus of osteomyelitis. **B, C:** Musculocutaneous flap in place 45 days postoperatively, with beginning of bone consolidation and remission of osteomyelitis. *F*, musculocutaneous flap.

CLINICAL RESULTS

Regarding the PL, disability from loss of foot eversion is minimal. Indeed, the loss of both these muscles is functionally and aesthetically inconsequential (Figs. 7 and 8).

SUMMARY

The EDL and the PL muscles can be combined to form a musculocutaneous flap that can be used to cover lower-third tibial defects.

References

1. Maquiera N. Estado atual dos retalhos mio-cutaneous. Presented at the XVIII Congresso Brasileiro de Cirurgia Plastica, Guarapari, 1981.
2. Mathes SJ, McCraw JB, Vasconez LO. Muscle transposition flaps for coverage of lower extremity defects: anatomic considerations. *Surg Clin North Am* 1974;54:1337.
3. Mathes SJ, Nahai F, eds. *Clinical atlas of muscle and musculocutaneous flaps.* St. Louis: Mosby, 1979.
4. Arnold PG, Hodgkinson DJ. Extensor digitorum turn-down muscle flap. *Plast Reconstr Surg* 1980;66:599.

CHAPTER 491 ■ EXTENSOR HALLUCIS LONGUS MUSCLE FLAP

M. PERS, S. MEDGYESI, AND B. KIRKBY

Situated in the anterolateral compartment just behind the tibialis anterior, the extensor hallucis longus muscle is often the muscle of choice to cover tibial defects with bare bone (Fig. 1). This is so because its belly extends farther distally than any other muscle, close to the anterior surface of the tibia (1–3).

ANATOMY

The tendon is easily recognized when the big toe is moved passively. Proximally, the muscle is closely connected with the tibialis anterior and the extensor digitorum longus. The extensor hallucis longus usually receives four small branches from the anterior tibial artery that enter its tibial aspect at approximately a 4-cm interval and a finger's breadth behind the tendon.

FLAP DESIGN AND DIMENSIONS

Because the muscle is rather thin, the size of the defect it covers should not be too large. If the muscle flap turns out to be smaller than expected, it sometimes can be supplemented with part of the powerful belly of the tibialis anterior muscle to cover denuded bone in the middle third of the tibia (see Fig. 2D). In the lower third, the peroneus brevis may serve as a supplement (Fig. 1).

OPERATIVE TECHNIQUE

The muscle is mobilized by freeing its distal extent from the deep attachments (Fig. 2). The muscle must be isolated by sharp and blunt excision, and finally the tendon is cut as far distally as needed. Great care should be taken to avoid pressure on the muscle after transfer, especially if it is passed behind the tibialis anterior tendon to reach the tibia. Sometimes resection of bone may give better space for transfer of the muscle.

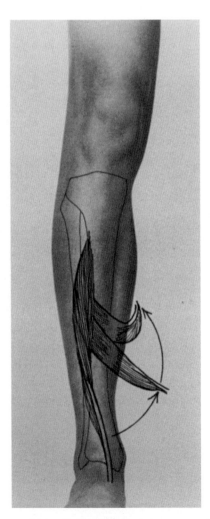

FIG. 1. Transposition of extensor hallucis longus muscle. Diagram shows arc of rotation.

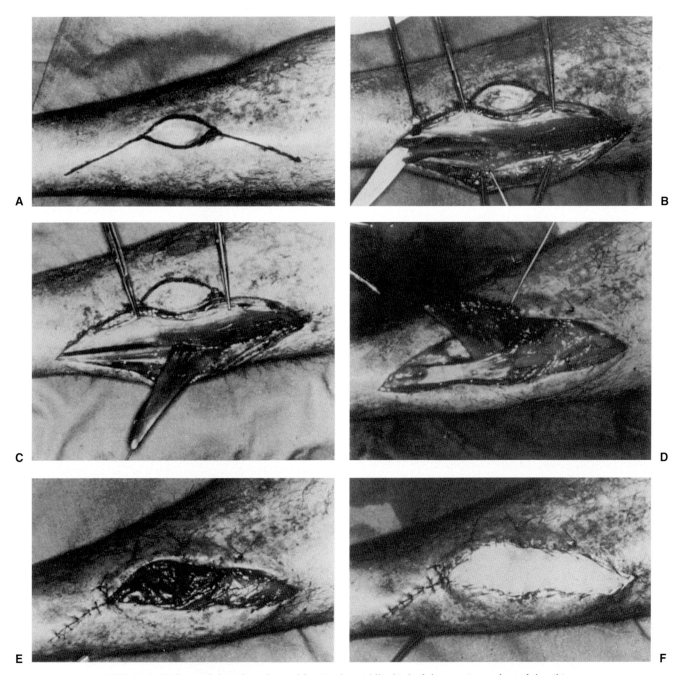

FIG. 2. A: Defect with bare bone located low in the middle third of the anterior surface of the tibia. Incision marked. **B:** Tape around extensor hallucis longus muscle located between tibialis anterior in front and extensor digitorum longus behind. **C:** The tendon cut. **D:** The scar has been excised and the muscle flap transferred. The tibialis anterior muscle provides a supplementary cover to the proximal part of the defect. **E:** The defect covered with muscle. **F:** Skin graft covers the muscle flap.

CLINICAL RESULTS

Transfer of the extensor hallucis longus muscle was carried out in 16 patients, our largest group of muscle transfers on the lower extremity. Most of the patients had previously sustained a compound fracture of the tibia and fibula. Infection was usually present in the soft tissue and bone. A small partial necrosis of muscle was observed in three patients. Too much tension, rather than infection, was responsible for this problem, but in one patient, heavy streptococcal infection caused total flap necrosis. Split-thickness skin grafts on the muscle flaps resulted in primary healing in most of the remaining 12 patients. There have been only minor functional deficits. In some patients, the distal ends of the cut tendon have been sutured to the tibialis anterior tendon.

SUMMARY

The extensor hallucis longus muscle flap is one of the most commonly used muscle flaps for tibial defects.

References

1. Pers M, Medgyesi S. Pedicle muscle flaps and their applications in the surgery of repair. *Br J Plast Surg* 1973;26:313.
2. Pers M. Muscle flaps in reconstructive surgery. In: Barron JN, Saad MN, eds. *Operative plastic and reconstructive surgery*, Vol. 1. London: Churchill-Livingstone, 1981;115–135.
3. Mathes SJ, Nahai F, eds. *Clinical applications for muscle and musculocutaneous flaps.* St. Louis: Mosby, 1982;577.

CHAPTER 492 ■ PERONEUS BREVIS MUSCLE FLAP

M. PERS, S. MEDGYESI, AND B. KIRKBY

The peroneus brevis muscle flap is a good alternative to a dorsalis pedis arterial island flap, especially when the defect is situated just proximal to the lateral malleolus (1–3).

ANATOMY

The muscle is the nethermost of the two muscles in the posterolateral compartment of the leg. It arises from the lower half of the lateral surface of the fibula and from the intermuscular septa. It lies between the extensor digitorum longus anteriorly and the flexor hallucis longus posteriorly. The muscle terminates in a short tendon that runs behind the lateral malleolus and then bends forward to end at the base of the fifth metatarsal bone.

In the area behind the lateral malleolus, the muscle is still fleshy and is crossed by the tendon of the peroneus longus. A common synovial sheath envelops the two tendons, which are covered by the superior peroneal retinaculum.

The blood supply is provided by small segmental branches, usually three to four in number, arising from the peroneal artery. Another set of nutrient vessels coming off the anterior tibial artery supplies the upper part of the muscle belly.

The nerve supply is from the superficial peroneal nerve, the lower stem of the common peroneal nerve that winds around the neck of the fibula. The muscle's function, in common with that of the peroneus longus, is to perform eversion and plantar flexion of the foot.

FLAP DESIGN AND DIMENSIONS

The muscle flap, nearly 10 cm long by 3 cm wide, can be swung forward to cover the upper half of the lateral malleolus and the adjoining part of the fibula (Fig. 1). A split-thickness skin graft provides the epithelial cover (Fig. 2). There will be no functional loss using this muscle flap if the peroneus longus is preserved intact.

OPERATIVE TECHNIQUE

The distal portion of the muscle belly can be felt immediately behind the lower third of the fibula in front of the Achilles ten-

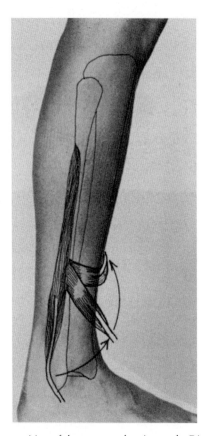

FIG. 1. Transposition of the peroneus brevis muscle. Diagram shows arc of rotation.

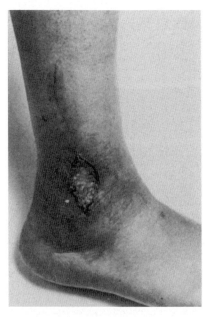

FIG. 2. The complete "take" of a split-thickness skin graft on the transposed peroneus brevis muscle. The site of the lesion is ideal for the use of the peroneus brevis muscle flap.

don. Access to the muscle is by a longitudinal incision along the posterior border of the lateral malleolus. The distal 10 to 12 cm of the muscular attachment to the fibula can be released without compromising the blood supply to the muscle flap.

Having cut through the superior peroneal retinaculum, the tendon is isolated. Damage to the peroneus longus tendon with its peritendineum, situated superficial to that of the brevis, must be avoided. The peroneus brevis tendon should be transected as far distally as possible.

CLINICAL RESULTS

We used the peroneus brevis muscle flap twice. In both instances, the patient had a complicated fracture of the lateral malleolus. The first patient was a 72-year-old man with a chronic ulceration, 3 cm long by 3 cm wide, with an underlying osteitis. The second patient was a 45-year-old woman with

a 2-cm-long by 3-cm-wide ulceration with exposed bone. In both patients, the peroneus brevis flap was successful.

SUMMARY

The peroneus brevis muscle flap can be used to cover defects just proximal to the lateral malleolus.

References

1. Pers M, Medgyesi S. Pedicle muscle flaps and their applications in the surgery of repair. *Br J Plast Surg* 1973;26:313.
2. Pers M. Muscle flaps in reconstructive surgery. In: Barron JN, Saad MN, eds. *Operative plastic and reconstructive surgery,* Vol. 1. London: Churchill-Livingstone, 1981;115–135.
3. Mathes SJ, Nahai F, eds. *Clinical applications for muscle and musculocutaneous flaps.* St. Louis: Mosby, 1982;577.

CHAPTER 493 ■ PERONEUS LONGUS MUSCLE FLAP

M. PERS, S. MEDGYESI, AND B. KIRKBY

The peroneus longus muscle can be used to fill cavities in the upper lateral part of the tibia (see Fig. 2). It can be used as an alternative to the coleus to cover smaller defects on the middle anterior surface of the leg (1–3). This relatively thick muscle has been satisfactorily used to fill a 6-cm defect in the tibial condyle.

ANATOMY

The peroneus longus muscle is located in the upper half of the anterolateral side of the leg in the superficial muscle layer. It arises from the head and upper part of the shaft of the fibula, the deep surface of the fascia, and the intermuscular septa. The relatively thick muscle belly terminates in a long tendon in the middle of the calf (Fig. 1). The peroneal artery gives off perforating branches to this muscle, usually three in number. The function of the muscle is eversion and plantar flexion of the foot.

OPERATIVE TECHNIQUE

To approach the muscle, an incision is made on the anterolateral surface of the leg. After dividing the tendon, the flap can safely be dissected to the upper third of its length (Fig. 2).

CLINICAL RESULTS

If the peroneus brevis (and tertius) is intact, foot eversion should not be impaired after peroneus longus transfer. We

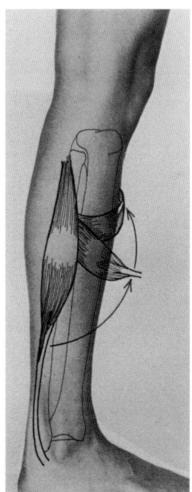

FIG. 1. Transfer of the peroneus longus muscle. Diagram shows arc of rotation.

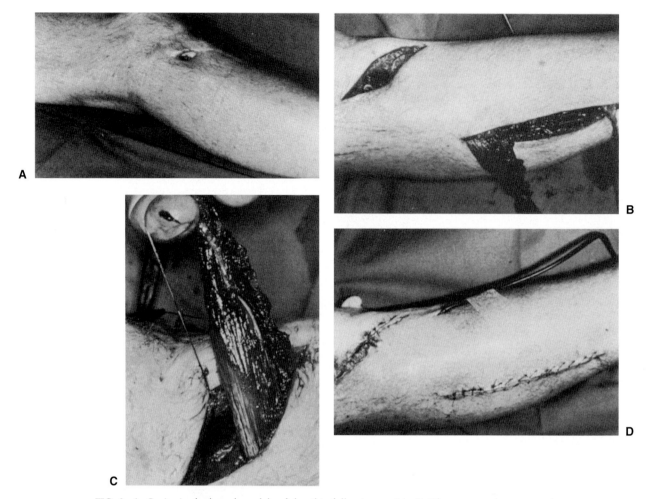

FIG. 2. A: Cavity in the lateral condyle of the tibia following osteitis. **B:** The peroneus longus muscle mobilized. **C:** The muscle flap ready to enter the cavity in the bone. **D:** Percutaneous transfixation suture keeps muscle in position; suction drainage and no dressing; small split-thickness skin graft to residual skin defect over transposed muscle.

used this relatively thick muscle to fill a 6-cm defect in the tibial condyle. The patient had sustained a comminuted fracture with subsequent osteitis. Several curettings of the cavity and transfers of bone chips had been undertaken without success. The patient had no loss of function. We have had no further opportunity to use this muscle.

SUMMARY

The peroneus longus muscle can be used to cover defects in the upper third of the leg.

References

1. Pers M, Medgyesi S. Pedicle muscle flaps and their applications in the surgery of repair. *Br J Plast Surg* 1973;313:1973.
2. Pers M. Muscle flaps in reconstructive surgery. In: Barron JN, Saad MN, eds. *Operative plastic and reconstructive surgery*, Vol. 1. London: Churchill-Livingstone, 1981;115–135.
3. Mathes SJ, Nahai F, eds. *Clinical applications for muscle and musculocutaneous flaps.* St. Louis: Mosby, 1982;565.

CHAPTER 494 ■ FREE GROIN FLAP

D. SERAFIN AND C. H. MANSTEIN

EDITORIAL COMMENT

Although the groin flap was the first unit applicable to transfer by microvascular surgery, the difficulty in execution has led to a choice of free muscle or musculocutaneous units.

Historically, the groin flap was one of the first flaps used in microsurgical composite-tissue transplantation (1,2). Once the anatomic basis for this flap was established, demonstrating a self-contained arteriovenous system (3), the flap was first employed as an alternative to the abdominal tubed pedicle flap. The next logical step was to transplant this vascularized donor tissue to a distant recipient site.

INDICATIONS

The greatest advantage of the vascularized groin flap is in the concealment of the donor deformity, even by a brief bathing suit. A defect up to 10 cm wide can easily be closed primarily. Flaps of greater dimension require a split-thickness skin graft to cover the donor defect, negating the primary advantage for selecting this flap as donor tissue.

A portion of the iliac crest may be included with the cutaneous portion if a segment of bone is required in reconstruction. Viability of the bone is maintained through its periosteal circulation. If the medial portion of the flap is excluded, the groin flap consists of non–hair-bearing tissue suitable for reconstruction in exposed areas.

The vascularized scapular flap (see Chap. 540), with its long vascular pedicle and vessel size of adequate external diameter, has replaced the vascularized groin flap as the donor tissue of choice when cutaneous cover alone is required in reconstruction.

ANATOMY

The vascular anatomy of the groin flap is well documented (3–5). Unfortunately, considerable vascular variability has contributed to unacceptably high flap failure rates (6). Anatomic dissections support these clinical observations.

The vascular basis for the vascularized groin flap is the superficial circumflex iliac artery. The external diameter of this vessel is approximately 1 mm. It arises as a separate branch from the femoral artery approximately two to three finger breadths inferior to the intersection of the femoral artery and inguinal ligament. The arterial length is usually quite short, often less than 1 cm (Fig. 1).

Frequently, a short distance from its origin from the femoral artery, the superficial circumflex iliac artery sends a muscle branch to the sartorius muscle. The artery then continues as a direct cutaneous artery laterally to terminate in multiple branches inferior to the anterior superior iliac spine. From this point laterally, the arterialized flap becomes a random one. It is not uncommon to find that the superficial circumflex iliac artery is duplicated, takes origin from a common trunk with the superficial inferior epigastric artery, or takes origin from the lateral circumflex femoral artery. Occasionally, the artery may be totally absent. When this occurs, the dominant blood supply to this cutaneous region is often from branches of the superficial inferior epigastric artery.

The venous drainage is more constant than the arterial blood supply. Frequently, small venae comitantes accompany the superficial circumflex iliac artery. Most often, however, these veins are too small in external diameter to be used in reestablishing venous continuity. The superficial drainage vein of the flap is most frequently employed. It has an external diameter of 1.5 to 2.5 mm and a length of 2 to 3 cm. It most frequently is found entering the termination of the greater saphenous vein just prior to its junction with the deep femoral vein in the fossa ovalis. Close to its junction to the saphenous vein, a valve system is almost always present.

Although the lateral cutaneous nerve of the thigh is often transected during dissection, the vascularized groin flap has not been successfully employed as a neurosensory flap.

FLAP DESIGN AND DIMENSIONS

Prior to flap dissection, a line corresponding to the course of the superficial circumflex iliac artery is outlined on the skin approximately 2.5 cm inferior to and parallel to the inguinal ligament. This line serves as a central axis of the flap. The flap then is outlined approximately 10 cm wide and 25 to 30 cm long. If a greater length of the flap is required, then a previous delay of the random portion is indicated.

OPERATIVE TECHNIQUE

By first determining the feasibility of transfer with a medial exploratory incision, there is the additional advantage of easy access to the contralateral groin with a minimum of dissection, reducing the length of the operative procedure. A medial curvilinear incision is first made overlying the femoral artery and vein (7) (Fig. 2A). A deeper dissection exposes first the superficial drainage vein at its junction with the saphenous bulb in the fossa ovalis. The dissection then is continued laterally and superiorly to the femoral artery, where the origin of the superficial circumflex iliac artery is identified (Fig. 2B). This medial dissection takes approximately 1 to 1½ hours. Because of the frequent finding of vascular variability, this maneuver allows assessment of the suitability of the vasculature prior to transfer and minimizes lost time. If the medial

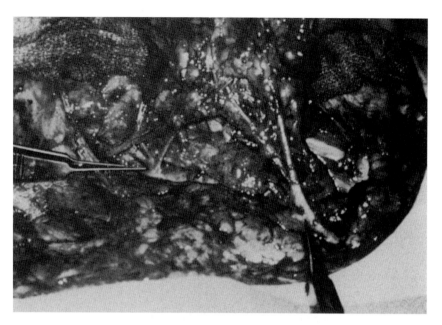

FIG. 1. Intraoperative photograph demonstrating origin of the superficial circumflex iliac artery from a common trunk (instrument left). Note the short arterial length, often less than 1 cm. The superficial drainage vein of the flap (instrument right) is more constant than the arterial blood supply. Note that the superficial drainage vein joins the termination of the greater saphenous vein just prior to its junction with the deep femoral vein in the fossa ovalis.

dissection reveals that the donor vasculature is unsuitable for anastomosis, then the other groin can be explored.

Once the flap has been deemed suitable for transfer and the vasculature is carefully dissected from the surrounding tissue through the medial incision, dissection then is begun laterally and proceeds in a medial direction (Fig. 3A). This portion of the dissection is quite rapid. Dissection proceeds in a loose areolar plane just anterior to the fascia lata of the thigh and the inguinal ligament. As the fascia overlying the sartorius muscle is encountered, dissection may proceed deep to this structure, where the muscular branch is identified and then ligated (Fig. 3B). Frequently, however, this is not necessary because this muscular branch is well visualized through the medial incision, making inclusion of the fascia overlying the sartorius unnecessary.

CLINICAL RESULTS

Disadvantages of the vascularized groin flap include primarily the variability of the donor arterial vasculature and the short length of the arterial pedicle. The short vascular pedicle length makes an end-to-side anastomosis to a recipient artery quite difficult without the use of an interpositional vein graft. This necessitates an additional anastomosis, with the added potential for thrombosis.

The flap may be quite thick, particularly in obese patients. Even in lean patients, the medial aspect of the flap often contains an excessive amount of adipose tissue that contributes to problems related to flap placement and positioning (Fig. 4).

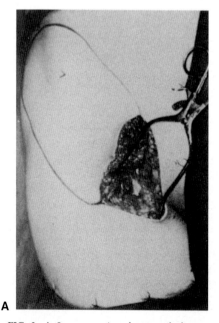

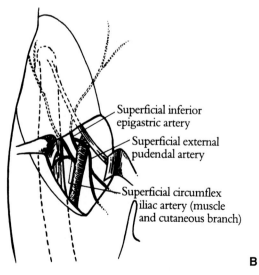

Superficial inferior epigastric artery

Superficial external pudendal artery

Superficial circumflex iliac artery (muscle and cutaneous branch)

FIG. 2. A: Intraoperative photograph demonstrating medial curvilinear incision used to assess the quality of the donor vasculature. B: Illustration depicting the superficial circumflex iliac artery as visualized through a medial curvilinear incision.

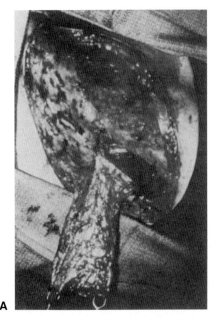
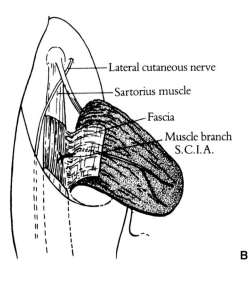

FIG. 3. **A:** Intraoperative photograph demonstrating lateral dissection. **B:** Illustration depicting the lateral dissection beneath the fascia overlying the sartorius muscle. Note the vessel branch of the superficial circumflex iliac artery.

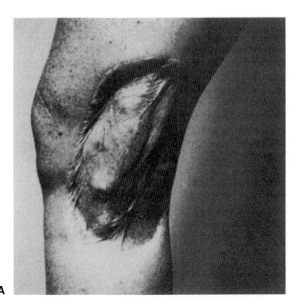
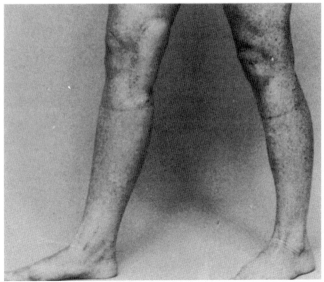

FIG. 4. **A:** Defect on the medial aspect of a patient's right knee subsequent to excision of a melanoma. **B:** Postoperative result following successful vascularized groin flap.

Finally, flap failure and morbidity statistics are significantly higher than with other cutaneous composite tissue used in microsurgical composite-tissue transfer. In an unpublished series consisting of approximately 90 patients, the failure rate of the vascularized groin flap was approximately 24% (8). This is approximately three to four times greater than flap failure rate statistics for other vascularized tissue employed at present in reconstruction of extensive defects. Today, an acceptable flap failure rate following microsurgical composite-tissue transfer should be in the range of 4% to 6%.

SUMMARY

The vascularized groin flap was the first cutaneous donor tissue employed in microsurgical composite-tissue transfer; however, transfer in many large series has been characterized by significant flap morbidity and failure.

References

1. Kaplan EN, Buncke HJ, Murray DE. Distant transfer of cutaneous island flaps in humans by microvascular anastomoses. *Plast Reconstr Surg* 1973;52:301.
2. Daniel RK, Taylor GI. Distant transfer of an island flap by microvascular anastomoses: a clinical technique. *Plast Reconstr Surg* 1973;52:111.
3. McGregor IA, Jackson IT. The groin flap. *Br J Plast Surg* 1972;25:3.
4. Taylor GI, Daniel RK. The anatomy of several free-flap donor sites. *Plast Reconstr Surg* 1975;56:243.
5. Harii K, Ohmori K. Free skin flap transfer. *Clin Plast Surg* 1978;3:111.
6. Serafin D, Georgiade NG, Smith DH. Comparison of free flaps with pedicled flaps for coverage of defects of the leg or foot. *Plast Reconstr Surg* 1977;52:492.
7. Serafin D, Georgiade NG. Microsurgical composite tissue transplantation. *Am J Surg* 1977;133:752.
8. Serafin D. Unpublished data. 1977.

CHAPTER 495 ■ MICROVASCULAR FREE TRANSFER OF A LATISSIMUS DORSI MUSCLE AND MUSCULOCUTANEOUS FLAP

R. M. BARTON AND L. O. VASCONEZ

The microvascular transfer of the latissimus dorsi muscle, with or without overlying skin, is perhaps the most reliable of all free-tissue transfers for the lower extremity, particularly involving wounds of the distal third of the tibia (1–3). The latissimus dorsi muscle is the largest muscle that can be transferred, and in most people, it can be sacrificed without significant loss of strength of the upper extremity. When taken with an overlying skin paddle less than 9 cm wide, the cutaneous defect can be closed primarily.

INDICATIONS

Several aspects of the latissimus dorsi make it amenable to free transfer to the lower extremity. The vascular pedicle is long, averaging 9 cm in length, with vessels of comparable size to those in the leg (2.5–4.0 mm). In nearly all patients, the nerve, artery, and vein arise in a common hilum. In addition, the length of the pedicle will often allow microsurgical anastomoses outside the zone of injury without the need for vein grafts.

ANATOMY

Studies of the intramuscular anatomy have demonstrated branching of the artery and vein into transverse and longitudinal segments, thus allowing harvesting of only part of the muscle for smaller defects (4) or splitting of the muscle to provide coverage for two defects (5). The latissimus dorsi has been transferred to restore motor function to the leg. If used for this purpose, careful preoperative planning is necessary to ensure that the motor nerve in the leg can be identified and is long enough to permit neural coaptation near the vascular pedicle of the flap (Fig. 1).

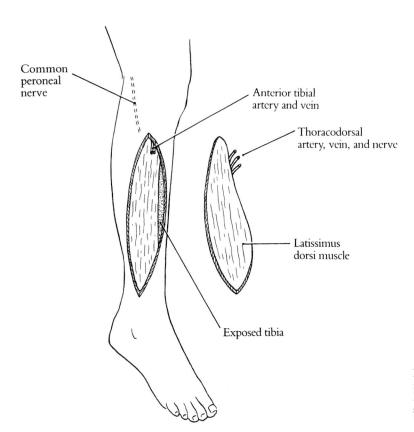

Common peroneal nerve

Anterior tibial artery and vein

Thoracodorsal artery, vein, and nerve

Latissimus dorsi muscle

Exposed tibia

FIG. 1. The latissimus dorsi muscle can be used as a free-muscle transfer for coverage of defects in the lower leg. The muscle then is covered with a split-thickness skin graft. Alternatively, a musculocutaneous flap can be used, but it is often unacceptably bulky.

FLAP DESIGN AND DIMENSIONS

The latissimus dorsi muscle can be reliably transferred using its entire bulk. When skin islands are included, they should be placed over musculocutaneous perforators, their location being determined by Doppler examination. In general, these perforators are more numerous over the proximal two thirds of the muscle. The "extended" latissimus dorsi flap, which may include the thoracolumbar fascia and overlying skin, is less reliable without a delay procedure.

The choice of ipsilateral or contralateral muscle may depend on the most favorable positioning of the patient in order to approach the medial or lateral aspect of the leg.

OPERATIVE TECHNIQUE

Occasionally, the zone of injury in the leg is so extensive that vein grafts are required to ensure that the microsurgical anastomoses are located in an area of uninjured vessels. A helpful technique, if exposure of the recipient vessels is difficult, is to attach the reversed segment of vein graft to the artery and vein as a loop. It is then much easier to divide the distal end of the loop and attach the muscle. In this way, the flap will not obscure exposure of the proximal anastomoses.

An alternative method has been used in rare circumstances to place the anastomoses outside the zone of injury. This method involves using the dorsalis pedis artery and saphenous vein as recipient vessels distal to the defect in the leg. This approach should be used with caution because of the potential of proximal vascular compromise. Although these vessels may be patent, the flow characteristics may not be sufficient to support the flap.

When transferring the muscle as a motor unit, it is helpful to take the tendinous insertion that will permit easier coaptation with the distal tendons in the leg. It is also advisable to place temporary sutures in the latissimus dorsi muscle at regular intervals before removing it from its donor site as a guide to restore the correct resting length when transferred to the leg.

Two problems encountered in patients with lower extremity trauma are hypercoagulability and increased spasm of the vessels. The phenomenon of hypercoagulability is poorly understood, but some form of prophylactic anticoagulation should be considered. A technique that has been helpful in minimizing vascular spasm is the application of 2% lidocaine (without epinephrine) prior to dissection of the periadventitial tissues. The use of a tourniquet, vessel loops instead of vessel clamps, and meticulous hemostasis also may help to prevent spasm.

End-to-side anastomoses have been shown to be as reliable as end-to-end repairs and are absolutely necessary for patients with one-vessel legs or for those in whom the blood flow to the distal extremity is tenuous. A technique has been described in which the thoracodorsal artery is harvested with a short segment of the subscapular artery in a T configuration. Although this requires an additional anastomosis, it has the theoretical advantage of not placing the suture line at the point of turbulent flow of the branch.

CLINICAL RESULTS

In many patients, the latissimus dorsi muscle with overlying skin produces a flap that is much bulkier than required, particularly for wounds of the distal leg. To produce a more cosmetically acceptable reconstruction, the muscle alone has been transferred, and a skin graft is applied after it has been tailored to the defect (Fig. 2). Postoperative edema of the flap is maximal at 3 to 5 days and begins to subside over the next several weeks. The leg should be elevated during the initial postoperative phase and should be wrapped with a compressive dressing when dependent. In noninnervated flaps, atrophy will gradually reduce the muscle bulk by approximately 25% to 50%.

A–C

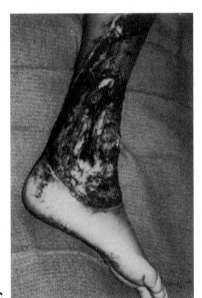
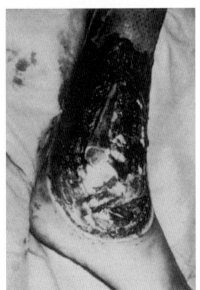
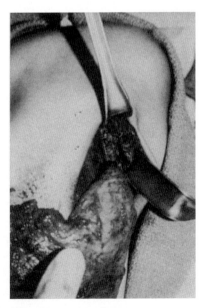

FIG. 2. A: A 7-year-old girl sustained a severe burn and crush injury to the ankle in a three-wheeler accident. Initial attempts at tangential excision and grafting were unsuccessful. **B:** Ultimately, a major debridement was required, leaving her with an open ankle joint and exposed tibia and fibula. **C:** A latissimus dorsi muscle flap was harvested through a short vertical incision along the posterior axillary line and transferred to the right-ankle area with anastomoses to the anterior tibial artery and vein. The muscle flap was covered with split-thickness skin grafts. *(Continued)*

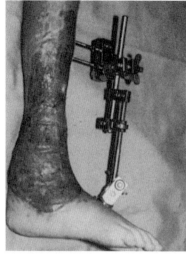
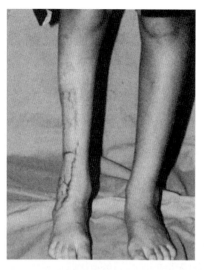
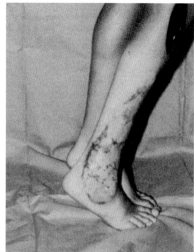

D–F

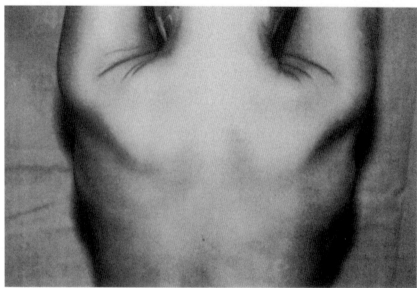

G

FIG. 2. *Continued.* **D:** At 1 month, the muscle flap and skin grafts have healed with no evidence of infection. **E, F:** One year postoperatively, the patient has resumed all normal activities. She lacks some ankle motion but has not required a fusion. She is pain free. **G:** The donor scar is virtually undetectable.

The timing of free-flap transfer to reconstruct major wounds of the lower extremity has been a subject of considerable discussion. Many surgeons believe there is a "golden period" of about 2 weeks from the time of injury when complications such as flap failure and recurrent infections will be at a minimum. If reconstruction during this period is not possible, it has been recommended that free-flap transfer be delayed at least 6 weeks; however, this is a subject for more critical analysis.

and it provides vessels of large size. In addition, the muscle can be reinnervated to restore muscle function.

SUMMARY

The latissimus dorsi is a large, dependable flap that fulfills many of the requirements for lower extremity reconstruction. Its versatility is demonstrated by the ability to provide coverage of large defects, or it can be tailored for smaller ones. A skin paddle can be included with orientation in any axis. The vascular pedicle is long enough to bridge the zone of injury,

References

1. May JW, Gallico GG, Lukash FN. Microvascular transfer of free tissue for closure of bone wounds of the distal lower extremity. *N Engl J Med* 1982;306:253.
2. Serafin D, Voci VE. Reconstruction of the lower extremity: microsurgical composite-tissue transplantation. *Clin Plast Surg* 1983;10:55.
3. Harii K. Reconstruction of the lower leg. In: Buncke HJ, Furnas DW, eds. *Symposium on clinical frontiers in reconstructive microsurgery.* St. Louis: Mosby, 1984.
4. Bartlett SP, May JW, Yaremchuk MJ. The latissimus dorsi muscle: a fresh cadaver study of the primary neurovascular pedicle. *Plast Reconstr Surg* 1981;67:531.
5. Tobin GR, Schusterman BA, Peterson GH, et al. The intramuscular neurovascular anatomy of the latissimus dorsi muscle: the basis for splitting the flap. *Plast Reconstr Surg* 1981;67:637.

CHAPTER 496 ■ FREE MUSCLE FLAPS WITH SPLIT-THICKNESS SKIN GRAFTS FOR CONTOURED CLOSURE OF DIFFICULT WOUNDS

J. W. MAY, JR., AND R. C. SAVAGE

A virtual explosion in available free-flap donor sites has occurred over the last decade (1,2). Most recently, the emphasis shifted from mere survival of free-tissue transfer to consideration of reconstructive and aesthetic refinements. The purpose of this chapter is to summarize the advantages that free-muscle flaps with split-thickness skin grafts provide in dealing with difficult wounds.

INDICATIONS

Recently, experimental and clinical evidence has firmly established the usefulness of local and distant muscle-flap coverage of chronic bony wounds compared with the historical options of random skin flaps, cross-leg flaps, and tubed pedicle "jump" flaps (3–8). It has been hypothesized that vascularized muscle flaps provide improved oxygen transport in concert with the direct delivery of host defense mechanisms, including phagocytes, immunoglobulins, and the complement system (7). This combination of factors and the ability to cover virtually any wound after thorough debridement are probably responsible for the recent improvement in the coverage of these difficult bony wounds.

The use of free muscle flaps, covered with a thick split-thickness skin graft from the buttock area, has many cosmetic and reconstructive advantages (9,10) (Fig. 1). The dissection of the donor muscle alone is easier, and the problems of location and design of the skin paddle over the muscle are avoided. When the muscle is grafted, there is no problem fitting the skin paddle to the recipient site without tension. Free muscle flaps can be tailored more effectively than free muscle-skin flaps in awkward locations, for example, heels (Fig. 2), and in wounds with unusual three-dimensional characteristics. Moreover, a muscle flap alone can more readily conform to fill all the recipient-site interstices. This elimination of dead space, combined with the delivery of well-vascularized tissue, effectively decreases bacterial counts and encourages the use of muscle flaps, especially compared with free skin flaps.

The latissimus dorsi muscle has become the "workhorse" of free-tissue transfer, for it satisfies most of the ideal donor-site characteristics (9,11–14). The entire latissimus dorsi muscle, for example, can be taken through a relatively short incision, most of which is concealed in the axilla (8). It possesses a long, flexible vascular pedicle of wide internal diameter. It is a broad, flat, pliable muscle with potential for durable coverage of defects of enormous size, yet its internal vascular anatomy allows for splitting the muscle (15) and for use of only part of the muscle when flaps of smaller size are required (16). In addition to the latissimus, the gracilis and rectus abdominis muscles also have many similar advantages, particularly for smaller wounds.

OPERATIVE TECHNIQUE

See the appropriate chapters of the various muscle flaps for details of dissection, etc. (Chaps. 495, 497, and 502.)

CLINICAL RESULTS

Thirty-five consecutive free latissimus dorsi muscle flaps covered with thick split-thickness skin grafts from the buttock area have been performed at the Massachusetts General Hospital, with the most common application being acute and chronic bony wounds of the distal lower extremity (Fig. 3). We have had a single flap loss due to infection 10 days postoperatively.

Skin-graft "take" on transferred muscle flaps is usually excellent. We have had only three partial graft losses requiring regraft procedures under local anesthesia in a series of 35 patients. Two of these failures were related to temporary venous obstruction of the flap.

When properly designed and inset, the muscle flap and skin graft should not require secondary debulking operations, so commonly needed following free-skin flap and skin-muscle flap transfers. Muscle flaps undergo a variable amount of shrinkage owing to both true atrophy and edema resolution. Experimental studies suggest that denervated muscle atrophies at a rate of 1% per day for approximately 60 days (17–20). It is our subjective clinical impression that free-muscle flaps, especially in a dependent location, undergo less than a 60% total volume reduction. In a single case of a muscle flap in a nondependent location, rapid shrinkage of more than 60% of the flap was seen within 2 months. These shrinkage factors must be considered in determining appropriate flap contouring at the initial procedure.

Proponents of skin-muscle flaps feel that a major advantage is the availability of a "skin marker" for postoperative color monitoring. Experienced observers of muscle flaps should be able to detect obstructive color changes by means of a "window" left at the edge of the skin graft. If any question arises, a small portion of the muscle can be cut and observed for bleeding. Furthermore, recent advances in thermocouple

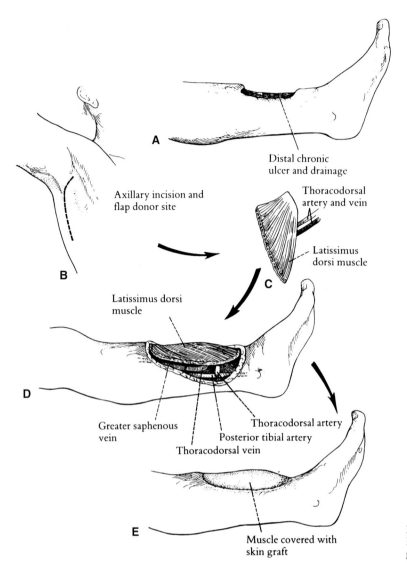

FIG. 1. Sequence of operative steps in transfer of free latissimus dorsi muscle flap with split-thickness skin graft. (From May et al., ref. 8, with permission.)

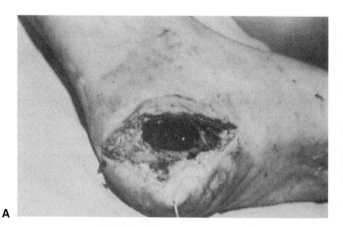
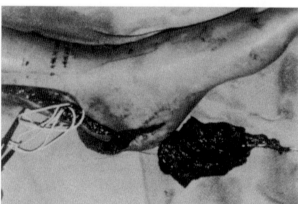

FIG. 2. A: Chronic draining wound of the left heel in a 35-year-old man who had a severely comminuted fracture of his os calcis. B: Contoured hemilatissimus dorsi muscle flap ready for transfer after further debridement of the heel. The subscapular-circumflex scapular T anastomosis was performed to the posterior tibial artery. An end-to-end venous repair was effected to the greater saphenous vein. Postoperatively, the patient was monitored clinically as well as with internal thermocouple monitors. An early venous thrombosis necessitated reoperation with anastomosis of the vein to the vena comitans of the posterior artery. (Continued)

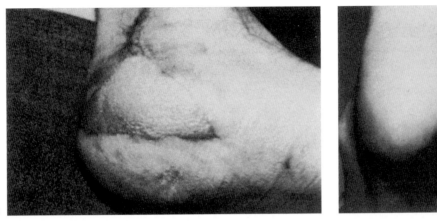
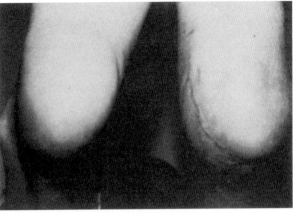

FIG. 2. *Continued.* C: Tailored muscle flap with split-thickness skin graft 6 months postoperatively. The patient walks without pain and has had no further drainage. D: Comparison with opposite heel 6 months postoperatively.

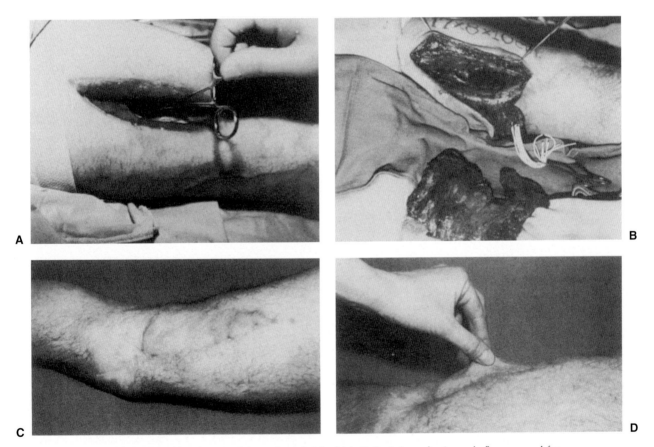

FIG. 3. A: Deep chronic wound, lower lateral right thigh. B: Latissimus dorsi muscle flap prepared for transfer, after femur debridement. Local thigh muscle flap reconstruction was not available because the zone of trauma had created marked anterior and posterior fibrosis. The thoracodorsal artery was repaired end-to-side to the popliteal artery, its vein end-to-end to a posterior popliteal vein. The postoperative course was uneventful except for a small donor-site seroma. C: Muscle flap and split-thickness skin graft 8 months postoperatively. The patient walks without assistance and is drainage free. D: Note the flexibility of healed transfer 8 months postoperatively.

temperature monitoring have been accurate in forecasting vessel occlusion (21).

SUMMARY

Free-muscle flaps with skin-graft coverage have added reconstructive and aesthetic refinements to the reconstructive surgeon's armamentarium. These flaps allow durable closure of difficult wounds with superior contour characteristics and minimal functional and cosmetic morbidity at the donor site.

References

1. Mathes SJ, Nahai F, eds. *Clinical atlas of muscle and musculocutaneous flaps.* St. Louis: Mosby, 1979.
2. Mathes SJ, Nahai F, eds. *Clinical applications for muscle and musculocutaneous flaps.* St. Louis: Mosby, 1982.
3. Stark WJ. The use of pedicled muscle flaps in the surgical treatment of chronic osteomyelitis resulting from compound fractures. *J Bone Joint Surg* 1946;28B:343.
4. Ger R. Muscle transposition for treatment and prevention of chronic posttraumatic osteomyelitis of the tibia. *J Bone Joint Surg* 1977;59B:784.
5. Serafin D, Georgiade N, Smith D. Comparison of free flaps with pedicled flaps for coverage of defects of the leg or foot. *Plast Reconstr Surg* 1977;59:492.
6. Chang N, Mathes S. A comparison of the effect of bacterial inoculation in musculocutaneous and random pattern flaps. *Plast Surg Forum* 1981;4:18.
7. Mathes SJ, Alpert BS, Chang N. Use of the muscle flap in chronic osteomyelitis: experimental and clinical correlation. *Plast Reconstr Surg* 1982;69:815.
8. May JW Jr, Gallico GG III, Lukash FN. Microvascular transfer of free tissue for closure of bone wounds of the distal lower extremity. *N Engl J Med* 1982;306:253.
9. May JW Jr, Lukash FN, Gallico GG III. Latissimus dorsi free muscle flap in lower extremity reconstruction. *Plast Reconstr Surg* 1981;68:603.
10. Gordon L, Buncke HJ, Alpert BS. Free latissimus dorsi muscle flap with split-thickness skin graft cover: a report of 16 cases. *Plast Reconstr Surg* 1982;70:173.
11. Maxwell GP, Stueber K, Hoopes JE. A free latissimus dorsi myocutaneous flap. *Plast Reconstr Surg* 1978;62:462.
12. Maxwell GP, Manson PN, Hoopes JF. Experience with 13 latissimus dorsi myocutaneous free flaps. *Plast Reconstr Surg* 1979; 64:1.
13. Watson JS. The free latissimus dorsi myocutaneous flap. *Plast Reconstr Surg* 1979;64:299.
14. Serafin D, Sabatier RE, Morris RL, Georgiade NG. Reconstruction of the lower extremity with vascularized composite tissue: improved tissue survival and specific indications. *Plast Reconstr Surg* 1980;66:230.
15. Tobin GR, Schusterman M, Peterson GH, et al. The intramuscular neurovascular anatomy of the latissimus dorsi muscle: the basis for splitting the flap. *Plast Reconstr Surg* 1981;67:637.
16. Bartlett SP, May JW Jr, Yaremchuk MJ. The latissimus dorsi muscle. A fresh cadaver study of the primary neurovascular pedicle. *Plast Reconstr Surg* 1981;67:631.
17. Tower SS. Atrophy and degeneration in skeletal muscle. *Am J Anat* 1935;56:1.
18. Guttman E. Effect of delay of innervation on recovery of muscle after nerve lesions. *J Neurophysiol* 1948;11:279.
19. Sunderland S, Ray LJ. Denervation changes in mammalian striated muscle. *J Neurol Neurosurg Psychol* 1950;13:159.
20. Guttman E, Selena J. Morphological changes in the denervated muscle. In: Guttman E, ed. *The denervated muscle.* Prague: Czechoslovak Academy of Sciences, 1962.
21. Cohn K, May JW Jr. Thermal energy dissipation: a laboratory study to assess patency in blood vessels. *Plast Reconstr Surg* 1982;70:475.

CHAPTER 497 ■ MICROVASCULAR FREE GRACILIS MUSCLE AND MUSCULOCUTANEOUS FLAP

R. T. MANKTELOW AND R. M. ZUKER

The gracilis muscle may be used for coverage of soft-tissue defects, for functional reconstruction in replacing missing skeletal musculature, and for facial reanimation in facial paralysis. When used for soft-tissue flap coverage, it may be transferred alone and a skin graft may be applied directly to the muscle, or it may be transferred with an overlying cutaneous island as a musculocutaneous flap. The gracilis muscle is well suited to small and medium-sized soft-tissue defects that cannot be adequately handled by simpler flap techniques. It will conform well to irregular contours (Fig. 1), can be split longitudinally at both ends to allow placement into cavities and awkwardly shaped spaces, and can be transferred in part or in whole. When transferring only a part of it, the transferred muscle will remain viable as long as the anterior margin of the muscle is transferred.

ANATOMY, FLAP DESIGN AND DIMENSIONS

See Chapter 329.

OPERATIVE TECHNIQUE

See Chapter 329.

Prior to removal of the muscle, the recipient site should be prepared so that ischemia time is minimized. The margins of the defect are excised back to healthy, viable tissue and the skin is elevated in order that the muscle can be tucked under the skin edges to provide a good skin-muscle junction.

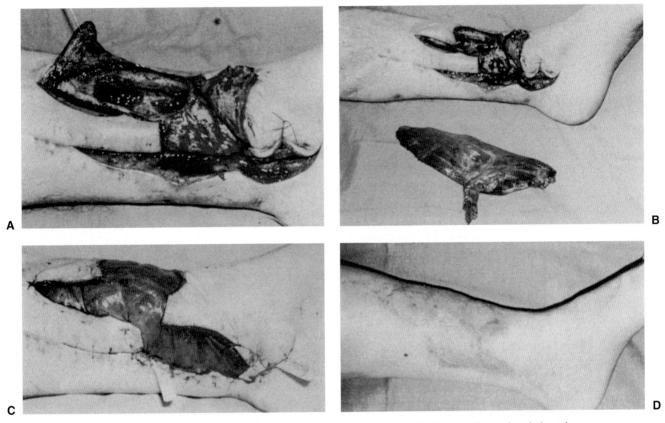

FIG. 1. **A:** Following a sequestrectomy of osteomyelitis in the distal third of the tibia, a deep hole and irregular soft-tissue defect are present. **B:** Gracilis muscle and defect. **C:** Muscle is revascularized, split into separate leaves, and inserted into the defect. **D:** Gracilis muscle with split-thickness skin graft applied directly, seen 1 year postoperatively.

The recipient vessels are evaluated under magnification. If dealing with an area of injury such as in the lower leg, it is important that the recipient vessels be proximal to the zone of injury. Otherwise, there is a strong tendency to vasospasm in the artery. In this location, end-to-side repairs are preferred, since the tendency to vasospasm is much less. Venous repairs to the venae comitantes are preferable and can be done in an end-to-side or end-to-end fashion.

The muscle is loosely tacked in place so that there will be no inadvertent shearing of the pedicle during the anastomoses. The artery and vein are positioned. Either can be repaired first, depending on the access to each. The deepest vessel is usually repaired first.

Repair of the largest vena comitans will usually provide a very adequate venous outflow tract. When patency is ensured, the muscle is then sutured under the skin margins with mattress sutures. The muscle may be trimmed proximally and distally as well as along the posterior margin.

One of the interesting features of the gracilis is the ease with which it may be stretched transversely to fill a defect that is wider than the muscle (Fig. 1). The usual 6-cm width of muscle can easily be spread to 9 to 10 cm following removal of some of the perimysium. A split-thickness skin graft is applied to the muscle and loosely tacked about the margins. A "window" (1 × 1 cm) is placed in the dressing and in the underlying skin graft, allowing for direct visualization of the muscle.

Fifty percent or more of the muscle bulk will atrophy. This provides a good-contour reconstruction of the anterior tibia, providing adequate padding without any excess bulk (Fig. 1D). The muscle will maintain sufficient pliability to tolerate the shear stresses produced by accidental bumps and blows to the anterior shin.

The flap is rarely used as a musculocutaneous flap. The reasons for this are that the skin usually provides excess bulk and most situations are best handled with a split-thickness skin graft applied directly to the muscle. See Chapter 329.

CLINICAL RESULTS

See Chapter 329.

SUMMARY

The gracilis can be used as a muscle or musculocutaneous flap to cover and fill defects of the lower extremity. It is usually used as a muscle flap and then covered with a split-thickness skin graft.

CHAPTER 498 ■ DEEP INFERIOR EPIGASTRIC ARTERY RECTUS MUSCULOCUTANEOUS FREE FLAP

G. I. TAYLOR, R. J. CORLETT, AND J. B. BOYD

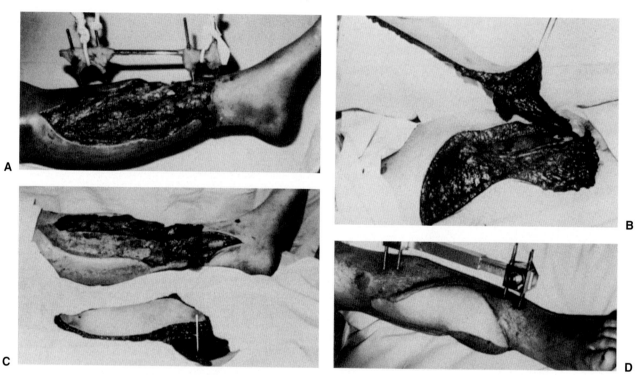

FIG. 1. A: A 21-year-old motorcyclist presented with a severe compound injury of his left leg. The skin defect extended from the knee to the ankle and was almost circumferential in the distal leg. There was an associated comminuted fracture of the distal tibia. Angiography revealed a patent posterior tibial artery. **B:** After repeated debridement of the wound and stabilization of the fracture with an external fixation device, the defect was closed with a free deep inferior epigastric artery thoracoumbilical flap. The flap measured 52 × 11 cm and included the entire rectus muscle. Note how thin the distal portion of the flap is in this obese patient. **C:** The flap was transferred to the leg and revascularized by end-to-side anastomoses to the posterior tibial vessels. Cancellous iliac bone grafts were packed around the fracture, and the skin flap was oriented longitudinally from the knee to the ankle. Additional split-thickness skin grafts were placed over the revascularized muscle. The donor site was closed directly in all layers, including the anterior rectus sheath. **D:** The flap healed without complication, and the tibia was united at 3 months. See Chapter 402 and Figure 1, in Chapter 498.

CHAPTER 499 ■ MICROVASCULAR FREE RECTUS ABDOMINIS MUSCLE FLAP FOR LOWER EXTREMITY RECONSTRUCTION

T. BENACQUISTA AND B. STRAUCH

EDITORIAL COMMENT

This is a workhorse and standard unit that, along with the latissimus, is one of the most commonly used muscles for reconstruction of the lower extremity. An advantage of the rectus abdominis is that the patient can be maintained supine for both the donor and recipient portions of the procedure. In addition, a long and large pedicle is provided, and the amount of muscle will cover large defects.

The rectus abdominis muscle flap has been used in the reconstruction of defects of the head and neck, chest and abdominal walls, perineum, and upper and lower extremities. It can be transferred either as a pedicled flap or as a microvascular free flap.

INDICATIONS

As a microvascular free flap to the lower extremity, this flap has gained enormous popularity. Harvesting of the rectus abdominis flap can be carried out rapidly and easily, and is usually accomplished simultaneously with exploration of the leg for recipient vessels. In addition, its vascular pedicle is quite constant, with a large-caliber artery, two sizeable venae comitantes, and of sufficient length to reach most recipient vessels without requiring the use of a vein graft (1).

The majority of free flaps for lower-extremity reconstruction are used to cover large wounds sustained from trauma, especially those with Gustilo type IIb and IIc tibial fractures (2). While some traumatic leg wounds can be closed with pedicled muscle flaps such as the gastrocnemius flap (upper third of the leg) or soleus flap (middle third of the leg), or with local fasciocutaneous flaps, most high-energy wounds require microvascular free flaps for adequate coverage (see Figs. 2 and 3).

Local flaps are inadequate, in that they are located in the area of injury, or are of sufficient bulk or length to reach the defect (3). Traumatic wounds of the lower third of the leg also require free-flap closure, as there is little or no local tissue in the distal leg. The rectus abdominis muscle, along with the latissimus dorsi muscle, has become a workhorse in treating these traumatic leg wounds, as well as wounds of the ankle or foot.

In the treatment of chronic osteomyelitis, free vascularized muscle flaps have also made a significant difference in obtaining stable, closed wounds in the lower extremity. Before the advent of free muscle flaps, the available treatment modalities, including debridement and closure with secondary intention, as well as local flap closure, resulted in high recurrence rates (4,5).

Limb salvage after excision of aggressive neoplasms is another indication for the use of free muscle flaps. Their use has been reported (6) to avoid amputation after excision of sarcoma in the lower extremity; seven of the 10 reported flaps were rectus abdominis flaps.

Perhaps the most challenging area of lower-extremity reconstruction is in patients with peripheral vascular disease. The addition of microvascular free-tissue transfer for revascularization of the extremities has led to increased limb salvage in this very complex patient population. Patients with diabetes and complex open wounds of the leg and foot have also benefited from free muscle flap closure of the wounds (6–9).

ANATOMY (FIG. 1)

The rectus abdominis muscle is a segmental muscle originating from the symphysis pubis and pubic crest, and inserting into the fifth, sixth, and seventh costal cartilages. It usually has three inscriptions and is enclosed in its rectus sheath, except for the area below the arcuate line.

The rectus muscle is a type III muscle, with a dual blood supply from the superior epigastric artery (which arises from the internal mammary artery) and from the inferior epigastric artery. The latter is the larger of the two and is the vessel used for microvascular transfer of the muscle. The superior epigastric artery is used for pedicled reconstructions of the breast and chest area.

The inferior epigastric artery arises from the external iliac artery just above the inguinal ligament. It then travels upward and medially toward the muscle, to enter on its lateral aspect below the arcuate line. It remains on the undersurface of the muscle, and divides into 2 to 3 branches that travel craniad above the rectus sheath, to anastomose with the superior epigastric vessels at the level of the umbilicus.

The average arterial length of the inferior epigastric pedicle is about 10 cm, and the diameter of the artery is about 2 to 3 mm. It is accompanied by two venae comitantes that average 3 mm in diameter.

OPERATIVE TECHNIQUE

A two-team approach is used to decrease operating time. A preoperative angiogram determines the recipient artery. The best choice is usually the posterior tibial artery, if it is available and uninjured (Fig. 2). This allows for the easiest positioning of the patient—supine and in a frog-leg position. It also allows the saphenous vein to serve as a recipient vein, if the venae comitantes are inadequate. In patients with periph-

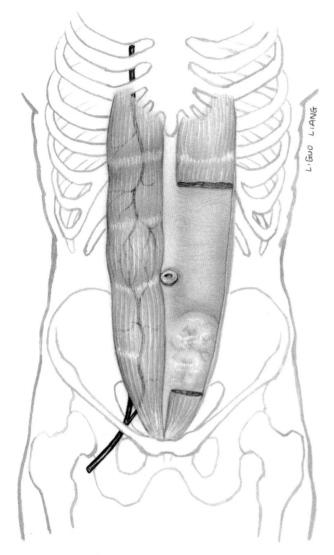

FIG. 1. Anatomy of the rectus abdominis muscle.

eral vascular disease, a preoperative angiogram and the vascular surgeon's bypass will determine the recipient vessel of choice. Even a prosthetic vascular bypass graft has served as a recipient vessel for the free muscle flap (10).

A paramedian incision is made, and the rectus abdominis muscle is dissected from its pubic origin to the rib insertion, preserving the rectus fascia to obtain a strong abdominal-wall closure and to prevent hernia formation. Endoscopic harvest of the rectus abdominis muscle has been shown to be possible in a cadaver and may be the means of decreasing donor-site morbidity (11). Only a part of the muscle may be necessary, and a segmental rectus abdominis free flap (Fig. 3) can be harvested for smaller wounds, especially about the foot and ankle (12).

The tendinous portion of the muscle is included, as it is useful in providing coverage for the pedicle during insetting of the flap. The muscle can be inset using either bolsters, if intact skin is present, or it is sutured to leg fascia. A split-thickness skin graft is used to cover the muscle. Musculocutaneous flaps are rarely used in lower-extremity reconstruction, as they are usually too bulky, and muscle covered with split-thickness skin graft has been found to be as durable.

Postoperatively, the leg is maintained in an elevated position. An external fixator allows for the best management of the extremity, as no splinting is necessary, and thus no external pressures are placed on the pedicle or the flap.

Monitoring of the flap is at the microsurgeon's preference. The initial bulkiness soon subsides and can be flattened more quickly with the use of an Ace bandage wrap, once the skin graft has healed. Over time, the contour of the flap improves dramatically, due to atrophy of the muscle. At times, revision of the flap may be necessary, especially around the ankle or foot, if shoe fit is affected (Figs. 2 and 3).

CLINICAL RESULTS

Most series report success rates of 90% or better in the transfer of the rectus abdominis muscle to the lower extremity, although these series usually group many muscle flaps together, as well as other types of free-tissue transfers. These success rates are quite consistent for microvascular tissue transfers to wounds resulting from trauma, chronic osteomyelitis, or after excision of malignant neoplasms (2–6).

Not unexpectedly, lower success rates have been reported when treating wounds resulting from peripheral vascular disease. The management of these patients is complicated by their concomitant medical problems, especially diabetes, decreased healing secondary to ischemia and the sequelae of diabetes, and the uncertain recipient vessels. A 73% success rate with free-flap transfer has been reported in 30 patients with atherosclerosis and complex lower-extremity wounds (9). In another series of 10 patients, an 80% limb-salvage rate was achieved (8), and a 93% limb-salvage rate was reported in a series combining free-tissue transfer with distal revascularization (7).

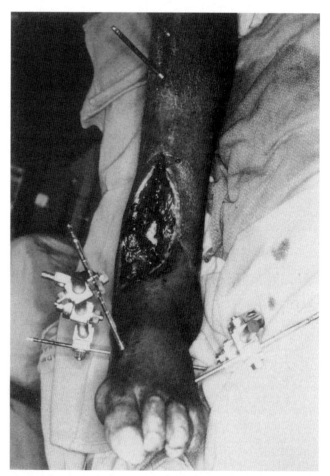

FIG. 2. Chronic open lower-extremity wound with open tibial-fibula fracture following multiple debridements.

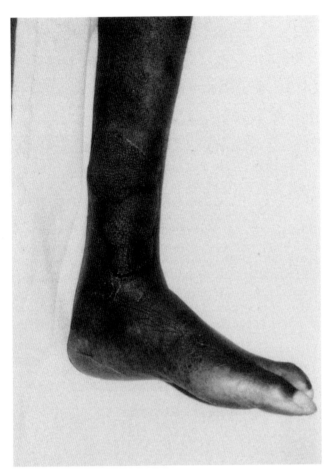

FIG. 3. Result 1 year after transfer of rectus abdominis free flap. No revisions were performed to obtain this smooth contour.

SUMMARY

The rectus abdominis muscle is easily dissected and highly reliable, with a consistent and large-caliber pedicle, and it is ideally suited to lower-extremity reconstruction. There is a high rate of limb salvage when it is used in microvascular free-tissue transfer, to cover defects of the lower extremity resulting from trauma, osteomyelitis, excision of malignant neoplasm, and peripheral vascular disease.

References

1. Reath DB, Taylor JW. Free rectus abdominis muscle flap: advantages in lower extremity reconstruction. *South Med J* 1989;82:1143.
2. Khouri RK, Shaw WW. Reconstruction of the lower extremity with microvascular free flaps: a 10 year experience with 304 consecutive cases. *J Trauma* 1989;29:1086.
3. Yaremchuck MJ. Acute management of severe soft tissue damage accompanying open fractures of the lower extremity. *Clin Plast Surg* 1986;13:621.
4. Eisenschenk A, Kern O, Lehnert M, Weber U. Free vascularized muscle flap transplantation in the treatment of chronic osteomyelitis. *Chir Organi Mov* 1994;79:139.
5. Gayle LB, Lineaweaver WC, Oliva A, et al. Treatment of chronic osteomyelitis of the lower extremities with debridement and microvascular muscle transfer. *Clin Plast Surg* 1992;19:895.
6. Heiner J, Rao V, Mott W. Immediate free tissue transfer for distal musculoskeletal neoplasm. *Ann Plast Surg* 1993;30:140.
7. Cronenwett JL, McDaniel MD, Zwolak RM, et al. Limb salvage despite extensive tissue loss: free tissue transfer combined with distal revascularization. *Arch Surg* 1989;124:609.
8. Greenwald LL, Comerota AJ, Mitra A, et al. Free vascularized tissue transfer for limb salvage in peripheral vascular disease. *Ann Vasc Surg* 1990;4:244.
9. Serletti JM, Deuber MA, Guidera PM, Herrera HR. Atherosclerosis of the lower extremity and free tissue reconstruction for limb salvage. *Plast Reconstr Surg* 1995;96:1136.
10. Berman BA, Zamboni WA, Brown RE. Microvascular anastomosis of a rectus abdominis free flap into a prosthetic vascular bypass graft. *J Reconstr Microsurg* 1992;8:9.
11. Bass LS, Karp NS, Benacquista T, Kasabian AK. Endoscopic harvest of the rectus abdominis free flap: balloon dissection of the fascial plane. *Ann Plast Surg* 1995;34:274.
12. Reath DB, Taylor JW. The segmental rectus abdominis free flap for ankle and foot reconstruction. *Plast Reconstr Surg* 1991;88:824.

CHAPTER 500 ■ LOWER-EXTREMITY MUSCLE PERFORATOR FLAPS

G. G. HALLOCK

The lower extremity is noteworthy as a challenging milieu for achieving wound healing and, even more, for obtaining even a facsimile of the original appearance. Although musculocutaneous flaps from this region were soon abandoned in favor of thinner muscle-only flaps, the same skin territories once again have become useful as muscle perforator flaps (Fig. 1), relying on the identical musculocutaneous perforators, but now without inclusion of the muscle. Not only is muscle function thereby preserved, but a superior aesthetic result with similar tissue also is possible, whether used as a local/regional flap or as a microsurgical tissue transfer.

INDICATIONS

Often, the selected donor site of a lower-extremity muscle perforator flap can be from the ipsilateral limb, which limits morbidity to the same extremity (1). The only prerequisite

Lower Extremity Muscle Perforator Flap Territories

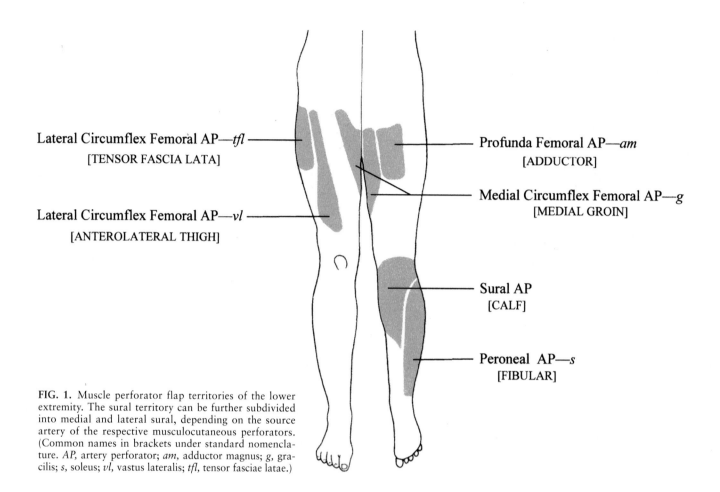

Lateral Circumflex Femoral AP—*tfl*
[TENSOR FASCIA LATA]

Lateral Circumflex Femoral AP—*vl*
[ANTEROLATERAL THIGH]

Profunda Femoral AP—*am*
[ADDUCTOR]

Medial Circumflex Femoral AP—*g*
[MEDIAL GROIN]

Sural AP
[CALF]

Peroneal AP—*s*
[FIBULAR]

FIG. 1. Muscle perforator flap territories of the lower extremity. The sural territory can be further subdivided into medial and lateral sural, depending on the source artery of the respective musculocutaneous perforators. (Common names in brackets under standard nomenclature. *AP*, artery perforator; *am*, adductor magnus; *g*, gracilis; *s*, soleus; *vl*, vastus lateralis; *tfl*, tensor fasciae latae.)

needed to sustain any cutaneous flap is that an adequate perforator (diameter 0.5 mm or greater or visibly pulsatile) can be found, allowing the creation of free-style local or free flaps (2) that do not necessarily rely on a named source vessel. However, to be more realistic, the precise localization of such a perforator can be quite variable, as anomalies tend to be the norm. For this reason, some guidelines for the harvest of the more commonly used lower-extremity muscle perforator flaps, all characterized by some anatomic consistency, are appropriate, as these are valuable alternatives, not just for the lower extremity. They have a versatile role throughout the body.

ANATOMY

Lateral Circumflex Femoral (Vastus Lateralis) Perforator Flap

Of interest, most described "freestyle free flaps" have focused on musculocutaneous perforators found in the anterolateral thigh region (2) (Fig. 2). Although Song et al. (3) originally described a septocutaneous flap from this same area, they noted that only a musculocutaneous perforator was present

on occasion. They may then have recorded the first "true" muscle perforator flap, although not yet called this. Rather, according to the standards set by the Canadian system (4), the proper nomenclature for this or any perforator flap should state the source vessel to the given territory and, secondarily, the muscle traversed by the chosen perforator(s) for further clarification, if necessary. Thus this rendition would now be called the lateral circumflex femoral artery perforator–vastus lateralis, LCFAP-vl flap. However, the original name, as introduced by Song et al. (3), as the "anterolateral thigh flap," understandably remains more established.

Many advocates (5,6) have stressed that the LCFAP-vl flap may be the "ideal" soft-tissue flap. More has been written about this versatile donor site than about any other muscle perforator flap (7). Certainly, at the least, it represents a "gold standard" with which all other alternative cutaneous flaps must be compared.

FLAP DESIGN AND DIMENSIONS

A line is drawn from the anterior superior iliac spine to the superior lateral border of the patella (Fig. 2) (8,9). This coincides with the lateral intermuscular septum between the vastus lateralis and rectus femoris muscles. At the midpoint of

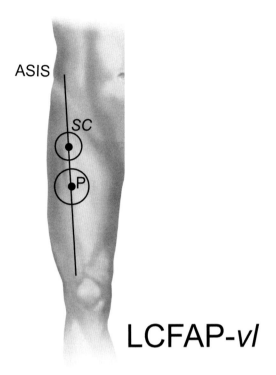

LCFAP-vl

FIG. 2. Perforators to the LCFAP-vl (i.e., "anterolateral thigh") flap can often be found within a circle with a radius of 3 cm, centered at point "*P*" on a line drawn between the anterior superior iliac spine (*ASIS*) and the superior lateral border of the patella. If absent, sometimes superior to this can be found a superior cutaneous perforating artery (*SC*).

this line, a circle with a radius of 3 cm is drawn. All quadrants of this circle are scanned, by using an audible Doppler. Most often, in the posterior inferior sector, a perforator can be identified (8,9). The desired LCFAP-vl flap boundaries can be centered about this perforator, although an eccentric design will accordingly adjust the length of the desired vascular pedicle.

OPERATIVE TECHNIQUE

The medial border of the LCFAP-vl flap is first incised down to the fascia lata. Identification of all perforators is easiest if the bloodless subfascial plane is entered, but a suprafascial dissection will preserve all fascia at the donor site. In about 15% of cases, a large septocutaneous branch is encountered exiting within the lateral intermuscular septum (5), but usually dissection must proceed over the vastus lateralis muscle before an adequate perforator is found. If the flap is very long, including a second, more distal, perforator, this better ensures perfusion to that area as well. The inclusion of multiple large perforators, if available, also provides a safety factor, in case one is inadvertently injured, and eliminates the risk of twisting about a single perforator.

Once all perforators have been selected, the flap can be redesigned, if necessary. The remaining boundaries can then be incised. The usual tedious intramuscular dissection of each perforator requires ligation or coagulation of all muscle side branches. This is usually continued back to the septum between the vastus lateralis and rectus femoris muscles, and to their origin from the descending branch of the lateral circumflex femoral vessels, which commonly resides there. Further proximal dissection ceases once attainment of a local flap has been accomplished, or if the pedicle length or caliber or both

are sufficient for use as a free flap. Donor-site closure, if larger than 8 to 10 cm, will require a skin graft.

Among the advantages of the LCFAP-vl flap are the following:

1. The skin territory is immense: a huge flap, sometimes including almost the entire anterior thigh, can be raised (although "turbocharging" perforators unrelated to the pedicle of the flap may be necessary to ensure total viability) (10);
2. Too long a vascular pedicle is sometimes a problem, but certainly vein grafts can usually be avoided when used as a free flap. If large side branches are maintained, a vascular "flow through" is another option (11), especially to "turbocharge" another perforator, or add another flap as a "sequential" flap;
3. Large-caliber vessels: even before reaching the lateral circumflex femoral vessels proper, vessel diameters that approach macrosurgery are obtainable;
4. Consistent anatomy: even though the exact site or type of perforator to this region can be extremely variable, almost always at least one adequate perforator will be found;
5. A supine position allows two-team flap harvest, sometimes even if the recipient site is the ipsilateral extremity;
6. As a consequence of the long potential vascular leash, a local flap can reach up to the umbilicus, groin, perineum, or trochanter and, if distal-based, even to the knee (12);
7. Combined flaps are possible, joining with vascularized fascia, nerve, muscle, and other thigh cutaneous/adiposal flaps, with numerous options as chimeric or conjoined flaps (5).

Among the disadvantages of the flap are the following:

1. Problems of contour: the flap is difficult to raise in an obese patient, and then can be very bulky, although immediate thinning has been described (13);
2. The donor-site scar: even a long, vertical scar of the thigh may be unacceptable, especially for women;
3. Absence of an adequate perforator: in the rare situation that no anterolateral thigh perforator can be found in the usual site, a prominent medial thigh perforator may exist for an alternative flap (14). A better option, if present, is to look for a superior cutaneous perforator artery (15), which will be found 5 to 8 cm above the midpoint of the line drawn from the ASIS to the superior lateral border of the patella (Fig. 2). One must be aware that this perforator does not necessarily arise from the descending branch of the lateral circumflex femoral vessels.

Lateral Circumflex Femoral (Tensor Fasciae Latae) Perforator Flap

On rare occasions, when no perforator can be found in the anterolateral thigh, dissection even more superiorly along the lateral intermuscular septum will reveal a perforator emanating via the tensor fasciae latae (TFL) muscle, which will allow another alternative thigh flap design (Fig. 3). Although described by Kimura (16) as a microdissected thin free flap, the major attribute of this lateral circumflex femoral artery perforator–tensor fasciae latae (i.e., LCFAP-tfl flap) is as a local flap for trochanteric wounds (17). The advantage as a perforator flap is that muscle function is preserved, which may be critically important for the ambulatory patient. But also the muscle itself can then be used as a backup flap for recidivism, common with patients with pressure sores in this area.

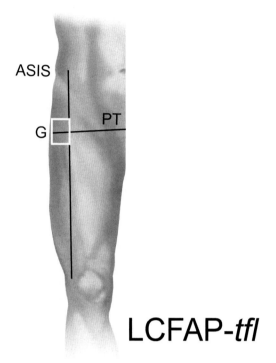

FIG. 3. A perforator to the LCFAP-tfl (i.e., tensor fasciae latae) flap will be found within a rectangle with one long side corresponding to a line drawn between the anterior superior iliac spine (*ASIS*) and the superior lateral border of the patella, and a parallel side tangent to the anterior prominence of the greater trochanter (*G*). The remaining sides connect the previous pair 4 cm above and below a line drawn from the pubic tubercle (*PT*) to the greater trochanter (*G*).

FLAP DESIGN AND DIMENSIONS

A line "x" drawn from the anterior superior iliac spine to the superior lateral border of the patella coincides with the lateral intermuscular septum superiorly between the tensor fasciae latae and rectus femoris muscles (Fig. 3) (17). A second line "y," perpendicular to this, is drawn from the pubis to the prominence of the greater trochanter. A rectangle is then constructed with sides 4 cm both above and below the "y" axis, and another pair parallel to the "x" axis, corresponding to the anterior prominence of the greater trochanter and the septum itself. This area is scanned by an audible Doppler, and a minimum of two perforators consistently can be found (17). Any flap boundaries must encompass this perforator, usually in an ellipsoid shape, with the major axis paralleling the "x" axis, to facilitate direct donor-site closure, if less than 9 cm wide.

OPERATIVE TECHNIQUE

The patient can be placed in a lateral decubitus or supine position. The distal edge of the flap is incised first down to the fascia lata. A suprafascial dissection then continues superiorly until an ideal perforator is encountered. The rest of the flap boundaries may then be incised to create an island flap. At this point, rotation may be possible as a local flap. If necessary, the perforator can be followed through the tensor fasciae latae muscle back to its origin from the ascending branch of the lateral circumflex femoral vessels, to extend reach and pedicle mobility, or to transfer as a free flap.

Among the advantages of this flap are the following: (a) the vascularized fascia lata may be combined as a

composite flap, if thick fascia is needed at the recipient defect (18,19); and (b) a local flap is the preferred option for trochanteric wounds.

Among the disadvantages are (a) the short pedicle: a pedicle length of 9 to 10 cm can be obtained only if dissection is completely back to the lateral circumflex femoral vessels. This is half the length possible with the LCFAP-vl flap; (b) a difficult dissection is involved: the usual tedious intramuscular dissection of any perforator flap is even more difficult involving the narrow window offered through the TFL; (c) pedicle fragility: the vascular pedicle is subject to tension, if stretched to reach a trochanteric defect, a risk enhanced by the forces of gravity if the patient is kept in a supine position.

Medial Circumflex Femoral (Gracilis) Perforator Flap

The gracilis musculocutaneous flap fell into disfavor because the usually longitudinally oriented skin paddle proved to be unreliable. Recent studies of the requisite gracilis musculocutaneous perforators have found usually one to three that arise from the proximal muscle in its midportion, with injection studies demonstrating staining of a skin area that actually parallels the groin crease (20–22). The anatomy otherwise is already extremely well known to the experienced surgeon, which facilitates creation of a medial circumflex femoral artery perforator—gracilis (i.e., MCFAP-g) flap. Moderate-sized flaps can be raised from the medial groin, and this donor site can easily be concealed by clothing, even if a skin graft is needed (23,24).

FLAP DESIGN AND DIMENSIONS

A line drawn from the pubic tubercle to the medial condyle of the femur along the medial thigh corresponds to the course of the often palpable or visible adductor longus muscle (Fig. 4). At a point 10 ± 2 cm below the pubic tubercle at the posterior edge of this muscle, the medial circumflex femoral pedicle enters the undersurface of the gracilis muscle (21,22). A semicircle with a radius of 7 cm, centered at that point and overlying the gracilis muscle, will include all possible perforators (20–22), which can be localized with an audible Doppler. The majority will be found in the upper half of that semicircle. The flap design must include these perforators, with a major axis paralleling the groin crease, staying toward the posterior thigh as much as possible, as this seems to be more reliably captured than the thigh skin anterior to the adductor longus muscle.

OPERATIVE TECHNIQUE

The donor limb is abducted with a bump under the flexed knee readily to expose the medial thigh. The distal boundary of the flap is incised first through the subcutaneous tissue and deep fascia to expose the gracilis muscle. The fascia is retracted cephalad over the gracilis muscle, to ascertain the presence of an adequate perforator. If one is found, the remaining flap boundaries are incised. Posteriorly, the flap can be raised at the level of the Scarpa fascia, to immediately thin it, until the posterior border of the gracilis muscle is reached. The remainder of the dissection must then be done in a subfascial plane, to ensure inclusion of all reasonable gracilis perforators, remembering that an inverse relation exists between perforator diameter and number (22). The usual intramuscular dissection is completed back to the medial circumflex femoral vessels.

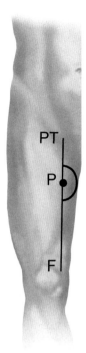

MCFAP-*g*

FIG. 4. A line is drawn from the pubic tubercle (*PT*) to the medial condyle of the femur (*F*). Centered at a point "*P*" on this line about 10 cm below the PT, a perforator to the MCFAP-g (i.e., medial groin) flap will often be found in a semicircle with a radius of 7 cm, as depicted.

Often, a sizeable septocutaneous branch between the adductor longus and gracilis muscles will be seen and should be retained. A branch of the greater saphenous vein will always be found anterior to the gracilis muscle and should be saved as an alternate venous outflow source in the event of later venous congestion. The MCF pedicle can be dissected under the adductor longus muscle back to the profunda femoris vessels as far as needed.

Among the advantages: (a) this is a local flap, and groin and perineum coverage is possible (25); (b) because any donor-site residue can be easily hidden by clothing, probably the aesthetic result is the best for any perforator flap; (c) as a chimeric flap, skin branches often diverge from major muscular branches, to allow simultaneous and independent transfer of both a cutaneous and gracilis muscle flap (26); (d) as a sentinel flap, inclusion of a small perforator flap with a gracilis muscle flap allows constant monitoring of the latter relying on capillary refill of the former (27); (e) the patient's supine position can allow a two-team flap harvest, especially if the recipient site is the contralateral extremity; and (f) the consistent anatomy allows the approach to the gracilis muscle and MCF pedicle already to be routine for the experienced surgeon.

Among its disadvantages, (a) the limited length of the short pedicle, even though slightly longer than for a strictly gracilis muscle flap, restricts reach as a local flap, and can make the anastomosis of a free flap awkward; (b) anomalies involving the frequency of diminutive perforators or even the total absence of perforators are relatively common, in which cases, this option will have to be abandoned; and (c) even in thin women, bulkiness or medial thigh fat deposits or both can be significant, although this could be a positive attribute for breast reconstruction.

Medial Sural (Gastrocnemius) Perforator Flap

The medial gastrocnemius musculocutaneous flap has long been abandoned, not only because of its excessive bulk but also because of the significant donor defect that accrued. Instead, as a muscle flap only, it has become a workhorse flap for coverage about the knee. However, if the same cutaneous territory is now taken as a muscle perforator flap, a reasonably thin local flap can achieve the same purpose, often leaving only a linear calf scar if less than 8 cm in width. Not only is muscle function preserved, but the muscle also remains as a "lifeboat" if any further problems are found (28). Even in the most obese individual, this can be a source of a relatively thin free flap, rivaled perhaps only by the forearm flaps, but in this case, no major limb vessel must be sacrificed. Based on the medial sural vessels, the medial sural artery perforator flap (i.e., MSAP flap) has been found always to be possible (29–31). This is in contradistinction to a lateral sural artery perforator flap where, not infrequently, no adequate musculocutaneous perforator can be found emanating from the lateral gastrocnemius muscle head (31). Unlike the other perforator flaps from the lower extremity, the MSAP flap can be accessed with the patient in either a prone or a supine position (32).

FLAP DESIGN AND DIMENSIONS

With the thigh abducted at the hip, and knee flexed and externally rotated, a line is drawn along the medial leg from the midpoint of the popliteal crease to the midpoint of the medial malleolus (Fig. 5) (29,33). A first major perforator usually can be found with an audible Doppler within the distal half of a circle with a radius of 2 cm, centered at a point along this line 8 cm from the popliteal crease (29,33). A second major perforator may be within a circle with a radius of 3 cm, whose center is on this line 15 cm from the popliteal crease (33). Some variation will be found in taller individuals. A flap designed on the first perforator will require the least dissection to reach the larger-caliber medial sural vessels that arise from the popliteal at the knee joint. This option may be a preferable choice if it is needed as a free flap (34). If the second perforator is chosen, the vascular pedicle can be longer, to allow extended reach as a local flap for knee coverage (29,35).

OPERATIVE TECHNIQUE

Depending on the location of the defect, the flap as marked can be harvested with the patient in either a prone or a supine position. A thigh tourniquet permits bloodless dissection. The anterior border of the flap is first raised through the deep fascia. Although a suprafascial dissection is possible, a subfascial approach most simply allows verification of the adequacy of a perforator. Sometimes, a third perforator may be found even more distally. The flap is redesigned according to the desired perforator.

All boundaries of the flap are then circumscribed. If a subcutaneous vein is identified at the proximal border of the flap, it is preserved for a secondary role in venous outflow later, if the flap otherwise becomes congested. The usual intramuscular dissection of the perforator proceeds back to the source vessel as far as desired. This can surprisingly be a very superficial dissection, as branches of the latter can be very near the outer (i.e., posterior) surface of the gastrocnemius muscle. A local flap can then be tunneled to reach the knee, or used according to routine as a free flap.

Among the advantageous attributes are (a) this is a local flap, with tissue in kind for knee or proximal leg defects;

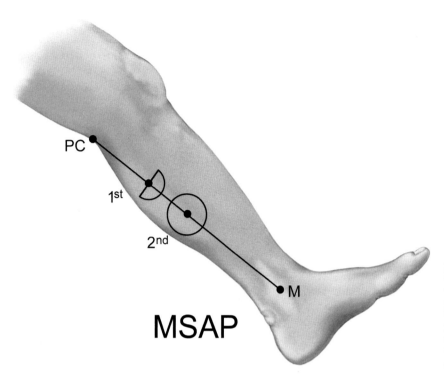

FIG. 5. A line is drawn from the midpoint of the popliteal crease (*PC*) to the prominence of the medial malleolus (*M*). If present, the first perforator to the MSAP flap (i.e., medial calf) will be within the distal half of a circle with a radius of 2 cm found 8 cm from the popliteal crease. A second perforator may be present within a circle with a radius of 3 cm located 7 cm below the center of the first circle.

TABLE 1

COMPARISON OF ATTRIBUTES OF LOWER-EXTREMITY MUSCLE PERFORATOR FLAPS

Flap	LCFAP-tfl	LCFAP-vl	MCFAP-g	MSAP
Anatomic anomalies	+++	++	−	+
Compound flaps				
Fascia	+++	+++	−	+
Muscle	−	+	++	+
Nerve (sensate)	−	++	−	+
Contour				
Bulky	+++	++	+	−
Thinness	−	+	++	++++
Donor site residue	+	−	+++	−
Ease of dissection	−	++	+	+++
Position				
Prone	−	−	−	+++
Supine	++	++	++	+
Size	++	++++	++	+
Vascular pedicle				
Length	+	++++	+	++
Caliber	+++	++++	++	++

(+), asset; (−), liability; LCFAP-*tfl*, lateral circumflex femoral artery perforator—*tensor fascia lata*; LCFAP-*vl*, lateral circumflex femoral artery perforator—*vastus lateralis*; MCFAP-*g*, medial circumflex femoral artery perforator—*gracilis*; MSAP, medial sural artery perforator.

(b) regarding tourniquet dissection, unlike the other major muscle perforator flaps of the lower limb, a tourniquet can be used to allow meticulous dissection, unencumbered by blood staining of tissue; (c) as to contour, a relatively thin cutaneous flap is possible, even in the obese; (d) the patient can be either supine or prone; and (e) the more distal the perforator chosen, the longer the potential pedicle.

Among the disadvantages: (a) anomalies may be found: usually, at least a single medial sural perforator exists, but not necessarily at the point marked for the first or second major perforator; and (b) even if primary donor-site closure is possible, a conspicuous scar results that may not be acceptable, especially for women.

SUMMARY

Lower-extremity muscle perforator flaps offer many advantages for lower- extremity coverage by using similar tissue, not only as straightforward local flaps but also as versatile free flaps. As with any muscle perforator flap, anatomic variations are the norm and must be anticipated; the dissection can be tedious; and the flap will be bulky and perhaps inappropriate in the very obese patient. Venous congestion is also always a concern with muscle perforator flaps, but those from the lower extremity have a distinct advantage in that a superficial vein can be included, and even should be sought out, to allow augmentation of venous outflow, if later found to be necessary.

The LCFAP-vl flap, better known as the "anterolateral thigh flap," remains the "ideal" donor site for soft-tissue flaps of the lower extremity, with which all others must be compared (Table 1). The LCFAP-tfl flap is a superb option for trochanteric defects. The MCFAP-g flap leaves the least donor-site residue. The MSAP flap is typically the thinnest available and is the only one of this group that can be harvested with the patient in a prone position. The lower-extremity muscle perforator flaps have allowed a whole new approach, not only for lower-extremity reconstruction but also throughout the body.

References

1. Hallock GG. Lower extremity muscle perforator flaps for lower extremity reconstruction. *Plast Reconstr Surg* 2004;114:1123.
2. Wei FC, Mardini S. Free-style free flaps. *Plast Reconstr Surg* 2004;114:910.
3. Song TG, Chen GZ, Song YL. The free thigh flap: a new free flap concept based on the septocutaneous artery. *Br J Plast Surg* 1984;37:149.
4. Geddes CR, Morris SF, Neligan PC. Perforator flaps: evolution, classification, and applications. *Ann Plast Surg* 2003;50:90.
5. Wei FC, Jain V, Celik N, et al. Have we found an ideal soft-tissue flap? An experience with 672 anterolateral thigh flaps. *Plast Reconstr Surg* 2002;109:2219.
6. Yildirim S, Gideroglu K, Akoz T. Anterolateral thigh flap: ideal free flap choice for lower extremity soft tissue reconstruction. *J Reconstr Microsurg* 2003;19:225.
7. Lutz DA, Hallock GG. Territories of perforator flaps by source vessel and subtype. (Appendix). In: Blondeel PN, Morris SF, Hallock GG, et al., eds. *Perforator flaps: anatomy, technique, and clinical applications*. St. Louis, MO: Quality Medical Publishing, 2006;1045.
8. Demirkan F, Chen HC, Wei FC, et al. The versatile anterolateral thigh flap: a musculocutaneous flap in disguise in head and neck reconstruction. *Br J Plast Surg* 2000;53:30.
9. Kuo YR, Jeng SF, Kuo MH, et al. Free anterolateral thigh flap for extremity reconstruction: clinical experience and functional assessment of donor site. *Plast Reconstr Surg* 2001;107:1766.
10. Koshima I, Yamamoto H, Moriguchi T, Orita Y. Extended anterior thigh flaps for repair of massive cervical defects involving pharyngoesophagus and skin: an introduction to the "mosaic" flap principle. *Ann Plast Surg* 1994;32:321.
11. Koshima I, Kawada S, Etoh H, et al. Flow-through anterolateral thigh flaps for one-stage reconstruction of soft-tissue defects and revascularization of ischemic extremities. *Plast Reconstr Surg* 1995;95:252.
12. Pan SC, Yu JC, Shieh SJ, et al. Distally based anterolateral thigh flap: an anatomic and clinical study. *Plast Reconstr Surg* 2004;114:1786.
13. Kimura N, Satoh K. Consideration of a thin flap as an entity and clinical application of the thin anterolateral thigh flap. *Plast Reconstr Surg* 1996;97:985.
14. Koshima I, Soeda S, Yamasaki M, Kyou J. The free or pedicled anteromedial thigh flap. *Ann Plast Surg* 1988;21:480.
15. Chen Z, Zhang C, Lao J, et al. An anterolateral thigh flap based on the superior cutaneous perforator artery: an anatomic study and case reports. *Microsurgery* 2007;27:160.
16. Kimura N, Satoh K, Hosaka Y. Tensor fasciae latae perforator flap. *Clin Plast Surg* 2003;30:439.
17. Ishida LH, Munhoz AM, Montag E, et al. Tensor fasciae latae perforator flap: minimizing donor-site morbidity in the treatment of trochanteric pressure sores. *Plast Reconstr Surg* 2005;116:1346.
18. Koshima I, Urushibara K, Inagawa K, Moriguchi T. Free tensor fasciae latae perforator flap for the reconstruction of defects in the extremities. *Plast Reconstr Surg* 2001;107:1759.
19. Deiler S, Pfadenhauer A, Widmann J, et al. Tensor fasciae latae perforator flap for reconstruction of composite Achilles tendon defects with skin and vascularized fascia. *Plast Reconstr Surg* 2000;106:342.
20. Thione A, Valdatta L, Buoro M, et al. The medial sural artery perforators: anatomic basis for a surgical plan. *Ann Plast Surg* 2004;53:250.
21. Lykoudis EG, Spyropoulou GC, Vlastou CC. The anatomic basis of the gracilis perforator flap. *Br J Plast Surg* 2005;58:1090.
22. Kappler VA, Constantinescu MA, Buchler U, Vogelin E. Anatomy of the proximal cutaneous perforator vessels of the gracilis muscle. *Br J Plast Surg* 2005;58:445.
23. Hallock GG. The gracilis (medial circumflex femoral) perforator flap: a medial groin free flap? *Ann Plast Surg* 2003;51:623.
24. Hallock GG. Further experience with the medial circumflex femoral gracilis perforator free flap. *J Reconstr Microsurg* 2004;20:115.
25. Hallock GG. The medial circumflex femoral gracilis local perforator flap: a local medial groin perforator flap. *Ann Plast Surg* 2003;51:460.
26. Hallock GG. The conjoint medial circumflex femoral perforator and gracilis muscle free flap. *Plast Reconstr Surg* 2004;113:339.
27. Hallock GG. Free-flap monitoring using a chimeric sentinel muscle perforator flap. *J Reconstr Microsurg* 2005;21:351.
28. Hallock GG. Sequential use of a true perforator flap and its corresponding muscle flap. *Ann Plast Surg* 2003;51:617.
29. Shim JS, Kim HH. A novel reconstruction technique for the knee and upper one third of lower leg. *J Plast Reconstr Aesthet Surg* 2006;59:919.
30. Chen SL, Chen TM, Lee CH. Free medial sural artery perforator flap for resurfacing distal limb defects. *J Trauma* 2005;58:323.
31. Hallock GG. Anatomic basis of the gastrocnemius perforator-based flap. *Ann Plast Surg* 2001;47:517.
32. Hallock GG, Sano K. The medial sural medial gastrocnemius perforator free flap: an "ideal" prone position skin flap. *Ann Plast Surg* 2004;52:184.
33. Kim HH, Jeong JH, Seul JH, Cho BC. New design and identification of the medial sural perforator flap: an anatomical study and its clinical applications. *Plast Reconstr Surg* 2006;117:1609.
34. Cavadas PC, Sanz-Gimenez-Rico JR, Gutierrez-de la Camara A, et al. The medial sural artery perforator free flap. *Plast Reconstr Surg* 2001;108:1609.
35. Hallock GG. The medial sural medial gastrocnemius peforator local flap. *Ann Plast Surg* 2004;53:501.

CHAPTER 501 ■ MICROVASCULAR FREE TRANSFER OF A COMPOUND DEEP CIRCUMFLEX GROIN AND ILIAC CREST FLAP

G. I. TAYLOR AND R. J. CORLETT

Use of free vascularized bone has greatly improved the success of large bone grafts, with bony union occurring at a similar rate to a double fracture in the same bone (1). These vascularized grafts also provide the opportunity to replace en bloc the involved soft tissues and to augment the blood supply to the distal part.

INDICATIONS

Large defects in the long bones of the lower limbs ideally are reconstructed with vascularized fibular grafts (2,3). However, it is not possible, to use the fibula in every case because it may be damaged in bilateral leg injuries or there may be a vascular anomaly that precludes its use. Furthermore, if a large skin defect exists, it may necessitate initial cover with a local muscle or musculocutaneous flap, a cross-leg flap, or a free skin flap. In these situations, a one-stage reconstruction using the deep circumflex iliac osteocutaneous flap may be prefer-

able, particularly if the bone defect is less than 8 cm (2,4,5) (see Fig. 1).

Size of the Bony Defect

Defects less than 5 cm can be treated with conventional nonvascularized bone grafts, provided the bed is well vascularized. If the skin cover is poor, if the vascularity of the bed is compromised by scar or vessel injury, or if the defect is in the distal third of the tibia, then a composite vascularized bone graft based on the deep circumflex iliac artery (DCIA) should be considered. An alternative solution would be a free muscle or musculocutaneous flap, combined with cancellous bone grafts.

Defects of 5 to 8 cm, especially if associated with soft-tissue loss, are the ideal indication for the iliac osteocutaneous flap. The bone can be used to bridge defects up to 14 cm. In these circumstances, however, an osteotomy is necessary to

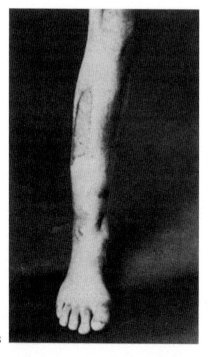
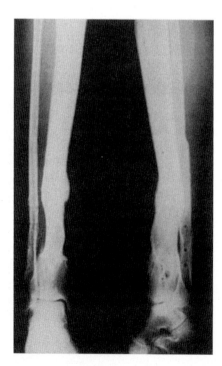

A,B

FIG. 1. **A:** A 21-year-old motorcyclist presented with a defect of the distal third of the tibia and unstable scarred soft tissues. An 8-cm segment of anterior iliac crest, together with overlying skin, was transferred to reconstruct the soft-tissue and bone defect, performed as a secondary procedure. The skin flap was thinned and no complications occurred. The follow-up is 6 years. **B:** The bone graft was united at 4 months and, as shown here, at 12 months had hypertrophied to the size of the tibia.

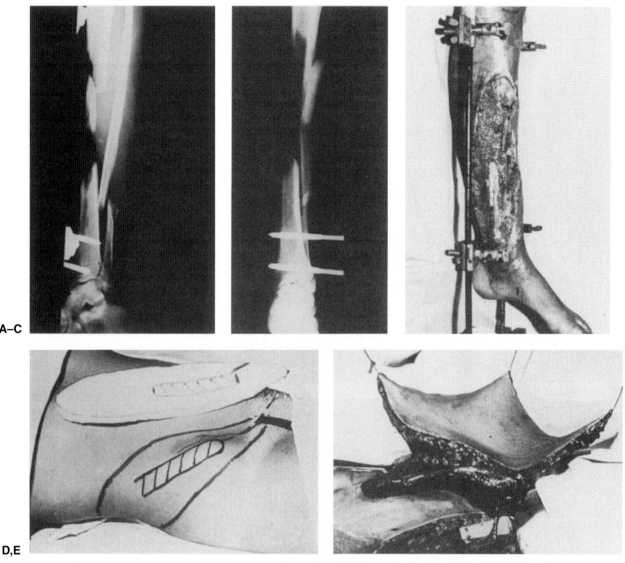

A–C

D,E

FIG. 2. A, B: A 19-year-old nurse sustained a severe compound wound to her left leg in an automobile accident. **C, D, E:** Three weeks later, a 14-cm curved iliac crest graft was used to repair the 12-cm defect in her tibia. The skin flap measured 30 × 11 cm. The deep circumflex iliac artery vessels were anastomosed to the posterior tibial vessels at the ankle. *(Continued)*

correct the curvature of the iliac crest, and a vascularized fibular graft is usually the better choice. The latter procedure may require initial skin cover, although the fibular flap is currently being modified to include additional muscle or skin to provide a one stage repair. When the bone defect exceeds 14 cm, the fibula is the flap of choice.

Associated Soft-tissue Loss

The osteocutaneous flap offers a one-stage repair of bone and skin. In some situations, the external oblique aponeurosis may be used to provide vascularized tendon grafts (6).

Site of the Defect

The shape of the iliac crest makes it the ideal graft for reconstructing the bones of the foot and the pelvic ring. Although the graft can be used to reconstruct the femur, it is difficult to maintain rigid fixation. The stresses on the graft are greater, and we therefore have confined the use of the iliac bone graft to the repair of tibial defects in most cases.

FLAP DESIGN AND DIMENSIONS

In an adult, it is possible to obtain a straight segment of bone 6 to 8 cm long from the anterior iliac crest. Beyond this point, the bone curves in two planes, causing a significant problem when reconstructing a long bone. The curvature of the graft extends outside the line of weight-bearing stresses, predisposing the graft to fracture. In two of our initial patients, this resulted in late stress fracture at the center of the bone graft after union had occurred at both ends (see Fig. 2).

To overcome this problem, a step or wedge osteotomy of the graft has been devised to straighten the curvature and has

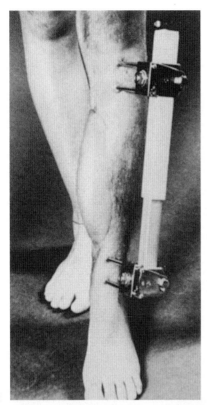
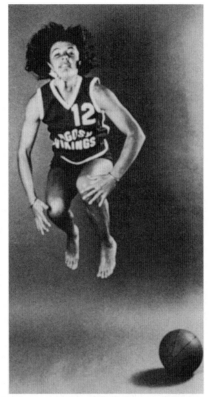

F,H

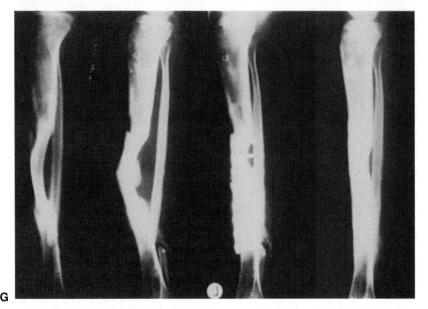

G

FIG. 2. *Continued.* F: The bone graft was secured in position with an external fixation frame shown at 6 weeks. G: At 6 months, bone union was evident, but at 13 months, a stress fracture occurred in the center of the graft that united spontaneously over a 1-month period. Unfortunately, the curvature of the graft had increased, and an osteotomy was required to straighten the bone. The graft united rapidly and by 2 years had hypertrophied to the size of the tibia. From left to right: union of the graft at 12 months, stress fracture that had united over 4 weeks (13 months), osteotomy and plate fixation to straighten the graft (18 months), hypertrophy and remodeling of the graft (2 years). H: The leg length is normal, there is a full range of knee and ankle movement, and the patient participates in all sporting activities.

resulted in a better alignment of the graft so that it lies within the weight-bearing stresses and has provided, in addition, an improvement in the cosmetic appearance of the limb. The largest defect bridged by this technique so far has been 14 cm (Fig. 3); however, the curvature of the bone is an advantage when reconstructing the longitudinal arches of the foot and the pelvis (Fig. 4).

OPERATIVE TECHNIQUE

Angiographic studies are recommended to define the suspect arteries (2). Any segment of artery without side branches,

especially if tapered or irregular in outline, must be regarded as abnormal and avoided at the affected level. In practice, this is achieved by dissecting the vessels in normal tissue and progressing toward the injured area. Angiograms also may show damaged vessels with a segmental block. In this situation, the vessel may be repaired at the same operation. The ascending branch of the DCIA is useful for this purpose.

As with the jaw (see Chap. 204), we use a model of an articulated pelvis with detachable iliac crests to select the hip whose curvature is best suited to the bone defect in question. This also helps to orient the vascular pedicle, and wherever possible, we prefer to perform the anastomoses end-to-side to the posterior tibial vessels at or above the ankle.

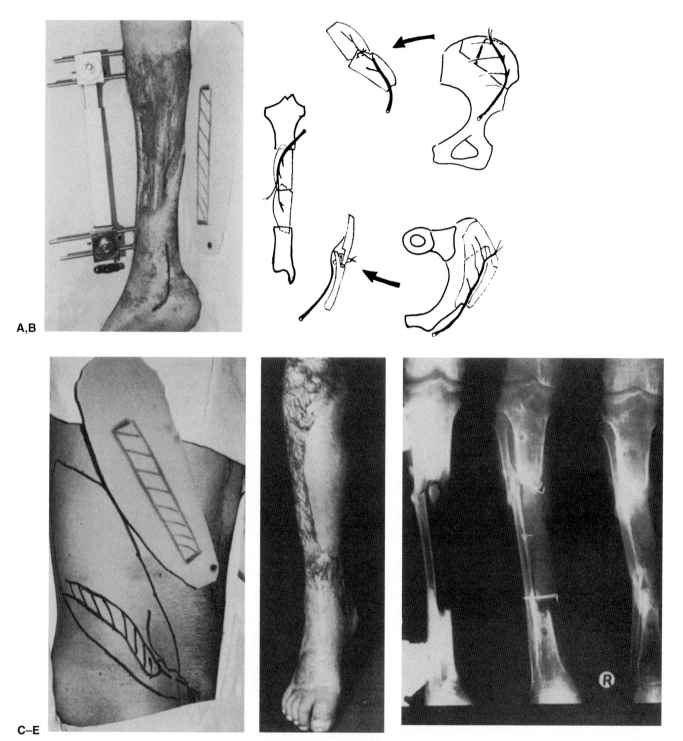

FIG. 3. A: A young motorcyclist presented with a compound leg wound and a 14-cm defect of the right tibia. **B:** Because of the complication of graft fracture seen in Fig. 2, it was decided to straighten the iliac crest graft at the time of transfer. This was achieved with a step osteotomy, with care taken to preserve the blood supply to the distal graft segment. **C:** The skin flap measured 32 × 12 cm. **D, E:** The result is shown at 6 and 18 months.

CLINICAL RESULTS

Most bone defects of the lower limb are the result of severe trauma, and the zone of tissue damage surrounding the defect may be quite extensive. Our early experiences using recipient vessels in this zone were disastrous. A high rate of complications awaits the uninitiated: vessel spasm, the difficult suture of edematous fragile vessels, and unrecognized venous thromboses. The long pedicle of the DCIA may bridge some of these injured areas but, if extensive, vein grafts are essential to permit anastomoses to normal vessels.

Our experience with vascularized iliac bone transfer to the lower limb currently totals 18 patients. The first four of these transfers were designed on the superficial circumflex iliac artery. Although this vessel supplies a large area of skin, its

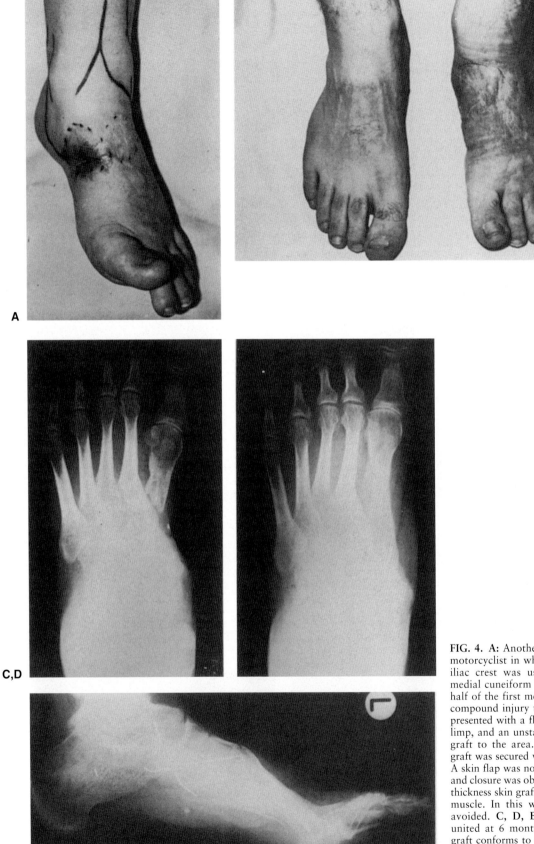

FIG. 4. A: Another case of a 19-year-old motorcyclist in whom a 6-cm segment of iliac crest was used to reconstruct the medial cuneiform bone and the proximal half of the first metatarsal bone, lost in a compound injury to the foot. The patient presented with a flail, shortened big toe, a limp, and an unstable split-thickness skin graft to the area. **B:** The revascularized graft was secured with transfixation wires. A skin flap was not included in the design, and closure was obtained by placing a split-thickness skin graft over the revascularized muscle. In this way, a bulky graft was avoided. **C, D, E:** The bone graft was united at 6 months. Note how the iliac graft conforms to the longitudinal arch of the foot.

bone supply is limited. The vessels are small and the pedicle is short. The remaining 14 transfers all have been designed on the DCIA, and we now use this pedicle exclusively.

Most of the patients referred to us had been considered for amputation, and the composite flap was therefore performed as a salvage procedure. Of the 18 transfers, two failed in the first quarter of our series as a result of avoidable anastomotic complications. One resulted from inadequate three-dimensional planning, and the other followed the selection of a traumatized recipient vessel.

Union of the bone was generally observed between 4 and 6 months. Our regimen has been to commence partial weight bearing at 6 weeks and to remove the external fixation at approximately 6 months. A protective caliper is worn for a further 6 months.

A supplementary bone graft was required in one patient for delayed union, and late stress fracture was seen in another two patients. Both fractures united rapidly, but one required an osteotomy for malunion.

SUMMARY

There are now a number of techniques available for the reconstruction of composite defects in the lower limb. The task of the reconstructive surgeon is to match the appropriate graft to the patient's needs. For defects less than 5 cm long, nonvascularized bone grafts may suffice if soft-tissue cover is adequate.

The deep circumflex iliac osteocutaneous flap offers a one-stage repair and is best suited for bone defects of up to 8 cm that are associated with large areas of soft-tissue loss. Beyond this size defect, the fibula is usually the graft of choice, although we have successfully bridged tibial defects of up to 14 cm with vascularized ilium.

CHAPTER 502 ■ INTERNAL OBLIQUE MUSCLE AND OSTEOMUSCULAR FLAP

W. M. SWARTZ AND S. S. RAMASASTRY

The internal oblique muscle flap has a thin, flat shape with excellent vascularity. The muscle has a blood supply independent of the iliac crest bone, an advantage in composite reconstruction (1). The vascular pedicle is 6 to 7 cm long and 1.5 to 3 mm in diameter, making the flap extremely reliable for free-tissue transfer. The donor site is well concealed, and there has been no morbidity following its use.

INDICATIONS

The internal oblique muscle is best used for medium-sized surface defects requiring a minimum of thickness. Such locations as the malleoli, pretibial areas, and dorsum of the foot requiring flaps of up to 10 × 15 cm are suitable for the internal oblique muscle. When covered with a split-thickness skin graft, this muscle atrophies to form thin, durable, well-vascularized soft-tissue cover.

ANATOMY

Based on the continuation of the deep circumflex iliac artery (DCIA), the iliac crest bone may be included with the internal oblique muscle flap, either intimately attached to the muscle or separated from it, depending on the presence of the ascending branch. It is this latter characteristic that makes the osteomuscular flap extremely versatile in composite-tissue reconstructions (Figs. 1 and 2) (1–3) (see Chap. 404).

FLAP DESIGN AND DIMENSIONS

For small defects such as an osteomyelitis cavity, the muscle flap can be positioned directly over the ascending branch to ensure maximal vascularity. Compound defects requiring up to 14 cm of iliac crest bone can be covered with the internal oblique osteomuscle flap, simultaneously providing both bone and soft-tissue coverage with minimal bulk (Fig. 3). An additional advantage of this procedure is that the muscle may be positioned independent of the bone, owing to its separate blood supply, the ascending branch.

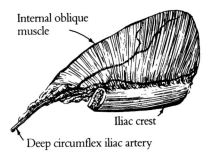

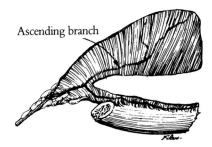

FIG. 1. The osteomuscular composite flap. The internal oblique muscle may be positioned independent of the iliac crest bone when the ascending branch is present.

OPERATIVE TECHNIQUE

An incision is made parallel to and slightly above the inguinal ligament and extended laterally beyond the anterior superior iliac spine. After incising the external oblique fascia, the internal oblique muscle is readily identified. Flap dissection is begun superiorly, splitting the muscle in the direction of its fibers. Care is taken to identify the transversus abdominis muscle, and this is easily noted by a change in the direction of the muscle fibers. Sharp dissection is required because muscle fibers interdigitate, particularly at its insertion along the rectus fascia.

The medial extent of the internal oblique muscle is reached, and dissection then is carried inferiorly. The muscle is then elevated, and the ascending branch of the DCIA is identified on the underside of the internal oblique muscle. In 65% of patients, the artery is found within 1 cm of the anterior superior iliac spine originating from the DCIA. In another 15%, it is found more medially (see Fig. 2). If the artery is not found as a separate entity, circulation to the muscle is maintained by identifying the DCIA at its origin with the common iliac artery and then tracing the artery distally to ensure its being included with the muscle. Once the ascending branch is identified, the desired muscle flap may be positioned directly over the artery to ensure its complete viability. Dissection then may proceed along the iliac crest, finally elevating the muscle on its vascular pedicle.

The entire length of the DCIA is used for the vascular pedicle, which usually measures between 6 and 7 cm long, with a vessel diameter of 1.5 to 3.0 mm. The vena comitans is some-

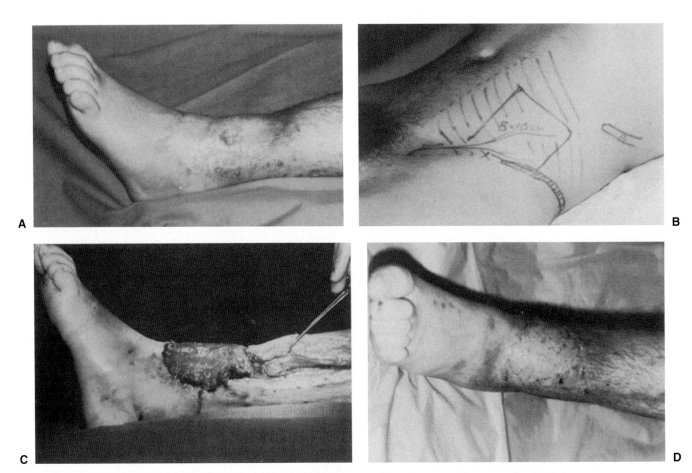

FIG. 2. Internal oblique muscle flap. **A:** Surface osteomyelitis with exposed bone over distal tibia in a 20-year-old man. **B:** An 8 × 10 cm internal oblique muscle flap based on the deep circumflex iliac artery. **C:** Muscle flap transferred to defect. Vascular anastomoses performed end-to-side to anterior tibial artery and vena comitans. **D:** One-year follow-up shows stable coverage with excellent contour. (From Ramasastry et al., ref. 1, with permission.)

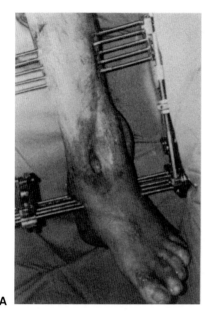
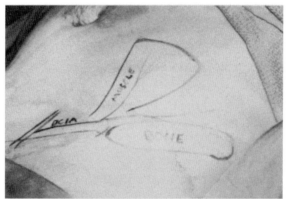
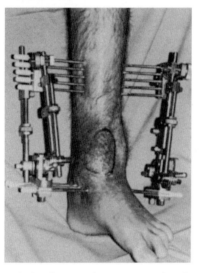
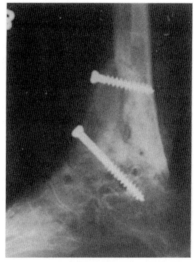

FIG. 3. Internal oblique osteomuscular flap. **A:** Chronic open infected nonunion following motorcycle accident in a 19-year-old man after an initial injury that measured 6 cm in length. **B:** A 6 × 4-cm internal oblique osteomuscular flap based on the deep circumflex iliac artery. The segment of the iliac crest measured 8 × 3 cm. **C:** Primary healing of the flap. The muscle flap had been covered at the time of transfer with a meshed split-thickness skin graft. (From Ramasastry et al., ref. 1, with permission.) **D:** Bone union achieved, 8-month follow-up. The patient is weight bearing without external support and has a completely healed wound.

what larger and lies anterior to the artery. Wound closure is easily obtained because the transversus abdominis muscle remains intact, and the external oblique fascia is closed over a suction drain. No skin is excised; so direct closure of the abdominal skin is easily performed (see Fig. 2).

Osteomuscular Flap

When the iliac crest bone is desired for composite reconstruction, the internal oblique muscle is initially left attached to the inner border of the iliac crest. Identification of the DCIA is carried out and traced to the anterior superior iliac spine. The ascending branch is easily identified at this time. The muscle flap then is dissected as previously described. The desired amount of iliac bone is cut using an oscillating saw, and the muscle and bone are isolated on the vascular pedicle of the DCIA. At the time of transfer, the muscle may be separated from the ilium, as reconstructive requirements dictate, provided the ascending branch is present as a separate vessel (see Fig. 1). Wound closure is achieved by suturing the transversalis fascia, the transversus abdominis muscle, the external oblique fascia, and the tensor fasciae latae to the new edge of the iliac crest after drilling holes through the bone to anchor the sutures.

CLINICAL RESULTS

The donor site is well concealed, and there has been no associated morbidity. To date, no hernia or abdominal wall weakness has occurred in any of our patients.

SUMMARY

The internal oblique flap can be used as a free muscle or osteomuscular flap and is particularly suited for small to medium-sized defects where bulk is undesirable.

References

1. Ramasastry S, Tucker J, Swartz W, Hurwitz D. The internal oblique muscle flap: An anatomic and clinical study. *Plast Reconstr Surg* 1984;73:721.
2. Taylor GI, Townsend P, Corlett R. Superiority of the deep circumflex iliac vessels as the supply for free groin flaps: experimental work. *Plast Reconstr Surg* 1979;64:595.
3. Taylor GI, Townsend P, Corlett R. Superiority of the deep circumflex iliac vessels as the supply for free groin flaps: clinical experience. *Plast Reconstr Surg* 1979;64:745.

CHAPTER 503 ■ MICROVASCULAR FREE TRANSFER OF FIBULA

A. J. WEILAND AND J. R. MOORE

In selected patients, free vascularized bone grafts offer significant advantages over conventional methods of treatment. A massive segment of bone can be detached from its donor site and transferred to a distant recipient site with preservation of the nutrient blood supply by microvascular anastomoses to recipient vessels.

INDICATIONS

With the nutrient blood supply preserved, osteocytes and osteoblasts in the graft can survive, and healing of the graft to the recipient bed will be enhanced without the usual replacement of the graft by creeping substitution. Thus, the surgeon can achieve a more rapid stabilization of bone fragments separated by a large defect without sacrificing viability. This is especially significant when the defect is situated in a highly traumatized or irradiated area with significant scarring and relative avascularity that preclude incorporation of conventional bone grafts (1–9).

ANATOMY

The nutrient artery of the fibula arises as a branch of the peroneal artery, which originates from the posterior tibial peroneal trunk. The peroneal artery gives off several periosteal branches before giving origin to the nutrient artery that supplies the medullary nutrient blood flow with the fibula. Penetration through the fibular cortex usually occurs at the middiaphysis, with a variation of 2.5 cm proximally or distally. The length of the nutrient artery external to the fibula ranges from 5 to 15 mm, and its diameter is between 0.25 and 1 mm (10,11).

The peroneal artery continues distally along the medial and posterior aspects of the fibular diaphysis and provides direct musculoperiosteal branches. Preservation of the medullary and periosteal blood supply to this straight cortical bone is, therefore, possible by isolation of the peroneal artery at its origin from the posterior tibial-peroneal arterial trunk (Figs. 1 and 2).

OPERATIVE TECHNIQUE

To clarify a description of the dissection technique, harvesting the fibula has been divided into eight steps. The procedure is performed with the patient supine and with the donor leg flexed approximately 135 degrees at the knee.

Step 1

A straight lateral skin incision is made along the line of the fibula from the neck as far distally as needed. The incision is carried through the skin and subcutaneous tissue to the fascia overlying the peroneus longus muscle.

Step 2

Elevation of anterior and posterior flaps is performed, as needed, to identify the interval between the peroneus longus and soleus muscles. The deep fascia then is incised over the entire length of the wound along this interval. The fibula is palpated periodically during the course of the dissection. Using a blunt elevator, the interval between the peroneus longus and soleus is developed. Using an extraperiosteal dissection technique, the peroneus longus and soleus are reflected from the fibular diaphysis anteriorly and posteriorly, respectively.

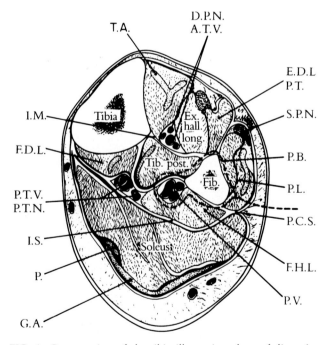

FIG. 1. Cross-section of the tibia illustrating plane of dissection (*dotted line*). (*TA*, tibialis anterior; *DPN*, deep peroneal nerve; *ATV*, anterior tibial vessels; *EDL*, extensor digitorum longus; *PT*, peroneus tertius; *SPN*, superficial peroneal nerve; *PB*, peroneus brevis; *PL*, peroneus longus; *PCS*, posterior crural septum; *FHL*, flexor hallucis longus; *PV*, peroneal vessels; *GA*, gastrocnemius aponeurosis; *P*, plantaris; *IS*, intermuscular septum; *PTV*, posterior tibial vessels; *PTN*, posterior tibial nerve; *FDL*, flexor digitorum longus; *IM*, interosseous membrane.)

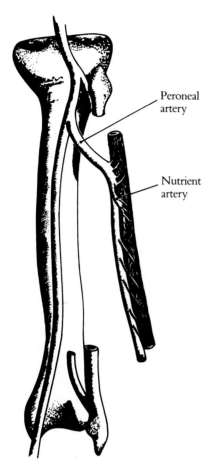

FIG. 2. This drawing demonstrates the fibula isolated on the peroneal artery. The nutrient artery is also illustrated.

(labels in figure: Peroneal artery; Nutrient artery)

Step 3

The lateral border of the fibula is now exposed. There are three perforators to the skin lying immediately posterior to the fascia overlying the soleus muscle. If skin is to be harvested with the fibula, these branches must be preserved. When the bone alone is to be transferred, these vessels should be ligated.

Step 4

Beginning proximally, the peroneus longus and brevis are elevated off the lateral border of the fibula, using a blunt elevator until the anterior crural septum is reached, staying close to bone. A 1-cm cuff of muscle is not left surrounding the fibula, as previously described. In the event that the vascularized graft fails, the cuff of muscle will become necrotic and serve as a nidus for infection. In addition, it will delay replacement of the graft by creeping substitution. The anterior crural septum is divided, and the extensor group of muscles (extensor digitorum longus, peroneus tertius, and extensor hallucis longus) is dissected off the interosseous membrane. The dissection continues until the anterior tibial artery and nerve have been identified and protected.

Step 5

The posterior crural membrane is divided the entire length of the graft. Using careful extraperiosteal dissection techniques, the soleus and flexor hallucis muscles are reflected off the posterior border of the fibula. The dissection continues until the peroneal vessels are encountered. The vessels must be left attached to the posterior surface of the intermuscular septum. Dissection is continued anteriorly and posteriorly for the length of graft required.

During the posterior dissection, any branches arising from the peroneal artery that will not be taken with the graft must be coagulated. Special care is taken not to damage the artery to the graft. In the distal third of the fibula, the peroneal artery lies directly on the posterior surface of the bone, and special care is taken to avoid damage to the artery during the osteotomy.

Step 6

The length of graft needed is measured and marked with methylene blue. All attempts should be made to preserve the distal 6 cm of fibula to maintain integrity of the lateral aspect of the ankle joint. If distal dissection is required in a child, a transfixion screw to preserve the integrity of the ankle mortise and to prevent possible proximal migration of the distal fibula should be employed. At the site of the distal osteotomy, the peroneal vessels should be identified and pushed medially off the intermuscular septum.

A hole is made in the septum sufficient to allow a 2.5-cm malleable retractor to be placed around the bone, protecting the vessels that lie posterior to the retractor. At this point, a Gigli saw may be passed and the distal osteotomy performed. A similar procedure is carried out at the proximal end of the graft. At this point, the distal limbs of the peroneal artery and veins are ligated at the site of the distal fibular osteotomy.

Step 7

Using a small bone hook in the medullary canal of the distal portion of the fibular graft to stabilize the fibula during the remaining portion of the dissection, the graft is retracted posteriorly, and division of the interosseous membrane is performed along the entire length of the graft. The graft then is carefully retracted anteriorly, and the tibialis posterior is dissected off the posterior aspect of the graft in the middle third, where it has remained attached to the fibula. This step is performed in a distal to proximal direction. The fibula is retracted anteriorly or posteriorly during this portion of the dissection, as needed, leaving the fibular graft isolated on its vascular pedicle proximally.

Step 8

Now that the fibula is completely dissected, the surgeon traces the peroneal artery proximally to its junction with the posterior tibial artery. A vessel loop is placed around the peroneal artery and vein. The fibula then is placed back in its bed until the recipient site is prepared. The tourniquet is deflated. Upon completion of the dissection of the recipient bed, the fibula is harvested and placed in the defect. After stable fixation is achieved, microvascular anastomoses of the artery and one vein are performed.

CLINICAL RESULTS

Our experience with the free vascularized fibular graft has encompassed its use in reconstruction following

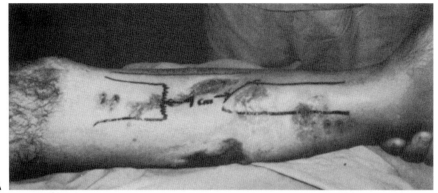

A

FIG. 3. A 22-year-old man was involved in a motorcycle accident, sustaining a fracture dislocation of the left hip, an intraarticular fracture of the left knee, and an open fracture of the left midtibia, with a 9-cm segmental bone loss. **A:** Six months after injury, he presented with a healed wound over the left leg.

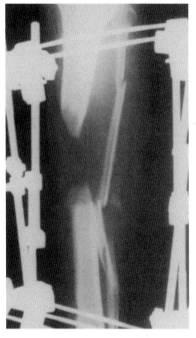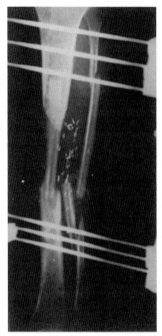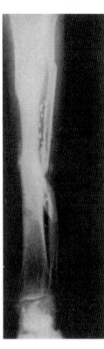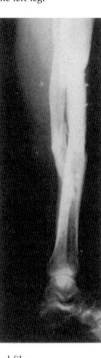

B–E

FIG. 3. **B:** Roentgenogram of the left leg demonstrating the bony defect. **C:** After a free vascularized fibular graft was performed, the patient's leg was placed in a Hoffmann device for 3 months, followed by a patellar tendon-bearing brace for an additional 3 months. **D,E:** At 6 months postoperatively, there was complete healing and hypertrophy of the vascularized fibular graft.

resection of low-grade malignant tumors and locally aggressive benign tumors, in addition to reconstruction of limbs following trauma (Fig. 3). The success rate was 90%, with only three failures (10%). Bony union occurred on an average of 3 to 5 months, with bony hypertrophy appearing in 4 to 9 months. The patients took 5 months on average to partial weight bearing and 12 to 15 months to full weight bearing.

Of secondary procedures, three (10%) required a bone graft, three (10%) underwent subsequent amputation, and two (6.6%) were of questionable viability. There has not been any donor-site morbidity associated with harvesting the fibula in any of our patients.

SUMMARY

The free vascularized fibula has dramatically altered the management of long-bone defects of the leg. Because it is living bone, it is more easily incorporated into the leg than "dead" bone grafts.

References

1. Taylor GI, Miller GDH, Ham FJ. The free vascularized bone graft: A clinical extension of microsurgical technique. *Plast Reconstr Surg* 1975;55:533.
2. Weiland AJ, Daniel RK, Riley LH Jr. Application of the free vascularized bone graft in the treatment of malignant and aggressive bone tumors. *Johns Hopkins Med J* 1977;140:85.
3. Weiland AJ, Daniel RK. Microvascular anastomoses for bone grafts in the treatment of massive defects in bone. *J Bone Joint Surg* 1979;61A:98.
4. Weiland AJ, Kleinert HE, Kutz JE, Daniel RK. Free vascularized bone grafts in surgery of the upper extremity. *J Hand Surg* 1979;4:129.
5. Chin-Tang H, Chi-Wei C, Kuo-Li S, et al. Free vascularized bone graft using microvascular technique. *Ann Acad Med Singapore* 1979;8:459.
6. Chung-Wei C, Zhong-Jia Y, Yean W. A new method of treatment of congenital tibial pseudarthrosis using free vascularized fibular grafts: A preliminary report. *Ann Acad Med Singapore* 1979;8:465.
7. Weiland AJ, Daniel RK. Congenital pseudarthrosis of the tibia: Treatment with vascularized autogenous fibular grafts. A preliminary report. *Johns Hopkins Med J* 1980;147:89.
8. Weiland AJ. Current concepts review: vascularized free bone transplants. *J Bone Joint Surg* 1981;63A:166.
9. Pho RWH. Malignant giant-cell tumors of the distal end of the radius treated by a free vascularized fibular transplant. *J Bone Joint Surg* 1981;63A:877.
10. Gilbert A. Free transfer of the fibular shaft. *Int J Microsurg* 1, 1979.
11. Restrepo J, Katz A, Gilbert A. Arterial vascularization to the proximal epiphysis and the diaphysis of the fibula. *Int J Microsurg* 1980;2:49.

CHAPTER 504 ■ TRANSPOSITION AND ROTATION SKIN FLAPS OF THE SOLE OF THE FOOT

J. W. CURTIN

The skin and subcutaneous tissues of the sole of the foot are unique; exact replacement of plantar skin is impossible, and substitution is difficult. Tissue brought to the sole of the foot from other parts of the body does not transform itself into normal plantar skin and consequently is subject to breakdown when weight bearing resumes, usually because the substituted tissue overlies a bony prominence and the covering flap taken from a distant site remains anesthetic. These artificially induced trophic changes lead to eventual breakdown.

When surgery is necessary to correct soft-tissue defects or lesions of the plantar aspect of the foot, the most ideal skin covering is adjacent plantar skin (Fig. 1). Previously delayed laterally based plantar flaps contain a fibrofatty pad that is specialized to resist weight bearing, and they afford protection by good permanent sensation (1,2).

INDICATIONS

When a tissue defect is encountered on the sole in an area where a bony prominence is not present, coverage can be achieved by either a full-thickness or a split-thickness skin graft. Depending on the clinical status, a split-thickness skin graft may be taken from the non-weight-bearing surface of the foot with good results and no problem with the donor site (3). Intelligent care of the anesthetic skin graft is important, but as long as some soft tissue underlies the graft, it usually will hold up quite well in weight bearing.

Past experiences with cross-leg and cross-plantar "functional flaps" have been less than satisfactory, because of prolonged cross-leg fixation, extended hospitalizations, and the disability of the donor site on the opposite leg or plantar surface of the foot (4,5).

Of patients with plantar conditions seen by me, most had ulcers of many years' duration beneath the metatarsal heads. Their incapacity was due to prolonged overtreatment; the original plantar wart was long gone, but painful keratosis and callus persisted. Plantar ulcerations are most commonly found in diabetic patients with peripheral neuropathy, diabetic small-vessel disease, and other metabolic disturbances.

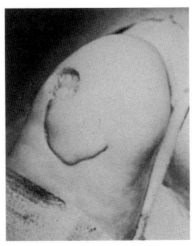 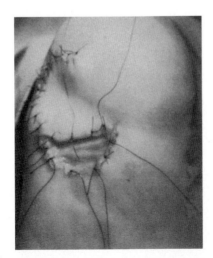 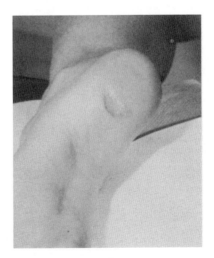

A–C

FIG. 1. **A:** Plantar ulcer and keratosis excised with outline of adjacent skin and subcutaneous tissue flap. **B:** Immediate rotation of plantar flap with split-thickness skin graft to the donor site. **C:** Patient has been walking on foot for 3 years.

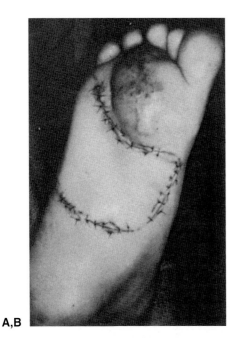
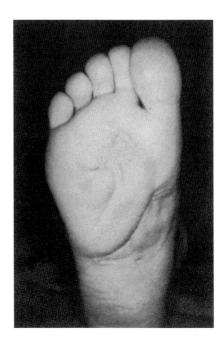

A,B

FIG. 2. **A:** Vascular tumor in a 3-year-old child with two previous unsuccessful operative attempts at removal. A delay procedure of a laterally based plantar pedicle flap. **B:** Surgical correction by excision of tumor, ligation of vessels, rotation of pedicle flap, and split-thickness skin graft to donor site.

FLAP DESIGN AND DIMENSIONS

Although a medially based plantar flap would seem more ideally designed as an axial flap, the resulting skin graft on the lateral donor area would be on the weight-bearing part of the foot. Therefore, laterally based flaps are preferred. It is usually necessary to carry out delay procedures on these laterally based flaps because they must be considered random flaps.

The bulk of the delayed laterally based plantar flap will consist of epidermis, dermis, and the specialized fibrofatty pad overlying the plantar fascia. The size of these flaps varies but will usually measure 5 × 6 cm or 6 × 8 cm, depending on the size of the anticipated surgical defect (Fig. 1 and see Fig. 6A).

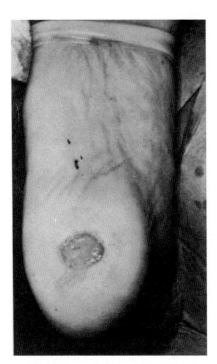
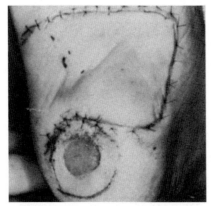
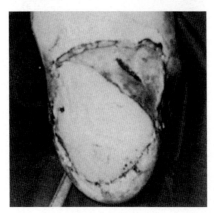

A–C

FIG. 3. **A:** A 59-year-old diabetic patient with plantar heel ulcer of 10 years' duration. **B:** A delay procedure of a laterally based plantar pedicle flap. **C:** Surgical correction with excision of ulcer, rotation of previously delayed laterally based plantar pedicle flap, and split-thickness skin graft to donor site.

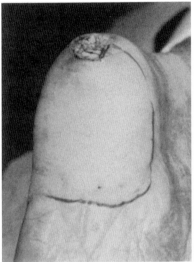
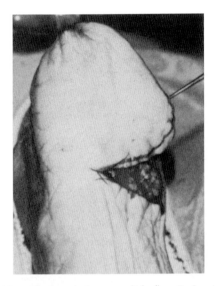
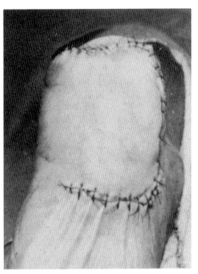

A–C

FIG. 4. **A:** Delay pattern of laterally based plantar pedicle flap. **B:** Surgical correction of persistent painful heel keratosis and rotation of pedicle flap to cover defect. **C:** Final result demonstrating primary suture of donor site.

OPERATIVE TECHNIQUE

My preferred method of delay is a skin and subcutaneous incision only without undermining of the flap and resuturing. This cuts off most of the peripheral feeders from three sides. I find that undermining the flap is a disadvantage, as considerable fibrosis of the flap is seen by the time of transfer 2 or 3 weeks later.

If the plantar flap were completely undermined and the circulation appeared so adequate that immediate transfer were possible, delay would not be necessary. However, my experience with the laterally based flap indicates that primary transfer is impossible and that delay is mandatory (Figs. 2 and 3).

When ulcers or calluses underlie a metatarsal head or os calcis, it is essential that plantar skin and subcutaneous tissue cover the surgical defect (Figs. 4–6). Frequently, when the plantar ulcer is beneath the head of the metatarsal, there is hyperextension of the metatarsophalangeal joints with associated hammer toes. The corrective operation should consist of ulcer excision, shaving or removal of the entire metatarsal head, or shortening of the metatarsal shaft (6) (Fig. 6). Sectioning of the extensor and flexor tendons to the affected toes is preferred as is closure of the surgical defect by rotation of a previously delayed laterally based plantar flap. The donor site, which will be on a relatively non-weight-bearing surface of the foot, will be covered by a moderately thick split-thickness skin graft (Fig. 6C, D).

These plantar flaps are somewhat inelastic, and the turn on the axis of rotation can be difficult. If dog-ears develop at the base of the flap, they are best left unattended surgically and probably will flatten on weight bearing (see Fig. 2B). Certainly

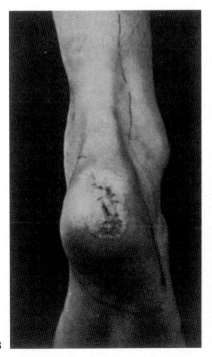
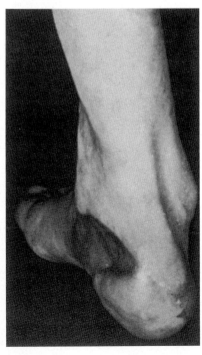

A,B

FIG. 5. **A:** An 18-year-old male patient exhibiting ulcer and surrounding keratosis of heel secondary to trauma of 5 years' duration. Note delay pattern of laterally based plantar flap. Also depicted is an alternative (but we feel hazardous) skin flap overlying Achilles tendon. **B:** Postoperative result after surgical excision of ulcer, rotation of previously delayed pedicle flap, and split-thickness skin graft to part of the donor site.

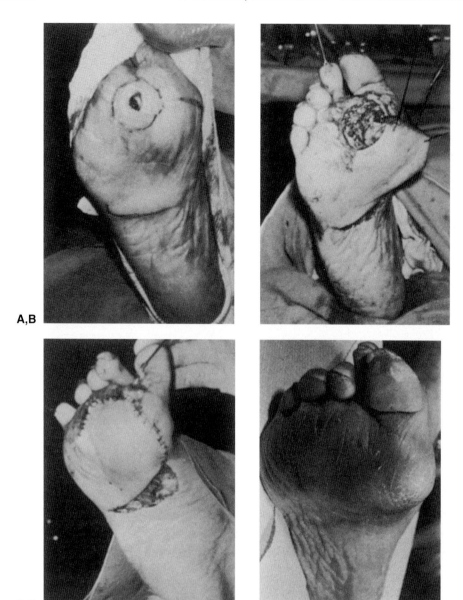

A,B

C,D

FIG. 6. A: Foot of a 63-year-old diabetic patient with plantar ulcer beneath heads of second and third metatarsals, hyperextension of metatarsophalangeal joints, and hammer toes of 6 years' duration. Note outline of delayed plantar flap. **B:** Excision of plantar ulcer with elevation and beginning rotation of previously delayed laterally based flap. **C:** Rotation of plantar flap to cover surgical defect. **D:** Final result after 18 months of weight bearing. A moderately thick skin graft was applied to the non-weight-bearing aspect of foot.

their removal at the time of rotation would be hazardous to the vascular supply of the flap.

CLINICAL RESULTS

Use of local plantar flaps in the weight-bearing areas of the foot brings in ideal structures of epidermis, dermis, and subcutaneous tissue. Experience with these patients refutes the notion that local flaps can be used only for small defects (5). Sensation returns rapidly in these local flaps, even when innervation has been sectioned (7). Their use results in superior weight-bearing surfaces with less restriction of the patient than when distant flaps are used.

SUMMARY

When the surgeon is confronted with complicated and intractable conditions on the plantar aspect of the foot, the use of local flaps, laterally based and previously delayed, affords ideal structures of epidermis, dermis, and subcutaneous tissue.

References

1. Curtin JW. Surgical therapy for Dupuytren's disease of the foot. *Plast Reconstr Surg* 1962;30:568.
2. Curtin JW. Fibromatosis of the plantar fascia. *J Bone Joint Surg* 1965;47A:1605.
3. Souther SG. Skin grafts from the sole of the foot: case report and literature review. *J Trauma* 1980;20:163.
4. Murray JE, Goldwyn R. Definitive treatment of intractable plantar ulcers. *JAMA* 1966;196:00.
5. Taylor GA, Hopson WLG. The cross-foot flap. *Plast Reconstr Surg* 1975;55:677.
6. Giannestras JJ. Shortening of the metatarsal shaft in the treatment of plantar keratosis. *J Bone Joint Surg* 1958;40A:61.
7. Freeman BS. Plantar flaps used for sole, heel lesions, *Texas J Med* 1968;64:64.
8. McFarlane RM. Hyperkeratosis and ulceration of the heel in the nonparaplegic patient. *Plast Reconstr Surg* 1962;29:674.

CHAPTER 505 ■ FASCIOCUTANEOUS CONE FLAP

W. CALDERÓN, P. ANDRADES, P. LENIZ, J. L. PIÑEROS, S. LLANOS, R. ROA, O. IRIBARREN, M. STEINER, AND D. CALDERÓN

The fasciocutaneous cone flap is a reliable and versatile option consisting of the combination of a rotation flap and a V-Y flap. The final shape of the repair is a cone, and the flap can be used to cover defects in various parts of the body (1–9).

INDICATIONS

The fasciocutaneous cone flap was initially designed to cover exposed bone in an open, lower-extremity fracture (Fig. 1). When osteomyelitis is present, a muscle flap is preferred; however, when no evidence of infection is found, this fasciocutaneous flap is indicated.

ANATOMY

The rotation and V-Y flaps are random-pattern fasciocutaneous flaps, with their blood supply coming from the deep arteries. Sensation to the flap is preserved.

FLAP DESIGN AND DIMENSIONS

The flap is elevated like a rotation flap, with a 1:1 width-to-length ratio. The donor site is covered with a V-Y fasciocutaneous flap, which has a 3:1 height-to-base ratio. The result is a cone-shaped flap (Fig. 2).

OPERATIVE TECHNIQUE

The primary defect is first covered by a rotation fasciocutaneous flap. A V-Y advancement fasciocutaneous flap is then designed to close the donor site. It is important to free the fascia all around the V-Y flap, to achieve the best advancement (Figs. 3 and 4).

CLINICAL RESULTS

Between June 2002 and March 2007, we operated on 100 patients with this technique. All were men, and patient ages

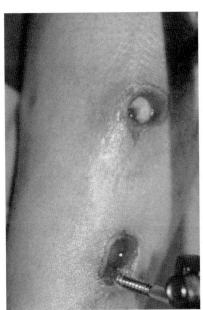 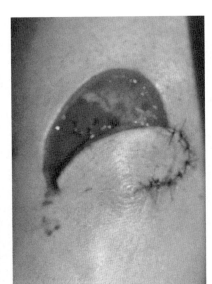 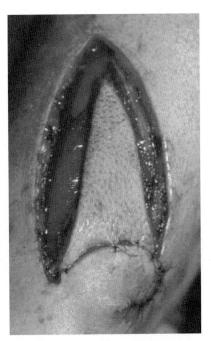

A–C

FIG. 1. **A:** Open wound with bone exposed. **B:** A rotation flap is rotated to cover the defect. **C:** A cone fasciocutaneous flap is elevated superiorly to close the defect created by the rotation flap.

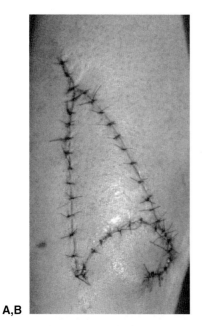
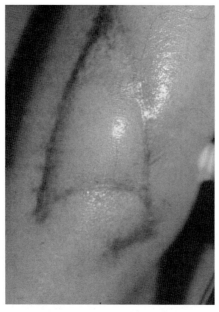

A,B

FIG. 2. **A:** Triangular flap elevated on fascial bed and advanced to fill the defect created by the rotation. **B:** AV-to-Y closure. **C:** Late postoperative photograph.

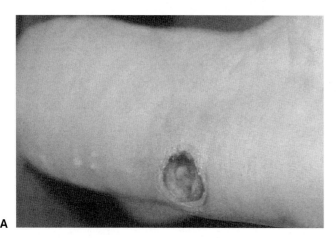

A

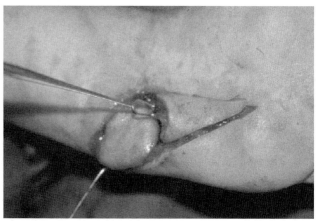

B

FIG. 3. **A:** A traumatic defect at the ankle. **B:** This is closed with a rotation flap and a sliding cone flap.

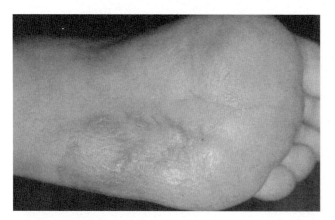

FIG. 4. A healed defect with a rotation flap and a cone flap on the sole of the foot.

ranged from 20 to 52 years. Initially, we began with open fractures of the distal lower extremity (tibia), and, because of good results, we subsequently treated other parts of the body with the same procedure (elbow, plantar region, big toe, arm, calvaria, and ankle). The cutaneous defects ranged from 0.5 to 3.5 cm^2. We experienced one necrosis of a V-Y flap and one necrosis of a rotation flap; both were repaired with split-thickness skin grafts.

SUMMARY

This cone-shaped flap, versatile for use at different physical locations, is especially practical when local physical characteristics are to be preserved.

References

1. Calderón W, Andrades P, Leniz P, et al. The cone flap: a new and versatile fasciocutaneous flap. *Plast Reconstr Surg* 2004;114:6.
2. Calderón W, Chang N, Mathes SJ. Comparison of the effects of bacterial inoculation in musculocutaneous and fasciocutaneous flaps. *Plast Reconstr Surg* 1986;77:785.

3. Fix RJ, Vasconez LO. Fasciocutaneous flaps in reconstruction of the lower extremity. *Clin Plast Surg* 1991;18:571
4. Hallock GG. Local fasciocutaneous flaps for cutaneous coverage of lower extremity wounds. *J Trauma* 1989;29:1240.
5. Hallock GG. Distal lower leg random fasciocutaneous flaps. *Plast Reconstr Surg* 1990;86:304.
6. Healy C, Tiernan E, Lamberty BG, Campbell RC. Rotation fasciocutaneous flap repair of lower limb defects. *Plast Reconstr Surg* 1995;95:243.
7. Masquelet A, Gilbert A. *Flaps in limb reconstruction*. London: Martin Dunitz, 1995.
8. Ponten B. The fasciocutaneous flap: its use in soft tissue defects of the lower leg. *Br J Plast Surg* 1981;34:215.
9. Tolhurst DE, Haesecker B, Zeeman RJ. The development of the fasciocutaneous flap and its clinical applications. *Plast Reconstr Surg* 1983; 71:597.

CHAPTER 506 ■ BIPEDICLE SKIN FLAP TO THE HEEL

N. I. ELSAHY

When there is deep tissue loss over the posterior heel, coverage should be accomplished by a flap. Local random pattern skin flaps are poorly vascularized and must be delayed before transposition. To improve the blood supply to a random pattern skin flap and to eliminate the need for delay, a local bipedicle skin flap may be used (1).

INDICATIONS

This bipedicle skin flap has been used to repair ulcers of the non-weight-bearing areas of the heel caused by pressure from a tight cast, immobilization in bed, direct trauma, and excision of a tumor or congenital sinus.

The vertical bipedicle flap has the following advantages:

1. It involves a simple one-stage operation.
2. It eliminates skin-graft complications over the defect, such as graft loss, hyperkeratosis, an unstable graft, and a painful scar.
3. It covers the defect with a thick layer of skin and subcutaneous tissue with good sensation, helping to prevent recurrence of the ulcer.
4. The donor area is placed well on the side of the foot, where a skin graft will "take" more easily and remain stable.

FLAP DESIGN AND DIMENSIONS

This bipedicle skin flap to the heel is an advancement flap. Its length is twice that of the defect and usually varies from 4 to 6 cm. The width of the flap should be at least half the length, that is, about 2 to 3 cm. The lateral incision should parallel the vertical long axis of the ulcer (see Fig. 1). Two bipedicle flaps, one on each side of the defect, may be used if the defect is too large to be closed with only one flap.

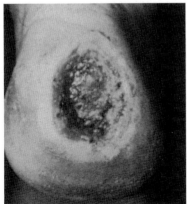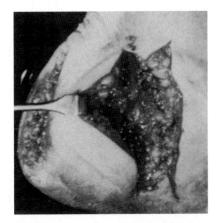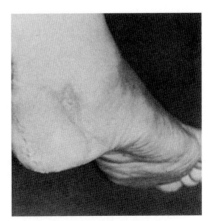

A–C

FIG. 1. **A:** Pressure ulcer in the posterior heel. The ulcer was deep to the bone, with destruction of the overlying periosteum. **B:** Incision in the lateral aspect of the foot, with V backcut made superiorly and inverted V backcut inferiorly to facilitate mobilization of the flap. **C:** Healed flap and donor site.

OPERATIVE TECHNIQUE

A backcut extension of the upper end of the lateral incision as a small V and of the lower end as an inverted V facilitates mobilization of the flap (Fig. 1B). The flap is then undermined, advanced, and sutured in place. The donor area is covered with a split-thickness skin graft.

CLINICAL RESULTS

This flap is not without complications. Skin necrosis at the suture line may occur, especially if the defect is large and the patient is diabetic or has peripheral vascular disease. There is no functional deficit from using this flap.

SUMMARY

A random pattern bipedicle skin flap can be used to cover heel defects.

Reference

1. Elsahy NI. The use of the bipedicle flap for the repair of ulcers in the non-weight-bearing areas of the heel. *Acta Chir Plast* 1978;20:34.

CHAPTER 507 ■ V-Y ADVANCEMENT FLAPS TO THE HEEL AND ANKLE

Y. MARUYAMA AND Y. IWAHIRA

EDITORIAL COMMENT

This presents a most helpful maneuver for the coverage of defects in the heel, with similar type of skin. It has the advantage of providing coverage "of the same kind" and avoids the problems of friction and insensitivity.

The V-Y advancement subcutaneous pedicle flap is useful for reconstruction of relatively small defects, especially in the lower leg. This flap, because of the attached local pedicle, provides comparatively safer applications than other flaps, even in the heel and ankle areas (1–3).

INDICATIONS

A difficult part of reconstructing ankle and heel defects is coverage of the exposed calcaneal tendon and bony prominence. Because of the location of such defects and the constant wearing of shoes, even small skin defects often present problems of healing. Past experiences with cross-leg flaps have provided less than satisfactory solutions, because of the prolonged immobility required and the resultant defect in the contralateral donor leg. There is also a problem with a satisfactory blood supply in these areas, using a conventional local flap.

The V-Y advancement flap has the advantages of short operating time in one stage; it does not require division of the pedicle, and color and texture matches are excellent. The remaining tissue can be effectively used, and skin grafting is not required at the donor site. Moreover, this local triangular flap, including fascia, with closure in a V-Y fashion, encourages a safe blood supply in the ankle region (1). For more reliable results, we limit this procedure to patients under 60 years of age without systemic vascular disease. The flap has also been reported for use in the facial region (4,5).

FLAP DESIGN AND DIMENSIONS

The triangular flap is designed to be 1.5 to 2 times as long as the diameter of the defect in the plane of advancement, and with its base equal to the perpendicular diameter of the defect (Fig. 1A). To facilitate a more distant advancement, the thickness of the layer of undermining between the distal and proximal portions of the flap is varied, taking every precaution to preserve the underlying subcutaneous structures. For flap survival and mobility, a ratio of 1:2 can be recommended. In our experience, flaps have been easily moved between 1.0 and 3.5 cm.

OPERATIVE TECHNIQUE

The incision is made, following a triangular design (Fig. 1A). We undermine the distal end of the flap in the subcutaneous layer as little as necessary. The opposite end of the flap,

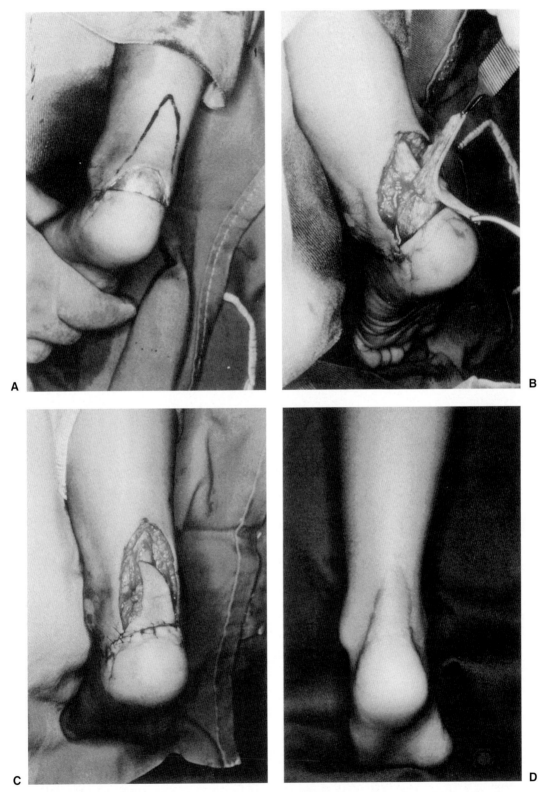

FIG. 1. **A:** A 7-year-old boy with a defect at the posterior heel. The V-Y flap is designed adjacent to the defect. **B:** Elevation of the flap, varying the thickness of undermining as little as possible to resurface the defect. **C:** Transposition of the flap. **D:** Appearance 1 year postoperatively. (From Maruyama Y, et al, ref. 1, with permission.)

consisting of a component with subcutaneous and fascial tissues, is deeply undermined under the fascia (Fig. 1B). Freeing is continued, until the flap moves into the defect with minimum tension (Fig. 1C). The pedicle, including the fascia, should be as broad and deep as possible, especially if undermining is close to the original wound. Blunt dissection is recommended. The flap is sutured with subcuticular 5–0 Vicryl at the advancing edge and at the V-Y junction (Fig. 1C).

CLINICAL RESULTS

Most of our cases healed without complications. The donor sites were all closed primarily (Fig. 1D). Superficial distal skin necrosis at the distal margin may occur; however, reepithelialization occurs within 2 weeks postoperatively. There has been no functional deficit, and the flaps have endured against constant friction for a long time.

SUMMARY

A V-Y advancement pedicle flap, including fascia, is used for reconstruction of soft-tissue defects in the heel and ankle region.

References

1. Maruyama Y, Iwahira Y, Ebihara H. V-Y advancement flap in the reconstruction of skin defects of the posterior heel and ankle. *Plast Reconstr Surg* 1990;65:786.
2. Iwahira Y, Maruyama Y. The design of a plantar flap with respect to plantar fissures. *Jpn J Plast Surg* 1992;35:293.
3. Colen LB, Replogle SL, Mathes Si. The V-Y plantar flap for reconstruction of the forefoot. *Plast Reconstr Surg* 1988;81:220.
4. Zook EG, Van Beek AL, Russell RC. V-Y advancement flap for facial defects. *Plast Reconstr Surg* 1980;65:786.
5. Argamaso RV. V-Y-S plasty for closure of a round defect. *Plast Reconstr Surg* 1974;53:99.

CHAPTER 508 ■ DEEPITHELIALIZED "TURNOVER" SKIN FLAP OF THE LOWER LEG AND FOOT

R. L. THATTE AND N. LAUD

EDITORIAL COMMENT

Anatomic knowledge of the septocutaneous vessels that are segmental branches from the three main arteries supplying the leg is the basis for these turnover flaps. The segmental septocutaneous vessels that arise at intervals from each of the three vessels into the leg, the last one approximately 10 cm above the medial malleolus, course through the intermuscular septum, perforate the fascia, and arborize on top of the fascia to supply the overlying skin and connect with vessels above and below. If only one of the septocutaneous vessels is maintained intact, then an independent territory can be outlined that can either be made into a proximally or distally based, flap or a "turnover" flap, as demonstrated in this chapter.

One-stage skin-flap coverage from local tissues is an ideal solution for complicated wounds in any part of the body. The one-stage random-pattern and axial-pattern deepithelialized "turnover" flaps of the lower leg and foot fulfill this expectation (1–4).

INDICATIONS

The turnover flap is a simple, quick, one-stage procedure and is particularly suitable for longitudinal defects on the lower leg, where the application of other local flaps is limited. Defects that need skin-flap coverage may have partly scarred skin on their periphery. The base of a turnover flap can be placed in such a scarred area as long as the area has intact tendons or muscles underneath it. When the flap turns over, it covers its own base. If the base area is scarred, the flap cover improves its quality; however, the flap should not be used if the base is undermined.

The turnover flap is especially useful when there is still a defect adjacent to a previously transferred flap. In actual practice, rotation or transposition of the existing flap skin to the adjacent area is a difficult maneuver, because any transferred skin flap is surrounded on all sides by scarring. This problem can be overcome by a deepithelialized turnover flap out of the existing flap skin (see Fig. 5).

The procedure reduces the risk of partial or major failures in the transfer of skin flaps of large dimensions around the whole circumference of the lower extremity (see Fig. 1). There also appears to be a strong possibility that the fascia in the

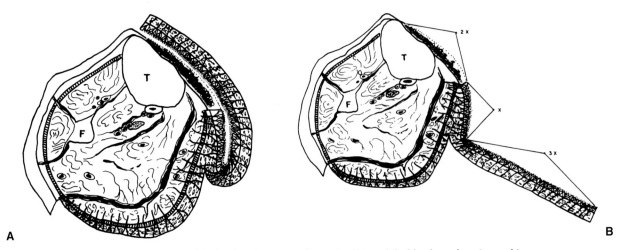

FIG. 1. A: Cross section of the leg showing a wound over the tibia and the blood supply to intact skin on the medial side of this wound. A deepithelialized flap is raised from the skin medial to the wound over the tibia. **B:** The flap turned over.

lower leg can be transposed or turned over to cover defects with exposed bone. When it comes to sacrificing tissue, the fascia might be a more appropriate choice than muscle (5).

ANATOMY

The principal blood supply to skin comes from the perforator vessels (6) (Fig. 1). A random-pattern flap survives mainly on the blood supply from these perforator vessels, the circulation in skin being carried forward by the intradermal anastomoses. The deepithelialized surface of the flap is the more vascular of its two surfaces because of exposed rich intradermal anastomoses. When the flap turns over, this surface advantageously faces the defect. In contrast, the raw undersurface of a conventional skin flap has a thin layer of fat covering it.

FLAP DESIGN AND DIMENSIONS

Figure 1 shows a complicated wound overlying the tibia and the blood supply of an area of skin on the medial side of the wound. A flap raised from this area with an adequate base-to-length

ratio (base unit = x, flap units = 3x) should survive (Fig. 1A), even if the surface of the flap, as well as its base, is deepithelialized. This is so because the technique of taking a medium-thickness skin graft leaves the intradermal anastomoses intact.

A deepithelialized turnover dorsalis pedis flap for a lateral malleolar defect has been recently reported (6,7), its advantage being that a dissection in front of the ankle is not needed to convert the flap into an island to facilitate its transposition. The deepithelialized turnover dorsalis pedis flap is also quite likely to be useful for defects in the lowest anterior surface of the leg. The dimensions of such a flap are about equal to the anterior half of the circumference of the lower leg (see Fig. 6).

OPERATIVE TECHNIQUE

Figure 1B shows the flap turned over on itself and covering the defect on the tibia. In the drawing (as well as in clinical practice), the area where the flap turns over on itself is a gentle curve, allowing unhindered circulation. The turned-over surface of the flap needs skin-graft cover. The defect left by flap transfer is covered by a split-thickness skin graft removed at the time of deepithelialization (Figs. 2–5).

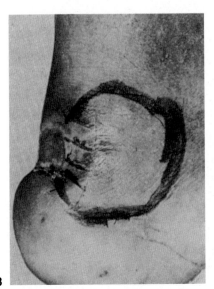
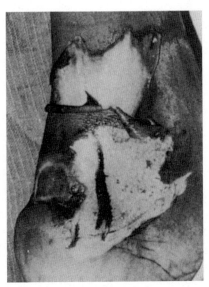

FIG. 2. A: An 18-year-old man was admitted to the hospital with a posttraumatic ulcer measuring approximately 2 cm in transverse diameter over the Achilles tendon. The ulcer had failed to heal following two attempts at split-thickness skin grafting, and skin flap cover was considered essential. **B:** An area approximately 4 cm in diameter was marked on the medial side of the ulcer. This was deepithelialized, and the skin was removed as shown. The line on the deepithelialized site shows the 1-cm² area that is left intact as the base of the flap. *(Continued)*

A,B

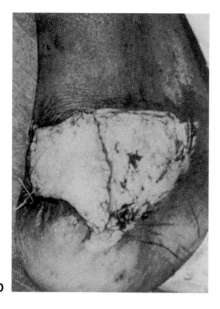
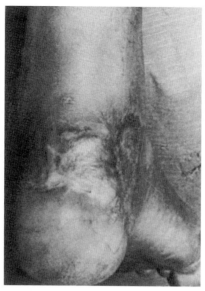

C,D

FIG. 2. *Continued.* C: The flap was turned over and sutured over the ulcer. The defect left by the flap transfer was covered by skin removed at the time of deepithelialization. The turned-over flap then was covered with a split-thickness skin graft from another location. D: A healed, stable area 6 months postoperatively.

CLINICAL RESULTS

In the 3 years of my experience, I have lost only one turnover flap of a total of 32 in the lower leg and foot. The failure was due to a faulty plan, according to which the base of the flap was undermined from the side of the chronic posttraumatic ulcer over which the flap turned over.

Seven out of a total of over 60 deepithelialized flaps executed in the upper and lower (2,5,7–9) extremities in the last 3 years have by now presented with discharging sinuses on their periphery. Of these, one sinus was confirmed to be due to osteomyelitis. In another patient, the discharge was occasional and minimal, and no active treatment was undertaken. In the remaining five patients, buried epithelium was responsible for the chronic discharge. The lesions were treated by placing a sinus probe in the discharging tract and excising the epithelial cyst and the tract by an incision placed over the probe. The wound was closed primarily and healed primarily in all five patients.

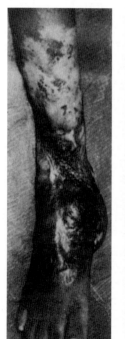
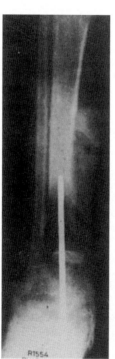
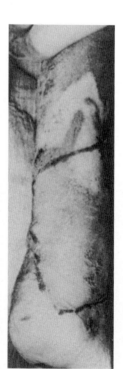
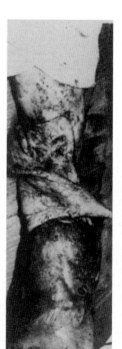
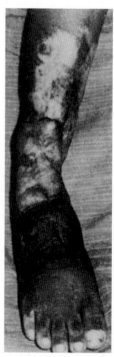

A–E

FIG. 3. A: A 9-year-old boy was admitted to the hospital with a dense adherent scar 9 cm vertically and 5 cm transversely in front of the ankle. There was a history of an avulsion-crush type of injury. B: X-ray showing fracture of the tibia and loss of the lower portion of the tibia. Skin-flap cover was considered essential prior to treatment of bony defect near the ankle. C: An area 9 cm vertically and 8 cm transversely was marked for deepithelialization on the lateral side of the leg and foot. D: A deepithelialized flap from this area being turned over. Flap size is 9 × 6.5 cm. E: Flap well settled 6 months postoperatively.

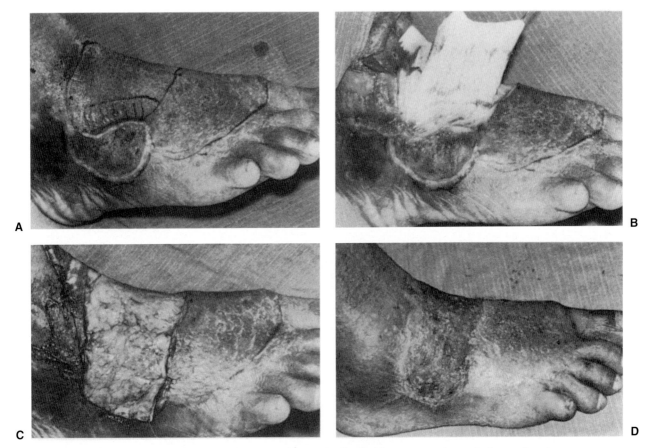

FIG. 4. **A:** A small area in the distal part of a cross-leg flap had become necrotic, producing an ulcer that measured 5 × 2.5 cm. An area 5 × 5 cm was marked out to the medial side of the ulcer over the dorsum of the foot, and the whole of this area was deepithelialized. **B:** The *cross-hatched area* (1 cm wide) shown in part *A* also was deepithelialized but was left attached to its bed as the base of the flap. **C:** The turnover flap was sutured over the ulcer, and all the raw surfaces were covered by a split-thickness skin graft. **D:** The graft "took" completely, and the area remained soundly healed when reviewed 3 months later. (From Thatter et al., ref. 7, with permission.)

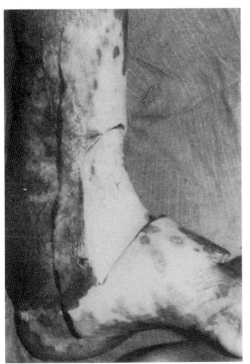

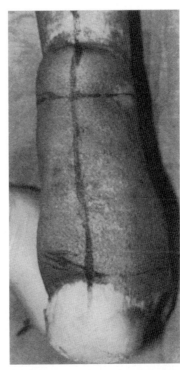

FIG. 5. **A,B:** Instead of achieving flap cover over the whole area at one time, a flap of approximately 250 cm^2 was first transferred on the posterior side of the leg from the opposite thigh in two stages (cross-thigh flap). *(Continued)*

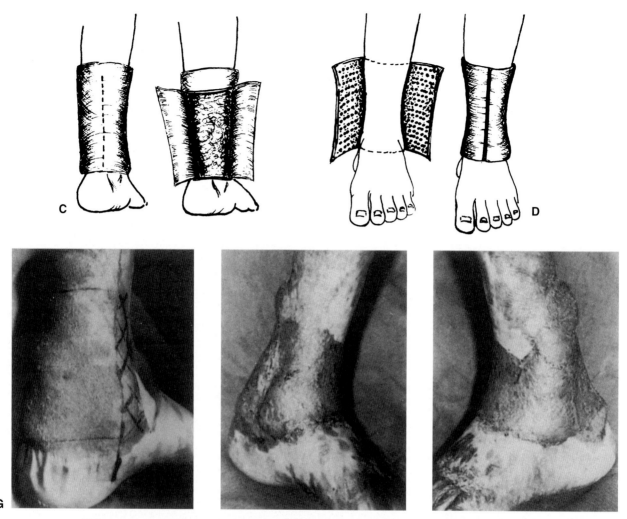

FIG. 5. *Continued.* **C,D:** This flap in its lower four fifths was then divided into two equal parts, each part to be turned over after deepithelialization, for a defect in front of the ankle. **E:** The base for the two turnover flaps was a long strip of about 2-cm width at its own periphery. The base of the turnover flap on one side is shown by cross-hatching. **F,G:** The flaps were turned over and sutured in the midline anteriorly. The turned-over flaps, as well as the defect left by the maneuver, were covered by a split-thickness skin graft. The final result, was a healed and stable area. Note that the bulk of the original flap has been shared, leading to a more pleasing appearance. Elastic support with bandages is not needed.

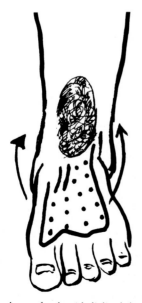

FIG. 6. Hypothetical use of a deepithelialized dorsalis pedis flap for defects on the anterior circumference of the lower leg.

SUMMARY

Notwithstanding the preceding complications, the deepithelialized turnover flap is valuable for defects in the lower leg and foot. Its application for salvage where losses have occurred in skin flaps during transfer is equally valuable. The procedure is quick and safe and can be executed in one stage.

References

1. Pakiam AI. The reverse dermis flap. *Br J Plast Surg* 1978;31:131.
2. Thatte RL. Random-pattern deepithelialized "turnover" flaps to replace skin loss in the upper third of the leg. *Br J Plast Surg* 1981;34:312.
3. Mahler D, Yanai E. The deepithelialized hinged flap. *Ann Plast Surg* 1981;7:298.
4. Thatte RL. One-stage random-pattern deepithelialized "turnover" flap in the leg. *Br J Plast Surg* 1982;35:287.
5. Daniel RK, Williams HB. The free transfer of skin flaps by microvascular anastomosis: an experimental study and reappraisal. *Plast Reconstr Surg* 1973;52:16.
6. Thatte RL, Patil D, Talwar P. Deepithelialized "turnover" axial-pattern flaps in the lower extremity. *Br J Plast Surg* 1983;36:327.
7. Thatte RL, Dhami LD, Patil UA. Deepithelialized turnover flaps for "salvage" operations. *Br J Plast Surg* 1983;36:178.

CHAPTER 509 ■ REVERSED DERMIS FLAP

A. I. PAKIAM

The reversed dermis graft has been used for coverage of small areas of devitalized tissue after debridement (1). The reversed dermis flap is a logical extension of the concept of the reversed dermis graft.

INDICATIONS

There are advantages in deepithelializing a flap and applying it dermis side down. While still kept alive by its pedicle, the numerous cut vessels of the dermal surface have a much greater potential for making sufficient anastomoses, particularly on poor beds, than the relatively avascular fatty undersurface of the conventional flap. Its use not only increases the number of possible flaps for repair of a given defect but simplifies flap repair in many instances. The reversed dermis flap is especially good for foot and ankle defects with exposed bone (2). It also has been used for reconstruction in many other areas of the body (2–12).

ANATOMY

A study of the blood supply of the skin demonstrates that the vessels at the subdermal level branch repeatedly as they approach the skin surface and, therefore, become smaller and more numerous. This difference is evident when one compares a skin graft taken at a more superficial level with one taken at a deeper level. The superficial graft site shows multiple, punctate, smaller bleeding vessels, whereas the thicker graft site demonstrates larger, fewer vessels. The former situation exposes more vessels for a vascular linkup of tissue transplants and aids in the "bridging" phenomenon, where small avascular areas may be covered successfully.

FLAP DESIGN AND DIMENSIONS

Two main types of flaps can be recognized: the direct bridge pedicle flap, used between adjacent digits or limbs or as distant flaps, and local turnover flaps, where the pedicle could remain intact by deepithelializing the skin bridge itself.

The established differences between axial and random flaps apply to reversed flaps. Whenever possible, an axially based flap should be used. Similarly, a local flap is preferable to a distant flap.

On the extremities, it would seem logical to use proximally or distally based turnover flaps. In larger defects, one may

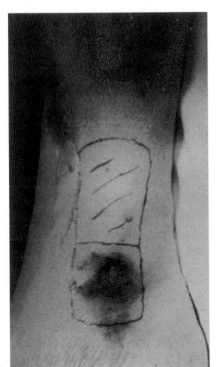
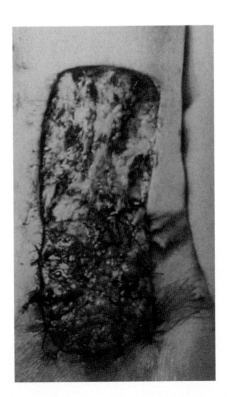

FIG. 1. A: Chronic painful ulcer of the medial malleolus with exposed bone. The *hatched area* is deepithelialized. B: After debridement, the defect was covered by a proximally based reversed dermis flap with a deepithelialized skin bridge in one stage. *(Continued)*

A,B

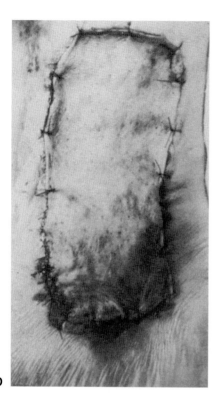
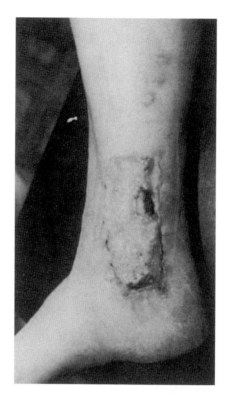

C,D

FIG. 1. *Continued.* **C:** Both the flap and the donor site are covered with a medium-thickness split-thickness skin graft. **D:** The result at 3 weeks. The small area of overgraft failure on the donor site will heal spontaneously. Pain has been relieved.

be faced with a near circumferential operated area with an attendant increased incidence of peripheral lymphedema with side flaps.

OPERATIVE TECHNIQUE

Because of a more rapid "take" of the flap, division is earlier than for conventional flaps. Because the flap usually involves just one stage, the procedure is less involved than either distant or free flaps.

The bases of flaps that are turned over 180 degrees are easily kinked, with disastrous results. Occasionally, epithelial cysts occur that may require excision (Fig. 1).

SUMMARY

The reversed dermis flap can be used to cover exposed ankle and foot defects. The possibilities of this flap are protean, and it is anticipated that more uses for this flap will be found in the future.

References

1. Hynes W. The skin dermis graft as an alternative to the direct or tubed flap. *Br J Plast Surg* 1954;7:97.
2. Pakiam AI. The reversed dermis flap. *Br J Plast Surg* 1978;31:131.
3. Braithwaite F. Closure of a tracheooesophageal fistula. *Br J Plast Surg* 1961;14:138.
4. Hasman L. Uzaver defektu bronchopleurokutannimi pistelemi dekortiko-vanym lalokem. *Acta Chir Orthop Traumatol (Czech)* 1967;34:6.
5. Clodius L, Smahel J. The reverse dermal-fat flap: an alternative cross leg flap. *Plast Reconstr Surg* 1973;52:85.
6. Maurice DG, Sharma DP. Repair of pharyngocutaneous fistula. *Br J Plast Surg* 1975;28:268.
7. Harashima T, Wadoa M, Inai T, Kakegawa T. A turnover deepithelialized deltopectoral flap to close fistulae following antethoracic oesophageal reconstruction. *Br J Plast Surg* 1979;32:278.
8. Leonard AG. Reconstruction of the chest wall using a deepithelialized "turn over" deltopectoral flap. *Br J Plast Surg* 1980;33:187.
9. Mahler D, Yanoi E. The deepithelialized hinged flap. *Ann Plast Surg* 1981;7:298.
10. Morris A McG. Rapid skin cover in hand injuries using the reverse dermis flap. *Br J Plast Surg* 1981;34:194.
11. Thatte RL. Random-pattern deepithelialized "turn over" flaps to replace skin loss in the upper third of the leg. *Br J Plast Surg* 1981;34:312.
12. Tomono T, Hirose T, Matsuo K, Matsui, T. A denuded "turn over" deltopectoral flap combined with a latissimus dorsi myocutaneous flap in the repair of extensive radionecrosis of the chest wall. *Br J Plast Surg* 1982;35:63.

CHAPTER 510 ■ FILLETED TOE FLAP

A. J. J. EMMETT

Neurovascular island flaps, particularly those of toe skin, offer readily available skin that can be turned onto the weight-bearing metatarsal head area (1–3). A patient whose ability to walk is limited by a chronically painful area on the sole is often happy to exchange the toe for a painless foot (3).

INDICATIONS

Repairs of the sole of the foot are complicated by the specialized requirements of the skin and subcutaneous tissue in that area. The firm adhesion of skin to plantar fascia limits skin mobility and makes it a firm gripping pad for heavy traction. The lobulated fat cells between the skin and plantar fascia give the skin in this area a resilience unlike most other skins. The rugose nature of the skin provides an ideal nonslip surface.

Sensation is the all-important factor, and over the long term, a flap must have adequate sensation for survival. It is well known that a flap transferred from the groin or abdomen to the sole of the foot is initially firm but later becomes floppy. Local flaps on the sole of the foot can be transferred from non-weight-bearing areas and a graft placed in the donor site. With dissection, these flaps tend to lose sensation to a degree, and they are limited in size. I have used this method in a number of patients to repair the chronic scarred painful area on the sole of the foot subsequent to repeated surgery or injury (see Fig. 3).

FLAP DESIGN AND DIMENSIONS

Generally, all the soft tissue of the toe is used in the flap, discarding the skeleton. Alternatively, one-half the toe skin on one neurovascular bundle could be used, grafting the resulting defect on the toe.

The neurovascular pattern of the foot (Figs. 1 and 2A) allows a toe flap to be hinged as far back as the plantar arch, although dissection deep to the toe flexors is involved. The big toe has been used as a neurovascular island for a heel defect (2), and the second and third toes have been used for heel repair (1). For replacement of a defect in the metatarsal head area, the toe may be hinged at the level of the transverse plantar ligament.

OPERATIVE TECHNIQUE

The toe is opened dorsally (Fig. 2A), and the soft tissues are dissected from the skeleton, identifying the neurovascular bundles (Fig. 2B). The toe skeleton then can be removed with or without the metatarsal head, depending on the foot and its requirements. The neurovascular bundles are identified

and mobilized, dividing the transverse ligament. The toe skin is freed, and excess skin at the base of the toe may be resected (Fig. 2C). The toe then is free to hinge into the defect (Fig. 3).

CLINICAL RESULTS

The lost toe presents a minor cosmetic disability, but it is well accepted after adequate discussion with the patient (see Fig. 3E). The flap has good circulation, and no vascular problems

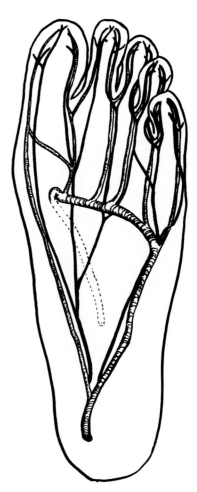

FIG. 1. The neurovascular anatomy of the foot, demonstrating that a flap can be filleted from the toe and transferred as far back as the heel. (From Emmett, ref. 3, with permission.)

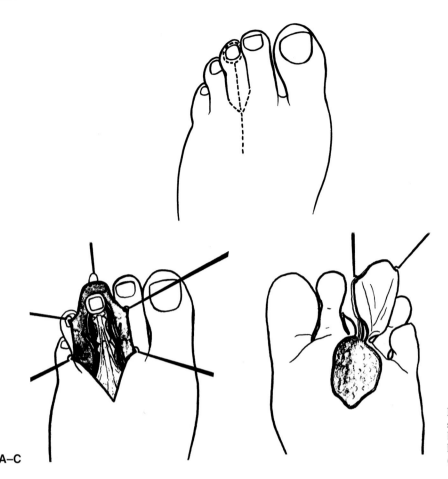

A–C

FIG. 2. **A:** The design of the flap. **B:** The toe is skeletonized on its neurovascular bundles. **C:** The bony structures, with or without the metatarsal head, are removed and the flap is transferred. (From Emmett, ref. 3, with permission.)

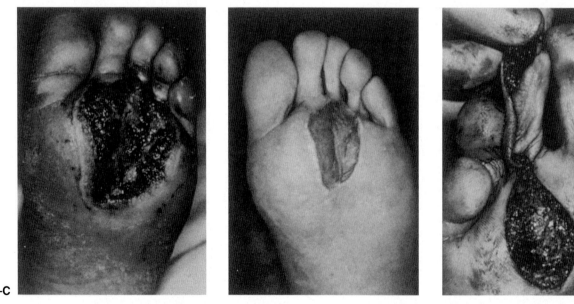

A–C

FIG. 3. **A:** An avulsion injury of the foot with loss of skin and fat. **B:** After a split-thickness skin graft had healed the wound and narrowed the defect, the patient was left with a painful area on walking. He needed replacement of the missing fat pad and skin. **C:** An example of a filleted toe flap after elevation and removal of the skeleton. *(Continued)*

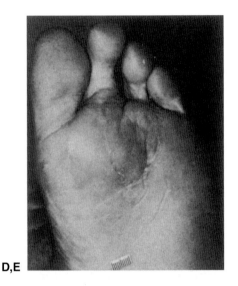
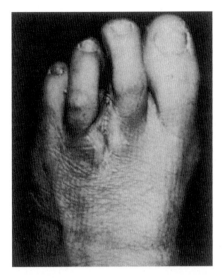

D,E

FIG. 3. *Continued.* **D:** A filleted toe flap was then used, producing a stable area that was not painful on walking. **E:** The donor site leaves a minor cosmetic deformity. (From Emmett, ref. 3, with permission.)

have been encountered. Healing and long-term survival of the flap are excellent.

SUMMARY

The filleted toe flap is an excellent way to provide durable, well-tolerated tissue to the sole of the foot.

References

1. Snyder GB, Edgerton MT. The principle of the island neurovascular flap in the management of ulcerated anaesthetic weight-bearing areas of the lower extremity. *Plast Reconstr Surg* 1965;36:518.
2. Kaplan I. Neurovascular island flap in the treatment of trophic ulceration of the heel. *Br J Plast Surg* 1969;22:143.
3. Emmett AJJ. The filleted toe flap. *Br J Plast Surg* 1976;29:19.

CHAPTER 511 ■ REVERSE ANTERIOR TIBIAL ARTERY FLAP

Y. P. PENG

EDITORIAL COMMENT

This is a very sophisticated flap for resurfacing the ankle and foot but fraught with difficulties. The arterial circulation is not reliable and must be checked before turning the flap down, either preoperatively with radiology or intraoperatively with release of tourniquet. The author has not reported how many cases he has abandoned. Venous congestion is an expected problem in this reverse flow flap.

The reverse anterior tibial artery flap is designed for foot and ankle resurfacing. Illustrated are the anatomy of the malleolar-, tarsal-, and metatarsal-level anastomoses between the anterior and posterior tibial artery system that perfuses the flap, the surgical technique, and measures to avoid complications.

INDICATIONS

Skin defects in the ankle and foot region have always been a difficult resurfacing problem (1–4). Free flaps are often indicated. The reverse anterior tibial artery flap was first designed for resurfacing the donor site of the big toe wrap-around flap (5,6). A long and thin flap (3 × 8 cm) was used to reconstruct the plantar surface of the big toe. The indications were subsequently extended for the reconstruction of larger defects on the dorsum of the foot and ankle.

This anterior tibial artery flap can be used in antegrade fashion to resurface proximal defects around the knee and proximal tibia. It can also be harvested as a free flap or as an osteocutaneous flap incorporating part of the bony tibia.

ANATOMY

Anatomy of the Anterior Tibia–Dorsalis Pedis–First Dorsal Metatarsal Artery

The anterior tibial artery supplies the skin of the anterolateral aspect of the leg. Multiple fasciocutaneous perforators traverse through the extensor and peroneal compartment to reach the skin in the proximal half of the leg (7–10). Proximally, the anterior tibial artery lies between the tibia and the tibialis anterior muscle (TA), close to the deep peroneal nerve. Pedicled flaps based on these perforators will require tedious dissection, if proximal dissection to the vascular pedicle is required.

We observed periosteal perforators that reach the skin in the plane between the tibia and the tibialis anterior muscle, lying on the periosteum of the bone (Fig. 1). On average, five to seven well-spaced periosteal perforators are found along the length of the tibia. These perforators were first mentioned by Crock and Morrison (10), and a periosteal flap based on

these perforators was successfully used to cover a tibial nonunion defect in 1992.

The anterior tibial artery gains a more superficial position distally, to lie between the tendons of the extensor hallucis longus (EHL) and the extensor digitorum longus (EDL) below the extensor retinaculum, before emerging as the dorsalis pedis artery in the ankle. The accompanying deep peroneal nerve has already given off its muscular innervations in its distal course. Thus raising the anterior tibial flap based on the distal periosteal perforators requires less dissection and better preserves vascularity and innervation of the limb. Because they are closely adherent to the periosteum of the tibia, segments of periosteum must be harvested to preserve these perforators.

The reverse-flow anterior tibial artery flap can be harvested and is vascularized by the anastomotic plexus between the anterior tibial and posterior tibial arterial system around the ankle and in the foot. The deep plantar artery, a branch of the dorsalis pedis artery, communicates with the deep plantar arch, a continuation of the lateral plantar artery, at the base of the first metatarsal. This forms the most-distal and most-significant anastomosis (level 1,

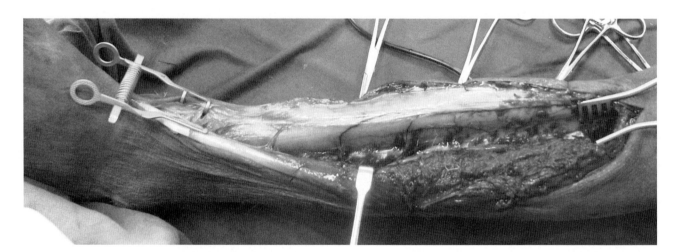

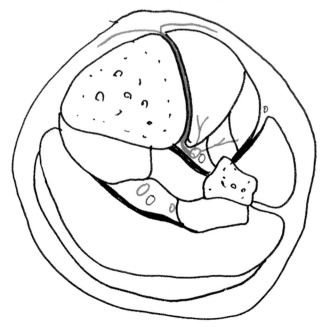

FIG. 1. Top: Periosteal perforators of the anterior tibial artery supplying the flap, with tibialis anterior muscle retracted laterally. Bottom: Cross section of leg illustrating relation of anterior tibial artery periosteal perforator with interosseous membrane and lateral surface of tibia.

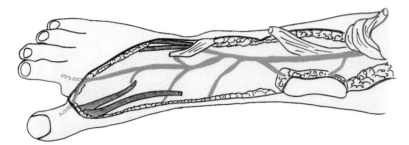

FIG. 2. Reverse anterior tibial flap anatomy. Schematic diagram illustrating the three levels of ankle anastomoses of anterior and posterior tibial systems supplying the flap.

metatarsal anastomosis). Arising 4 cm proximal to the deep plantar artery are the medial and lateral tarsal branches of the dorsalis pedis artery (level 2, tarsal anastomosis). The medial and lateral malleolar branches originate a further 2 cm proximally (level 3, malleolar anastomosis). The tarsal branches are covered by the muscle of the extensor hallucis brevis muscle, which can be used as a landmark (Fig. 2).

FLAP DESIGN AND DIMENSIONS

Preoperatively, the patient should be assessed to determine the presence of both anterior and posterior tibial artery systems. A clinically palpable posterior tibial and dorsalis pedis pulse is a reliable and simple way. In electing to use this technique to resurface a dorsal foot wound after trauma, an angiogram of the foot can be done preoperatively to ascertain the integrity of the deep plantar artery, which forms a direct communication of the two systems.

The anterior tibial artery is outlined by joining the midpoint between the tibial tuberosity and fibular head proximally and the midpoint between the medial and lateral malleolus distally. To resurface a dorsal foot or toe defect, the flap is designed centered on the lower third of the artery, where the artery is superficial, with the pivot point clearly marked. Longer flaps allow more perforators to be harvested and facilitate primary closure of the donor site, if the flap is less than 3 cm wide. The cutaneous vascular territory of the anterior tibial artery has been demonstrated to reach 2 cm medial to the anterior border of the tibia (10). It will be prudent to restrict the medial margin to the anterior border of the tibia, to minimize the exposure of the bone.

For the reverse-flow flap to be successful, it is of vital importance that the design of the flap take into consideration the following points. First, the deep plantar artery should be preserved, as this forms the most distal level of anastomosis. Second, the pivot point of the reverse anterior tibial flap must be determined before the procedure. It is a good measure to add another 1 cm of pedicle length for tension-free transposition, with the ankle adopting its natural posture of slight plantar flexion. To resurface the most distal and plantar aspect of the big toe, the malleolar and tarsal anastomoses can be sacrificed to increase pedicle length. Third, after islanding the flap, it is prudent to clamp temporarily the anastomosis intended for ligation, as well as the proximal anterior tibial artery, and to release the tourniquet to check for flap vascularity. If the flap cannot be adequately supplied in this situation, it can be converted to a free anterior tibial artery flap, or the flap can be replaced, and an alternative flap can be raised.

OPERATIVE TECHNIQUE

The flap is harvested from the fibular side, carrying out a subfascial dissection to the interval between the tibialis anterior muscle and the tibia. Retracting the tibialis anterior muscle laterally will expose the periosteal perforators (Fig. 1, top). These originate from the posteromedial surface of the anterior tibial artery and must be freed from their attachments to the interosseous membrane (Fig. 1, bottom). As the periosteal perforators are closely adherent to the tibia, it is safe to harvest the underlying segment of periosteum together with the perforators, to prevent damage. The muscular branches of the anterior tibial artery are ligated. The dissection is carried out distally, to expose the first branches of the ankle anastomotic network, the medial and lateral malleolar arteries.

The island flap is then passed under the distal tendons of the TA and EHL to avoid tenting of the artery that runs below these tendons. Access to cover the distal foot and ankle structures is thus accomplished (Fig. 3).

CLINICAL RESULTS

Thirty-three foot and ankle reconstructions with the described technique were performed. The size of the flaps ranged from 6 cm^2 to 45 cm^2. The number of perforators per flap ranged from one to four. Primary closure of the anterior tibial flap donor site was achieved with smaller flaps. The remaining cases required full-thickness skin-graft coverage of the anterior compartment muscles. All the flaps survived (100%); however, two cases had distal-tip necrosis. In the earlier cases, a portion of the flaps developed postoperative venous congestion, which resolved with elevation and release of sutures. Modifications to minimize venous congestion included lower-limb elevation, immobilizing the ankle in a neutral position, as well as attention to preventing tension in the pedicle.

SUMMARY

The reverse anterior tibial flap is a useful option for foot and ankle resurfacing. The principal perfusion for retrograde flow is the lateral plantar artery at the deep plantar artery, supplemented by anastomosis around the ankle joint. In properly selected cases with no previous damage to the ankle and midfoot blood supply, the flap-survival rate is excellent. It is therefore prudent to ensure preoperatively that both anterior and posterior tibial systems are patent, before proceeding with this reconstruction. In our experience, little donor-site morbidity occurs with careful patient selection. However, postoperative management should take into account the not-insignificant problem of venous congestion.

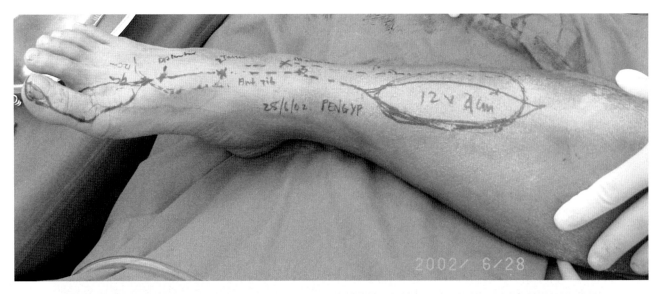

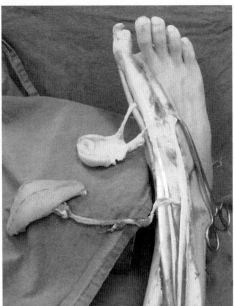

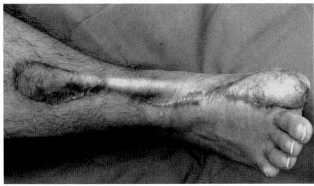

FIG. 3. Simultaneous reconstruction of thumb avulsion injury with a free big-toe wrap-around flap and a pedicled reverse-flow anterior tibial artery flap for the donor site.

References

1. Foucher G, Binhammer P. Plea to save the great toe in total thumb reconstruction. *Microsurgery* 1995;16:373.
2. St-Laurent JY, Lanzetta M. Resurfacing of the donor defect after wrap around toe transfer with a free lateral forearm flap. *J Hand Surg* 1997;22A:9137.
3. Hamilton RB, O'Brien BM, Morrison WA. The cross toe flap. *Br J Plast Surg* 1979;32:213.
4. Samson MC, Morris SF, Tweed AEJ. Dorsalis pedis flap donor site: acceptable or not? *Plast Reconstr Surg* 1998;102:1549.
5. Dong JS, Peng YP, Zhang YS, et al. Reverse anterior tibial artery flap for reconstruction of foot donor site. *Plast Reconstr Surg* 2003;112:1604.
6. Serafin D. The anterior tibial artery flap: discussion by Yousif, N.J. In: *Atlas of microsurgical composite tissue transplantation*. Philadelphia: WB Saunders, 1996;459.
7. Wee JTK. Reconstruction of the lower leg and foot with the reverse-pedicled anterior tibial flap: preliminary report of a new fasciocutaneous flap. *Br J Plast Surg* 1986;39:327.
8. Satoh K, Yoshikawa A, Hayashi M. Reverse-flow anterior tibial flap type III. *Br J Plast Surg* 1988;41:624.
9. Rocha JFR, Gilbert A, Masquelet A, et al. The anterior tibial artery flap: anatomic study and clinical application. *Plast Reconstr Surg* 1987;79:396.
10. Crock JG, Morrison WA. Case report: a vascularized periosteal flap: anatomical study. *Br J Plast Surg* 1992;45:474.

CHAPTER 512 ■ MEDIAL PLANTAR FLAP

R. E. SHANAHAN

Skin defects of the plantar surface of the heel pose a difficult problem for the reconstructive surgeon. In the absence of subcutaneous tissue, split-thickness skin grafts tend to break down under the influence of pressure and constant shearing forces, and distant flaps lack sensation and tend to be bulky.

INDICATIONS

The plantar concavity or non-weight-bearing region of the sole has sufficient surface area to cover the entire plantar surface of the heel. Because the plantar concavity derives its sensory innervation from the fourth and fifth lumbar nerve roots, innervated flaps from this region are capable of restoring sensation to heel surfaces that are anesthetic as a result of lesions of the first and second sacral nerve roots. The medial plantar artery and nerve can be used in designing a plantar transposition flap that is both arterialized and innervated (1,2).

ANATOMY

The medial plantar artery is the lesser of two terminal branches of the posterior tibial artery. It arises behind the origin of the abductor hallucis muscle and courses deep to the plantar fascia between the abductor hallucis and the flexor digitorum brevis muscles. It gives branches to each muscle and finally terminates in small digital branches to the medial two or three toes. Throughout its course, it supplies the skin of the medial two thirds of the plantar concavity through direct cutaneous branches and through musculocutaneous branches by way of the abductor hallucis. All branches originate deep to the plantar aponeurosis (Fig. 1).

The medial plantar nerve arises from the tibial nerve behind the medial malleolus. It accompanies the medial

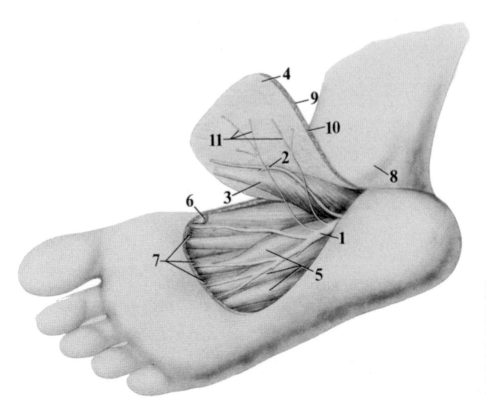

FIG. 1. Anatomy of the medial plantar artery. *1,* Medial plantar nerve; *2,* medial plantar artery; *3,* abductor hallucis; *4,* plantar aponeurosis; *5,* flexor digitorum brevis; *6,* tendon of the abductor hallucis; *7,* divided branches of the medial plantar artery; *8,* medial malleolus; *9,* skin; *10,* subcutaneous tissue; *11,* plantar cutaneous branches of the medial plantar nerve.

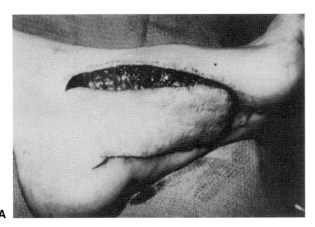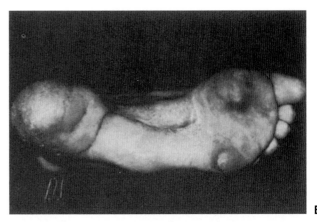

FIG. 2. A: Heel ulcer resulting from injury to the first and second sacral nerve roots. B: Postoperative result 3 years later. (From Shanahan, Gingrass, ref. 1, with permission.)

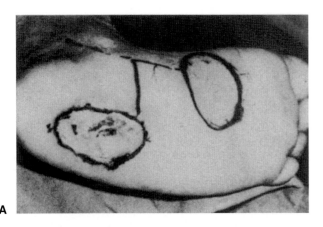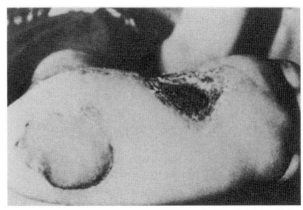

FIG. 3. A: A 5 × 6-cm plantar heel defect. B: Early postoperative result using a medial plantar neurovascular island flap. (From Harrison, Morgan, ref. 2, with permission.)

plantar artery and terminates in one proper digital and three common digital nerves. It provides motor branches to the abductor hallucis, the flexor digitorum brevis, and the medial lumbricals. Sensory branches perforate the plantar fasciae and are distributed to the skin of the medial two thirds of the plantar concavity. The plantar cutaneous fascicles can be separated from the remainder of the nerve by perineurial dissection. The greater saphenous vein and the venae comitantes provide venous outflow.

OPERATIVE TECHNIQUE

The presence of a patent medial plantar artery should be verified using a Doppler device or arteriography. The surface design of the flap may be varied according to need. Dissection is begun distally. After the skin incision is deepened through the plantar fascia, the digital branches of the artery are divided. As dissection is carried proximally, the plantar cutaneous nerve branches are identified and separated from the medial plantar nerve by perineurial dissection using magnification, and the arterial branches to the flexor digitorum brevis are divided. Finally, as the artery and nerve branches pass proximally beneath the abductor hallucis, this muscle must be divided near its insertion in order to achieve mobility of the flap. If further mobility is desired, the proximal attachments of the plantar fascia and the origin of the abductor hallucis

also may be divided (Fig. 2). Although the base of the flap need not be wide, an effort should be made to preserve the greater saphenous vein along with its plantar tributaries. It may be necessary to mobilize the vein by dividing the dorsal tributaries. After the flap is transferred, the donor area is resurfaced with a split-thickness skin graft.

The principle of using the medial plantar artery and nerve has been further amplified (2) by designing a neurovascular island flap for covering a 5 × 6 cm plantar heel defect. Figure 3 illustrates the design, execution, and early postoperative result of this innovative procedure.

SUMMARY

The medial plantar flap provides a method of covering skin defects of the plantar surface of the heel. It has the advantages of being an arterialized sensory flap and is of good quality for the special requirements of the plantar surface.

References

1. Shanahan RE, Gingrass RP. Medial plantar sensory flap for the coverage of heel defects. *Plast Reconstr Surg* 1979;64:295.
2. Harrison DH, Morgan BDG. The instep island flap to resurface plantar defects. *Br J Plast Surg* 1981;34:315.

CHAPTER 513 ■ LATERAL CALCANEAL ARTERY SKIN FLAP

L. C. ARGENTA

EDITORIAL COMMENT

Of the local flaps around the ankle, this is probably the most reliable, although its usefulness is limited.

The lateral calcaneal artery skin flap is an extremely reliable flap for providing sensate coverage for the posterior heel in one stage (1). The extended form of the flap reaches the plantar portion of the heel. Because it includes a random area, however, it is not as reliable as the shorter version.

ANATOMY

The lateral calcaneal artery skin flap is an axial-pattern flap that contains the lateral calcaneal artery, lesser saphenous vein, and sural nerve (Fig. 1). The lateral calcaneal artery is an almost constant terminal branch of the peroneal artery. Occasionally, it can be present as the terminal branch of the posterior tibial artery. The artery, paralleled by one or two small veins, is located in the subcutaneous tissue at the level of the lateral malleolus, within 1 cm lateral to the gastrocnemius tendon. From this point, the artery slowly descends into a deeper plane to lie immediately over the extensor retinaculum covering the peroneus longus and peroneus brevis tendons.

The artery usually bifurcates at this point, and the tributaries branch distally toward the plantar surface of the heel and toward the head of the fifth metatarsal bone. In most

cases, discrete branches of these vessels persist almost to the head of the fifth metatarsal. In approximately 20% of patients, a rete plexus forms over the retinaculum and spreads distally.

The sural nerve lies anterior to the artery and parallels it. It is almost uniformly within 10 mm of the artery (see Fig. 3).

The Doppler probe has been most useful in determining the patency of the calcaneal artery. In persons who have been exposed to significant trauma or in cases of severe atherosclerosis, it is important to determine directional flow, since retrograde flow may occur. Directional Doppler scans or digital occlusion of the dorsalis pedis and posterior tibial vessels can be used to determine directional flow. In patients in whom the extremities have been exposed to severe trauma, an angiogram is necessary to ensure that at least one other vessel to the foot remains intact.

Studies on patients with atherosclerosis demonstrated that the peroneal artery is usually the last vessel of the trifurcation to be significantly compromised (2–5). In fact, patients with severe atherosclerosis may have a significantly enlarged calcaneal artery that functions as a collateral vessel because of occlusion of the remaining infrapopliteal vessels.

The peroneal artery is rarely involved, even in patients with severe diabetes, although diabetics have more severe atherosclerotic disease in the infrapopliteal major vessels than nondiabetics. In my experience, diabetics have suffered fewer complications with the axial portion of the flap than nondiabetics. When the extended portion of the flap has been employed, however, the risk of complications and infection has been higher than in nondiabetics.

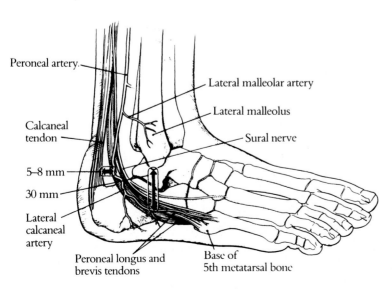

FIG. 1. The anatomy of the lateral foot and ankle region. (From Grabb, Argenta, ref. 1, with permission.)

1467

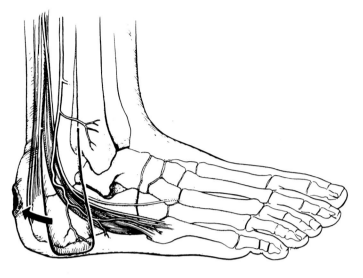

FIG. 2. The short total axial version of the lateral calcaneal artery skin flap is localized directly over the artery. The course of the artery has been previously marked out with the aid of a Doppler device. The dimensions of the flap are determined by the size of the defect. (From Grabb, Argenta, ref. 1, with permission.)

FLAP DESIGN AND DIMENSIONS

The proximal 8 cm of the flap, that is, the vertical distance between the lateral malleolus and the plantar surface of the heel, is completely axial. The flap can be extended up to 6 cm more distally by including a random portion of tissue proximal to the base of the fifth metatarsal.

The position and course of the calcaneal artery is marked on the skin (Fig. 2). With the leg dependent, the course of the lesser saphenous vein is also marked out. The length and width of the desired flap are planned in reverse, using a cloth pattern over the defect and transposing it to lie over the previously demarcated artery.

The pedicle of both versions of the flap lies immediately above the level of the lateral malleolus. The base of the flap is usually left intact and optimally should be at least 4 cm wide. On occasion, the flap can be elevated as an island, but care must be taken to avoid trauma to the lesser saphenous vein during rotation. Because this is an axial-pattern flap, the distal portion may be wider than the proximal end if necessary.

The short version of the flap (Figs. 2 and 3) encompasses the vertical distance between the lateral malleolus and the plantar heel. If there is an excessive amount of callous or slightly greater length is required, the flap can be gently curved distally, maintaining the previously marked artery as close to the center of the flap as possible.

When a larger amount of tissue is necessary to cover areas of the plantar heel, the flap can be extended to include a random area (Fig. 4). In this case, the flap curves distally in the direction of the base of the fifth metatarsal. Dissections of adult cadavers have revealed that the lateral calcaneal artery is usually 30 mm below the tip of the malleolus. The curve of the extended flap must be such as to incorporate the vessel as close as possible to its center.

OPERATIVE TECHNIQUE

Axial-Pattern Flap

Dissection is most easily begun at the lateral aspect of the calcaneal tendon and is carried down distally to the periosteum of the os calcis. The plane is then developed, leaving the periosteum intact. The anterior incision is made immediately behind the lateral malleolus and carried down through the subcutaneous tissues. The flap is mobilized in a retrograde fashion.

The neuromuscular structures lie in the deep surface of the subcutaneous tissues and can be visualized if the dissection is too superficial. Optimally, the vessels are never exposed and therefore not traumatized.

Dissection is carried out in a retrograde fashion to the level of the lateral malleolus. The Doppler probe can be used intra-

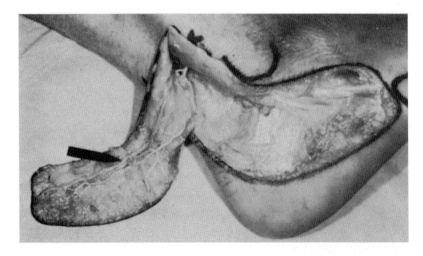

FIG. 3. The undersurface of the cadaver dissection of the calcaneal artery skin flap. The sural nerve (arrow) parallels the calcaneal artery. In practice, these vessels need never be visualized, since extensive dissection may traumatize them. (From Grabb, Argenta, ref. 1, with permission.)

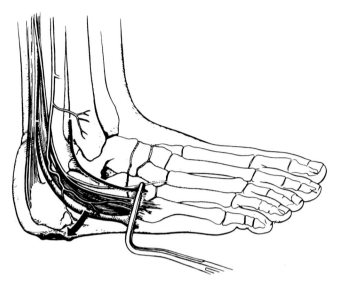

FIG. 4. The long version of the calcaneal artery flap includes a distal random area. This flap is useful for coverage of plantar foot defects. (From Grabb, Argenta, ref. 1, with permission.)

operatively when the tourniquet is avoided to ensure that the vessel is incorporated within the flap. Immediately above the malleolus, the calcaneal artery begins to plunge to a deeper level. A minimal amount of dissection can facilitate rotation, but deeper dissection may be perilous.

Rotation to the defect is then performed, and the flap is inset. No deep sutures are used. A small silicone drain is left in the bed of the lesion, especially if underlying bone has been removed. A split-thickness skin graft is placed over the donor defect and immobilized with a tieover dressing.

Postoperatively, the patient is kept in bed with the leg elevated for 5 to 7 days. This prolonged elevation minimizes skin graft loss as well as dehiscence of the flap secondary to edema.

Extended Flap

Initial dissection is identical to that for the short flap. Three to 5 mm anterior to the lateral calcaneal tendon, the dissection leaves the periosteal plane and continues distally on the lateral aspect of the abductor digiti minimi muscle and the peroneal retinaculum overlying the peroneus longus and peroneus brevis tendons. This flap is dissected, leaving the distal end of the flap uncut.

Once total undermining has been accomplished, an atraumatic vascular clamp is placed across the distal end of the flap and fluorescein is given intravenously. In approximately 60% of all nondiabetic patients, there is adequate fluorescence immediately so that the flap can be divided and rotated. In cases where fluorescein does not reach the distal margin, the flap is sutured back into place and the distal end is divided in stages. Division is begun 5 to 7 days after the first operation.

It is important that the patient remain in bed after the initial operation while waiting for the delay procedures.

When the extended flap is rotated, the donor defect is again covered with a split-thickness skin graft. I have not allowed patients to place full weight on the heel that has been covered with an extended flap for a period of 6 weeks to avoid shear. During this period, a splint is important to maintain a 90-degree position of the foot.

CLINICAL RESULTS

This flap has proven effective and reliable even in older patients with atherosclerotic occlusive disease and diabetes. If the calcaneal artery has been present on Doppler examination and has antegrade flow, there have been no significant complications with the short version of the flap. Similarly, when the extended version of the flap has been adequately delayed, there have been few complications.

Postoperative infection, especially in diabetics, has been the most frequent complication. Prophylactic antibiotics have not significantly decreased the incidence of these effects. Shearing of the flap from the underlying bed has been observed if ambulation is begun prior to complete healing.

Two of my patients have undergone amputations of toes and a portion of the foot several years after the lateral calcaneal artery flap because of progressive diabetes. In both patients, there has been no evidence that the flap was compromised.

All the patients who have had sensation in the distribution of the sural nerve have maintained sensation postoperatively and have been able to discriminate pinprick and pressure within the flap. I have experienced no breakdown of the transposed flap despite frequent trauma in the heel area.

This operation, to my knowledge, has been performed on two children. The location of the vessels and technique have been similar to those in adults.

SUMMARY

The lateral calcaneal artery skin flap can be used to provide sensory skin coverage to the heel in one stage. Occasionally, the extended form of the flap may need a delay procedure to cover the plantar aspect of the heel.

References

1. Grabb WC, Argenta LC. The lateral calcaneal artery skin flap (the lateral calcaneal artery, lesser saphenous vein, and sural nerve skin flap). *Plast Reconstr Surg* 1981;68:723.
2. Wessler S, Schlesinger MJ. Studies in peripheral arterial occlusive disease: I. Methods and pathologic findings in amputated limbs. *Circulation* 1953; 7:641.
3. Conrad MD. Large and small artery occlusion in diabetics and nondiabetics with severe vascular disease. *Circulation* 1967;36:83.
4. Haimovici, H. Patterns of arteriosclerotic lesions of the lower extremity. *Arch Surg* 1967;95:918.
5. Barner HB, Kaiser GC, Willman VL. Blood flow in the diabetic leg. *Circulation* 1971;43:391.

CHAPTER 514 ■ PLANTAR ARTERY-SKIN-FASCIA FLAP

R. S. REIFFEL

When resurfacing defects on the plantar surface of the foot, consideration must be given to the specialized nature of the missing tissue. Restoration may be more desirable than a skin graft (1–7). The thick and unyielding nature of plantar skin makes rotation of a wide-based flap difficult. The design of an arterialized flap eliminates any constraints on the size of the skin pedicle and permits reliable transfer of large amounts of skin and subcutaneous tissue. Moreover, incorporation of nerves in the pedicle maintains sensibility in the reconstructed part (8).

INDICATIONS

Defects on the plantar aspect of the calcaneus can be covered easily with a proximally based flap (see Fig. 4). With greater flap rotation, defects on the posterior surface of the calcaneus, including the level of insertion of the Achilles tendon, also can be reliably covered. The distally based flap can be used to cover defects over the metatarsal head region (see Fig. 5); however, this flap cannot provide sensory coverage because it is distally based.

ANATOMY

Arterial Supply

The posterior tibial artery supplies three main plantar vessels. The lateral plantar artery crosses the foot in the plane between the flexor digitorum brevis and the quadratus plantae muscles (Fig. 1). In roughly the central third of the foot, it turns in a medial direction, passing deep to the oblique head of the adductor hallucis muscle to form the plantar arch. The termination of the plantar arch is the deep plantar artery, which passes between the first and second metatarsals to reach the dorsalis pedis artery. Connections also exist between the plantar arch and the medial plantar artery. Common digital arteries originate from the plantar arch and supply the toes. Small vessels perforate the overlying flexor digitorum brevis muscle and plantar fascia in a vertical direction to connect the lateral plantar artery with the overlying skin.

The medial plantar artery courses distally superficial to the quadratus plantae and deep to the abductor hallucis and

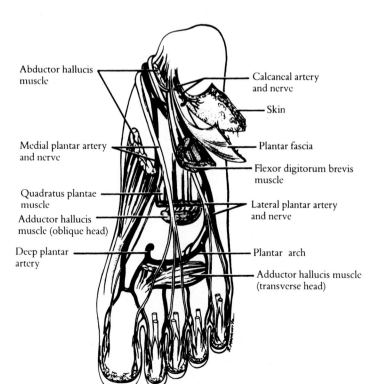

FIG. 1. The lateral plantar nerve and artery cross the foot between the flexor digitorum brevis and quadratus plantae muscles, sending perforating branches through the plantar fascia to the skin of the central third of the foot. The calcaneal artery courses in a posterior direction to supply the posterior third of the foot. The deep plantar artery connects the dorsalis pedis artery with the plantar arch, which also receives a major supply from the lateral plantar artery and a minor supply from the medial plantar artery.

1470

flexor digitorum brevis muscles. After connecting with the plantar arch, it terminates in the big toe.

The calcaneal artery perforates the flexor digitorum brevis muscle and plantar fascia near their origin from the os calcis. Thereafter, while passing in a posterior direction, it branches to supply the weight-bearing calcaneal skin.

Nerve Supply

The lateral plantar, medial plantar, and calcaneal nerves follow the same course as that described for the equivalent arteries, with one exception. The lateral plantar nerve supplies only the lateral one and one-half toes, with the medial plantar nerve supplying the remainder.

FLAP DESIGN AND DIMENSIONS

The fact that blood may reach the lateral plantar artery either antegrade from the posterior tibial artery or retrograde from the plantar arch makes the design of two lateral plantar artery skin-muscle-fascia arterialized flaps possible.

Proximally Based Flap

If the artery is divided distally just before it becomes the plantar arch, a proximally based flap may be designed whose point of rotation is located just anteromedial to the os calcis (Fig. 2). A 10-cm-long, 7-cm-wide flap can be designed easily. The pos-

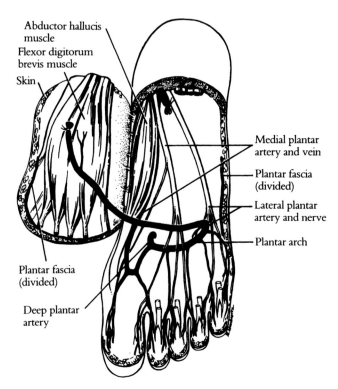

FIG. 3. Distally based flap. The lateral plantar artery is divided just anterior to the calcaneus. The lateral plantar nerve is left in situ. The flexor digitorum brevis muscle and plantar fascia are divided as before. Deep dissection in the region of the plantar arch should be avoided. Exposure of the deep structures in this diagram is for explanatory purposes only.

terior margin of the flap is generally the defect to be reconstructed. The lateral margin should be on the side of the foot, off the weight-bearing surface. The medial margin curves sharply back toward the medial malleolus, making the skin pedicle narrow. Special care should be taken not to extend the distal margin of the flap onto the metatarsal head weight-bearing skin. The secondary defect, either closed primarily or resurfaced by a split-thickness skin graft, is located between the calcaneal and metatarsal head weight-bearing areas.

Distally Based Flap

Division of the lateral plantar artery near its origin from the posterior tibial artery allows the design of a second flap whose blood supply is retrograde from the plantar arch (Fig. 3). The flap may be designed with the same dimensions as previously described, with care being taken to plan the medial and lateral incisions slightly on the sides of the foot, off the weight-bearing surface. In addition, the tip of the flap (posterior skin incision) must not extend onto the calcaneal weight-bearing area. The skin pedicle is kept narrow. With a rotation point overlying the plantar arch, the flap may be used to resurface defects of the metatarsal head region (see Fig. 5). The secondary defect lies once again in a non-weight-bearing area, anterior to the calcaneus.

OPERATIVE TECHNIQUE

Prior to ligation of the lateral plantar artery either proximally or distally, patency of both the dorsalis pedis and posterior tibial arteries must be established. One should, either by

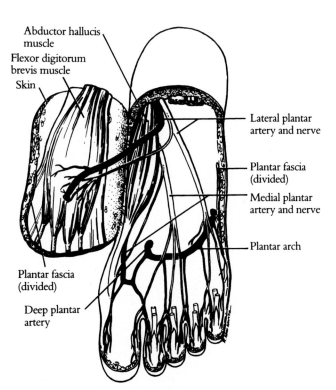

FIG. 2. Proximally based flap. The lateral plantar artery is divided just proximal to the plantar arch. The branches of the lateral plantar nerve that supply the flap are split longitudinally from the remainder of that nerve. The flexor digitorum brevis muscle and plantar fascia are divided proximally from the calcaneus and distally at the level of the skin incision, which is located just proximal to the metatarsal head weight-bearing region.

manual palpation or with the aid of a Doppler flowmeter, ascertain that neither pulse disappears when the other vessel is manually occluded. In doubtful cases, an arteriogram may be helpful. If both of the preceding vessels are not patent, surgical division of the lateral plantar artery may interrupt the only collateral blood supply to a major portion of the foot and is, therefore, inadvisable.

Excision of the lesion or pressure sore, including all infected or desiccated bone, and lowering of bony prominences such as the anterior lip of the calcaneus are performed first.

Whether a proximally or distally based flap is planned, dissection always commences with the lateral incision, in the middle third of the foot. The skin and subcutaneous tissues are sharply incised. After the underlying plantar fascia has been divided parallel to the skin incision, the undersurface of that fascia is bluntly explored for any identifiable perforating vessels. Once any vessel is found, no matter how small, it should be bluntly traced proximally to the lateral plantar artery. If one encounters the long toe flexor tendons, the plane of dissection is too deep.

Once the lateral plantar artery has been identified, it is mobilized in association with the overlying plantar fascia and skin (Fig. 4B). Blunt dissection along the artery will expose its accompanying venae comitantes and the lateral plantar nerve, all of which must be preserved.

To achieve flap mobility, the numerous fibrous septa attaching the plantar fascia to the metatarsals must be divided. Traction on the flap tightens the septa and allows their easy palpation. After blunt dissection along the neurovascular bundle to protect the artery and nerve, the septa are carefully divided. The skin incision is elongated, further flap rotation is achieved, and more septa are identified and divided. The plantar fascia and the flexor digitorum brevis muscles must be divided both at their origins from the calcaneus and at the level of the distal transverse skin incision (see Fig. 2).

In the case of a proximally based flap, the lateral plantar artery is divided between ligatures just before it turns medially to become the plantar arch. In the case of a distally based flap, that same vessel is divided just anterior to the calcaneus (see Fig. 3). On some occasions, when only a small amount of flap rotation is required, it may be possible to mobilize and stretch the vessel sufficiently to make its division unnecessary. In such cases, division should be avoided (Fig. 5). All the vascular connections between the lateral plantar artery and the overlying skin are preserved. Deep muscular branches are divided between small stainless steel hemostatic clips. In the case of a proximally based flap, the lateral plantar nerve may be split longitudinally. Perforating branches may therefore be included with the overlying flap while sensibility of the lateral toes is preserved. Because retrograde nerve pathways do not exist, no branches of the nerve are included with the distally based flap.

The processes of elongating the skin incision, protecting the neurovascular pedicle between, dividing the fibrous septa, and rotating the flap are continued until the flap can be transferred into its desired position without any tension. The skin pedicle can be made as narrow as necessary to eliminate tension or dog-ear formation, as the flap is of an axial nature.

The skin is closed over a low-vacuum, soft suction catheter. If the secondary defect cannot be closed primarily without tension, it is covered with a split-thickness skin graft.

The suction catheter is removed after 2 to 3 days or when drainage decreases to 5 to 10 ml in any 24-hour period. Elevation of the foot is maintained for 1 week if no skin graft was required or for 2 weeks if grafting was necessary. Ambulation on crutches is begun at that point. Progressive weight bearing is begun, culminating in full weight bearing 1 or 2 weeks later, as tolerated.

CLINICAL RESULTS

If the preoperative analysis of the vascular system has been accurate, and if care is taken not to injure the lateral plantar artery during the process of flap elevation, no flap ischemia should be expected. Diabetics with small-vessel disease may

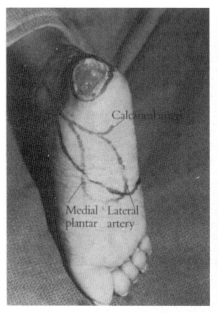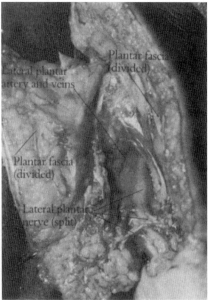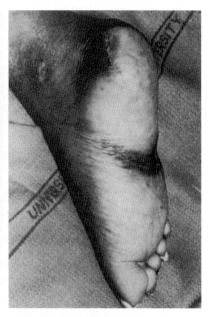

A–C

FIG. 4. A: A medium-sized posteroinferior pressure sore in a 55-year-old woman. The skin incisions and vascular supply are outlined. **B:** Lateral view of undersurface of flap. The plantar fascia and flexor digitorum brevis muscle have been divided and the neurovascular pedicle exposed. The lateral plantar artery has been ligated and the nerve split longitudinally. **C:** Appearance at 1 month. The secondary defect has been closed primarily; no skin graft was required. (From Reiffel, McCarthy, ref. 8, with permission.)

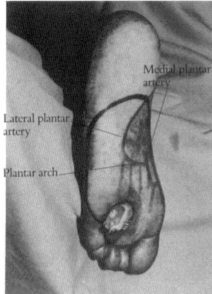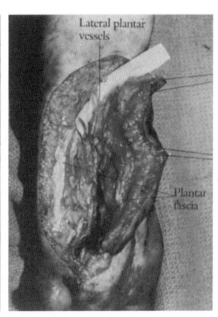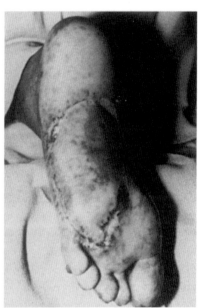

A–C

FIG. 5. **A:** One week after debridement of an infected ulcer in a 37-year-old patient with lepromatous leprosy. Oblique view shows lateral skin incision to be slightly on side of foot, off the weight-bearing surface. (From Reiffel and McCarthy, ref. 8, with permission.) **B:** The plantar fascia has been divided and the lateral plantar vessels identified. **C:** Oblique view at 3 weeks. Ulcer is closed and infection is gone. Skin-grafted secondary defect is on non-weight-bearing portion of foot.

exhibit delayed healing of incisions and skin grafts, but no hematomas, infections, wound breakdowns, or instances of necrosis should be expected unless surgical technique has been improper.

Neuroma symptoms in ambulatory patients may be troublesome at first, but they diminish with time and with desensitization training. Special insoles may be added temporarily to the shoe to redistribute pressure away from the nerve. No loss of stability seems to result from division of the plantar fascia. The long-term effect of division of one of the major pathways of blood to the plantar arch, especially with the possible formation of atherosclerosis in the remaining pathways, is not known.

SUMMARY

The plantar artery flap is an axial flap that can be used to provide durable cover for plantar and calcaneal defects. The proximally based flap is innervated, whereas the nerve must be divided in order to mobilize the distally based flap.

References

1. Mir y Mir L. Functional graft of the heel. *Plast Reconstr Surg* 1954; 14:444.
2. Snyder GB, Edgerton MT. The principle of the island neurovascular flap in the management of ulcerated anesthetic weight-bearing areas of the lower extremity. *Plast Reconstr Surg* 1965;36:518.
3. Kaplan I. Neurovascular island flap in the treatment of trophic ulceration of the heel. *Br J Plast Surg* 1969;22:143.
4. Buntine JA. Repair of the sole. *Med J Aust* 1970;1:520.
5. McCraw JB. Selection of alternative local flaps in the leg and foot. *Clin Plast Surg* 1979;6:227.
6. Buncke HJ, Colen LB. An island flap from the first web space of the foot to cover plantar ulcers. *Br J Plast Surg* 1980;33:242.
7. Shanahan RE, Gingrass RP. Medial plantar sensory flap for coverage of heel defects. *Plast Reconstr Surg* 1979;64:295.
8. Reiffel RS, McCarthy JG. Coverage of heel and sole defects: a new subfascial arterialized flap. *Plast Reconstr Surg* 1980;66:250.

CHAPTER 515 ■ MEDIAL PLANTAR FLAP

D. MARTIN, B. GOROWITZ, J. M. PERES, AND J. BAUDET

The authors modify the classic medial plantar flap by shifting its vascular supply, to create reverse flow in the lateral plantar artery and vein. This flap is useful for covering defects in the distal weight-bearing areas of the foot over a wide range.

INDICATIONS

This modified flap, because of its wider arc of rotation, is suitable for a variety of local defects, extending the range of flap coverage and allowing it to reach the tips of the toes. It provides excellent cover for the distal weight-bearing areas of the foot when a classic flap cannot be used, due to anatomic anomalies and/or in the presence of an unreliable flap blood supply (1–9).

ANATOMY

The classic medial plantar artery derives its main blood supply from the medial plantar artery, a terminal branch of the posterior tibial artery. In our modification, reverse blood flow is created from the lateral plantar artery, after dividing the posterior tibial artery just proximal to its distal bifurcation. Survival of the reverse flow is ensured by the rich anastomoses that usually occur between the dorsalis pedis and lateral plantar arteries. Venous return is also lengthened by a similar reverse flow pattern (Fig. 1).

FLAP DESIGN AND DIMENSIONS

The flap modification, although not changing typical flap dissection, allows the transfer of the pedicled flap distally. The authors call this procedure a "reverse flow Y-V pedicle extension of the flap." The idea is to raise the flap distally on a branch of the Y-like vascular bifurcation of the posterior tibial artery. Sectioning the trunk at the bifurcation turns the Y into

a V vascular pattern, allowing distal mobilization of the flap on the remaining branch of the V. The distal range of flap transfer can reach twice the length of the unmodified flap. The arterial blood supply is provided by reverse flow through the attached remaining branch of the V, and venous drainage is also ensured (Fig. 2).

OPERATIVE TECHNIQUE (FIG. 3)

First, the main trunk of the posterior tibial artery is traced to its bifurcation into the medial plantar and lateral plantar arteries, after releasing the abductor muscle of the big toe. Then, the flap is raised in the usual fashion. It is relatively easy, after dislocating the plantar flexor, to isolate the lateral plantar pedicle. After clamping the posterior tibial artery to evaluate flow, it is divided just proximal to the bifurcation. Finally, the vascular bundle of the lateral plantar pedicle is isolated from its accessory nerve, and enough further dissection is carried out to allow the reverse flow artery island flap to be transferred to its desired site (Figs. 4 and 5).

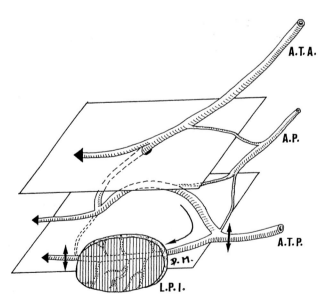

FIG. 1. Medial view of the vascular network of the right foot. *AP* = peroneal artery; *ATA* = anterior tibial artery; *ATP* = posterior tibial artery divided proximal to its bifurcation; *LPI* = medial plantar flap. (From Martin et al, ref. 5, with permission.)

REVERSE FLOW Y-V

PEDICLE EXTENSION OF A FLAP

1/ Normal flow
2/ Reverse flow
   consecutive
   to the section
   of the trunk of
   a vascular
   bifurcation
3/ The distal range
   of transposition
   of the flap (X)
   can reach twice
   the length AB

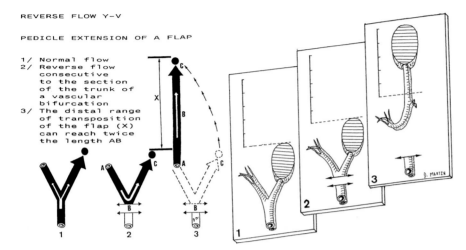

FIG. 2. Reverse flow Y-V pedicle extension or elongation of flap. 1, normal flow; 2, reverse flow after section of the common trunk at the vascular bifurcation; 3, distal range of flap transfer (X); the reach is twice the length of AB. (From Martin et al, ref. 5, with permission.)

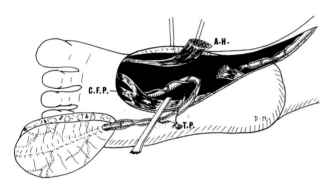

FIG. 3. Medial plantar flap with lateral plantar pedicle. AH, abductor hallucis; CFP, flexor digitorum brevis; TP, sectioned tibialis posterior artery.

A–C

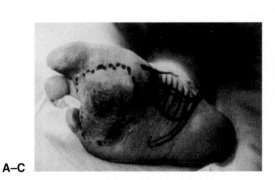
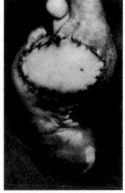
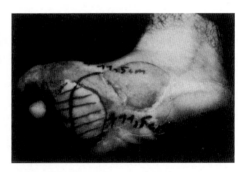

FIG. 4. Patient with electrical burn of the forefoot and exposure of second metatarsal head. A: Outline of medial plantar flap. B: Postoperative view on day 3. C: Result at 1 year, showing 11.5-cm flap advancement.

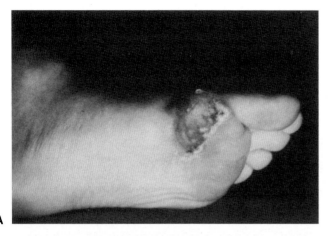

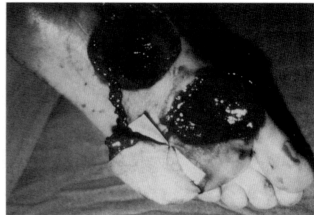

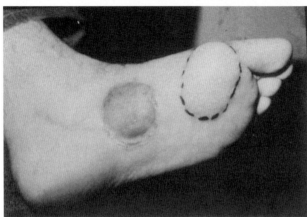

FIG. 5. **A:** Scar tissue in first metatarsal head region subsequent to skin avulsion. **B:** Perioperative view of medial plantar flap based on lateral plantar pedicle. **C:** Result at 6 months.

SUMMARY

A modified medial plantar flap, based on the lateral plantar artery and vein with reversed flow, can cover any area of the foot.

References

1. Torii S, Namiki Y, Mori R. Reverse-flow island flap: clinical report and venous drainage. *Plast Reconstr Surg* 1987;79:600.
2. Amarante J, Martins A, Reis J. A distally based median plantar flap. *Ann Plast Surg* 1978;20:468.
3. Amarante J, Martins A, Reis J. A distally based median plantar flap (letter). *Plast Reconstr Surg* 1987;81:137.
4. Martin D. Le lambeau sous-mental. *Ann Chir Plast Esthet* 1990;35:480.
5. Martin D, Gorowitz B, Peres JM, Baudet J. Le lambeau plantaire interne a pedicule plantaire externe. *Ann Chir Plast Esthet* 1991;36:544.
6. Martin D, Legaillard P, Bakhach J, et al. L'allongement pediculaire en YV a flux retrograde: moyen pour doubler l'arc de rotation d'un lambeau sous certaines conditions. *Ann Chir Plast Esthet* 1994;39:403.
7. Panconi B, Vidal L, Bovet JL, et al. Utilisation du lambeau plantaire interne pour la couverture des pertes de substance du talon. *Ann Chir Plast Esthet* 19885;30:78.
8. Baker GL, Newton ED, Franklin JD. Fasciocutaneous island flap based on the medial plantar artery: clinical applications for leg, ankle and forefoot. *Plast Reconstr Surg* 1990;85:47.
9. Shanahan RE, Gingrass RP. Medial plantar sensory flap for coverage of heel defects. *Plast Reconstr Surg* 1979;64:2295.

CHAPTER 516 ■ LATERAL SUPRAMALLEOLAR FLAP

A. C. MASQUELET AND M. C. ROMAÑA

The lateral supramalleolar flap, raised on the lateral aspect of the lower leg, is very useful for covering defects involving the lower leg, ankle, and foot.

INDICATIONS

This reliable and versatile flap has many possibilities. It can be used as a rotation flap with a distal hinge (peninsular flap), which is a quick and easy procedure for covering the distal quarter of the medial aspect of the leg. A proximally-based pedicled flap has a limited arc of rotation, but is sufficient for covering defects in the ankle area. Used as a distally-based pedicled flap, it has a wide range that includes the whole dorsum of the foot, the medial and lateral arches, and the entire heel region. However, although the flap is not advocated for the weight-bearing area of the heel (the skin of the flap is rather thin and delicate), among the best indications for its use are defects of the posterior aspect of the heel, and resurfacing of a stump resulting from a transmetatarsal amputation. A distally-based pedicle flap with a compound pedicle comprising the vascular axis and a band of subcutaneous fascial tissue can be used for distal defects as far as the base of the toes. The lateral supramalleolar flap can be used as a sensory flap by suturing the superficial peroneal nerve to a nerve at the recipient site.

The advantages of the flap are those of any pedicled flap: the rapid and reliable procedure provides an excellent alternative to a free flap in many instances. The principal disadvantages are the division of the superficial peroneal nerve and the scar resulting from skin grafting on the lateral aspect of the leg. Usually, the donor site is quite acceptable, but may be a problem in young women.

ANATOMY (FIG. 1)

The vascular supply is provided by the anastomotic arcade of the ankle. The key anatomic vascular structure is the perforating branch of the peroneal artery, which pierces the interosseous membrane at the distal tibiofibular angle, just proximal to the anterior tibiofibular ligament (1). It anastomoses at a variable level with the anterior lateral malleolar

artery arising from the anterior tibial artery, courses on the anterior tibiofibular ligament, and then descends to the level of the sinus tarsi, where it anastomoses with the lateral tarsal artery and small branches issuing from the lateral plantar artery. Between its emergence from the interosseous membrane and tibiofibular ligament, the perforating artery gives off one or two ascending branches to the skin of the distal half of the lateral aspect of the leg, which constitutes the territory of the flap.

The perforating branch of the peroneal artery is accompanied by small venae comitantes. The branch is sometimes very large and, in some cases, may replace the distal part of the anterior tibial artery. In other rare cases, the perforating branch anastomoses with the anterior tibial artery that courses on the anterior tibiofibular ligament. For these reasons, an arteriogram is always needed preoperatively.

The cutaneous branches issuing from the perforating branch run anteriorly to the fibula and anastomose with the vascular network that accompanies the superficial peroneal nerve. This enters the subcutaneous tissue at the junction of the middle and distal thirds of the leg, and divides into medial and lateral branches at the level of the ankle joint.

These constant anatomic considerations allow clarification of the different varieties of the lateral supramalleolar flap—the territory of all varieties remains the same. The rotation flap maintains continuity of the perforating branch, and no

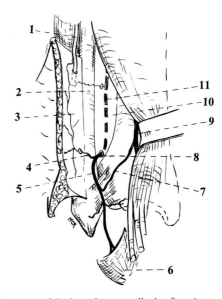

FIG. 1. Anatomy of the lateral supramalleolar flap. *1*, superficial peroneal nerve; *2*, fibula; *3*, territory of the flap; *4*, cutaneous branch for the flap; *5*, ramus perforans; *6*, extensor brevis muscle; *7*, anterior malleolar artery; *8*, emergence of the ramus perforans; *9*, tibialis anterior artery; *10*, interosseous membrane; *11*, peroneal artery.

vascular dissection is required. The pivotal point of the flap is the emergence of the branch through the interosseous membrane. The rotation flap may be a peninsular flap with a distal skin hinge, or an island flap with a very short pedicle that need not be dissected. In both cases, the rotation cannot exceed 90 degrees.

A proximally-based pedicled flap is based on the anterior lateral malleolar artery, when this vessel is suitable. The perforating branch is ligated and severed just proximal to the cutaneous branches to the flap, and just distal to the anastomosis with the anterior lateral malleolar artery. In this case, the flap is supplied by the anterior lateral malleolar artery and through the skin branches issuing from the perforating branch.

A distally-based island pedicled flap is based on the perforating branch, which is ligated and divided just proximal to the cutaneous branch, and released as far as the sinus tarsi that constitutes the pivot point of the pedicle (2). The length of the pedicle is approximately 7 cm; the venae comitantes are sufficient to ensure venous return. When the perforating branch is interrupted in its course distal to the cutaneous branch to the flap, the skin paddle is designed proximally on the lower half of the leg, and the flap is supplied by a subcutaneous fascial pedicle. In this case, the pivot point is the emergence of the perforating branch.

It is also possible to combine a subcutaneous fascial pedicle in continuity with the vascular axis of the perforating branch, until it reaches the sinus tarsi. The flap is designed at the middle of the leg, and the pedicle is approximately 15 cm in length (3). This procedure is valuable for small and very distal defects of the extremity.

FLAP DESIGN AND DIMENSIONS

The boundaries of the largest flap are proximally, the middle of the leg; anteriorly, the crest of the tibia; posteriorly, the fibula; and distally, the emergence of the perforating branch. This latter point is identified on the skin by the depression in the lower part of the tibiofibular space, which can be palpated with a finger. Whatever the dimensions, the design of the flap should include this landmark, as the outline of the flap is traced 2 to 3 cm distal to the landmark. Flap dimensions vary according to the proximal limit; the largest flap is about 20 × 8 cm.

OPERATIVE TECHNIQUE

We begin with the standard distally-based pedicled flap. The patient is supine with a sandbag under the ipsilateral buttock. A tourniquet is applied. The design of the flap, as described above, should include the landmark of emergence of the perforating artery distally. A line of incision is drawn anterior to the lateral malleolus and reaches the depression of the sinus tarsi on the lateral aspect of the hindfoot (Fig. 2).

The skin, including the fascia, is incised in continuity along the anterior margin of the flap, and anterior to the lateral malleolus. A posterior skin hinge is maintained. The pedicle is first exposed, lying deep to the extensor retinaculum, which is incised. The muscles of the extensor compartment are gently retracted, exposing the lower part of the tibiofibular space, in order to identify the vascular structures, chiefly, the cutaneous branch to the flap. The perforating branch is ligated and severed just proximal to the cutaneous branch (Fig. 3). It is sometimes necessary to incise the membrane in order to free the perforating branch. The anastomosis with the anterior lateral malleolar artery is ligated and divided.

Then, the posterior margin of the flap is incised, including the fascia. The superficial peroneal nerve is severed proximally,

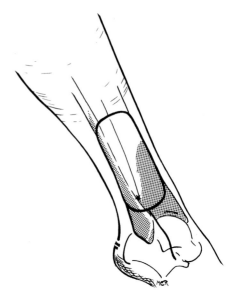

FIG. 2. Design of the flap. The distal landmark should include the emergence of the ramus perforans issuing from the peroneal artery (*star*). Distal incision is performed to the sinus tarsis, to expose the flap pedicle.

and its proximal end is buried in the muscles; the fascial septum, which attaches the flap to the fibula, is progressively released from proximal to distal. At the level of the course of the cutaneous branch to the flap, the septum is subperiosteally released to protect the supplying branches (Fig. 4).

The pedicle is isolated with its surrounding loose areolar tissue, until it reaches the sinus tarsi (Fig. 5).

The posterior edge of the fascia of the extensor digitorum brevis muscle should be divided, in order to avoid compression of the pedicle when it is turned. Closure of the donor site is performed by suturing the peroneal and extensor muscles together. A split-thickness skin graft is applied immediately or a few days later.

For a rotation flap, no dissection or ligature is required in what is a rapid and reliable procedure. The design of the flap should include the tendon of emergence of the perforating branch.

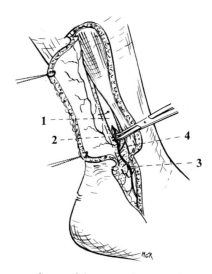

FIG. 3. Ramus perforans of the peroneal artery is ligated and severed just proximal to the cutaneous branch supplying the flap. *1*, interosseous membrane; *2*, cutaneous branch supplying the flap; *3*, flap pedicle; *4*, anterior malleolar artery. This latter inconstant vascular axis may be used as the supplying pedicle for a proximally-based flap.

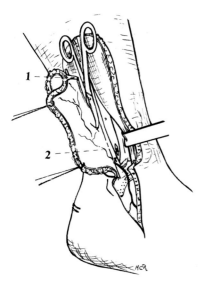

FIG. 4. Release of the flap from the fibula; the septum is incised. *1*, septum; *2*, cutaneous branch.

A distally-based island flap with subcutaneous fascial pedicle is useful when the perforating artery is viable at its emergence, but is interrupted distally. In this case, the pivot point of the pedicle is related to the emergence of the perforating branch. The subcutaneous fascial pedicle is subdermally dissected to 2 cm in width (Fig. 6). If the perforating artery is viable until the sinus tarsi, it can be dissected in continuity with the subcutaneous fascial pedicle. The total pedicle length is about 15 cm when a small flap is raised at the middle of the leg (Fig. 7).

A proximally-based island flap can be utilized when the defect is around the ankle joint. The flap can be raised on the anterior lateral malleolar artery. The territory of the flap is the same as that of a distally-based flap.

CLINICAL RESULTS

More than 60 lateral supramalleolar flaps have been used by our group, with practically all the regions of the foot involved.

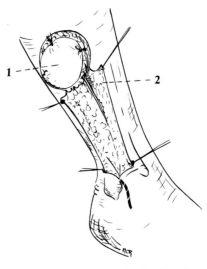

FIG. 6. Variation of the lateral supramalleolar flap. The skin paddle is designed at the middle third of the leg. A subdermal dissection allows raising a subcutaneous fascial pedicle. *1*, skin paddle; *2*, subdermal dissection. Two flaps are elevated to delimit the subcutaneous fascial pedicle. Pedicle length can be increased by freeing the vascular pedicle beyond the emergence of the ramus perforans.

The best indications for use of this flap were defects involving the dorsum of the foot and the posterior aspect of the heel, which require supple skin (Fig. 8). The postoperative course should be managed very cautiously. The foot should be elevated for 5 days postoperatively, and walking is allowed only progressively to avoid flap congestion. An immediate venous congestion of the flap will result from any operative errors. Compressive garments can be used after complete healing.

We would emphasize the following several important points. The flap is not suitable for resurfacing the weight-bearing area of the heel. The rotation flap is very useful for covering defects of the distal quarter of the leg; a peninsular subcutaneous fascial flap can be used to avoid the skin graft at the donor site.

Sensibility of the flap can be restored by suturing the peroneal nerve to a nerve at the recipient site. This procedure is valuable, if the flap is designed in the lower part of the leg, which is supplied by the superficial peroneal nerve.

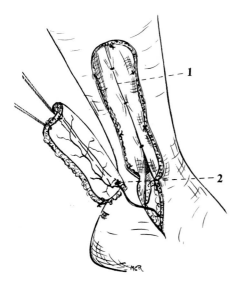

FIG. 5. The flap and its pedicle are raised. *1*, extensor and peroneal muscles are sutured together to provide a well-vascularized bed for the graft; *2*, stump of the severed ramus perforans.

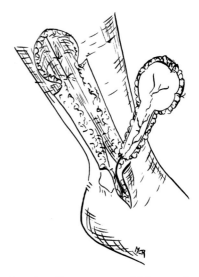

FIG. 7. Arc of rotation allows coverage of defects on the dorsal aspect of the MP joints.

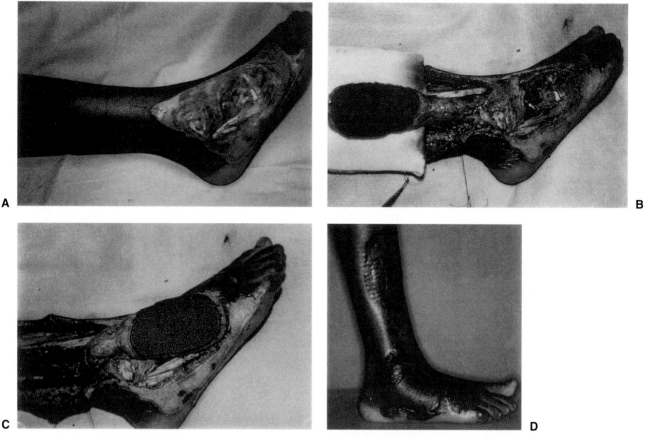

FIG. 8. Clinical case. A: Avulsion of the dorsum of the foot. B: Elevation of flap with a subcutaneous fascial pedicle. The pivot point of the pedicle in this case is the emergence of the ramus perforans. C: Flap at the recipient site. D: Final result.

SUMMARY

The lateral supramalleolar flap, often offering an alternative to a free flap, is reliable and versatile. It can be used for a variety of defects in the foot, ankle, and lower part of the leg.

References

1. Romaña MC, Masquelet AC. Vascularization of the inner border of the foot: Surgical applications. *Surg Radiol Anal* 1988;11:177.
2. Masquelet AC, Romaña MC. The medialis pedis flap: a new fasciocutaneous flap. *Plast Reconstr Surg* 1990;85:765.
3. Ishikura N, Heshiki T, Israkada S. The use of a free medialis pedis flap for resurfacing skin defects of the hand and digits: results in five cases. *Plast Reconstr Surg* 1995;95:100.

CHAPTER 517 ■ SURAL FLAP

A. C. MASQUELET

The sural flap has gained popularity by proving its validity for reconstruction around the ankle and foot. Its main advantages are an extensive mobility and versatility, without sacrificing important arteries. The safe and relatively short technical procedure is easily transmitted to young surgeons. Most of the reported complications can be avoided by a careful selection of indications and a rigorous technique. In the past, this flap had several nomenclatures: neurocutaneous flap, distally based superficial sural artery flap, reverse sural island flap, and lesser saphenous sural veno-neuro adipofascial flap. Nevertheless, *sural flap* is a simple description that is now well accepted.

INDICATIONS

Elective indications for the sural flap concern the posterior aspect of the heel and Achilles tendon, the anterior and lateral aspects of the ankle, the dorsum of the foot, the lateral aspect of the hindfoot, and the anterior crest of the lower third of the leg (1–3).

Relative indications of the sural flap are coverage of the totality of the heel and of defects of the medial aspect of the lower leg. These two areas are not too distant from the pivot point, but their coverage might involve kinking of the pedicle, or the flap might provoke partial arterial insufficiency or a difficulty in venous return.

ANATOMY

The sural artery issues from the popliteal artery (1,4,5). It joins the sural nerve coursing between the two heads of the gastrocnemius and follows the lateral edge of the Achilles tendon. The sural artery is intimately connected with the sural nerve and plays an important role in supplying the skin of the lower and middle posterior leg. It terminates with the lateral supramalleolar branch of the fibular artery and posterior tibial artery. A pair of comitant veins travel with the sural artery.

The sural nerve descends in close association with the lesser saphenous vein, coursing posterior to the lateral malleolus, to innervate the lateral side of the foot and the fifth toe. The vascularization of the nerve is ensured by the sural artery in the proximal third of the leg and by an arterial fascial plexus issuing from the perforators of the fibular artery.

Approximately four to eight perforators arise from the fibular artery, pierce the crural fascia, and give rise to several branches that join adjacent perforators, forming an interconnecting vascular suprafascial plexus that extends from the proximal part of the leg to the posterior margin of the lateral malleolus. A larger perforator is located approximately 5 cm proximal to the lateral malleolus (Fig. 1). After giving off the anterior perforator that pierces the interosseous membrane, the distal portion of the fibular artery gives off a posterior lateral malleolar branch and more distally, the lateral calcaneal artery.

FLAP DESIGN AND DIMENSIONS

Considering the anatomic structures involved, the flap pedicle includes superficial and deep fascia, sural nerve, lesser saphenous vein, and sural artery. The lesser saphenous vein is generally used to determine the axis of the pedicle (3). The pivot point of the pedicle is the main perforator, located 5 cm proximal to the lateral malleolus, as it is the most reliable. The two more distal perforators issuing from the posterior lateral malleolar and lateral calcaneal branches are likely to provide a pivot point for the pedicle (6). Nonetheless, dissection is more risky at this level, and the width of the pedicle is limited.

The standardized sural flap is designed as follows. The skin island is designed on the posterior aspect of the calf at the junction of the two heads of the gastrocnemius. The pivot point of the pedicle and the source supplying the flap is the most reliable perforator. The pedicle is a strip of adipofascial tissue, including subdermal tissue, lesser saphenous vein, sural nerve, and deep fascia (1,3,4,7). The ratio of length to width of the pedicle is approximately 4:1.

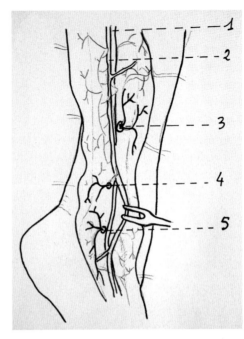

FIG. 1. The suprafascial courses of the sural nerve and the lesser saphenous vein. The deep course of the fibular artery demonstrates the emergence of the perforators. The larger perforator, which is usually the pivot point of the pedicle, is located approximately 5 cm proximal to the lateral malleolus. *1*, Sural nerve; *2*, lesser saphenous vein; *3*, the larger perforator; *4*, perforator from the posterior malleolar branch; *5*, perforator from the lateral calcaneal artery.

Some points should be reemphasized. The pivot point is approximately 5 cm proximal to the lateral malleolus and posterior to the fibula. The axis of the pedicle is oblique and can be located precisely by the course of the lesser saphenous vein. The length of the pedicle is determined by the arc of rotation required. However, a reliable adipofascial pedicle should not exceed the ratio of 4:1 (i.e., if the pedicle length is 12 cm, the width is about 3 cm). The design of the skin island is in continuity with the pedicle. The dimensions of the flap can reach 15 cm in length and 12 cm in width.

OPERATIVE TECHNIQUE

A prone position is indicated only when the defect is located at the posterior aspect of the heel or the lateral aspect of the ankle. In other cases, the patient lies in a supine position, the ipsilateral buttock slightly elevated. Flexion and adduction of the hip and flexion of the knee allow raising the flap in a rather comfortable position while the whole anterior aspect of the ankle and the medial side of the leg remain easily accessible.

The flap is outlined approximately at the junction of the two heads of the gastrocnemius. The precise location of the skin paddle depends on the length of pedicle required. The pivot point of the pedicle is about three finger-breadths proximal to the tip of the lateral malleolus. The line of incision is traced over the course of the sural nerve and lesser saphenous vein, which may have been identified previously with Doppler ultrasound (Fig. 2).

A distal transverse short debridement, resulting in an H-shaped incision, allows the raising of two skin flaps to isolate the adipofascial pedicle. In cases of a thick subcutaneous layer, it is advisable to leave a thin layer of adipose tissue connected with the two skin flaps. The pedicle is isolated by two parallel incisions, fascia included, before raising the flap (Fig. 3).

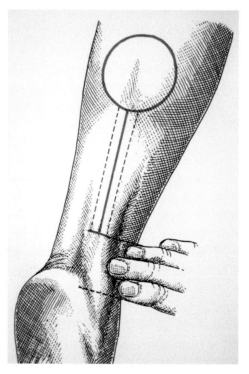

FIG. 2. Flap design and landmark of the pivot point.

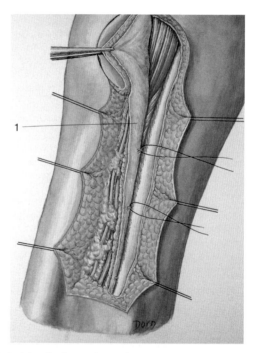

FIG. 4. Raising the flap and its pedicle including the fascia. Small perforators from the fibular artery should be ligated and severed. These proximal perforators can be used as pivot points for a more proximally designed flap. *1*, Deep fascia.

Once the pedicle is isolated, the flap, with fascia included, is raised. Small arteries arising from the fibular artery should be ligated and divided within the adipofascial pedicle. Note that these small perforators can be used as a pivot point for a more proximal pedicled flap (8), with the aim of covering any part of the middle third of the leg (Fig. 4). The arc of rotation allows easy coverage of the posterior aspect of the heel. The skin bridge is incised to bury the pedicle. The donor site and the exposed aspect of the pedicle are covered with a split-thickness skin graft (Fig. 5).

The postoperative course should be carefully evaluated. Excessive pressure on the pedicle or on the flap must be avoided. An external device, with pins in the distal tibia and foot, is a reliable procedure that facilitates postoperative compliance, allows maintenance of the ankle joint and permits easy changing of the dressing (3). Slight elevation of the lower extremity is possible, avoiding any contact of the flap that could result in partial or total necrosis.

CLINICAL RESULTS

Although the sural artery flap has received favorable judgments in the literature, the clinical success rate has been diversely reported. The rate of complications ranges from 5% to 36%, and includes partial or complete necrosis of the flap, infection, hematoma, delayed healing, and skin-graft necrosis on the flap margins (2–5,7,9). Venous congestion and arterial insufficiency may be obvious explanations for complications. However, technical errors are often the main causes, especially

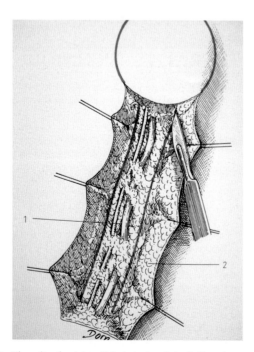

FIG. 3. The adipofascial pedicle is isolated, including the nerve and vein. *1*, Sural nerve and vein; *2*, subdermal dissection.

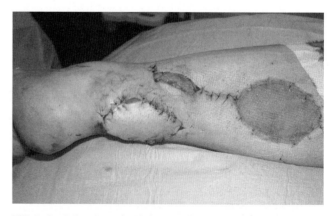

FIG. 5. Recipient site and pedicle covered with split-thickness skin graft.

among inexperienced surgeons, and can easily be avoided if the following possible causes of trouble are kept in mind.

- The flap has been designed in a much too proximal location or the adipofascial pedicle is not large enough.
- The lesser saphenous vein and the sural nerve are not included in the pedicle.
- The twisting of the base of the pedicle at the pivot point is too tight.
- The flap or the connections between the flap and the pedicle are angulated at the recipient site.
- The flap has been placed at the recipient site before deflating the tourniquet, which causes difficulties in flap reperfusion.
- The pedicle is passed subcutaneously through retractile tissue, which leads to hyperpressure on the pedicle.
- It may be difficult to suture the flap to the surrounding fibrous tissue because of the thickness of the subcutaneous layer of the flap.
- Technical guidelines to avoid the surgical mistakes or conditions mentioned should be emphasized.
- The lesser saphenous vein and arterial perforator should be identified by Doppler ultrasound. If the lesser saphenous vein cannot be located, this may be an indication for a delay in the procedure (10).
- The ratio of length to width of the pedicle should not exceed 4:1.
- The pedicle should be long enough to allow loose twisting.
- The use of a tourniquet must be carefully assessed in arteriosclerotic patients.
- The flap should be placed without angulation. For this reason, repair of the weight-bearing area of the heel is a risky indication. Conversely, the repair of the totality of the heel may require an excision of the greater tuberosity of the calcaneus to avoid flap angulation.
- It is preferable to incise the skin bridge between the pivot point and the recipient site. The use of a "skin tail" overlying the pedicle seems to improve venous return but limits rotation of the pedicle (9). Flap transposition through a subcutaneous tunnel with the aid of an intraoperative soft-tissue expander has been proposed (11).
- The skin-to-skin suture of a bulky flap implies performance of extensive mobilization of the recipient area and planning the design of the flap initially larger than the defect.
- The postoperative course is facilitated by the use of an external device or a posterior plaster splint, providing a posterior chamber to avoid excessive pressure.

COMORBIDITY

Age alone is not a risk factor by itself. The risk factors mentioned include diabetes mellitus, venous insufficiency, and peripheral arterial disease (3). If all three factors are present, the risk of a necrotic flap is very high. However, comorbidity with any of these diseases should not present an absolute contraindication, but one should understand that association of one or two risks with a technical error will lead to unavoidable necrosis.

SUMMARY

With respect for the technical guidelines, and despite the limitations implied by the risk factors of comorbidity, the sural artery flap is a valuable tool for reconstruction of the lower extremity. In many cases, it remains the last alternative to an amputation.

References

1. Masquelet AC, Romaña MC, Wolf G. Skin island flaps supplied by the vascular axis of the sensitive superficial nerves: anatomic study and clinical experience in the leg. *Plast Reconstr Surg* 1992;89:1115.
2. Raveendran S, Perera D, Happuharachchi T, Yoganathan V. Superficial sural artery flap: a study in 40 cases. *Br J Plast Surg* 2004;57:266.
3. Baumeister SP, Spierer R, Erdmann D, et al. A realistic complication analysis of 70 sural artery flaps in a multimorbid patient group. *Plast Reconstr Surg* 2003;129:129.
4. Almeida MF, da Costa PR, Okawa RY. Reverse-flow island sural flap. *Plast Reconstr Surg* 2002;109:583.
5. Hollier L, Sharma S, Babigumira E, Klebuc M. Versatility of the sural fasciocutaneous flap in the coverage of lower extremity wounds. *Plast Reconstr Surg* 2002;110:1673.
6. Zhang FH, Chang SM, Lin SQ, et al. Modified distally based sural neuroveno-fasciocutaneous flap: anatomical study and clinical applications. *Microsurgery* 2005;25:543.
7. Akhtar S, Hameed A. Versatility of the sural fasciocutaneous flap in the coverage of lower third leg and hind foot defects. *J Plast Reconstr Aesthet Surg* 2006;59:839.
8. Ozalp T, Masquelet AC, Bégué T. Septocutaneous perforators of the peroneal artery relative to the fibula: anatomical basis of the use of pedicled fasciocutaneous flaps. *Surg Radiol Anat.* 2006;28:548.
9. Noack N, Hartmann B, Kuntscher M. Measures to prevent complications of distally based neurovascular sural flaps. *Ann Plast Surg* 2006;57:37.
10. Kneser U, Bach A, Polykandriotis E, et al. Delayed reverse sural flap for staged reconstruction of the foot and lower leg. *Plast Reconstr Surg* 2005;116:1910.
11. Buluç L, Tosun B, Sen C, Sarlak A. A modified technique for transposition of the reverse sural artery flap. *Plast Reconstr Surg* 2006;117:2488.

CHAPTER 518 ■ DORSALIS PEDIS FLAP

L. T. FURLOW, JR.

The dorsalis pedis flap consists of the skin, subcutaneous tissue, and the most superficial layer of fascia of the dorsum of the foot supplied by the dorsalis pedis artery through its subcutaneous branches between the first and second toe long extensor tendons. Sensory innervation can be maintained through the superficial and deep peroneal nerves. My experience with the dorsalis pedis flap is as a local attached flap, either as an island or with a skin bridge, for foot and ankle coverage (1). It has found more use as a free flap owing to its thinness and its potential for reestablishment of sensation through neurorrhaphy (2–4).

INDICATIONS

The dorsal pedis flap is useful for coverage of defects of the medial and lateral aspects of the foot and the front and both sides of the ankle. It has provided excellent cover for both malleoli. Although the saphenous veins are long enough, the dorsalis pedis artery may have to be lengthened by a graft to permit the flap to cover heel or Achilles tendon defects (5). Distal foot coverage by basing the flap on the perforating branch of the dorsalis pedis with reverse flow from the posterior tibial artery supplying the flap was described recently (6).

Disadvantages of the flap include a relatively difficult and tedious dissection, during which it is distressingly easy to dissect the flap from its artery, and a sensory deficit of the entire dorsum of the foot. There is a potential for healing problems in the donor site if complete paratenon cover of the extensor tendons is not maintained to ensure skin graft "take."

If the foot is not supplied by both the posterior tibial and dorsalis pedis arteries, the flap should not be used. After flap elevation, the dorsalis pedis is required for flap survival and the posterior tibial artery is required for foot survival. Unfortunately, these requirements remove the dorsalis pedis flap from consideration in the large number of ischemic ulcerations about the foot with which we are faced.

ANATOMY

The dorsalis pedis flap is classified as an axial flap, which it is not. It must be emphasized that the dorsalis pedis flap is a random subcutaneous flap resting on but only tenuously connected to its axial artery, the dorsalis pedis (Fig. 1).

The dorsalis pedis artery is the extension of the anterior tibial that enters the foot beneath the extensor retinaculum of the ankle, where it lies immediately on the tarsal bones. From proximal to distal in the tarsal region, the dorsalis pedis gives off the lateral tarsal artery, the medial tarsal artery or arteries, and the arcuate artery, which courses laterally at approximately the tarsometatarsal level. Unfortunately, all these branches course deep to the extensor tendons of the foot and so cannot be elevated with the flap.

As the dorsalis pedis artery reaches the first intermetatarsal space, it dips plantarward through the interosseous muscles to join the plantar arch and gives off its terminal branch, the first dorsal metatarsal artery, to the first web space. The origin of the first dorsal metatarsal artery is the most important variable in the arterial anatomy of the flap (Fig. 2). In about 80% of feet, the first dorsal metatarsal artery arises superficially or just within the interosseous muscle, but in the other 20% it is given off more deeply in the intermetatarsal space and must rise back through the interosseous musculature to supply the web space (2,3). The tiny branches of the dorsalis pedis artery that directly supply the flap have been studied (4).

There are three routes of venous return for the flap. The greater and lesser saphenous veins form the dorsal venous arch within the substance of the flap and course toward the medial and lateral malleoli, respectively. Either of these veins may be preserved if a skin pedicle is left, or the flap will survive on the dorsalis pedis venae comitantes.

The first web space area of the flap is supplied by the deep peroneal nerve, which accompanies the dorsalis pedis artery, becoming superficial at its terminal bifurcation. The remainder of the dorsal skin of the foot is supplied by the superficial peroneal nerve through its medial and intermediate dorsal cutaneous branches.

The critically important pedestal of tissue connecting the dorsalis pedis artery and the flap lies between the extensor hallucis longus tendon and the extensor digitorum longus tendon to the second toe. The extensor hallucis brevis muscle and tendon course obliquely through this pedestal superficial to the dorsalis pedis-first dorsal metatarsal artery and deep peroneal nerve.

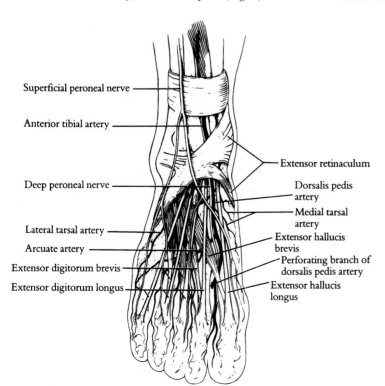

FIG. 1. Pertinent anatomy encountered in flap dissection.

Superficial peroneal nerve

Anterior tibial artery

Deep peroneal nerve

Lateral tarsal artery

Arcuate artery

Extensor digitorum brevis

Extensor digitorum longus

Extensor retinaculum

Dorsalis pedis artery

Medial tarsal artery

Extensor hallucis brevis

Perforating branch of dorsalis pedis artery

Extensor hallucis longus

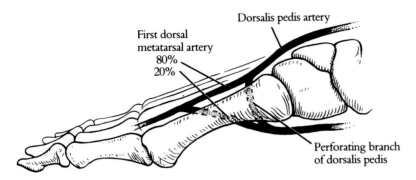

FIG. 2. Variations in the origin and course of the first dorsal metatarsal artery.

It is important to establish the proximal patency of both the posterior tibial and dorsalis pedis arteries by palpation or Doppler examination. Because pulsation of the dorsalis pedis may be transmitted distally through its plantar arch anastomosis, pulsation or flow must be demonstrated in four circumstances: (1) With the dorsalis pedis pulse finger-occluded on the dorsum of the foot, pulsation should be felt just proximal in the vessel. (2) Pulsation in the dorsalis pedis should be palpable when the posterior tibial artery is finger-occluded. These two maneuvers indicate patency of the anterior tibial artery. (3) When the dorsalis pedis is finger-occluded, pulsation in the posterior tibial artery should be palpable, indicating its patency. (4) It is of interest but not critical to flap or foot survival to note whether pulsation is present in the dorsalis pedis distally when it is finger-occluded over the dorsum of the foot, indicating strong flow from the plantar arch through the perforating branch. This maneuver would of course be critical if the flap were to be distally based on retrograde flow through the perforating branch of the dorsalis pedis artery (6).

FLAP DESIGN AND DIMENSIONS

The flap may include the skin of the entire dorsum of the foot extending from the web spaces to the extensor retinaculum and across the entire breadth of the dorsum of the foot. The flap may be elevated with the proximal skin pedicle to include either the greater or lesser saphenous veins or as an island. The maximum flap size is approximately 12 × 12 cm. Coverage requirements usually allow use of a smaller flap that should be centered over the dorsalis pedis artery in the proximal end of the intermetatarsal space.

I have been quick to delay the flap, primarily under three circumstances:

1. If the first dorsal metatarsal artery cannot be elevated with the flap.
2. If skin more than 2.5 cm from the dorsalis pedis artery, particularly in the lateral direction, is required.
3. I am more likely to delay an island flap than one with a proximal skin pedicle.

OPERATIVE TECHNIQUE

The weak link of the dorsalis pedis flap is the vascular supply between the axial dorsalis pedis artery and the subcutaneous flap. Because of the tenuous nature of this connection, necrosis of all or a part of the flap is quite possible in the presence of a bounding dorsalis pedis pulse. Every precaution must be taken to avoid elevating the flap from the dorsalis pedis artery, which is distressingly easy to do, and to preserve the tiny connecting vessels within the soft tissue between the extensor hallucis longus and extensor digitorum longus tendons (Fig. 3).

The dissection is done under tourniquet control, but the limb is elevated without wrapping so that some blood will remain in the vessels to be dissected. Five or six wraps of an Ace bandage around the knee will limit the thigh blood coming through the femoral medullary canal beneath the tourniquet.

Although others begin elevation of the flap medially or proximally, I prefer to begin in the first web area by elevating the distal-medial corner of the flap and identifying and dividing the first dorsal metatarsal artery (Fig. 4). The tie on the flap end of the vessel is left long and is used to elevate the flap. The superficial fascia overlying the extensor tendons is elevated with the flap, leaving a filmy layer of paratenon over the extensor tendons. The first dorsal metatarsal artery is followed into the intermetatarsal space, as necessary into the interosseous muscle, until the perforating branch of the dorsalis pedis artery is found. Elevation of the lateral portion of the flap is carried proximally, leaving paratenon on the extensor tendons. All soft tissue between the extensor hallucis longus and extensor digitorum longus tendon margins and the first dorsal metatarsal artery must be elevated with the flap, including the extensor hallucis brevis tendon, which is divided and left within the flap.

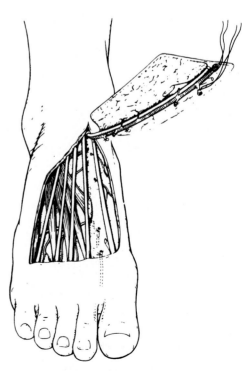

FIG. 3. The flap elevated, supplied by fine vessels from the dorsalis pedis artery between the extensor hallucis longus and second toe extensor digitorum longus tendons.

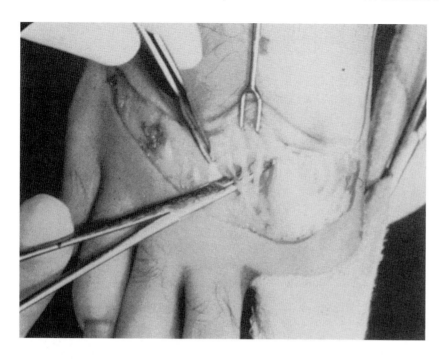

FIG. 4. Distal identification of first dorsal metatarsal artery and deep peroneal nerve.

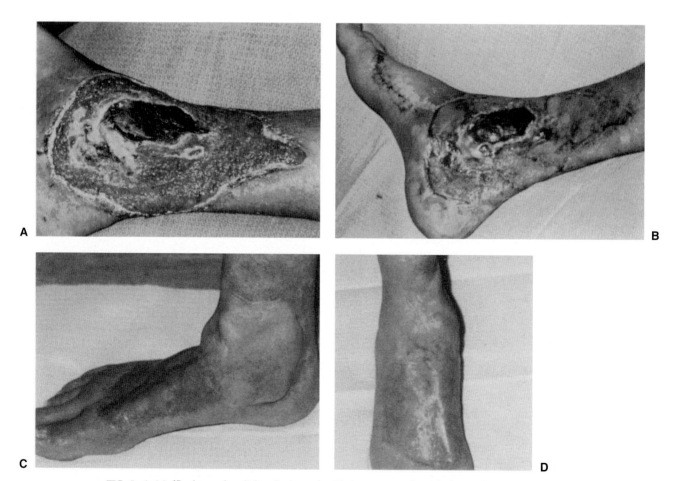

FIG. 5. A: Muffler burn of medial malleolus and ankle in a motorcyclist. The bone of the medial malleolus was burned. He had a palpable dorsalis pedis pulse, and the posterior tibial pulse was identified by Doppler examination. B: One week after flap delay and grafting of defect margins. C,D: Appearance 9 1\2 years after coverage with a dorsalis pedis flap.

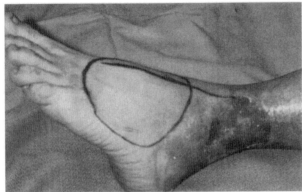
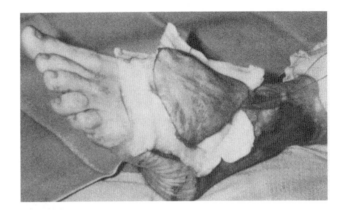

A,B

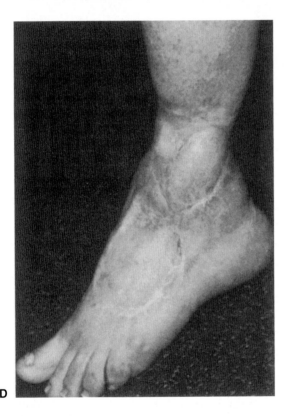
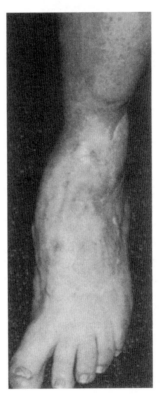

C,D

FIG. 6. A: In 1971, prior to the first free flap transfer, this 55-year-old woman was the first patient to undergo dorsalis pedis flap elevation. She had a medial ankle ulcer recurrent after multiple previous skin graftings, a contralateral AK amputation, and an ipsilateral elbow flexion contracture. B: The dorsalis pedis flap was elevated as an island and transferred primarily. There was some marginal flap loss, primarily the skin from the lateral aspect of the foot, but this area was skin-grafted. C,D: Appearance 14 years later, with no further ulcerations.

When the perforating branch of the dorsalis pedis is reached, all three vessels at the junction, the proximal feeding dorsalis pedis, the perforating branch, and the first dorsal metatarsal artery, are identified before the perforating branch is ligated and divided. Again, the tie on the proximal (flap) end is left long and used to elevate the flap; the flap is thus lifted on its artery rather than away from it.

Flap dissection is continued proximally, dissecting the dorsalis pedis artery and the deep peroneal nerve from the underlying tarsal bones and preserving the maximum amount of soft tissue available between the extensor hallucis longus and extensor digitorum longus tendons. As the arcuate and tarsal branches of the dorsalis pedis artery are encountered, they are dissected to the point where they pass beneath the extensor tendons before being divided to ensure the maximum number of connecting vessels between the dorsalis pedis artery and the flap. The extensor hallucis brevis muscle belly is divided where it passes beneath the second toe extensor digitorum longus tendon, leaving its tendon and distal muscle in the flap.

If the flap is to be left attached by a skin pedicle, a saphenous vein, or the superficial peroneal nerve, these are dissected at the proximal end of the flap. If the flap is to be elevated as

an island, these structures are divided as encountered. It may be necessary to incise the lower portion of the extensor retinaculum for adequate mobilization of the dorsalis pedis pedicle proximal to the flap.

When flap delay is indicated, the distal dissection is carried proximally until the perforating branch of the dorsalis pedis can be ligated and divided and from medially and laterally to the margins of the extensor hallucis longus and extensor digitorum longus tendons, leaving the tissue between the tendons undissected and a portion of the proximal skin intact. Final elevation of the flap is scheduled for 1 week later. This interval is adequate for the delay phenomenon but permits easy finger dissection of the previously elevated portions of the flap before significant fibrous tissue forms in the wound.

If the flap is elevated as an island, I prefer to divide the skin between the pedicle and the defect to be covered rather than passing the flap beneath the skin bridge. If necessary, this incision can be left unsutured and grafted with the donor defect.

Before grafting the donor defect of the dorsum of the foot, any rents in the paratenon must be closed carefully to cover all exposed tendon. The remaining portion of the extensor hallucis brevis muscle belly may be helpful for tendon coverage (Figs. 5 and 6).

SUMMARY

The dorsalis pedis flap should be considered as a random subcutaneous flap resting on an underlying axial artery. It has been very useful for difficult coverage problems of the foot and ankle area but has been used more often as a free flap because of its thinness; the presence of two sensory nerves for reinnervation; and because extensor tendons, metatarsi, and toes can be transferred with it.

References

1. McCraw JB, Furlow LT Jr. The dorsalis pedis arterialized flap. *Plast Reconstr Surg* 1975;55:177.
2. Gilbert A. Composite tissue transfers from the foot: Anatomic basis and surgical technique. In: Daniller A, Strauch B, eds. *Symposium on microsurgery.* St. Louis: Mosby, 1976. Chap. 25.
3. May JW Jr, Chait LA, Cohen BE, O'Brien BM. Free neurovascular flap from the first web of the foot in hand reconstruction. *J Hand Surg* 1977;2:387.
4. Man D, Acland R. The microarterial anatomy of the dorsalis pedis flap and its clinical applications. *Plast Reconstr Surg* 1980;65:419.
5. Caffee H, Hoefflin S. The extended dorsalis pedis flap. *Plast Reconstr Surg* 1979;64:807.
6. Ishikawa K, Isshiki N, Suzuki S, Shimamura S. Distally based dorsalis pedis island flap for coverage of the distal portion of the foot. *Br J Plast Surg* 1987;40:521.

CHAPTER 519 ■ DORSALIS PEDIS MYOFASCIAL FLAP

T. I. A. ISMAIL

EDITORIAL COMMENT

This is a brilliant modification of the dorsalis pedis flap. Very similar to the radial forearm fascial flap, the dorsalis pedis can be used with fascia alone. This militates against many of the skin problems that were associated with the dorsalis pedis flap. The flap can be used either as a pedicle flap, as described by Ismail, or as a free flap.

The dorsalis pedis myofascial flap, composed of the deep fascia of the dorsum of the foot and underlying extensor digitorum brevis muscle, is a reliable and safe local flap with minimal donor-site morbidity.

INDICATIONS

Defects in the lower half of the leg and malleolar region are difficult and common problems facing the plastic surgeon. Several flaps have been described (1–7) for their management. The dorsalis pedis myofascial flap has many advantages. The donor site can be closed primarily without skin grafting. This is a very safe and well-vascularized flap.

It is used to supply coverage for small- and moderately-sized defects over both the medial and lateral malleoli. The flap can be carried up to cover defects in the lower half of the leg. It can also potentially be used as a free flap to supply thin coverage over areas such as the dorsum of the hand. In addition, the flap can be used to cover the Achilles tendon, either by direct rotation, or by passage through a hole in the interosseous membrane. The extensor tendons of the toes may be included, to supply vascularized tendon grafts.

The flap is contraindicated when either anterior or posterior tibial arterial pulsations are not palpable. Such a situation will limit its use in some traumatic defects with damage to either vessel.

ANATOMY

The flap consists of the deep fascia of the dorsum of the foot, with a thin layer of fat over it, and the extensor digitorum brevis muscle on its undersurface. It is supplied by the dorsalis pedis artery and drained by its venae comitantes. It extends from the web space up to the extensor retinaculum. The extensor digitorum brevis muscle is not an essential part of the flap, but its inclusion is believed to augment flap vascularity and to facilitate the dissection and elevation of the dorsalis pedis artery.

FLAP DESIGN AND DIMENSIONS

Patency of the anterior tibial and posterior tibial vessels is mandatory for flap harvesting. The skin incision starts between both malleoli and descends to the base of the second toe. Proximal extension of the incision into the leg may be needed if the flap is to be carried to the lower half of the leg. The flap surface area can oblige defects of 80 cm^2 or more, and its size can be increased, if the deep fascia and extensor digitorum brevis muscle are spread in a bilobed manner (Fig. 1).

OPERATIVE TECHNIQUE

A bloodless field using a tourniquet is essential. The skin is undermined medially and laterally in the subdermal plane,

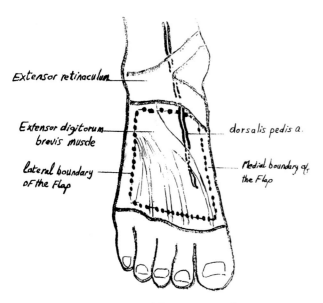

FIG. 1. Illustration of flap anatomy and extent.

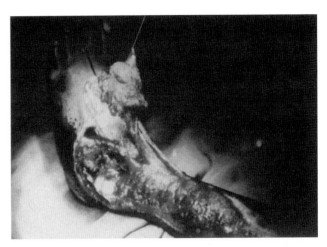

FIG. 3. Dorsalis pedis myofascial flap on its way to cover exposed cartilage at the lateral malleolus.

preserving one lobule of fat on its undersurface. The skin is reflected medially and laterally 0.5 cm beyond the flap margins. The desired amount of deep fascia on the dorsum of the foot is elevated with the dorsalis pedis artery and its venae comitantes, after its ligation at the base of the first metatarsal space.

The flap is elevated from distal to proximal, ligating the deep and side branches of the dorsalis pedis artery. The extensor digitorum brevis muscle is commonly included on the undersurface of the deep fascia. If the flap is to be carried to the lower leg, the extensor retinaculum must be cut and the dorsalis pedis artery (now the anterior tibial artery) is mobilized for a suitable distance, indicated by the site of the defect. Now, the flap is passed through a subcutaneous tunnel to the malleolar defect, or rotated into the leg defect.

The flap is spread over the defect and covered by a split-thickness skin graft. The donor site on the dorsum of the foot is closed primarily with a small suction drain.

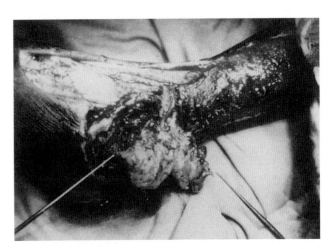

FIG. 4. Flap and extensor digitorum brevis muscle are spread in a bilobed fashion to cover the defect.

CLINICAL RESULTS

Currently, the flap has been used in 20 cases without a single failure (Figs. 2–5). Minimal complications may occur, such as

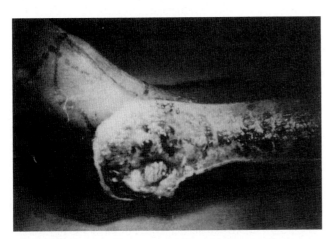

FIG. 2. Defect of the lateral malleolus and lower leg, with exposed ankle joint.

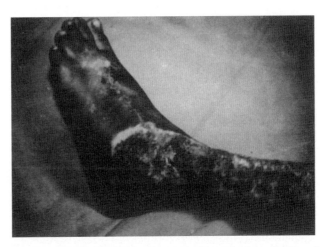

FIG. 5. Full take of the skin graft over the flap and primary healing of the donor site.

delayed healing of the donor site, widening of the scar, hypopigmentation of the donor site, and hypothesia of the dorsum of the foot. Such complications have been well-tolerated by patients.

SUMMARY

The dorsalis pedis myofascial flap, consisting of the deep fascia of the dorsum of the foot with the extensor digitorum brevis muscle, is a simple, safe, and reliable local flap. It is used to cover defects over both malleoli and the lower half of the leg, with minimal donor-site morbidity.

References

1. Ismail TIA. The dorsalis pedis myofascial flap. *Plast Reconstr Surg* 1990;86:573.
2. Morrison WA, Shen TY. Anterior tibial artery flap: anatomy and case report. *Br J Plast Surg* 1987;40:230.
3. Landi A, Soragni O, Monteleone, M. The extensor digitorum brevis muscle island flap for soft-tissue loss around the ankle. *Plast Reconstr Surg* 1985; 75:892.
4. Townsend PLG. An inferiorly based soleus muscle flap. *Br J Plast Surg* 1979;31:210.
5. Pontén B. The fasciocutaneous flap: its use in soft tissue defects of the lower leg. *Br J Plast Surg* 1981;34:215.
6. Donski PK, Fogdestam I. Distally based fasciocutaneous flaps from the sural region. *Scand J Plast Reconstr Surg* 1983;17:191.
7. Amarante J, Costa H, Reis J, Soares R. A new distally based fasciocutaneous flap of the leg. *Br J Plast Surg* 1986;39:338.

CHAPTER 520 ■ MEDIALIS PEDIS FLAP

A. C. MASQUELET AND M. C. ROMAÑA

The medialis pedis flap is a fasciocutaneous flap raised on the medial aspect of the foot. Initially developed as an island pedicled flap for coverage of elective areas of the foot (1,2), it also has been used as a free flap for resurfacing restricted areas of the foot, and skin defects of the hand and digits (3).

INDICATIONS

For certain indications, no other flap is better: use of the dorsalis pedis implies a heavy arterial sacrifice; the medial plantar flap is not pliable enough; and the lateral supramalleolar flap is too thick and too big. We think that the free flap should be reserved for areas where a sensory flap is not mandatory; it also can be very useful in the hand for large defects, when other conventional flaps, because of their bulk, are not suitable. The flap has restricted, but elective, indications on the foot: it can be used to cover the tip of the medial malleolus and the area of insertion of the Achilles tendon; defects of the medial aspect of the heel (calcaneum) may also be easily covered by this flap. The length and caliber of the vessels allow its application as a free flap, and it

can be oriented specifically for tissue repairs in the hands and fingers (3).

Among its advantages, the medialis pedis flap is very thin, compared to other free or local flaps raised from the foot. Unlike many conventional free and pedicled flaps, it can be used for small-sized defects. It also provides a good color and texture match for finger repairs. The thinness of the flap allows good recovery of protective sensation, although the flap is not sensory.

A principal disadvantage is that a skin graft is usually required for donor-site closure.

ANATOMY (FIG. 1)

The flap is supplied by a constant and reliable cutaneous artery arising from the medial plantar artery (1). At the level of the plantar vault, the medial plantar artery divides into a superficial and a deep branch. The superficial branch emerges from the septum between the abductor hallucis and flexor digitorum brevis muscles. It gives off 2 to 4 cutaneous branches destined for the plantar arch and constitutes the arterial axis of the medial plantar flap.

The deep branch has not been well explored. It arises from the medial plantar artery near its origin, and also divides into two branches—a lateral branch that penetrates into the sole of the foot and anastomoses with the deep plantar arch; and a medial branch that is of interest for the flap under discussion. This branch follows the medial aspect of the bones of the foot, to reach the base of the first metatarsal and to anastomose with the first plantar metatarsal artery. The medial branch

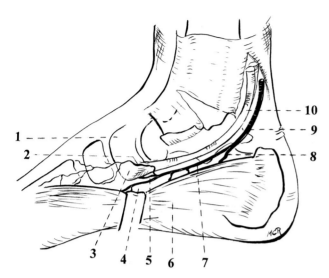

FIG. 1. Diagram of vascular anatomy. *1*, navicular bone; *2*, cutaneous branch supplying the medial aspect of the foot; *3*, tubercle of the navicular bone; *4*, superficial branch of the medial plantar artery; *5*, deep branch of the medial plantar artery; *6*, abductor hallucis muscle; *7*, medial plantar artery; *8*, lateral plantar artery; *9*, posterior tibial artery; *10*, tibialis posterior tendon.

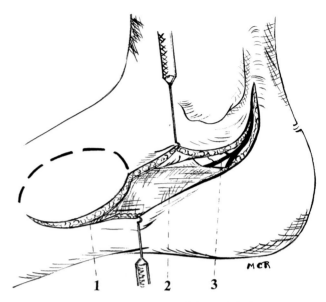

FIG. 2. Elevation of the flap; origin of the medial plantar artery is identified. The fascia covering the abductor hallucis muscle is incised in line with the skin incision. The insertion of the tibialis posterior tendon and the tubercle of the navicular bone should be included in the design.

crosses the terminal part of the tibialis posterior tendon, on which it lies just behind the tuberosity of the navicular bone. It then takes an oblique course parallel to the medial aspect of the foot. At the level of the distal end of the tibialis posterior tendon, the artery gives off several cutaneous branches supplying a cutaneous area from the navicular bone to the mid-shaft of the first metatarsal, which constitutes the territory of the medialis pedis flap.

Among possible variations, the cutaneous branches sometimes arise from the trunk of the medial plantar artery. This variation is not important, as a constant landmark is the passage of the cutaneous branch on the tibialis posterior tendon, just behind the tubercle of the navicular bone. The pedicle of the flap is always dissected up to the origin of the medial plantar artery.

FLAP DESIGN AND DIMENSIONS

The flap is outlined on the medial border of the foot, including the tuberosity of the navicular bone and the slight depression that identifies the distal part of the tibialis posterior tendon. The proximal end of the flap can be extended proximally beneath the medial malleolar; the distal end extends to the mid-shaft of the first metatarsal bone. Flap size clinically ranges from 2 × 3 cm to 5 × 10 cm.

OPERATIVE TECHNIQUE

Raising the flap is performed under tourniquet. Arteriograms may be mandatory to assess flow-through of the main distal trunks. Through a retro-malleolar incision, the terminal portion of the tibialis posterior artery is first exposed just proximal to the posterior edge of the abductor hallucis muscle. The plantar border of the flap is incised with fascia included (Fig. 2). The subcutaneous veins are ligated and severed; they should be spared for anastomosis at the recipient site, when the flap is

used as a free flap. On the dorsal border of the flap, only the skin is incised, to spare a dorsal hinge of fascia.

The flap is progressively raised and retracted from plantar to dorsal. The dissection in depth is performed close to the tubercle of the navicular and the tendon of the tibialis posterior bones. Dissection is pursued until the deep branch plunging under the navicular is seen. Then, the abductor hallucis muscle is retracted (Fig. 3) and detached from the inner border of the foot. The flap remains attached by its dorsal hinge.

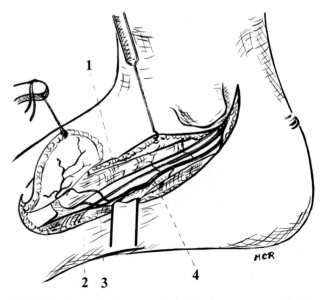

FIG. 3. The flap is progressively raised from posterior to anterior. The abductor hallucis muscle is retracted. The vascular branches are identified. The release of the pedicle implies ligation of the deep and superficial branches of the medial plantar artery distal to the cutaneous branch supplying the flap.

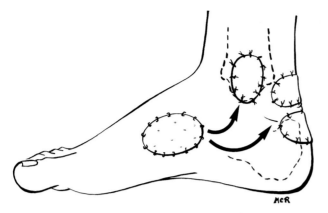

FIG. 4. Arc of rotation of the flap. Medial aspect of the posterior tuberosity of the calcaneum also can be covered.

Retraction of the abductor hallucis allows exposure of the vascular axis.

The superficial branch of the medial plantar artery, the pedicle to the abductor hallucis, and the distal portion of the deep branch of the medial plantar artery are successively ligated and divided. At last, the dorsal hinge of the flap is cut, and the pedicle is released as far as the division of the posterior

tibial artery. The donor site is immediately covered with a split-thickness skin graft.

CLINICAL RESULTS

The arc of rotation provided by the medial plantar artery allows coverage of defects of the medial malleolus and the heel. Division of the lateral plantar pedicle dramatically increases the arc of rotation of the flap. The flap is mandatory when a thin, supple, and hairless flap is needed. In the foot, the medial aspect of the heel, the medial malleolar, and the distal insertion of the Achilles tendon are all sites for elective indications (Fig. 4). The flap is not indicated in the weight-bearing area and posterior aspect of the heel. The precise location of the cutaneous branch (just behind the tuberosity of the navicular bone) allows the raising of small and reliable flaps, very useful for small defects that are otherwise difficult to manage (Fig. 5).

SUMMARY

The medialis pedis flap has restricted, but elective, indications for defects of the foot and for other areas where a very supple coverage is required.

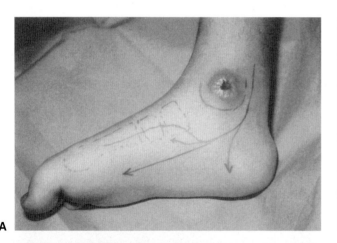

A

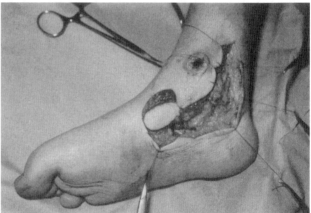

B

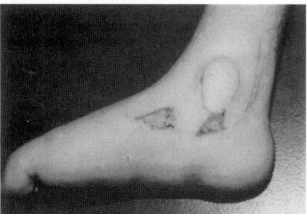

C

FIG. 5. A: Recurrent ulceration of the medial malleolar area in spina bifida. Note marking of the vascularization. B: Elevation of the medialis pedis flap. C: Final result.

References

1. Romaña MC. Masquelet AC. Vascularization of the inner border of the foot: surgical applications. *Surg Radiol Anat* 1988;11:177.

2. Masquelet AC, Romaña MC. The medialis pedis flap: a new fasciocutaneous flap. *Plast Reconstr Surg* 1990;85:765.
3. Ishikura N, Heshiki T, Tsukada S. The use of a free medialis pedis flap for resurfacing skin defects of the hand and digits: results in five cases. *Plast Reconstr Surg* 1995;95:100.

CHAPTER 521 ■ LOCAL FASCIOCUTANEOUS FLAPS FOR DORSAL FOOT AND ANKLE COVERAGE

G. G. HALLOCK

Undelayed cutaneous flaps from the fascial plexus of the lower leg may be used as a simple means of coverage for adjacent defects of the dorsal foot and ankle.

INDICATIONS

Substantial defects involving the ankle or dorsum of the foot are usually treated most expeditiously by microsurgical tissue transfer (1). However, if the resultant morbidity is unacceptable, a source of vascular inflow or exit is unavailable, or because of patient disagreement, a dorsal foot or ankle fasciocutaneous flap may be a simpler alternative. Of course, sufficient local tissue must still be available as a donor, and the multiple perforators of the deep fascia must have remained undisturbed by the original injury or disease.

ANATOMY

The deep fascia of the dorsum of the foot, although not as thick as the crural fascia, nevertheless is a distinct layer, except at the ankle where it tends to blend with the extensor retinaculum (2). All three major leg arteries contribute to the confluence of perforators nourishing this deep fascia, which has longitudinally-oriented perfusion. Periodic direct perforators, ascending and descending malleolar or tarsal branches, and their terminal vessels are included (Fig. 1), as well as collaterals from the proximal plantar subcutaneous plexus of the sole (3).

Although this confluence of perifascial vessels makes the boundaries of skin territories on the dorsal foot relatively indistinct, the branches of the posterior tibial vessels dominate in their supply to the posteromedial ankle and foot. The anterior tibial vessels, the terminating dorsalis pedis, and the first dorsal metatarsal vessels (4) supply the peroneal to the posterolateral region, and the remaining central portion. Any proximally-based flap will have the additional advantage of being sensate if a cutaneous nerve branch is included.

FLAP DESIGN AND DIMENSIONS

One boundary of any chosen local dorsal foot or ankle flap will coincide with the defect to be covered (Fig. 2). A length:width ratio not exceeding 1.8:1 allows undelayed flap

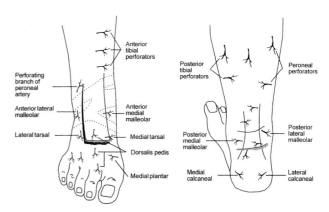

FIG. 1. Diagram of typical distribution of multiple perforators to the region of the dorsal foot and ankle. Note contributions from all three major lower-limb source vessels. A proximally-based flap overlying the anterior tibial-dorsalis pedis axis can be used to cover medial or lateral malleolar defects. It will rely on an interconnecting network with more proximal fascial perforators (left). A bipedicled flap, shown in a horizontal orientation (right), captures perforators from two directions (medial and lateral), which otherwise might be sparse over the Achilles tendon. (Diagram courtesy of Carol Varma, medical illustrator at the Lehigh Valley Hospital, Allentown, Pennsylvania.)

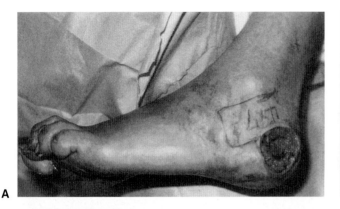

A

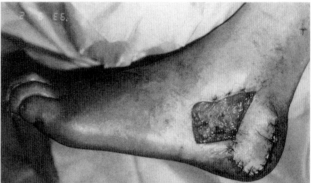

B

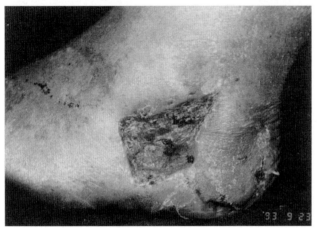

C

FIG. 2. **A:** Following diabetic coma, this male patient developed a full-thickness pressure sore over the lateral heel. Because of bone exposure after debridement, vascularized coverage was proposed, with a 7 × 4 cm proximally-based local flap, intended to capture the territory of the lateral calcaneus branches, but without their specific identification. **B:** Flap inset without tension. **C:** Viable flap in the early stage of healing, demonstrating how the mandatory skin graft at the donor site can have an unaesthetic result.

transfer, without risk of necrosis, if the circulation is otherwise normal (2). Any choice should lie preferentially over the course of one of the major leg source vessels to ensure that a fascial perforator is captured in the base of the flap. The long flap axis is drawn parallel to the known longitudinal orientation of the microcirculation. When based proximally, the flap will be potentially sensate, and a subcutaneous vein can be included to enhance venous outflow.

Since underlying tendons are numerous and easily exposed in any donor site from this region, sometimes a distally-based flap offers the potential of reduced donor-site morbidity (Fig. 3) (5). It must also be noted that the extensor retinaculum must be kept with the deep fascia at the ankle area, to avoid injuring the fascial plane. This may not be an option in patients with compromised vascularity and marginal antegrade inflow. In these cases, a vertical or horizontal bipedicle flap to maximize the number of perforators may be elected at the expense of less freedom in flap mobility (Fig. 3) (6).

OPERATIVE TECHNIQUE

Once the flap boundaries have been marked, the margin furthest from the flap base should be raised first to identify the plane under the deep fascia. Rapid and bloodless dissection toward the flap pedicle should follow until inset without tension is possible. A small backcut in the deep fascia, avoiding any vascular structures, can facilitate this. Paratenon, if exposed, is carefully preserved, or tendons are buried under adjacent soft tissue to enhance the take of a skin graft, invariably required to close the donor site. Postoperative immobilization and bedrest are obviously important to ensure healing and must be enforced.

CLINICAL RESULTS

Intrinsic local flaps of the dorsum of the foot include the extensor digitorum brevis muscle flap (7) and the dorsalis pedis and lateral calcaneal cutaneous flaps (8,9). Elevation of the first two can compromise circulation of the foot by sacrificing a named source vessel; the latter flap often has no single distinct artery, but rather multiple terminal branches, often also becoming a Pontén-type of flap that depends on multiple fascial perforators (2).

Extrinsic skin territories in the leg can be used as distally-based flaps to resurface the foot or ankle, without sacrifice of a source vessel. However, they may be multistaged procedures and can cause significant cosmetic donor-site morbidity (10). Acceptable donor-site morbidity must also be considered before using any of the local Pontén-type intrinsic flaps as well (Fig. 2). Therefore, a free flap might be a better selection and remains an appropriate choice if insufficient local tissue is unavailable (1).

Nevertheless, for small defects, the morbidity and risk of failure involved in microsurgical transfer can be avoided entirely by using the simple local flap described. For the polytrauma patient with compromised vascularity, these Pontén-type fasciocutaneous flaps may be the only alternative to limb amputation.

SUMMARY

A "random," local, fasciocutaneous flap from the dorsum of the foot or ankle can often solve the problem of covering small defects, without resorting to a free flap.

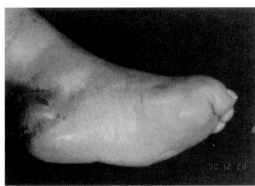
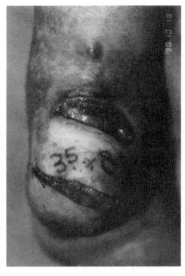
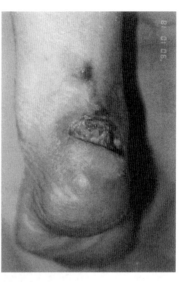

A–C

FIG. 3. **A:** Necrotic pressure sore involving the Achilles tendon in a pareparetic woman who also had significant atherosclerotic peripheral occlusive disease. **B:** A more caudal 8 × 3.5-cm horizontal bipedicled fasciocutaneous flap was raised and transferred superiorly, capturing inflow from both sides of the Achilles tendon. **C:** This allowed successful healing and avoidance of limb amputation in a difficult situation.

References

1. Hallock GG, Rice DC, Keblish PA, Arangio GA. Restoration of the foot using the radial forearm flap. *Ann Plast Surg* 1988;20:12.
2. Hallock GG. Fasciocutaneous flap skin coverage for the dorsal foot and ankle. *Foot Ankle* 1991;11:274.
3. Hidalgo DA, Shaw WW. Anatomic basis of plantar flap design. *Plast Reconstr Surg* 1986;78:6227.
4. Pontén B. The fasciocutaneous flap: Its use in soft tissue defects of the lower leg. *Br J Plast Surg* 1981;34:215.
5. Ishiskawa K, Isshiki N, Hoshino K, Mori C. Distally based lateral calcaneal flaps. *Ann Plast Surg* 1990;24:10.
6. Hallock GG. Bipedicled fasciocutaneous flaps in the lower extremity. *Ann Plast Surg* 1992;29:397.
7. Hing DN, Buncke HJ, Alpert BS. Applications of the extensor digitorum brevis muscle for soft tissue coverage. *Ann Plast Surg* 1987;19:530.
8. Smith AA, Arons JA, Reyes R, Hegstad SJ. Distal foot coverage with a reverse dorsalis pedis flap. *Ann Plast Surg* 1995;34:191.
9. Grabb WC, Argenta LC. The lateral calcaneal artery skin flap (the lateral calcaneal artery, lesser saphaenous vein, and sural nerve skin flap). *Plast Reconstr Surg* 1981;68:723.
10. Lagvankar SP. Distally-based random fasciocutaneous flaps for multi-staged reconstruction of defects in the lower third of the leg, ankle, and heel. *Br J Plast Surg* 1990;43:541.

CHAPTER 522 ■ ANTEROLATERAL THIGH FLAP

T. BÉGUÉ AND A. C. MASQUELET

EDITORIAL COMMENT

This is another flap that can be useful for reconstruction in the lower extremity when there are few other alternatives.

The anterolateral thigh is a useful and reliable septocutaneous flap for free-flap transfer. Its dimensions are easily applicable for large defects of the lower limb that involve the distal third of the leg, dorsum of the foot, and plantar sole (1–7).

INDICATIONS

The anterolateral thigh flap is a wide, fasciocutaneous flap elevated on a perforating artery issuing from the lateral circumflex artery. Vascularized by a direct vascular bundle, with two terminal branches following the main axis of the flap, it is easy to elevate for free-flap transfer. As its pedicle is long enough to allow its use in areas where recipient-site vessels are distant from the defect to be covered, the main indications are cutaneous defects of the distal leg, including the distal fourth of the leg, the ankle, the heel, and the forefoot. Its most successful utilization is for large defects exposing tendons, nerves, and even bone and joints, on the dorsum of the foot. Large heel defects, including those of the plantar sole, may also be covered by this flap. There are no indications for its use in the upper extremity, as the subcutaneous fat tissue makes the flap too thick for this recipient site.

The main advantages are reliability of vascularization of the skin paddle in the mid-flap, and the large dimensions of tissue that can be elevated. Its main inconvenience is that the donor site cannot be closed directly in the majority of flaps designed. The cosmetic aspect of a skin graft on the anterolateral thigh may be unacceptable to some patients.

ANATOMY

The arterial and venous blood supply of the flap comes from branches issuing from the femoral artery and returning to the femoral vein. The artery at the origin is the lateral thigh circumflex artery. One of the collateral branches of this vessel is the descending branch of the circumflex artery, which leaves the lateral-thigh circumflex artery on its lateral side, gliding beneath the rectus femoris and in front of the vastus lateralis muscles. At this level, the muscular branches to the different segments of the quadriceps leave the main axis of the artery, which courses downward and laterally. The cutaneous branch follows this intermuscular space, lying on the vastus lateralis muscle. The vessel crosses the anterolateral thigh aponeurosis and divides into two axial cutaneous branches (proximal and distal), which have a longitudinal axis and give off many cutaneous branches to the skin paddle.

The cutaneous branch of the descending circumflex artery has a regular caliber of 1 mm at its origin, and the length of the pedicle averages 5 cm.

The venous pattern of the flap has the same axis, parallel to the arterial system all the way from the skin to the intermuscular space between the vastus lateralis and rectus femoris muscles. At this level, the anatomy is more variable. In most cases, the vein remains with the artery, going up to the lateral circumflex vein and then to the femoral vein. In the remaining cases, the vein goes more medially, with a transverse axis to the superficial lateral femoral vein, ending in the greater saphenous vein proximal to the femoral vessel.

Nerve distribution comes from cutaneous nerves issuing from the anterolateral aspect of the thigh and entering the flap near its anterosuperior border. No anastomosis to produce sensibility is reliable, as the nerves are too small and are randomly distributed.

FLAP DESIGN AND DIMENSIONS

Used as a free-flap transfer, flap length and width are designed to meet the required dimensions of the recipient-site defect. The flap is elevated on the anterolateral aspect of the thigh, with an axis joining the anterosuperior iliac spine to the superolateral angle of the patella. The center of the flap corresponding to the perforating vascular bundle through the aponeurosis is at the junction of the upper and middle thirds (Fig. 1). From that point, flap design must maintain a 2:1 length:width ratio. The maximal length available is 30 cm, and the maximal width is 15 cm. For direct closure of the donor site, after subcutaneous release of the flap margins, the largest available dimensions are 8 cm in length and 4 cm in width.

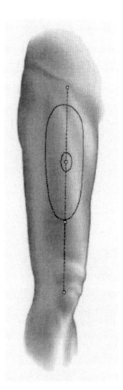

FIG. 1. Skin landmarks (anterosuperior iliac crest, lateral border of patella) and emerging vascular bundle at junction of proximal third and distal two-thirds.

OPERATIVE TECHNIQUE

Measurements at the recipient site are recorded, so that the length and width of the anterolateral thigh flap can be properly designed. The center of the skin paddle on the lateral aspect of the thigh is determined by the emerging cutaneous branches of the descending branch of the lateral circumflex artery. If in doubt, detection of the vessel by Doppler flowmetry may be useful. The flap is centered and designed according to the emerging point of the artery (Fig. 1). Depending on the case, the flap can be drawn more proximal or distal from this point. In any event, the emerging point must be included in the flap design.

To perform an easy dissection, the patient is placed in the supine position with a sandbag under the buttock. Moderate internal rotation of the limb allows greater facility of dissecting. The distal part of the flap is elevated first, with dissection going deep to the aponeurosis. (We used to fix the aponeurosis to the skin to avoid dissection between these tissues.) The intermuscular space between the rectus femoris (medially and anteriorly) and the vastus lateralis muscles (laterally and posteriorly) is identified. The posterior and anterior borders of the flap are then raised, leaving in place the intermuscular space and perforating vessels coming through it.

At that point, the vascular pedicle is identified by retracting the rectus femoris muscle medially. The main artery and vein are isolated and elevated from the vastus lateralis behind them. Then, the intermuscular space is freed, with ligature of the accessory perforating vessels coming through it to the distal cutaneous portion of the flap. Sometimes, the vascular bundle does not lie on the vastus lateralis, but passes through a thin layer of the muscle. Careful dissection of the vastus lateralis allows the elevation of the vascular pedicle. The skin paddle and emerging cutaneous vascular pedicle through the intermuscular space are elevated (Fig. 2).

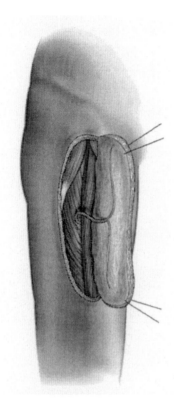

FIG. 2. Complete dissection of the flap and its pedicle emerging from intermuscular space with fatty tissue.

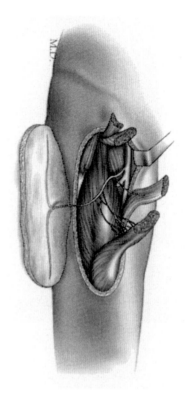

FIG. 3. Medial dissection and muscular vessels to be ligated for a longer vascular pedicle; only the rectus femoris and sartorius should be retracted. (From Bégué et al, ref. 2, with permission.)

If a longer vascular pedicle is required, dissection can be done medially beneath the rectus femoris muscle, by retracting it and ligating the muscular vessels (Fig. 3). The pedicle length will be 10 cm, and the diameter at its origin averages 1.8 mm. Dissection is done simultaneously for the artery and vein. If extended medially to the rectus femoris muscle, venous anatomic variations may be encountered, as previously mentioned.

However, the flap is thick enough for all pressure-sore areas to be covered.

SUMMARY

The anterolateral thigh flap is a useful septocutaneous flap for free transfer and is especially useful for large defects of the lower limb.

CLINICAL RESULTS

Most of the cases we have treated with the anterolateral flap have involved free-flap transfers for coverage of defects of the foot and ankle (2). In some cases, the flap may be used as a rotation flap for coverage of defects around the trochanteric area, like pressure sores. In these cases, the same operative procedure is used, with rotation along the vascular pedicle in a clockwise direction for the left limb and in a counterclockwise direction for the right limb, which allows sufficient coverage of the trochanteric area.

Used in whatever clinical situation, we remind the surgeon of the thickness of the flap; the anterolateral aspect of the thigh has a large amount of subcutaneous fat. Therefore, the flap is not suitable for areas where a thin skin flap is required.

References

1. Baird RD, Cope JS. On the terminations of the circumflex veins of the thigh and their relation to the origins of the circumflex arteries. *Anat Rec* 1933; 57:325.
2. Bégué T, Masquelet AC, Nordin JY. Anatomical basis of the anterolateral thigh flap. *Surg Radiol Anat* 1990;12:311.
3. Koshima I, Kukuda H, Utonomiya R, Soeda S. The anterolateral thigh flap: variations in its vascular pedicle. *Br J Plast Surg* 1989;42:260.
4. Masquelet AC, Romaña MC. Vascularisation tejgumentaire des membres et applications chirurgicales. *Rev Chir Orthop* 1988;74:669.
5. Salmon M. *Les artères de la peau.* Masson: Paris, 1936.
6. Song YG, Chen GZ, Song YL. The free thigh flap: a new free flap concept based on the septocutaneous artery. *Br J Plast Surg* 1984;37:149.
7. Xu DC, Zong SZ, Kong JM, et al. Applied anatomy of the anterolateral femoral flap. *Plast Reconstr Surg* 1988;82:305.

CHAPTER 523 ■ POSTERIOR CALF FASCIOCUTANEOUS FLAP WITH DISTAL PEDICLE TO RECONSTRUCT ANKLE DEFECTS

D. LE NEN, W. HU, AND C. LEFEVRE

EDITORIAL COMMENT

Our anatomic knowledge of the intermuscular perforators or so-called septocutaneous vessels allows us to design a fasciocutaneous flap, whether proximally or distally based or even as an island flap, as one septocutaneous vessel is maintained alongside the flap. The limiting factor is that the lowest septocutaneous vessel usually arises about 6 cm above the malleolus.

A distally-based, posterior-calf fasciocutaneous flap can be used to cover large ankle defects with exposed bones and joints.

INDICATIONS

Coverage of a major ankle defect with exposed bones or joints after acute injury remains a difficult problem. Local flaps are not usually indicated, and the choices for coverage are a cross-leg flap or a free flap. Since its introduction in 1983 (1), a distally-based fasciocutaneous flap from the sural region has been used with a high rate of success for large ankle defects (2). Reports of the flap based posteriorly or laterally for reconstruction of the distal third of the leg, ankle, and heel have shown variable success (3–5). Among its advantages, the flap is relatively wide and reliable. It can be harvested without functional loss and is easily dissected. In addition, it is rapidly elevated, does not require microvascular anastomosis, and provides a good cosmetic result.

Among the disadvantages are the necessity for a two-stage procedure. Also, the saphenous nerve must be sacrificed. A twist at the base required by flap design may compromise the vascular supply, and the extensive fasciocutaneous pedicle decreases the arc of rotation. Coverage of more distal defects cannot be achieved, because this flap does not reach the forefoot.

ANATOMY

The flap receives its arterial blood supply distally in various ways: from a branch of the peroneal artery (6), the saphenous venous plexus (6), and the fasciocutaneous network (3).

FLAP DESIGN AND DIMENSIONS

After division of the saphenous nerve and vein (see Fig. 2), the flap should be elevated from proximal to distal, including the fascia. The distal limits of flap viability, indicating the maximal survivable length, lie about 10 cm above the medial malleolus and 12 cm above the lateral malleolus.

OPERATIVE TECHNIQUE

A posterior-calf fasciocutaneous flap was designed, outlined, and elevated to cover an ankle defect with skin loss and loss of all lateral tendons, ligaments, capsule, distal fibula, and lateral third of the talus, tibia, and calcaneus (Figs. 1 and 2). In this patient, the branch of the peroneal artery was not available because of the wide lateral defect, and the saphenous nerve was already damaged. After elevation, the flap was turned back over the ankle and easily reached the distal edge of the defect (Fig. 3). The donor site was not grafted at this time.

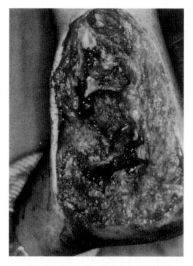

FIG. 1. The ankle defect involved skin, all lateral tendons, ligaments, capsule, distal fibula, and lateral third of the talus, tibia, and calcaneus. (From Le Nen et al, ref. 2, with permission.)

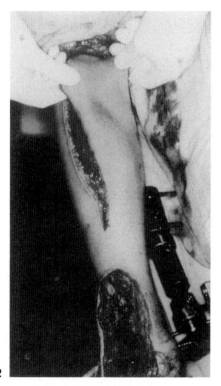
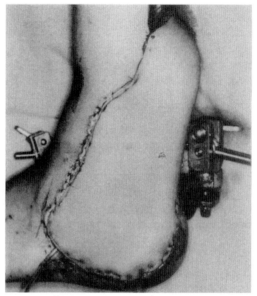

2   **3**

FIGS. 2,3. A posterior-calf fasciocutaneous flap with distal pedicle was elevated and turned back over the ankle. The distal part of the defect was easily covered by the flap. (From Le Nen et al, ref. 2, with permission.)

CLINICAL RESULTS

Wound healing was complicated by a small area of necrosis at the distal margin, which was excised after 10 days. The defect healed spontaneously by scar epithelialization, without advancement of the flap or skin graft. The donor site was cov-

ered 21 days postoperatively by a split-thickness skin graft, which healed with no problems. At this time, the pedicle was divided.

After 3 months, an iliac crest bone graft was screwed laterally onto the tibia to prevent ankle instability. On 2-year follow-up, the patient remained free of osteomyelitis, with an excellent cosmetic result; however, the range of motion was poor (Fig. 4).

SUMMARY

A modified medial plantar flap, based on the lateral plantar artery and vein with reversed flow, can cover any area of the foot.

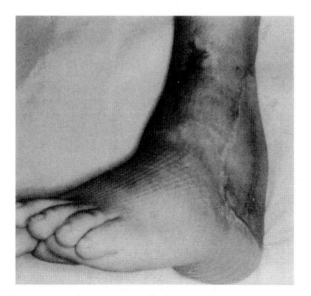

FIG. 4. Ten months postoperatively, the cosmetic result was excellent. (From Le Nen et al, ref. 2, with permission.)

References

1. Donski PK, Fogdestam I. Distally based fasciocutaneous flap from the sural region: a preliminary report. *Scand J Plast Surg* 1983;17:191.
2. Le Nen D, Riot O, le Noach JF, et al. Use of a posterior calf fasciocutaneous flap with distal pedicle to reconstruct a huge ankle defect. *Arch Orthop Trauma Surg* 1992;111:291.
3. Greco JM, Simons G, Darsonval V, et al. Le lambeau fasciocutane jambier externe a pedicle distal. *Ann Chir Plast Esthet* 1986;31:109.
4. Le Huec JC, Chauveaux D, Bovet JL, et al. Intérét du lambeau fasciocutané sural à base distal pour la couverture des pertes de substance du tiers inférieur de jambe. *Rev Chir Orthop* 1988;74(Suppl. II):324.
5. Tolhurst DE. Surgical indications for fasciocutaneous flaps. *Ann Plast Surg* 1984;13:495.
6. Casey R, Darsonval V. Les lambeaux fasciocutanés pedicules à la jambe. In: *Encyclopedia medicale, chirugicale, techniques chirurgicale, et chirurgie reparatrice.* Masson: Paris, 1986;4–11.

CHAPTER 524 ■ FLEXOR DIGITORUM LONGUS MUSCLE FLAP

R. GER

The flexor digitorum longus, a modest-sized muscle, can be used to supplement other muscles, the soleus above or the abductor hallucis below, when large defects require coverage. By itself, the muscle is ideal both for closing small soft-tissue defects and for filling a small but deep osteomyelitic lesion. In the latter situation, larger muscles are unsuitable, and using a small isolated portion of these muscles may be hazardous (1–7).

ANATOMY

Arising from the middle two fourths of the posteromedial surface of the tibia, the moderate-sized muscle belly gives way to its tendon that runs along most of the posterior surface of the muscle. The tendon crosses the tendon of the tibialis posterior behind the medial malleolus. The neurovascular supply from the posterior tibial nerve and vessels reaches the muscle at the junction of the upper and middle thirds of the leg.

OPERATIVE TECHNIQUE

The muscle is easily exposed through a vertical incision placed 1 in (2.5 cm) behind the posterior border of the subcutaneous surface of the tibia and running from the junction of the proximal and middle thirds of the leg to the medial malleolus (Figs. 1–3). The long saphenous vein and saphenous nerves lie anterior to the incision. The deep fascia is incised, and the muscle belly is recognized lying at a deeper level than the soleus muscle. It is easiest to mobilize the muscle from below, where the tendon can be divided as it crosses the tendon of the

tibialis posterior. The distal part of the divided tendon can be sutured to the underlying tibialis posterior tendon to retain a considerable portion of the muscle's function. An alternative method is to dissect the muscle belly off its long tendon, leaving the latter intact.

CLINICAL RESULTS

Functional deficits are minimal. Presumably, the flexor digitorum brevis, the substantial slip from the flexor hallucis longus as the latter is crossed by the tendon of the flexor digitorum longus, and the quadratus plantae help to compensate for any functional loss.

SUMMARY

The flexor digitorum longus muscle can be used alone to cover small leg defects or in conjunction with other muscles to cover larger defects.

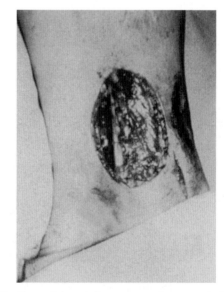

FIG. 1. The flexor digitorum longus occupying an excised ulcer bed, its tendon still intact. A varicosed branch of the long saphenous vein has been removed through the small anterior incision.

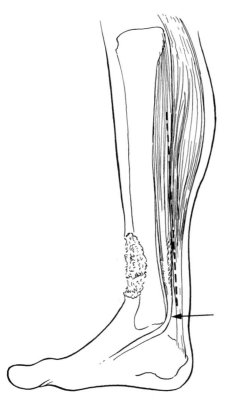

FIG. 2. The flexor digitorum muscle is seen lying anterior to the superficial calf muscles. The ulcer is situated in the distal third of the anteromedial area of the leg. The line of incision is depicted by the dotted outline.

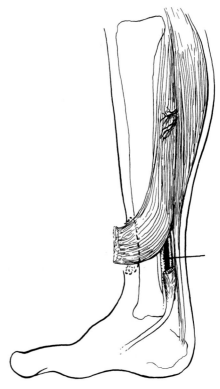

FIG. 3. The mobilized muscle is rotated into the excised defect. The main neurovascular supply is situated in the proximal third of the leg. The *arrow* indicates the posterior tibial vessels.

References

1. Ger R. The operative treatment of the advanced stasis ulcer: a preliminary communication. *Am J Surg* 1966;111:659.
2. Ger R. The management of pretibial skin loss. *Surgery* 1968;63:757.
3. Ger R. Operative treatment of the advanced stasis ulcer using muscle transposition: a follow-up study. *Am J Surg* 1970;120:376.
4. Ger R. The technique of muscle transposition and the operative treatment of traumatic and ulcerative lesions. *J Trauma* 1971;2:502.
5. Ger R. Surgical management of ulcerative lesions of the leg. *Curr Probl Surg* Mar 72:1.
6. Ger R. The management of stasis ulcers of the leg where the tendocalcaneus is exposed. *Plast Reconstr Surg* 1977;60:337.
7. Mathes SJ, Nahai F, eds. *Clinical applications for muscle and musculocutaneous flaps.* St. Louis, Mosby, 1982;563.

CHAPTER 525 ■ ABDUCTOR DIGITI MINIMI MUSCLE FLAP

R. GER

EDITORIAL COMMENT

The usefulness of this flap is limited by the relative smallness of the muscle unit.

The abductor digiti minimi muscle is used to cover defects of the heel and the lateral surface of the ankle joint and lower leg (1–3). Its posterior bulk is surprisingly large and considerably bigger than that of the abductor hallucis.

ANATOMY

This muscle has a wide posterior origin from both processes (tubercles) and the intervening bone of the calcaneus and the

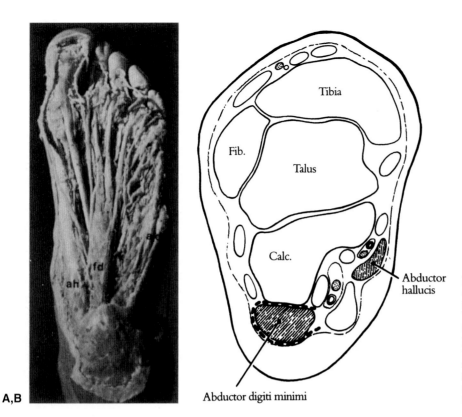

A,B

Tibia

Fib.

Talus

Calc.

Abductor
hallucis

Abductor digiti minimi

FIG. 1. A: The flexor digitorum brevis (fd) is flanked by the abductor digiti minimi (ad) and abductor hallucis (ah) muscles. Note the double insertion of the abductor digiti minimi into the base of the fifth metatarsus and into the proximal phalanx of the fifth toe. The digital vessels and nerves are well seen. **B:** Coronal section of the ankle joint showing the relative sizes of the abductor digiti minimi and abductor hallucis muscles near their origins. (From Ger, ref. 1, with permission.)

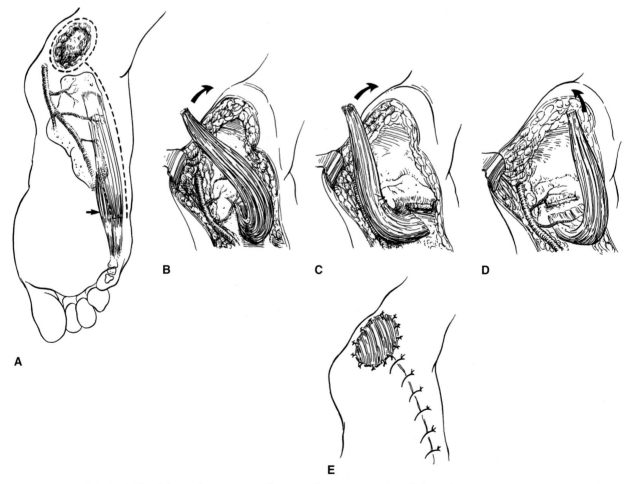

A

B

C

D

E

FIG. 2. A: The abductor digiti minimi with its vascular supply. An ulcer of the heel is excised as depicted by the *oval dotted outline*. The *longitudinal dotted line* exposes the muscle. The abductor digiti minimi tendon is dissected free from the adjoining flexor digiti minimi brevis tendon and muscle (*arrow*). **B:** The muscle is rotated superiorly without disturbing its bony origin. **C:** The muscle is rotated superiorly with partial separation of its bony origin. **D:** The muscle is completely detached from its broad origin for maximal mobilization. **E:** The muscle occupies and is sutured to the edges of the defect.

1502

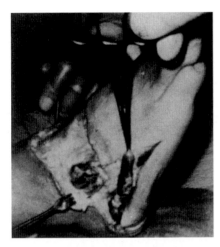

FIG. 3. The abductor digiti minimi is dissected free, its distal tendon having been severed. The extensor digitorum brevis is seen lying in situ.

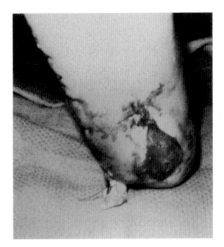

FIG. 4. The muscle is occupying an excised heel defect prior to skin-graft application.

adjacent thick fascia (Figs. 1, 2 and see also Fig. 1 in Chapter 529). The wide muscle belly narrows to a tendon near the base of the fifth metatarsal. The final insertion of the muscle is into the lateral side of the proximal phalanx of the little toe, in common with the flexor digiti minimi brevis. Variations may occur on the way to this insertion. The overlying thickened fascia, the calcaneometatarsal band or lateral cord that inserts into the base of the fifth metatarsal, may contain muscle fibers and constitute the abductor metatarsi quinti. Sometimes, there are two separate muscle bellies that stop and start opposite the base of the fifth metatarsal. The neurovascular supply from the lateral plantar nerve and vessels enters the muscle well toward its origin.

OPERATIVE TECHNIQUE

This muscle is exposed by an incision just above the lateral border of the foot that runs from the heel to the head of the fifth metatarsal. The tendon is divided near its insertion, and the muscle is dissected proximally where it requires separation from the flexor digiti minimi brevis. The lateral plantar vessels and nerves lie well to the medial border of the muscle between it and the flexor digitorum brevis (Fig. 3).

Because the main vessels and nerve enter the muscle from the medial side, the dissection should first proceed along the lateral border of the muscle to its calcaneal origin. Along the medial border of the muscle, dissection proceeds until the neurovascular bundle is identified. The muscle can be maximally mobilized by severing its broad calcaneal origin and leaving it attached by its neurovascular pedicle only (Fig. 4).

CLINICAL RESULTS

Intrinsic muscles of the sole of the foot are concerned mostly with the maintenance of the longitudinal or transverse arches. The functional deficiency following loss of this muscle is not clinically discernible.

SUMMARY

The abductor digiti minimi muscle can be separated from both its origin and its insertion and used to cover defects of the heel and lateral ankle.

References

1. Ger R. The surgical management of ulcers of the heel. *Surg Gynecol Obstet* 1975;140:909.
2. Ger R. The management of chronic ulcers of the dorsum of the foot by muscle transposition and free skin grafting. *Br J Plast Surg* 1976;29:199.
3. Mathes SJ, Nahai F, eds. *Clinical applications for muscle and musculocutaneous flaps.* St. Louis: Mosby, 1982.

CHAPTER 526 ■ ABDUCTOR HALLUCIS BREVIS MUSCLE FLAP

R. GER

This muscle can be used to cover defects over the heel and medial aspect of the ankle joint and medial malleolus (1–6). In combination with other muscles, it also can be used to cover defects of the dorsum of the foot and lower end of the tibial shaft.

ANATOMY

The abductor hallucis arises from the medial process (tubercle) of the calcaneus and the surrounding fascia. The fleshy belly gives rise to a tendon at about the midfoot (medial cuneiform-first metatarsal articulation) that inserts into the medial side of the proximal phalanx of the big toe in common with the tendon of the medial portion of the flexor hallucis brevis. The neurovascular supply from the medial plantar nerve and vessels arises proximally about two to three fingerbreadths behind the navicular tuberosity (Fig. 1; also Figs. 1 and 2A, Chap. 50; Fig. 1A, Chap 527; and Fig. 4, Chap 528.)

OPERATIVE TECHNIQUE

The muscle is exposed by an incision that lies just above the medial border of the sole of the foot and curves from the heel to the ball of the big toe (Fig. 2). The tendon is divided proximal to the metatarsophalangeal joint and dissected proximally. It is usually possible to separate the tendon from the adjacent flexor hallucis brevis, but sometimes the tendon and muscle of the abductor fuse with the flexor hallucis brevis and sharp dissection is required.

Because the neuromuscular bundle enters from the lateral side, the medial border of the muscle is first mobilized until the calcaneal origin is reached. The lateral border is then immobilized until the neurovascular bundle is located. As in the case of the abductor digiti minimi, the muscle can be stripped off the calcaneus, depending on the amount of mobilization required (Fig. 3).

CLINICAL RESULTS

Functional deficits are not clinically apparent. The muscle is a supporter of the medial longitudinal arch, and it would seem that the numerous other supporting structures of this arch are sufficient to compensate for loss of this muscle.

SUMMARY

The abductor hallucis muscle can be used to cover defects from the heel to the area of the medial malleolus. Used with other muscles, it can cover defects of the dorsum of the foot and ankle.

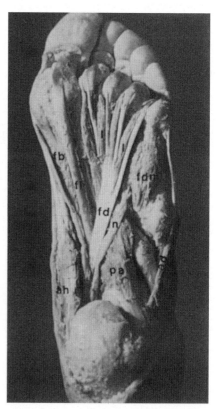

FIG. 1. The abductor hallucis (*ah*) with the medial plantar neurovascular structures and the tendon of the flexor hallucis longus (*fl*) on its medial side. The abductor digiti minimi (*ad*) on the lateral aspect of the foot. The flexor digitorum longus tendon (*fd*) and the lateral plantar nerve (*n*) are running mediolaterally across the sole of the foot. The flexor hallucis brevis (*fb*), flexor digiti minimi brevis (*fdm*), plantar accessories (*pa*), and lumbrical (*l*) muscles are also seen. (Dissections performed by A. DiLandro.)

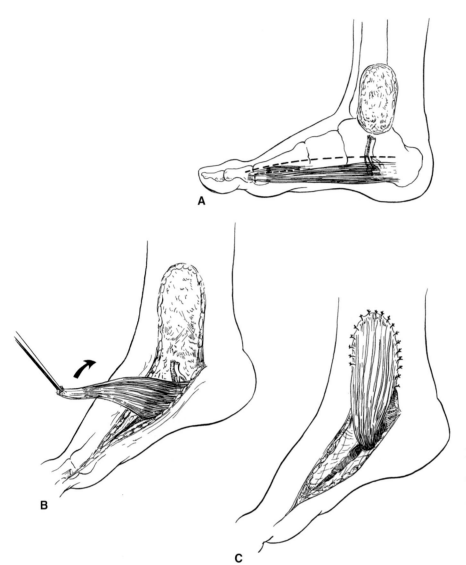

FIG. 2. A: The abductor hallucis and its blood supply. The line of incision for exposure is indicated, and a medial malleolar ulcer is depicted. **B:** The muscle has been divided at its tendinous junction and is about to be rotated into the defect created by the excised ulcer. **C:** The muscle is sutured to the skin edges of the excised defect.

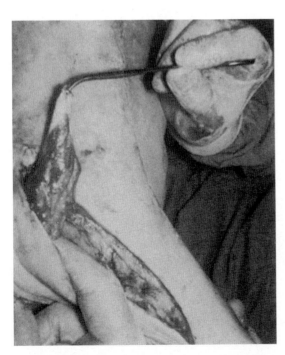

FIG. 3. The mobilized abductor hallucis is rotated superiorly to cover an underlying defect.

References

1. Ger R. The management of pretibial skin loss. *Surgery* 1968;63:757.
2. Ger R. Operative treatment of the advanced stasis ulcer using muscle transposition: A follow-up study. *Am J Surg* 1970;120:376.
3. Ger R. The technique of muscle transposition and the operative treatment of traumatic and ulcerative lesions. *J Trauma* 1971;2:502.
4. Ger R. The surgical management of ulcer of the heel. *Surg Gynecol Obstet* 1975;140:909.
5. Ger R. The management of chronic ulcers of the dorsum of the foot by muscle transposition and free skin grafting. *Br J Plast Surg* 1976;29:199.
6. Mathes SJ, Nahai F, eds. *Clinical applications for muscle and musculocutaneous flaps.* St. Louis: Mosby, 1982;594.9

CHAPTER 527 ■ FLEXOR DIGITORUM BREVIS MUSCLE FLAP

R. GER

The flexor digitorum brevis muscle is used exclusively to cover defects of the heel (1–3).

ANATOMY

This muscle has a relatively narrow origin from the medial process (tubercle) of the calcaneum but a substantial origin from the plantar aponeurosis. The belly gives rise to four tendons just beyond the metatarsophalangeal joints that run deep to the divisions of the plantar aponeurosis. Opposite the bases of the proximal phalanges, the tendons split to allow the passage of the tendons of the flexor digitorum longus and then insert into the sides of the middle phalanges. The neurovascular bundles to the digits and the lumbricals run between the tendons. The muscle is covered by the thick plantar aponeurosis and is flanked by the abductors hallucis and digiti minimi muscles. The neurovascular supply to the muscle arises proximally from the lateral plantar nerve and vessels as they pass laterally deep to the muscle (see Fig. 1A).

OPERATIVE TECHNIQUE

The muscle is exposed by a midline incision on the plantar aspect of the foot (Fig. 1 and see Fig. 1 in Chap. 525). The

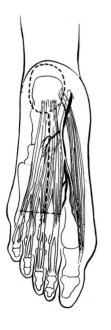
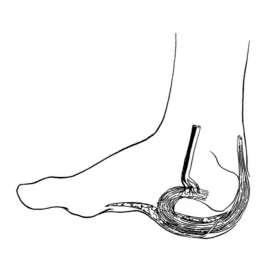

A,B

FIG. 1. **A:** The flexor digitorum brevis and the abductor hallucis muscles are depicted with the medial plantar vessels between them. The *oval dotted line* indicates the excised heel ulcer, and the *longitudinal dotted line* indicates the incision required to expose the flexor digitorum brevis. The *transverse dotted line* indicates the division at the muscles and tendinous junctions. **B:** The muscle belly is turned on itself to cover the heel defect.

plantar aponeurosis is incised and reflected medially and laterally, and the muscle is identified deep to the fascia. The musculotendinous junctions are severed, and the muscle is turned back on itself proximally (Fig. 1). Mobilization proceeds until the muscle covers the calcaneus, taking care not to injure the underlying lateral plantar nerve and vessels.

CLINICAL RESULTS

Functional deficits are not seen, since the flexor digitorum longus flexes the joints of the toes.

SUMMARY

The flexor digitorum brevis muscle can be used to cover heel defects.

References

1. Bostwick J III. Reconstruction of the heel pad by muscle transposition and split-skin graft. *Surg Gynecol Obstet* 1976;143:972.
2. Hartrampf CR Jr, Scheflan M, Bostwick J III. The flexor digitorum brevis muscle island pedicle flap: A new dimension in heel reconstruction. *Plast Reconstr Surg* 1980;66:264.
3. Mathes SJ, Nahai F, eds. *Clinical applications for muscle and musculocutaneous flaps*. St. Louis: Mosby, 1982;598.

CHAPTER 528 ■ FLEXOR HALLUCIS BREVIS MUSCLE FLAP

R. GER

The medial portion of the flexor hallucis brevis is suitable for use in conjunction with the abductor hallucis for lesions of the dorsum of the foot (1–5). The whole muscle can be used by itself to fill defects in the anteromedial sole of the foot, such as perforating ulcers (mal perforans).

ANATOMY

This muscle arises by a pointed tendon from the contiguous surfaces of the plantar surface of the cuboid and medial cuneiform. Medial and lateral portions of the muscle develop and insert into either side of the base of the proximal phalanx of the big toe, a sesamoid bone developing in each tendon and articulating with the head of the first metatarsal. Each portion is joined by another tendon of insertion, the medial by that of the abductor hallucis and the lateral by the adductor hallucis. The tendon of the flexor hallucis longus straps the muscle belly down to the first metatarsal (Fig. 1). The nerve supply from the first digital nerve enters the muscle near its origin. The blood supply is from the medial plantar and first plantar metatarsal vessels.

OPERATIVE TECHNIQUE

The incision is the distal portion of that used for exposing the abductor hallucis. The muscle is easily recognized as it lies against the plantar aspect of the first metatarsal. Either the medial portion or the whole muscle can be used. The medial portion can be used in conjunction with the abductor hallucis (Figs. 2 and 3). In this instance, the conjoint tendon of insertion into the medial side of the first phalanx is divided, and the muscles are mobilized proximally. Because the flexor hallucis longus tendon lies on the middle of the muscle, it demarcates each portion. It is therefore simple to split the muscle along the line of the tendon. Both the medial portion and the abductor hallucis are reflected proximally as far as necessary. If the whole muscle is to be used, it is detached at its origin and mobilized distally, reflecting the tendon of the flexor hallucis longus laterally to facilitate this dissection. During this dissection, the nerve supply to the muscle is sacrificed (Fig. 4).

CLINICAL RESULTS

There are no discernible functional deficits, as the flexor hallucis longus will flex the metatarsophalangeal joint.

SUMMARY

The flexor hallucis brevis muscle can be used in its entirety for anteromedial defects. The medial portion can be used with the abductor hallucis brevis for dorsal foot defects.

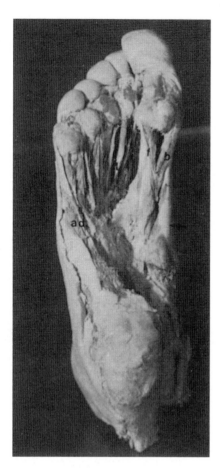

FIG. 1. The two portions of the flexor hallucis brevis (fb) can be seen; the medial portion is joined by the distal portion of the abductor hallucis (*arrow*). The lumbricals (l) and the abductor digiti minimi (ad) are also seen.

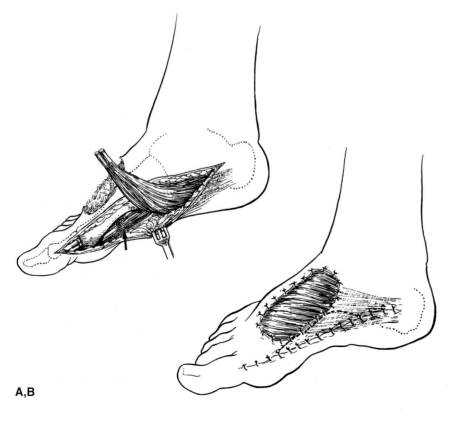

FIG. 2. A: The conjoint medial portion of the flexor hallucis brevis and abductor hallucis muscles has been exposed through an incision along the medial border of the sole of the foot and is being rotated onto the dorsum of the foot to cover an ulcer. The lateral portion of the flexor hallucis brevis is in situ (*arrow*). B: The muscles are occupying the defect. Depending on the proximity of the ulcer to the incision, the latter can be placed to include the medial border of the ulcer or it can be placed some distance away. Wherever placed, a narrow skin bridge between the ulcer and the incision should be avoided.

A,B

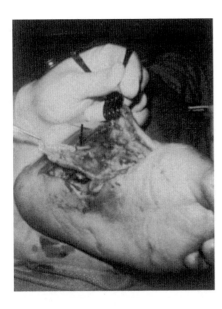

FIG. 3. The mobilized abductor hallucis and flexor hallucis brevis muscles rotated on themselves to fill a plantar defect. At this level, the abductor hallucis is represented by its tendon only (*arrow*).

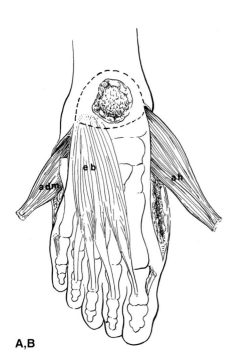
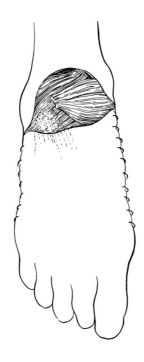

A,B

FIG. 4. A: The mobilized abductor digiti minimi (adm) and conjoined abductor hallucis and flexor hallucis brevis muscles (ah). The extensor digitorum brevis (eb) is undisturbed. The ulcer over the anterior aspect of the ankle joint is depicted as well as the lines of excision. **B:** The abductors have been rotated into the defect. The extensor digitorum brevis does not require mobilization.

References

1. Ger R. The management of pretibial skin loss. *Surgery* 1968;63:757.
2. Ger R. Operative treatment of the advanced stasis ulcer using muscle transposition: A follow-up study. *Am J Surg* 1970;120:376.
3. Ger R. The technique of muscle transposition and the operative treatment of traumatic and ulcerative lesions. *J Trauma* 1971;2:502.
4. Ger R. The management of chronic ulcers of the dorsum of the foot by muscle transposition and free skin grafting. *Br J Plast Surg* 1976;29:199.
5. Mathes SJ, Nahai F, eds. *Clinical applications for muscle and musculocutaneous flaps.* St. Louis: Mosby, 1982;594.

CHAPTER 529 ■ EXTENSOR DIGITORUM BREVIS MUSCLE FLAP

R. GER

EDITORIAL COMMENT

This muscle should be thought of for relatively small defects on the dorsum of the foot.

The extensor digitorum brevis is not of great use because of its limited mobility. Nevertheless, at times it may be used to cover a defect in the region of the lateral malleolus and anterior ankle.

ANATOMY

This small muscle arises mainly from a small anterior area of the lateral surface of the calcaneus close to the calcaneocuboid articulation. The muscle belly runs forward and medially to end in four tendons at the level of the tarsometatarsal joints. The three lateral tendons join and insert with the tendons of the extensor digitorum longus to the lateral three toes. The most medial tendon is sometimes called the extensor hallucis brevis, because it forms a somewhat distinct slip and inserts into the base of the proximal phalanx of the big toe. The vascular supply is a branch of the lateral tarsal artery that arises from the dorsalis pedis, enters the deep surface of the muscle, and then anastomoses with several other arteries (see Fig. 1A).

OPERATIVE TECHNIQUE

The muscle can be exposed by a curved incision that is placed over the muscle and runs from just below the crease of the ankle for approximately 4 in (10 cm) (Fig. 1 and see Fig. 3 in Chapter 525). The four tendons are divided, and the muscle is reversed on itself.

CLINICAL RESULTS

Functional deficits are minimal, since the extensors hallucis and digitorum longus are more effective extensors.

SUMMARY

The extensor digitorum brevis can sometimes be used to cover defects around the lateral malleolus.

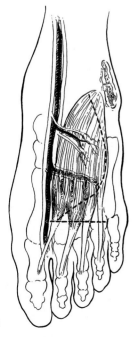
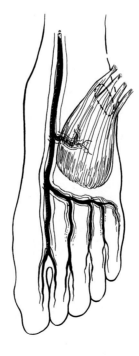

A,B

FIG. 1. **A:** Extensor digitorum brevis muscle supplied by branches of the dorsalis pedis vessels. The curved dorsal incision over the lateral part of the muscle is indicated by the *dotted line*. Distally, the transverse *dotted line* marks the division of the muscle at the musculotendinous junctions. **B:** The muscle is reversed on itself to cover the excised ulcer over the lateral malleolus.

CHAPTER 530 ■ FLEXOR HALLUCIS BREVIS MUSCLE FLAP

K. T. MAHAN

EDITORIAL COMMENT

This is a good flap for coverage of plantar ulcerations, if the muscle is still viable.

The flexor hallucis brevis muscle flap can be particularly useful for providing muscle coverage below the first metatarsal head. This flap, as well as other intrinsic muscle flaps of the foot, rotated and used to provide muscle coverage, is limited in its coverage area by a small arc of rotation (1–5).

INDICATIONS

The flexor hallucis brevis flap can be used for managing ulcerations on the plantar and medial sides of the foot. The flap is not a first choice of treatment, but can be used when ulcers fail to respond to conservative therapy. The procedure involves excision of the ulcer, filling the defect with the muscle, and applying a split-thickness skin graft over the muscle, as necessary. The most common indication is sub first metatarsal-head ulceration. This frequently occurs in conjunction with neuropathy associated with diabetes mellitus.

ANATOMY

The flexor hallucis brevis has a Y-shaped fibrotendinous origin within the foot. A medial component originates from the tendon of the tibialis posterior and the medial cuneiform. The lateral origin begins on the lateral side of the foot, including the lateral cuneiform and cuboid, the peroneal tendons, and the short and long bifurcate ligaments. The body of the muscle then runs beneath the first metatarsal, where, distally, it divides into medial and lateral heads. The lateral head inserts on the plantar plate, the medial aspect of the fibular sesamoid, and the base of the proximal phalanx, where it joins with the fibers of the adductor hallucis. The medial head is somewhat larger and inserts on the medial aspect of the plantar plate and on the lateral aspect of the tibial sesamoid, as well as on the base of the proximal phalanx medially, in conjunction with fibers from the abductor hallucis.

Muscle innervation comes from the first proper digital nerve of the big toe, a branch of the medial plantar nerve. The vascular supply comes from the first plantar metatarsal artery, forming from the junction of the lateral and deep plantar arteries. It generally enters from the lateral side of the muscle in the mid-body region.

OPERATIVE TECHNIQUE

The incisional approach is from the plantar aspect of the foot, in order to have full and complete visualization of the flexor hallucis brevis. This can be done through a straight linear incision or a zig-zag anti-tension line approach (Fig. 1). An incision is made in the deep fascia, and the tendon of the flexor hallucis longus is retracted laterally. From this point forward, the approach will depend on whether the surgeon wishes to rotate the flap proximally or distally. Bone resection may be necessary if there is underlying osteomyelitis or exostoses.

The sequence of events for distal rotation follows. The incisional approach is made back into the mid-foot area, in order to identify the origins of the flexor hallucis brevis. These are sharply transected, and the muscle flap is lifted gently and reflected distally (Fig. 2). Care must be taken to ensure that the muscular artery is initially preserved. If the arc of rotation allows for enough muscle to fill the sub first metatarsal space, then the divided origins of the muscle are sutured into place on the plantar plate. If there is inadequate rotation, a muscular artery can be divided and the flap rotated far more distally. In either event, the flap can be sutured into place, and the incisional approach closed or covered with a skin graft. This reduces the mechanical effects caused by bone protrusion, as well as providing additional space for the muscle flap. Another alternative is for the skin to be closed primarily over the muscle flap, although this can create excessive tension (Fig. 3).

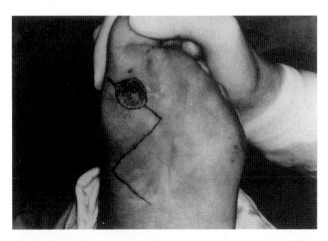

FIG. 1. A sub first metatarsal ulceration in a diabetic patient. Note zig-zag anti-tension line approach. (From Mahan, Feehery, ref. 5, with permission.)

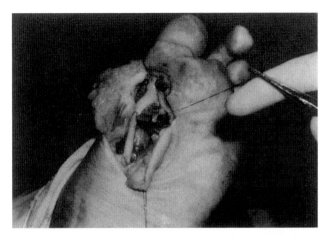

FIG. 2. Detachment of the origins of the flexor hallucis brevis and pivoting of muscle on its arc of rotation. (From Mahan, Feehery, ref. 5, with permission.)

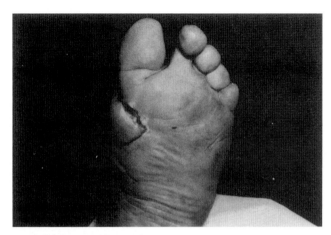

FIG. 3. Plantar aspect of the foot 3 weeks postoperatively, demonstrating superficial dehiscence caused by tension of the primary closure. Nonetheless, the wound went on to complete healing and has not broken down since the time of surgery, about 6 years previously. (From Mahan, Feehery, ref. 5, with permission.)

CLINICAL RESULTS

Postoperatively, the patient is managed in non-weight-bearing in a posterior splint for approximately 3 weeks. Return to weight-bearing begins at this point, with partial weight allowed. Neuropathic patients are graduated to full weight-bearing more slowly.

A caveat is that, if the mechanical imbalances in the foot have not been addressed, the flap will ultimately fail. For example, a diabetic neuropathic patient who has a plantar-flexion deformity of the first metatarsal is likely to have ulceration through the muscle flap. Care should be taken to rebalance the foot with an orthotic or shoe modification. Some loss of hallux purchase will occur with the sacrifice of the flexor hallucis brevis. This is not too important in apropulsive patients, such as neuropathic diabetics. Additional stabilization can be created by suturing the plantar plate and flexor hallucis brevis tendons to the flexor hallucis longus.

The flexor hallucis brevis muscle flap has a limited, but important, role in the management of ulcerations in the foot. Because of foot mechanics, the first metatarsal area is a common site for ulceration. Patients who have been resistant to conservative therapy respond well to this muscle flap as a permanent form of coverage.

SUMMARY

The flexor hallucis brevis muscle flap is useful for ulcerations beneath the first metatarsal. It has a limited arc of rotation and one primary blood supply.

References

1. Weaver J, Porter MC. Surgical repair of the foot with muscle transposition. *JAPMA* 1988;78:254.
2. Ger R. The surgical management of ulcers of the heel. *Surg Gynecol Obstet* 1975;140:909.
3. Ger R. Newer concepts in the surgical management of lesions of the foot in a patient with diabetes. *Surg Gynecol Obstet* 1984;158:213.
4. Ger R. Muscle transposition in the management of perforating ulcers of the forefoot. *Clin Orthop* 1983;175:186.
5. Mahan KT, Feehery RV. Flexor hallucis brevis muscle flap. *J Foot Surg* 1991;30:284.

CHAPTER 531 ■ CROSS-FOOT SKIN FLAP

G. A. TAYLOR

Reconstruction of the weight-bearing portion of the plantar surface of the foot is an ongoing challenge to the ingenuity of the plastic surgeon (1).

INDICATIONS

The cross-foot flap may be used for reconstruction of weight-bearing and friction-bearing plantar skin defects up to 5 × 8 cm. The contralateral instep donor site provides histologically similar skin.

ANATOMY

The cross-foot flap (2,3), as a "functional graft of the heel," is a random-pattern flap of the distant direct type (4) raised from the plantar instep of the contralateral foot. The plantar skin differs significantly from the skin of the other parts of the body. The epidermis is much thicker (up to 1.4 mm) and consists of well-defined classic layers of stratum corneum through stratum germinativum, with the former particularly well developed. Pigment cells are rare, and sebaceous glands and hair follicles are absent. The dermis is thicker (up to 3 mm), with more regularly aligned collagen bundles and less ground substance (5). The extension of the collagen bundles into the subcutis and plantar fascia binds the plantar skin to the skeleton for traction, at the same time producing a "shock-absorbing" system of closed fat loculations. These characteristics are best developed over the metatarsal heads, the heel, and the lateral aspect of the sole (the weight-bearing region), and gradually fade out toward the periphery.

Although not so distinctive as in the weight-bearing areas, these features are still well developed in the non-weight-bearing or instep portion of the sole of the foot (Fig. 1). The instep skin is supplied by two branches of the medial plantar artery that perforate on either side of the underlying abductor hallucis muscle and by small perforating vessels that represent the musculocutaneous circulation through that muscle (6).

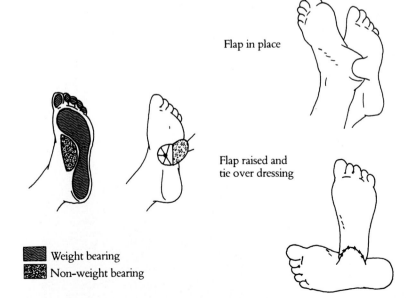

Flap in place

Flap raised and tie over dressing

■ Weight bearing
▓ Non-weight bearing

FIG. 1. (*Left*) The donor area for a cross-instep flap. (*Center*) The flap is outlined on the instep of the donor foot using a pattern and raised, applying a split-thickness skin graft to the donor defect. (*Right*) The feet can be placed either parallel (*above*) or at 90 degrees (*below*) when the flap is sutured in place. (From Taylor, Hopson, ref. 7, with permission.)

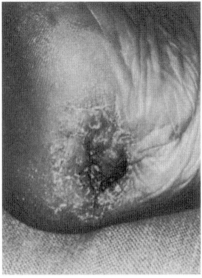
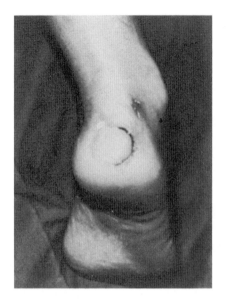

A,B

FIG. 2. **A:** A 37-year-old woman with a full-thickness defect on her posterior heel from a tight cast applied for a fractured medial malleolus. Preoperative hyperkeratotic scar on the right heel. **B:** Postoperatively, the patient has a soft and completely healed and stable skin flap, with no evidence of hyperkeratosis. (From Taylor, Hopson, ref. 7, with permission.)

FLAP DESIGN AND DIMENSIONS

A random-pattern flap of skin can be raised from this area without a delay procedure and without encountering circulation problems if the following guidelines are followed (Figs. 1 and 2). The flap can be up to 5 × 8 cm large and based either medially or laterally depending on the size, shape, and location of the defect to be covered on the affected foot.

Preoperative planning should be done with the patient supine in bed to ensure a comfortable leg position. The feet may be positioned parallel or at 90 degrees to one another.

OPERATIVE TECHNIQUE

The defect is patterned and the flap is designed and marked according to the preoperative plan. The flap is raised in the natural plane of dissection deep to the subcutaneous tissue, and the defect is covered with a split-thickness skin graft, usually taken from the opposite instep and secured with a tieover dressing (Fig. 3).

After the flap is sutured in place, leg fixation is applied using Elastoplast, flannel bandage, plaster of Paris, or threaded Steinmann pins transfixing the tibiae.

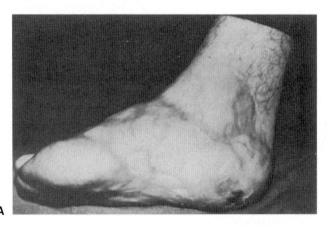
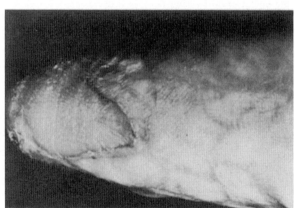

A   **B**

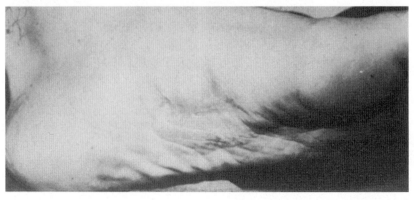

FIG. 3. **A:** Preoperatively, there was a persistent ulcer on the weight-bearing prominence of the os calcis. This patient had sustained a severe crush and avulsion injury of his right foot 7 to 10 years previously when it was caught beneath the wheel of a train. The defect had been repaired with a combination of full- and split-thickness skin grafts. **B:** The well-padded recipient area has remained healed postoperatively. (From Taylor, Hopson, ref 7, with permission.) **C:** The donor site on the opposite instep postoperatively.

C

Postoperatively, the patients' knees and hips usually can be moved through a reasonable range of motion without disturbing the flap.

The pedicle is divided in 2 to 3 weeks without a definitive insetting procedure. Ambulation is begun without weight bearing at 3 to 4 weeks, with weight bearing commencing at 4 to 5 weeks (7).

CLINICAL RESULTS

The largest reported experience with the use of this flap has been 16 patients, with no problems in the reconstructed foot and only one troublesome donor-site scar that was excised secondarily (3). Recently, a cross-foot flap using an arterialized dorsalis pedis flap from the dorsum of the foot for coverage of defects of the opposite lateral malleolus was described (8).

SUMMARY

The cross-foot skin flap replaces pressure-bearing skin with histologically similar skin. The cross-foot position is a comfortable one, and the donor site is particularly inconspicuous.

References

1. Sommerlad BC, McGrouther DA. Resurfacing the sole: long-term follow-up and comparison of techniques. *Br J Plast Surg* 1973;31:107.
2. Mir y Mir L. Functional graft of the heel. *Plast Reconstr Surg* 1954;14:444.
3. Mir y Mir L. Follow-up clinic. *Plast Reconstr Surg* 1975;55:702.
4. Grabb WC, Myers MB eds. *Skin flaps.* Boston: Little, Brown, 1975;145, 151.
5. Bloom W, Fawcett DW eds. *A textbook of histology,* 9th ed. Philadelphia: Saunders, 1968.
6. Harrison DH, Morgan DG. The instep island flap to resurface plantar defects. *Br J Plast Surg* 1981;34:315.
7. Taylor GA, Hopson WL. The cross-foot flap. *Plast Reconstr Surg* 1975;55:677.
8. Cervino AL, Thottam H. Cross-foot flap for ankle coverage. *Ann Plast Surg* 1979;2:72.

CHAPTER 532 ■ CROSS-THIGH FLAP

H. TRAMIER

The fragility and lack of mobility of the skin and subcutaneous tissue of the leg and foot make skin defects in this region especially serious. In many cases, flap coverage from a distance is required.

The cross-leg flap has been used since the nineteenth century; however, surgeons soon became aware that the posterior part of the leg, a rather narrow area used most commonly for this flap, had very fragile circulation. The flap also resulted in prolonged discomfort for patients (1). It became evident that there was a need for using other territories of the leg as donor sites.

INDICATIONS

There are problems involved in using the cross-thigh flap (2–9). The flap is contraindicated for older patients and those without supple joints. The sensory requirements of the recipient defect must be taken into account. The thinner the flap, the better the return of sensation.

ANATOMY

The vascular system of the skin of the lower leg is apparently different above and below the knee (10). The skin below the knee is vascularized mainly by the perforating arteries coming from the deep trunk, each one providing the nutritional supply of an important cutaneous area. Normally, small anastomoses exist between the larger vessels, but generally they are insufficient to compensate for the loss of several perforating arteries. Delaying the flap will allow the development of small anastomoses, but their state will remain precarious. Venous drainage of the lower limb is ensured principally by the two large longitudinal saphenous veins, at least one of which must remain intact (11).

The thigh, however, is supplied by arteries that are long and large, although few. Large-diameter subdermal anastomoses are especially scarce in the inferolateral third of the thigh, although dermal anastomoses are numerous in the anterior and medial areas and in a band of tissue separating the posterior and lateral regions.

In the anterior thigh, a wealth of large transverse vessels permits a certain amount of undermining without risk, except in the upper area. Transecting large vessels presents little drawback because of the number of subdermal and dermal anastomoses. In the lateral region, large arteries are scarce, the subdermal anastomotic network is rich, and the dermal network less so. Undermining at this level causes few problems if it is not too extensive.

Posteriorly, the upper half possesses long, large arteries with numerous anastomoses. In the lower half, however, the arteries are shorter and thinner with poor subdermal anastomoses. Superficial venous drainage is provided by a rich subcutaneous network. Thus, the good cutaneous vascularity of the thigh provides the best donor site for taking a flap from the lower limb.

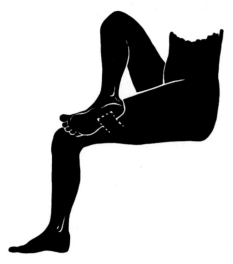

FIG. 1. The cross-thigh flap can easily be designed to cover ankle and foot defects.

FLAP DESIGN AND DIMENSIONS

Once the exact extent of the defect is determined, the flap size, donor site, and orientation must be carefully designed (11). Gillies advised sitting on the floor beside the patient to find the best position and the ideal "cross-leg." This notion is still valid in determining the best flap location and the best position for the lower limbs (Fig. 1).

OPERATIVE TECHNIQUE

First Stage (Delay)

Depending on the length of the skin defect redrawn on the thigh, the flap is extended by the distance separating the donor site from the recipient site—at least 2 cm. Three sides of the flap are cut, including the superficial fascia of the thigh. The flap is then sutured in place.

Second Stage (Flap Transfer)

On the eighth day, the flap is transferred. After the defect is prepared, the thigh flap is elevated and sutured in place. Elasticized tape is used to immobilize the legs in the correct position (Fig. 2).

Third Stage (Pedicle Division)

This is performed after 2 weeks of immobilization and involves cutting the pedicle from the flap, which has been thickened by edema.

Fourth Stage (Insetting)

The flap is inset a week later. The donor site is grafted either at this point or earlier during the second stage. The flap margin is trimmed and sutured without tension to the remaining edge of the defect.

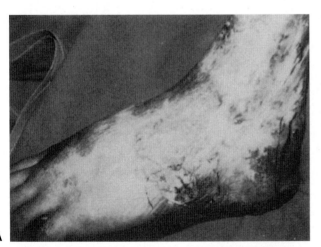

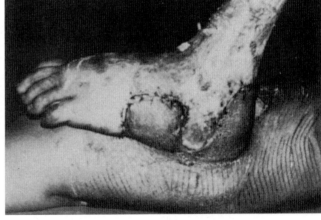

A   B

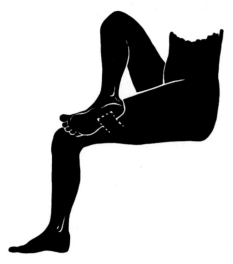

C

FIG. 2. **A:** Defects of both the heel and lateral surface of the foot outlined. **B:** Just prior to stage III (division of the pedicle). The elasticized tape used to immobilize the legs has been removed. **C:** Postoperative result.

Variations in Shape

By changing the position of the two limbs as well as the direction of the flap and the location of its pedicle, all the skin of the thigh can be used without difficulty. As many different techniques as patients may be imagined. Two simultaneous flaps can be used in various combinations to cover one or more defects on the leg or foot (9).

CLINICAL RESULTS

The good vascularity of the thigh as well as the proper surgical precautions reduce the risk of flap necrosis. Small pressure sores may appear on the donor thigh in patients who are not well supported, but they are of little consequence because of the thickness of the muscles of the anterior part of the thigh. A simple excision of the injured tissues solves this problem. The position may not be tolerated, especially by obese patients.

SUMMARY

The cross-thigh flap is a reliable technique that gives the patient little discomfort. It provides an important source of tissue for covering skin defects of the leg and foot. More than one skin flap can be used simultaneously.

References

1. Ombredanne L, Jeambrau E, Nove-Josserand P. *Chirurgie reparatrice et orthopedique.* Paris: Masson, 1920;97–100.
2. Pierre M, Jouglard JP. La réparation des pertes de substance de la plante du pied. *Marseilles Chir* 1966;00:328.
3. Mladick RA, Pickrell KL, Thome FL, Royer JR. Ipsilateral thigh flap for total plantar resurfacing. *Plast Reconstr Surg* 1969;43:198.
4. Tramier H. Les pertes de substances traumatiques de la plante du pied: Approche anatomo-chirurgicale. *Prix Acad Med* 1969.
5. Tramier H, Jouglard JP. Le "cross-thigh flap": une interessante source de tissu dans la chirurgie du pied. *Ann Chir Plast* 1976;21:285.
6. Fumas DW. The cross-groin flap for coverage of foot and ankle defects in children: case report. *Plast Reconstr Surg* 1976;57:246.
7. Wexler MR, Abu-Dalu X, Rousso M. The lotus position: bilateral cross-thigh flap for simultaneous coverage of both feet. *Plast Reconstr Surg* 1978;61:784.
8. Drabyn GH, Avedian L. Ipsilateral buttock flap for coverage of a foot and ankle defect in a young child. *Plast Reconstr Surg* 1979;63:422.
9. Di Piro EM, Moser MH. Cross-thigh flap for bimalleolar defect. *Plast Reconstr Surg* 1979;44:91.
10. Salmon M. *Artères de la peau.* Paris: Masson, 1936.
11. Goumain AJM, Pellegris M, Scnegas J. Technique des autoplastics cutanées jambières par lambeau hétérolateral. *Rev Chir Orthop* 1969; 55:131.

CHAPTER 533 ■ CROSS-GROIN SKIN FLAP

D. W. FURNAS

> ### EDITORIAL COMMENT
>
> Although this procedure is meritorious for keeping the scar hidden in the groin crease, the extreme nature of the flexion and long period of immobilization required would reserve this procedure for those situations in which a free-tissue transfer cannot be accomplished.

The cross-groin skin flap is an excellent means of gaining coverage of defects of the foot and ankle area in children (1). The child's short lower limbs and supple joints make this pedicle sequence possible.

INDICATIONS

The ease with which children tolerate the cross-leg flap has been previously reported (2) (Fig. 1). The groin flap offers more tissue than either a cross-leg flap or a cross-thigh flap, and the donor defect is much easier to handle, particularly when it can be closed directly (3). In a child, the positioning and immobilization for a cross-groin flap are no more difficult than for a cross-thigh flap. A cross-groin flap is probably not useful for defects that are any appreciable distance above the ankle, but the flap is an excellent means for covering soft-tissue defects of the distal portion of the lower limb in children.

OPERATIVE TECHNIQUE

McGregor's landmarks are used to design the flap (4,5), and a Doppler probe is used to verify the position of the superficial circumflex iliac artery. The Doppler probe is also used in monitoring the delay incisions for expeditious separation of the flap (6) (Figs. 2 and 3).

SUMMARY

The cross-groin skin flap is useful for covering soft tissue defects of the distal portion of the lower limb in a child.

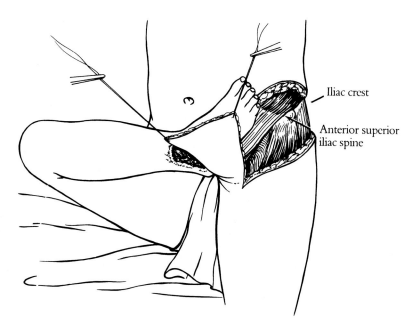

FIG. 1. Cross-groin flap in position on ankle defect. (The position can be maintained by plaster of Paris, a Hoffman device, or bone screws and a custom-made acrylic bar.) (From Furnas, ref. 1, with permission.)

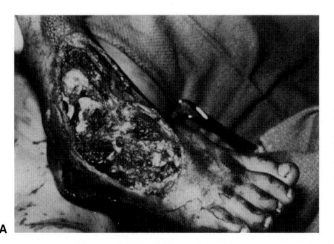

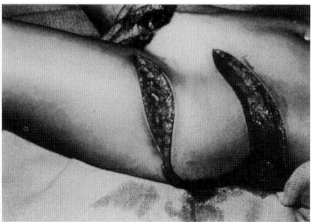

A

B

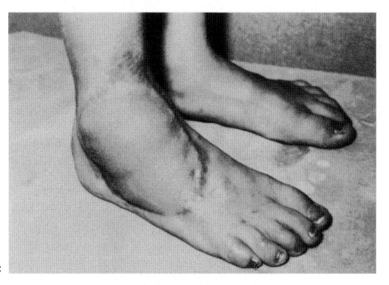

C

FIG. 2. A: A 7.5 × 15-cm avulsion-abrasion injury that destroyed the skin, tendons, joint capsule, and bone, exposing the ankle and tarsal joints, in a 6-year-old girl. Segments of the peroneal and the extensor digitorum communis tendons were lost. **B:** The cross-groin flap, 8 × 16 cm, elevated and ready for transfer. The distal edge of the flap was halfway between the anterior superior iliac spine and the posterior superior iliac spine. The donor site and the raw surface of the flap were covered with split-thickness skin grafts. The flap was divided and inset on the 12th postoperative day after several preliminary delay incisions. These incisions were made at the site that had the most prominent Doppler signal. **C:** The flap 5 months postoperatively. Two months after the injury, the child could walk with a barely perceptible limp; however, a progressing eversion of her foot necessitated an extensor hallucis longus transfer, with a split tibialis transfer. (From Furnas, ref. 1, with permission.)

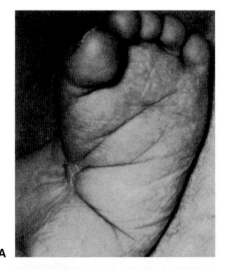
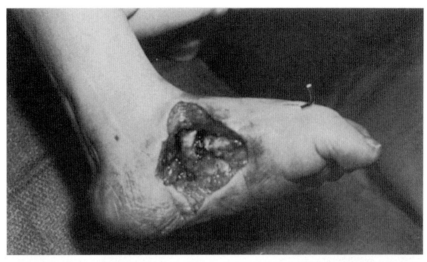

A

B

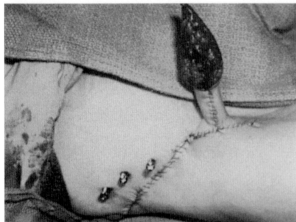
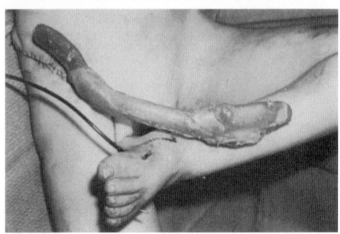

C

D

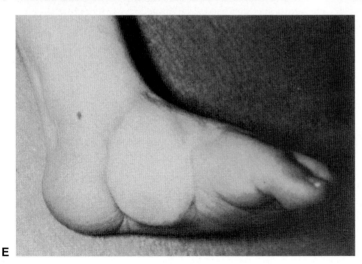

E

FIG. 3. A: This 6-year-old boy with a meningomyelocele was confined to a wheelchair. He had a left clubfoot with a cicatricial deformity secondary to complications from previous foot surgery, which resulted in a severe adduction contracture of the midfoot that prevented him from walking with braces. Surgical release of the adduction deformity was planned by the orthopedists. A cross-groin flap was plotted for closure of the resulting defect. B: At surgery, the adduction contracture of the foot was released and the foot was secured with pins. C: A right groin flap, 7 cm wide and 15 cm long, was elevated and tubed. Woodruff screws were inserted into the right iliac crest and into the tibia. D: The defect of the foot was held in apposition to the pedicle while an acrylic bar was fashioned to form a bridge between the iliac screws and the groin screws. The flap was then sutured into position. E: Serial delay incisions were carried out, guided by the Doppler arterial signal, and on the 12th postoperative day, the pedicle was divided and the acrylic bridge and screws were removed. On the 14th day, final inset of the flap was carried out. This view shows the patient 3 months after surgery, when he was fitted for braces and began training with them.

References

1. Furnas DW. The cross-groin flap for coverage of foot and ankle defects in children. *Plast Reconstr Surg* 1976;57:246.
2. Argamaso RV, Lewin ML, Baird AD, et al. Cross-leg flaps in children. *Plast Reconstr Surg* 1973;51:662.
3. Harii K, Ohmori K. Free groin flaps in children. *Plast Reconstr Surg* 1975;55:588.
4. McGregor I, Jackson I. The groin flap. *Br J Plast Surg* 1972;25:3.
5. Smith PJ, Foley B, McGregor IA, Jackson IT. The anatomic basis of the groin flap. *Plast Reconstr Surg* 1972;49:41.
6. Karkowski J, Buncke HJ. Simplified technique for free transfer of groin flaps by use of a Doppler probe. *Plast Reconstr Surg* 1975;55:682.

CHAPTER 534 ■ BUTTOCK SKIN FLAP

G. A. DRABYN AND J. F. NAPPI

Reconstruction of ankle and foot defects with exposure of deep structures has required major and complicated procedures to secure adequate coverage and a functional limb. Cross-leg flaps were the standard form of coverage until the advent of free composite-tissue transfer. Anyone who has done cross-leg flaps is well aware of the magnitude of potential complications (1,2). In children, the postural restrictions often result in anxiety and fear, and free flaps in children are often difficult undertakings. Many of these drawbacks can be avoided by the use of an ipsilateral extremity flap (3–6). It has been our preference to use the ipsilateral buttock flap to resurface ankle and foot defects in children (7).

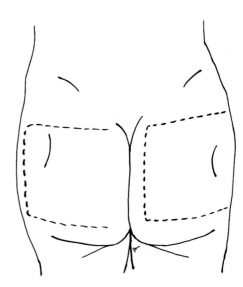

FIG. 1. Flap design.

INDICATIONS

The ipsilateral buttock flap offers several advantages over the cross-leg flap in a child. (1) *Size:* this is an extremely large random-pattern flap. (2) *Protection:* the flap offers adequate soft tissue for padding and bulk. (3) *Comfort:* the patient is immobilized in a position of relative comfort and may ambulate with crutches a few days postoperatively. (4) *Ipsilaterality:* there is avoidance of potential complications with the normal leg. (5) *Donor site:* the scars are well hidden, and unsightly scars on the opposite leg are avoided. (6) *Anxiety:* children are much less prone to anxiety with fewer postural restrictions.

Children, with their tendency toward supple joints, generally tolerate well immobilization of the knee in full flexion for

a period of 2 to 3 weeks, with rapid return of full motion. Therefore, this flap should be limited to use in children.

FLAP DESIGN AND DIMENSIONS

The buttock flap is a random-pattern flap that may be based either medially or laterally, depending on the location of the defect to be resurfaced (Fig. 1). Flap length is generally 25 cm and width is 20 cm, although the dimensions vary according to the sizes of the defect and the child. The inferior limits of the flap are kept 3 and 4 cm above the gluteal fold.

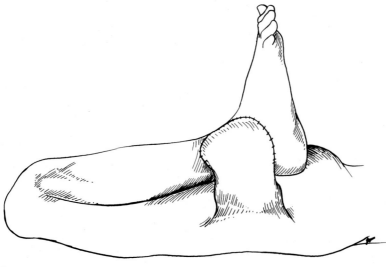

FIG. 2. Contoured flap applied to defect.

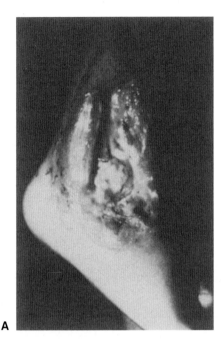

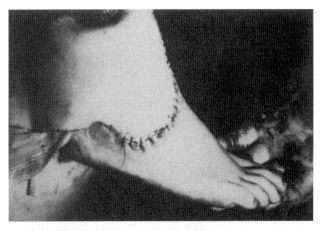

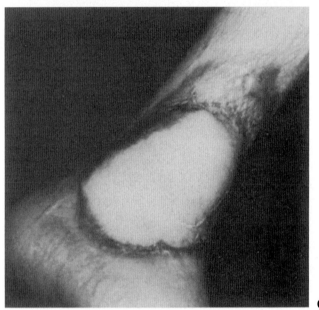

FIG. 3. Posttraumatic defect in a 6-year-old child. **A:** Open wound of foot and ankle. **B:** Buttock flap applied to wound. **C:** Flap 6 weeks postoperatively.

OPERATIVE TECHNIQUE

The flap is delayed by making the upper and lower transverse incisions and undermining the flap between them above the gluteal fascia. The flap then is completely elevated 2 to 3 weeks later (following debridement of the defect), the knee is flexed, and the flap is contoured and applied to the defect (Figs. 2 and 3). The donor site is covered with a split-thickness skin graft.

Immobilization may be accomplished in a variety of ways, but it should maintain rather rigid fixation of knee flexion. In the past, an Orthoplast splint was designed preoperatively and custom fit with padding. More recently, Hoffmann external fixation (with pins in the femur and tibia) has been used and seems to offer several advantages.

The flap is divided (in one or more stages) and inset in 2 to 3 weeks. The patient then begins vigorous range-of-motion exercises with the knee.

CLINICAL RESULTS

The major disadvantage of this flap is the need for immobilization of the knee in full flexion for a 2 to 3 weeks. Another major disadvantage is the random pattern of this flap, which necessitates delay. Although complications are infrequent, one should consider flap separation due to inadequate immobilization, flap necrosis due to inadequate delay or pedicle torsion, and loss of full range of motion of the knee.

SUMMARY

The ipsilateral buttock flap can be effectively used to cover defects of the ankle and foot in children.

References

1. Bennett JE, Kahn RA. Surgical management of soft-tissue defects of the ankle-heel region. *J Trauma* 1972;12:696.
2. Dalton RLG. Complications of the cross-leg flap operation. *Proc R Soc Med* 1972;65:626.
3. Drabyn GA, Avedian L. Ipsilateral buttock flap for coverage of a foot and ankle defect in a young child. *Plast Reconstr Surg* 1979;63:422.
4. Mladick RA, Pickrell KL, Thome FL, Royer JR. Ipsilateral thigh flap for total plantar resurfacing. *Plast Reconstr Surg* 1969;43:198.
5. Wilensky RJ, Grabb WC. Soft-tissue coverage of the lower extremities. *Mich Med* 1975;74:591.
6. Shubailat GF, Ajluni NJ, Shahateet MA. Repair of a lower leg defect with an ipsilateral gracilis myocutaneous flap. *Plast Reconstr Surg* 1979;64:560.
7. Shubailat GF, Ajluni NJ, Kirresh BS. Reconstruction of heel with ipsilateral tensor fascia lata myocutaneous flap. *Ann Plast Surg* 1979;4:323.

CHAPTER 535 ■ IPSILATERAL GRACILIS MUSCULOCUTANEOUS FLAP

G. F. SHUBAILAT

Use of the gracilis musculocutaneous flap in reconstruction of the ipsilateral ankle and lower leg region adds yet another alternative to the limited choice of methods available (1).

INDICATIONS

The ipsilateral gracilis musculocutaneous flap can be used to cover ankle and foot defects in certain thin, young patients.

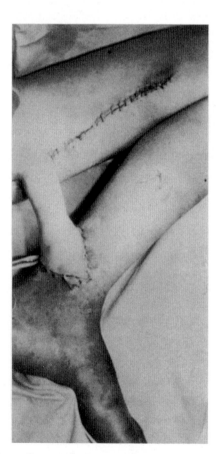

FIG. 1. A gracilis musculocutaneous flap applied to an ipsilateral ankle defect.

The operation is in two stages only. The other limbs and trunk are spared. Only the knee joint is immobilized for 3 weeks, with no resultant stiffness in selected patients. Easy nursing care is possible with the use of this flap.

ANATOMY

The detailed anatomy of the gracilis muscle is described in Chapter 421 (2).

FLAP DESIGN AND DIMENSIONS

In thin, young patients, if the knee can be fully flexed, the anterior arc of rotation can reach the anterior, medial, and posterior aspects of the lower leg and ankle (Fig. 1).

CLINICAL RESULTS

Hematoma formation under the flap, causing circulatory embarrassment, is best prevented by adequate drainage. Partial loss of the distal end of the flap due to ischemia can be avoided if the viability of the flap is confirmed by fluorescein. Infection, if it occurs, is usually secondary to inadequate circulation in the flap.

SUMMARY

An ipsilateral gracilis musculocutaneous flap occasionally can be used to cover ankle and foot defects in selected thin, young patients.

References

1. Shubailat GF, Ajluni NJ, Shahateet MA. Repair of a lower leg defect with an ipsilateral gracilis myocutaneous flap. *Plast Reconstr Surg* 1979; 64:560.
2. Mathes SJ, Nahai F, eds. *Clinical atlas of muscle and musculocutaneous flaps.* St. Louis: Mosby, 1979.

CHAPTER 536 ■ GASTROCNEMIUS MUSCULOCUTANEOUS CROSS-LEG FLAP

C. L. PUCKETT AND J. F. REINISCH

Because of its low surgical and psychological morbidity, the ipsilateral gastrocnemius musculocutaneous flap has been offered as a superior alternative to the standard cross-leg skin flap for coverage of defects of the middle third of the lower extremity. This flap, along with other local muscle flaps and free flaps, has significantly reduced the need for cross-leg skin flaps in recent years; however, the gastrocnemius flap can be used in a cross-leg manner when other means of local tissue reconstruction are unavailable or rejected by the patient (1).

or, by themselves, would not provide sufficient coverage, (2) inadequate expertise or facilities for microsurgical reconstruction, and (3) previous free-flap failure or poor recipient vessels for free-tissue transfer.

The gastrocnemius musculocutaneous flap can provide coverage for defects in the middle third of the leg; however, its use as a cross-leg flap expands its range of coverage to include most of the lower extremity, including the foot (Fig. 1). Its large size and its predictable vascularity allow it to cover most of the opposite extremity without extreme positioning.

INDICATIONS

Its basic indication is any situation in which one would have formerly used a standard cross-leg skin flap. Examples include (1) large tissue defects where local flaps have been destroyed

FLAP DESIGN AND DIMENSIONS

Because of proximity, the medial gastrocnemius flap is selected for cross-leg transfer. This flap carries the skin over the muscle as well as distal skin to a point 5 cm proximal

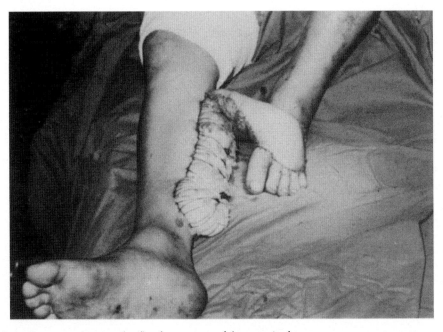

FIG. 1. Gastrocnemius cross-leg flap for coverage of the opposite foot.

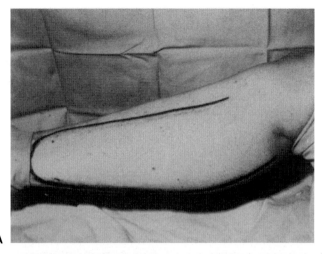

A

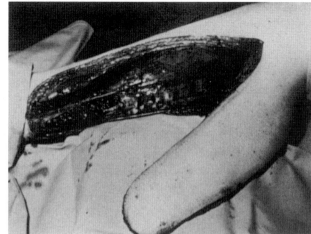

B

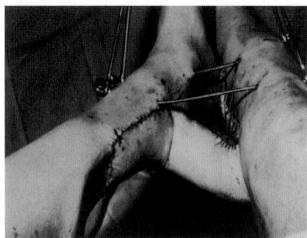

C

FIG. 2. Coverage of a chronic nonhealing wound following gunshot wound to lower extremity. **A:** Outline of medial gastrocnemius flap. **B:** Elevation of the flap including the underlying medial head of the gastrocnemius muscle and deep fascia. The soleus muscle and cut edge of the lateral head are seen in the base of the wound. **C:** Coverage of the defect of the opposite leg and cross-leg pin fixation.

to the medial malleolus. The width of the flap extends from the posterior midline to the medial border of the tibia (see Fig. 2A).

OPERATIVE TECHNIQUE

A plane between the gastrocnemius muscle and the underlying soleus muscle is developed, exposing the plantaris tendon, which is left intact. The medial head of the gastrocnemius is separated from the lateral head and the distal skin is elevated with its deep fascia intact to provide vascularity to the skin (Fig. 2B). The saphenous vein is protected. The vascular pedicle of the flap enters proximally and is not visualized.

Because the flap is too bulky to be tubed, skin grafts are required to cover both the donor defect and the exposed undersurface of the flap. The flap is inset, and the legs are secured either with pins (Fig. 2C) or plaster. The flap can be divided between 1½ and 4 weeks following surgery. The fluorescein test is useful in determining the time of division. Occasionally, a partial division (delay) of the pedicle under local anesthesia is necessary before final division.

SUMMARY

Despite the advent of free-flap transfer and a variety of muscle flaps, we find the cross-leg gastrocnemius flap a valuable occasional adjunct in lower extremity reconstruction.

Reference

1. Furnas DW, Anzel SH. Two consecutive repairs of the lower limbs with a single gastrocnemius musculocutaneous cross-leg flap. *Plast Reconstr Surg* 1980;66:137.

CHAPTER 537 ■ GASTROCNEMIUS MUSCULOCUTANEOUS V-Y ADVANCEMENT FLAP

P. C. LINTON

The gastrocnemius musculocutaneous V-Y advancement flap can be used to reconstruct the Achilles tendon while simultaneously closing an overlying skin and soft-tissue defect (1).

INDICATIONS

The massive gastrocnemius musculocutaneous V-Y advancement flap is clearly not a flap for all applications. The major indication would be in those few patients in whom restoration of active ankle plantar flexion must be combined with reconstruction of a significant soft-tissue defect. The patient whose case is presented had a 4.5 × 7 cm skin and Achilles defect and good passive ankle flexion (see Fig. 3).

ANATOMY

The blood supply to the skin of the entire posterior calf to 5 cm above the medial malleolus and 7 cm above the lateral malleolus is primarily from vessels that perforate the fascia of the underlying medial and lateral gastrocnemius muscles (2). Distal to the muscle bellies, these perforators run superficial to the Achilles tendon. The muscles are each supplied by a single neurovascular pedicle arising from the popliteal artery high in the popliteal space and entering the proximal muscle belly just distal to their tendinous origins on the femur. This neurovascular bundle is stretchable to at least 4.5 cm when the muscle origins are detached (3), allowing distal mobilization of the functioning musculocutaneous unit, simultaneous reconstruction of Achilles tendon integrity, active ankle plantar flexion, and soft-tissue coverage in the distal posterior ankle.

OPERATIVE TECHNIQUE

The technique consists of detachment of the proximal gastrocnemius origins, separation of the distal confluence of soleus-gastrocnemius at the proximal Achilles tendon, advancement of the musculocutaneous unit over the soleus bed, and distal tendon repair (Figs. 1 and 2).

The area of the distal square or rectangular defect is transferred to the proximal V-shaped donor defect, and because of the excess tissue here, primary closure should be possible as a V-Y. The skin island must be tacked to the fascia with particular care distally in the tendinous region because it is here that the greatest risk of devascularization exists. To facilitate closure, the proximal portion of the skin island should be designed as a long, narrow V, taking care to start the point of the V at or distal to the popliteal flexion crease in order to prevent flexion contracture. Access to the neurovascular pedicle and muscle origins proximally should be through a Z incision in the popliteal area for the same reason (Fig. 3C).

Following surgery, the knee should be splinted at 90 degrees to relieve all tension on the neurovascular leash and on the Achilles repair. Gradual knee extension is allowed after soft-tissue healing has occurred.

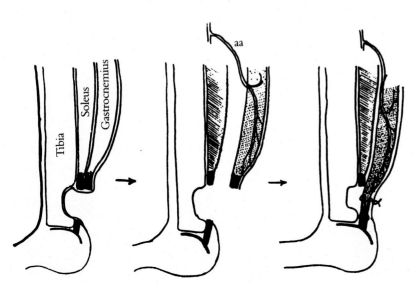

FIG. 1. Schema of operation. (From Linton, ref. 1, with permission.)

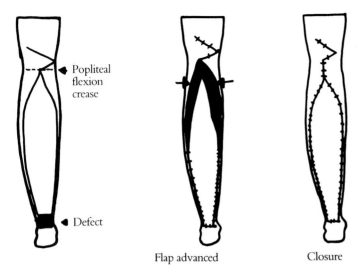

Popliteal
flexion
crease

◄ Defect

Flap advanced

Closure

FIG. 2. Operative design. (From Linton, ref. 1, with permission.)

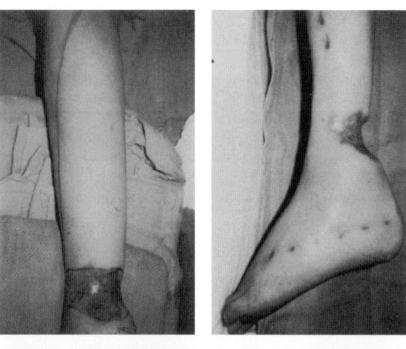

A,B

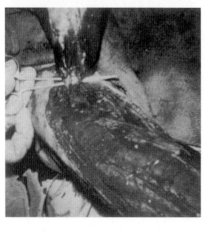

C–E

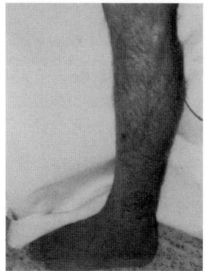

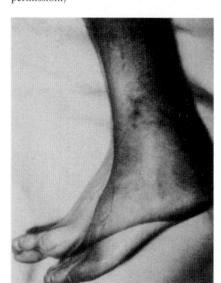

FIG. 3. A,B: Preoperative defect. C: Flap raised on its neurovascular pedicles. D,E: Postoperative result with 20 degrees of active range of motion. (From Linton, ref. 1, with permission.)

CLINICAL RESULTS

In my patient, nearly 6 months elapsed before full knee extension was achieved. No complications or functional deficits resulted, and at 1 year the patient was walking with virtually no limp (1).

SUMMARY

The gastrocnemius musculocutaneous V-Y advancement flap can be used simultaneously to reconstruct defects of the Achilles tendon and overlying skin and soft tissue.

References

1. Linton PC. The combined medial and lateral gastrocnemius musculocutaneous V-Y island advancement flap. *Plast Reconstr Surg* 1982;70:490.
2. McCraw JB, Dibbell DG, Carraway JH. Clinical definition of independent myocutaneous vascular pedicles. *Plast Reconstr Surg* 1977;60:3.
3. Dibbell DG, Edstrom LE. The gastrocnemius myocutaneous flap. *Clin Plast Surg* 1980;7:45.

CHAPTER 538 ■ MICRONEUROVASCULAR FREE TRANSFER OF A DORSALIS PEDIS FLAP TO THE HEEL

L. A. SHARZER

Skin coverage of weight-bearing areas such as the heel is a controversial problem in reconstructive surgery. It is well known that coverage with skin grafts may be adequate and well tolerated in the intelligent, motivated patient. Nevertheless, many patients require flap coverage. It was previously shown that the provision of sensation to the insensate heel can prevent recurrent breakdown (1–4).

INDICATIONS

Most reports of the dorsalis pedis neurovascular island flap involve reconstruction of the hand (5–7). In these, a two-point discrimination of 10 to 20 mm is usual. The dorsalis pedis flap has been used in lower-extremity reconstruction of the same leg as an island flap (8,9) or in the opposite leg as a free flap. Only one author has discussed its use as a free neurovascular flap to a weight-bearing area of the other foot (7). The three patients achieved a 10- to 20-mm two-point discrimination.

ANATOMY

The vascular anatomy is described in Chapter 518.

Cutaneous sensation is supplied to the dorsal foot skin by means of the superficial peroneal nerve. The superficial peroneal nerve, one of the two terminal branches of the common peroneal nerve, arises high in the leg between the tibialis and the peroneus longus muscles. It passes distally between the extensor digitorum longus and the peronei to the distal third of the leg, where it pierces the deep fascia on its way to the dorsum of the foot. Whereas it is rarely necessary to dissect a very long nerve pedicle, it is possible to do so. This is particularly useful if the recipient-site nerve is far from the heel. In the distal third of the leg, the superficial peroneal nerve bifurcates to form the medial and intermediate dorsal cutaneous nerves (Fig. 1A). These nerves cross the ankle joint superficial to the extensor retinaculum. It is here that they are encountered during the elevation of the flap.

FLAP DESIGN AND DIMENSIONS

The vascular anatomy and technique of elevation of the dorsalis pedis flap are as described in Chapter 518. A few considerations are necessary when the flap is being used to provide sensory skin over the heel (Fig. 1). Pretransfer delay of the flap is rarely necessary for a dorsalis pedis flap used in this manner. The defects are often not large enough to require an augmented flap, and the weight-bearing area is almost always of a size that can be covered by an undelayed flap. If the entire plantar defect is larger than the flap, the non-weight-bearing areas usually can be covered by skin grafts.

Preoperative arteriography is routine and should be performed on both the donor and recipient legs. It is important to assess the quality, location, and patency of the dorsalis pedis artery as well as the collateral circulation. In the recipient leg, the location, continuity, and patency of all vessels must be determined. Mere presence of pulses may be unreliable because of reverse flow by means of plantar anastomoses.

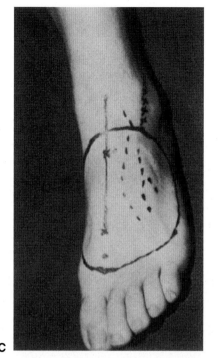
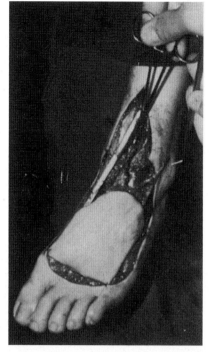
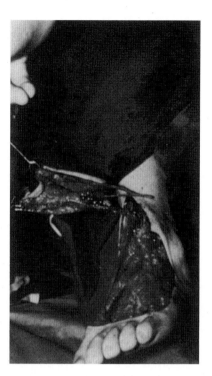

A–C

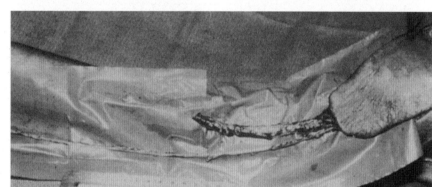

D

FIG. 1. A: Outline of neurovascular dorsalis pedis flap (*solid line*, dorsalis pedis artery; *broken line*, superficial draining veins; *x's*, superficial peroneal nerve). **B:** Dissected flap. (Hemostat points to vascular pedicle and probe to nerve pedicle.) **C:** Deep aspect of flap. (Note the nerve and vascular pedicles.) **D:** Note the long vascular pedicle and very long nerve pedicle that can be obtained.

Generally, the posterior tibial artery and the sural nerve are the recipient structures of choice. They are located near the heel, allowing relatively short pedicles. The vessels are of good caliber, and the nerve is a pure sensory nerve. Furthermore, the sensory consequences of sural nerve division are not serious. The nerve can be traced high in the leg, if necessary, to reach a normal fascicular pattern.

OPERATIVE TECHNIQUE

Elevation of a neurovascular dorsalis pedis flap begins similarly to a standard dorsalis pedis flap (Fig. 1B–D). When the distal incision is made, the terminal branches of the superficial peroneal nerve are found as they cross to the toes and are divided. As the lateral portion of the flap is elevated, these nerve branches may be used as a guide to locate the one or two main trunks of the superficial peroneal nerve proximally in the foot.

After making the distal, medial, and lateral incisions of the flap, the medial portion is dissected toward the vascular pedicle and the distal portion toward the penetrating branch of the dorsalis pedis artery. As the lateral portion of the flap is elevated, the nerves are usually found at the proximal lateral

corner. Further dissection of the proximal edge of the flap toward the vascular pedicle is then limited, depending on the length of the nerve required. The skin only may be incised and then with a longitudinal incision made proximally in the leg. The leg skin is then elevated off the extensor retinaculum to allow as much proximal dissection of the superficial peroneal nerve as required. Once adequate length has been obtained and the nerve is divided, the remainder of the flap dissection can proceed (Fig. 1D). The retinaculum is divided, and the vascular pedicle is traced into the anterior tibial vasculature as far proximally as necessary. The donor site is closed with a skin graft.

After transfer, the flap is usually tacked in place and the vascular anastomoses are carried out either end-to-side or end-to-end. The sural nerve is divided as far distally as possible, at a point where normal fascicular structures are noted. The superficial peroneal nerve is divided so that it will fit comfortably without redundancy or tension, and a careful microscopic anastomosis is carried out.

Postoperative management requires continuous elevation of the flap, which generally means that the patient remains in the prone position for the first postoperative week. Dependency of the leg is not allowed for 3 weeks, and partial weight bearing is begun at 6 weeks and is increased as

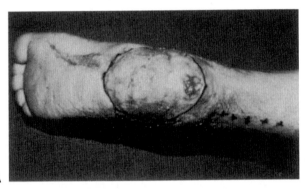
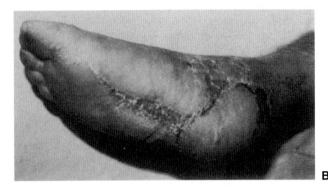

FIG. 2. **A:** Recurrent breakdown of the heel. **B:** Postoperative appearance of the heel covered by dorsalis pedis neurovascular free flap.

tolerated. The evolution of sensibility in the flap is assessed by following an advancing Tinel's sign.

SUMMARY

The dorsalis pedis free flap can provide stable skin coverage over the heel with protective tactile sensation (Fig. 2).

References

1. Snyder GB, Edgerton MT. The principles of the island neurovascular flap in the management of ulcerated anesthetic weight-bearing areas of the lower extremity. *Plast Reconstr Surg* 1965;36:518.
2. Kaplan I. Neurovascular island flap in the treatment of trophic ulceration of the heel. *Br J Plast Surg* 1969;22:143.
3. Maquiera NO. An innervated full-thickness skin graft to restore sensibility to finger tips and heels. *Plast Reconstr Surg* 1974;53:568.
4. Lister GD. Use of an innervated skin graft to provide sensation to the reconstructed heel. *Plast Reconstr Surg* 1978;62:157.
5. Daniel RK, Terzis JK, Midgley RD. Restoration of sensation to an anesthetic hand by a free neurovascular flap from the foot. *Plast Reconstr Surg* 1976;57:275.
6. Ohmori K, Harii K. Free dorsalis pedis sensory flap to the hand with microneurovascular anastomoses. *Plast Reconstr Surg* 1976;58:546.
7. Robinson DW. Microsurgical transfer of the dorsalis pedis neurovascular island flap. *Br J Plast Surg* 1976;29:209.
8. Kobus K, Licznerski A, Stepniewski J, Charles W. Management of island and free dorsalis pedis flaps in surgery of the lower extremities. *Acta Clin Plast* 1980;22:138.
9. McCraw JB, Furlow LT. The dorsalis pedis arterialized flap: A clinical study. *Plast Reconstr Surg* 1975;55:177

CHAPTER 539 ■ FREE PARIETOTEMPORALIS FASCIAL FLAP

J. UPTON AND C. M. RODGERS

The anatomy, flap design, and operative technique of this flap are described in Chapter 306.

INDICATIONS

Our most common use has been to provide stable coverage with minimal bulk over localized defects in the extremities in difficult regions. In the lower extremity, the free parietotemporalis fascial flap can be used for coverage of small pretibial defects, exposed Achilles tendons, and exposed extensor tendon and/or bone in the dorsum of the foot (Fig. 1).

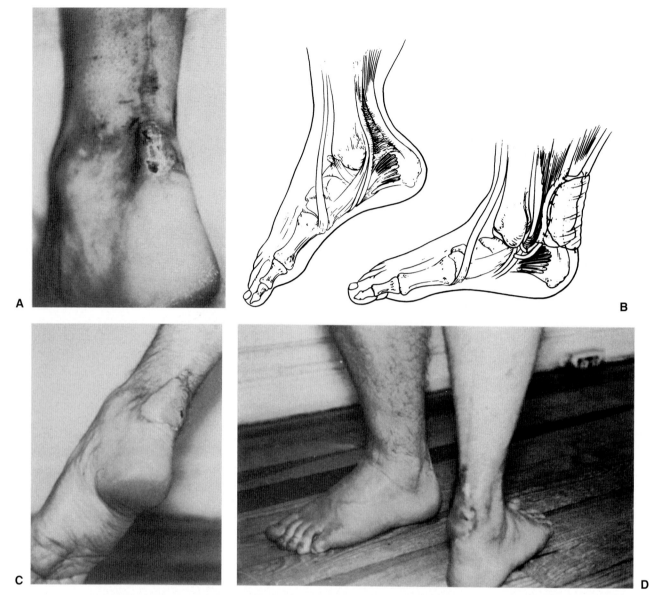

FIG. 1. A: Professional ballet dancer who, while performing in December 1981, ruptured his Achilles tendon. Following a primary repair with tendon graft by an orthopedic surgeon, his wound dehisced, became infected, and failed to heal. By the fall 1982, he was unable to walk because of pain. Following multiple debridements, his wound healed spontaneously. B: Reconstruction consisted of thorough excision of scar tissue and release of the Achilles tendon from the peroneus longus and brevis tendons as well as from the posterior joint capsule. The superficial temporal vessels of the flap were joined end-to-side into the posterior tibial artery and end-to-end into one vena comitans. Then the vascularized flap was wrapped completely around the Achilles tendon, obliterating a potential space and providing external coverage. The areolar side of the flap faced the Achilles tendon as a gliding surface. A split-thickness skin graft completed the external skin coverage. C,D: Within 6 weeks, the patient had regained enough motion to ambulate without assistance. In 5 months, he was teaching in a professional dance studio.

CHAPTER 540 ■ FREE SCAPULAR FLAP

L. FONSECA DOS SANTOS AND A. GILBERT

The scapular flap, based on the cutaneous branches of the subscapular artery, has become a favored donor site for free vascularized tissue transfer (1–7).

INDICATIONS

The free scapular flap has the advantages of strong skin and a thin subcutaneous pedicle. It is especially good for defects about the heel and ankle.

ANATOMY

The subscapular artery, a branch of the axillary artery, divides rapidly into an inferior branch, the thoracodorsal artery, and a posterior branch, the circumflex scapular artery (Fig. 1). It runs between the teres major and minor to reach the lateral side of the scapula. The circumflex scapular artery divides into several branches. The first of these vascularizes the subscapular muscle and runs between the muscle and the deep side of the scapula.

There are then two branches that supply the supraspinatus and infraspinatus and the teres major and minor. This whole vascular system gives a rich blood supply to the lateral side of the scapula. Finally, the subscapular artery takes a downward turn and goes toward the tip of the scapula along its lateral side, turning into bony muscular and cutaneous branches.

The main branch to the skin starts from the circumflex scapular artery at the level where it reaches the side of the scapula. Then it extends over toward the infraspinatus to divide shortly into two or three branches.

The subscapular artery was always present in our anatomic studies of 70 cases. In one clinical case, the artery could not be found. Its diameter varies between 0.8 and 2.0 mm from the lateral side of the scapula. If the trunk of the circumflex scapular artery is used, the diameter can reach 3 mm. The artery is usually accompanied by two veins, of which only one has a significant diameter (2–3 mm).

The circumflex scapular artery usually emerges at a point two fifths of the distance between the spine of the scapula and its lower angle. The artery can be felt quite easily in thin patients, or it can be identified with a Doppler probe.

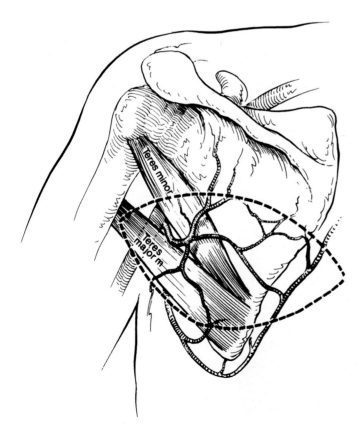

FIG. 1. The circumflex scapular artery as it arises from the axillary artery and emerges between the teres major and minor muscles.

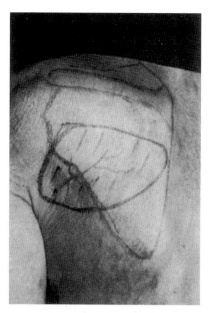

FIG. 2. The flap outlined in the lower scapular region.

FLAP DESIGN AND DIMENSIONS

The flap is then drawn horizontally or diagonally, with the pedicle on its lateral extremity (Fig. 2). The pedicle is located on the lateral side of the flap for two reasons: (1) the cutaneous branches run toward the midline and (2) the subcutaneous fat in the axillary area is very thick. The cutaneous territory of this flap is not yet well defined. It extends at least to the midline of the back and has been successfully raised to a length of 30 cm.

OPERATIVE TECHNIQUE

The arm is maintained in 90 degrees of abduction during elevation of the flap. The flap is elevated just above the fascia of the infraspinatus muscle. Once half the flap is raised, the vascular pedicle can be identified as it emerges at the lateral edge of the muscle. At this point, it is still possible to modify the lateral part of the incision to correct a possible error in planning.

The rest of the incision is completed. The flap remains attached only to its vascular pedicle. This dissection is the most delicate part of the surgery, because there are multiple branches and the difficulty increases with depth. The dissection progresses slowly, each branch being tied separately. Vascular clips can be used to gain time. Up to the appearance of the subscapular branch, the pedicle measures about 6 to 8

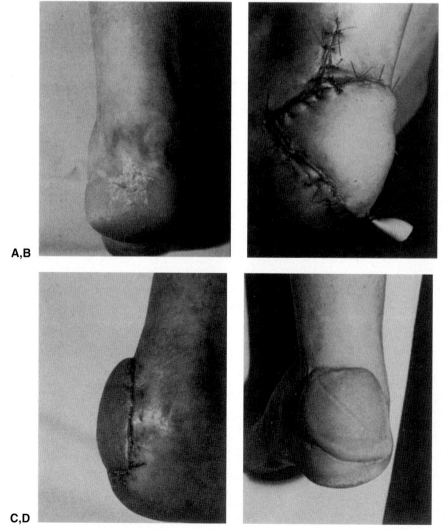

A,B

C,D

FIG. 3. A: Unstable scar of the heel in a 42-year-old woman. B: Immediately after resection and coverage with the scapular flap. C,D: Two months postoperatively the flap is thin and does not need defatting.

cm. Beyond that, the dissection requires a wider area that is rarely justified.

The donor site can be closed primarily, undermining the edges if necessary. A suction drain is left in place.

CLINICAL RESULTS

Between 1979 and 1982, 32 free scapular skin flaps have been performed (Fig. 3).

SUMMARY

The free scapular skin flap has become an ideal donor site for reconstruction of leg and ankle defects.

References

1. Fonseca dos Santos L. *Le lambeau scapulaire et l'artère cutanée scapulaire*. Paris: Mémoires de la Laboratoire Anatomique de la Faculté du Médicine, 1980.
2. Hamilton SG, Morrison W. The scapular free flap. *Br J Plast Surg* 1982;35:2.
3. Mayou B, Whitby D, Jones B. The scapular flap: anatomical and clinical study. *Br J Plast Surg* 1982;35:8.
4. Marcondez-Nassif T, Vidal L, Bovet JL, Baudet J. The parascapular flap: a new cutaneous microsurgical free flap. *Plast Reconstr Surg* 1982;69:591.
5. Gilbert A, Teot L. The free scapular flap. *Plast Reconstr Surg* 1982;69:601.
6. Urbaniak J, Koman L, Goldner R, et al. The vascularized cutaneous scapular flap. *Plast Reconstr Surg* 1982;69:772.
7. Barwick W, Goodkind D, Serafin D. The free scapular flap. *Plast Reconstr Surg* 1982;69:778.

CHAPTER 541 ■ MICRONEUROVASCULAR FREE INFERIOR GLUTEAL ARTERY PERFORATOR (IGAP) FASCIOCUTANEOUS FLAP FOR ACHILLES TENDON DEFECTS

C. PAPP AND C. WINDHOFER

The fasciocutaneous infragluteal (FCI) free flap is a viable option in repair of acute rupture of the Achilles tendon with combined skin, soft-tissue, and tendon defects. When used for reconstruction, it provides protection against rerupture and allows full weight-bearing, with good range of motion of the ankle.

INDICATIONS

Repair of an acute rupture of the Achilles tendon usually undergoes an uneventful course. However, some cases may be complicated by infection or rerupture with soft-tissue loss. In these cases, there is often a need for secondary reconstruction (1–5). The fasciocutaneous infragluteal free flap is sensate, giving the patient the advantage of avoiding skin breakdown due to repetitive trauma in the region (6).

The FCI free flap described is not used only for Achilles tendon reconstruction. We also obtain acceptable results when it is used as a free flap for breast reconstruction or augmentation (7). We also have used it as a free flap for defects of the lower extremity. It can be used as a transposition flap to reconstruct defects in the gluteal and perineal regions, as well as for vaginal reconstruction. The length of the vascular pedicle (up to 18 cm) and the ability to raise subcutaneous tissue with the skin island make the FCI an attractive alternative for reconstruction with these indications.

ANATOMY

The blood supply of the FCI flap is an end branch of the inferior gluteal artery (IGA). It is important to note that the blood supply of this flap does not perforate the gluteal muscle at any point. The IGA supplies the skin of the posterior thigh region, the majority of the blood supply to the lower two thirds of the gluteus maximus muscle, and it supplies perforators to the overlying skin (8). The inferior gluteal artery perforator (IGAP) flap is supplied by these perforators (9,10). The fasciocutaneous posterior thigh flap, described by Hurwitz et al. (11), is also supplied by the descending branch of the IGA. One branch of this vessel, which courses around the lower border of the gluteus maximus muscle and ascends to the subcutaneous and fascial tissue of the gluteal crease region, provides the blood supply of the FCI. An epifascial and subdermal vascular plexus supplied by this cutaneous branch ensures optimal vascularization of both the subcutaneous and fascial structures in the flap area (12,13).

Sensory innervation of the inferior gluteal region is provided by the inferior cluneal nerves, branches of the posterior femoral cutaneous nerve. These nerves course around the lower border of the gluteus maximus muscle together with the cutaneous branch of the IGA. On the basis of 118 anatomic preparations, we were able to show the close relation between the femoral cutaneous nerve and the descending branch of the

IGA. The nerve formed a loop around the vessel in 29% of the dissections. The descending branch of the IGA was present in 91%, and the cutaneous branch was a constant finding. When the descending artery was absent, this cutaneous branch came from the medial or lateral femoral circumflex artery of the thigh or from a perforator of the deep femoral artery (13).

Another anatomic consideration that is vital to this flap is the fascial network in the area. The sheets of the gluteal fascia and the fascia lata of the thigh converge at the gluteal crease. Where these fascial structures meet, the so-called "raphe" is fixed to the ischial tuberosity by the ischiocutaneous ligament. The subcutaneous tissue is firmly anchored between the dermis and the gluteal fascia. Vertical tension is maintained right through the fascia to the intramuscular septa of the gluteus muscle. This special architecture of the connective tissue makes the skin of this region particularly resistant to mechanical stress (8).

FLAP DESIGN AND DIMENSIONS

The most important landmark for designing the flap is the gluteal crease. The flap is positioned over the crease in a transverse fashion (Fig. 1). The dimensions of the skin island depend on the dimensions of the soft-tissue defect over the Achilles tendon. The FCI can be safely raised up to 26 × 8 cm. It is important to include the gluteal fascia, as well as the proximal portion of the fascia lata. Temporary flap design should be done preoperatively with the patient in the standing position. A duplex Doppler ultrasound preoperatively can be obtained, to confirm the presence of the descending branch of the IGA. The position of the vessel can be marked on the skin. This allows the surgeon to redesign the flap intraoperatively, if necessary.

OPERATIVE TECHNIQUE

With the patient in a prone position, the first step is to perform debridement of the Achilles defect. This allows precise definition of the extent of the defect before reconstruction is initiated. After this is done, the flap can be harvested. If necessary, the flap can be redesigned, based on the vessel that was located by ultrasound preoperatively. When harvesting the flap, the first step in finding the vessels and sensory nerve is to incise the lateral margin. A lateral-to-medial dissection is the safest approach. At this point, the skin, subcutaneous tissue, and fascia are dissected en bloc from the gluteal muscle. The

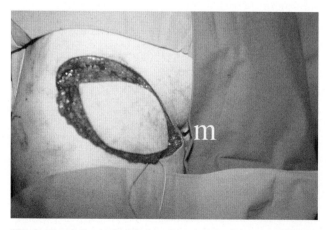

FIG. 1. Flap design in the left gluteal crease region after incision of the skin. Vessel loop winds around the posterior femoral cutaneous nerve on the lower border of the flap. Marking the nerve avoids injuring it in further preparation. *m*, Medial aspect of the left gluteal crease.

gluteal muscle fibers run obliquely, and the descending branch of the IGA supplying the flap, as well as the nerve, can be found at the inferomedial border of the muscle.

As the fascia is dissected from the muscle fibers, care must be taken to include the intramuscular septae within the fascial layer of the flap. This provides additional fascial thickness and strength for the tendon repair. During the dissection of the fascia from the muscle, the myocutaneous perforators from the IGA are encountered and may be ligated.

When the border of the gluteus muscle is reached, care is taken in dissection of the neurovascular supply. Once the neurovascular structures are identified, the medial and inferior margins of the flap are incised to raise the flap completely on its neurovascular pedicle. During the medial dissection, it is important to avoid injuring the bursa over the ischial tuberosity while elevating the ischiocutaneous ligament, and lifting the perimysium of the ischial crural musculature laterally. In our experience, resection of the bursa over the ischial tuberosity leads to long-term problems in sitting.

Once the skin and subcutaneous tissues of the flap are completely free from the surrounding tissue, the pedicle can then be further dissected. To isolate the pedicle, the gluteal muscle is retracted superiorly, and the vessel is dissected free to the level of the infrapiriform foramen. At this point, the artery and vein can be divided. Below the foramen, in most cases, a more prominent branch of the inferior gluteal artery to the gluteus maximus originates. This branch can be ligated before it perforates the muscle. Ligating the branch allows one to achieve an additional 2 to 3 cm of pedicle length. The mean length of the vascular pedicle prepared in our institution was 16 cm.

When dissecting the vascular pedicle at the inferomedial border of the gluteus muscle, the posterior femoral cutaneous nerve runs with the vessel. As our anatomic investigations have shown, the posterior femoral cutaneous nerve beneath the gluteus maximus muscle often forms tight loops around the vessels supplying the flap or around a branch of these vessels. This often requires a microscopic division of the epineurium, so that the vascular pedicle can be pulled through this gap. As the posterior femoral cutaneous nerve courses to the posterior thigh, it gives off the inferior cluneal nerves, branches that provide sensation to the flap (Fig. 2). During incision of the subcutaneous tissue, care should be taken to avoid injury to the posterior femoral cutaneous nerve, but the vessel to the posterior thigh is ligated as the dissection proceeds.

It should be noted that, in 118 anatomic preparations investigated, a variant of the blood supply was observed in only 10 cases. In these instances, the cutaneous branch to the fascia was supplied either by a circumflex femoral artery or by a perforator of the deep femoral artery. Such variations, however, were not encountered in any of our 110 operative cases. After the flap is harvested, the wound is carefully repaired in layers. The flap is transferred, and the Achilles tendon is reconstructed first. The fascial part of the flap is rolled into a tube and sutured in a circular fashion to the distal and proximal edges of the tendon stump. This wraparound method enables stability in both partial and total Achilles tendon reconstructions.

The arterial anastomosis is performed end-to-side, and the veins are usually anastomosed end-to-end. This prevents circulatory problems in the foot, particularly in older patients with peripheral vascular disease. The cluneal branch from the posterior femoral cutaneous nerve is coapted to a branch of the sural nerve to restore sensation. Finally, the skin and subcutaneous tissue are sutured in place.

CLINICAL RESULTS

In our series, 13 patients underwent repair of the Achilles tendon defect with the FCI. In 11 of our 13 patients, the Achilles

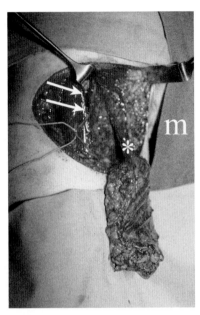

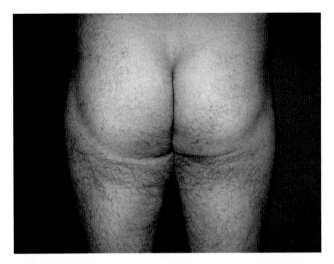

FIG. 3. Donor-site scar in the left gluteal crease, 66 months after flap raising.

FIG. 2. Raised FCI flap with neurovascular pedicle (*), in relation to gluteus maximus muscle (*arrows*, lower border of the muscle). The posterior femoral cutaneous nerve is looped and isolated from the vascular pedicle. *m*, Medial aspect of the gluteal crease.

tendon was reconstructed with good function of the ankle joint. One diabetic patient required below-the-knee amputation, because of gangrene elsewhere in the extremity. Despite the need for amputation, the Achilles-tendon repair was able to tolerate full weight. The second patient without a full recovery was an obese female, who had arthritis of the knee and hip joint. Despite full weight bearing of the Achilles tendon and acceptable motion in the ankle joint, total recovery did not take place, because of pain in the other joints of the leg. The other patients have returned to work, with no restrictions in activities of daily living. It is also worth mentioning that seven patients are able to pursue sporting activities, such as climbing, jogging, cycling, and tennis, without restrictions. Minor complications, such as donor-site seroma, were managed conservatively and did not affect final outcome.

In six patients, sensory innervation of the flap was accomplished by coaptation to the sural nerve. In the other cases, the patients reported deep sensation of pressure. After a mean follow-up period of 66 months, recipients were able to recognize stress caused by pressure (Fig. 3).

To achieve a better aesthetic result, we performed liposuction in nine patients, to contour the flap. We believe that primary liposuction is possible in younger patients with healthy vessels; otherwise, a delay of 4 to 6 months is warranted. Three patients in our group were satisfied with the flap, despite the bulkiness, and they declined liposuction. In the other two cases, liposuction was not required because of satisfactory aesthetic results.

SUMMARY

In our experience, the FCI, based on the end branch of the descending branch of the IGA, has been a viable option for functional and sensate Achilles-tendon repair, when soft-tissue reconstruction is also necessary. It has a dependable anatomy and reproducible results.

References

1. Deiler S, Pfadenhauser A, Widmann J, Stützle H. Tensor fasciae latae perforator flap for reconstruction of composite Achilles tendon defects with skin and vascularized fascia. *Plast Reconstr Surg* 2000;106:342.
2. Sylaidis P, Fatah MFT. A composite lateral arm flap for the secondary repair of a multiply ruptured Achilles tendon. *Plast Reconstr Surg* 1995;96:1719.
3. Inoue T, Tanaka I, Imai K, Hatoko M. Reconstruction of Achilles tendon using vascularised fascia lata with free lateral thigh flap. *Br J Plast Surg* 1990;43:728.
4. Lee IW, Yu IC, Shieh SJ, et al. Reconstruction of the Achilles tendon and overlying soft tissue using antero-lateral thigh free flap. *Br J Plast Surg* 2000;53:574.
5. Wei FC, Chen HC, Chuang CC, Noordhoff MS. Reconstruction of Achilles tendon and calcaneus defects with skin-aponeurosis-bone composite free tissue from the groin region. *Plast Reconstr Surg* 1988;81:579.
6. Papp C, Todoroff BP, Windhofer C, Gruber S. Partial and complete reconstruction of Achilles tendon defects with the fasciocutaneous infragluteal free flap. *Plast Reconstr Surg* 2003;112:777.
7. Papp C, Windhofer C, Gruber S. Breast reconstruction with the fasciocutaneous infragluteal free flap (FCI). *Ann Plast Surg* 2007;58:131.
8. Lanz T, Wachsmuth W. *Praktische anatomie, Bein und Statik*, vol. I/part 4. Berlin: Springer Verlag, 1938.
9. Allen RJ. Perforator flaps in breast reconstruction. In: Spear SL, Little JW, Lippman ME, et al., eds. *Surgery of the breast: principles and art.* Philadelphia: Lippincott-Raven, 1998.
10. Guerra AB, Allen RJ, Levine JL, Erhard HA. Inferior gluteal artery perforator flap. In: Blondeel PN, Morris SF, Hallock GG, et al., eds. *Perforator flaps: anatomy, technique and clinical applications.* St. Louis: Quality Medical Publishing, 2006.
11. Hurwitz DJ, Swartz WM, Mathes SJ. The gluteal thigh flap: a reliable, sensate flap for closure of buttock and perineal wounds. *Plast Reconstr Surg* 1981;68:521.
12. Frick A, Baumeister RGH, Wiebecke B. Microvasculature of the inferior gluteal flap. *Eur J Plast Surg* 1993;16:30.
13. Windhofer C, Brenner E, Moriggl B, and Papp C. Relationship between the descending branch of the inferior gluteal artery and the posterior femoral cutaneous nerve applicable to flap surgery. *Surg Radiol Anat* 2002;24:253.

CHAPTER 542. Scapular and Parascapular Flaps *J. Baudet, T. Nassif,*
J. L. Bovet and B. Panconi
www.encyclopediaofflaps.com

CHAPTER 543 ■ MICRONEUROVASCULAR SKIN AND OSTEOCUTANEOUS FREE RADIAL ARTERY FLAP

E. BIEMER AND W. STOCK

The radial artery flap can be used as a free flap to cover defects in the foot and lower extremity. It provides thin, pliable skin that can provide sensation through anastomoses with the antebrachial cutaneous nerves. By incorporating a portion of vascularized radius, the flap also can be used as a free osteocutaneous flap (Fig. 1).

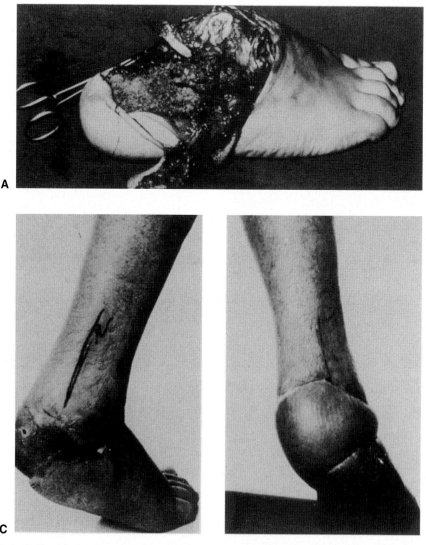

FIG. 1. A: Total foot amputation that was successfully replanted. **B,C:** An area of local necrosis at the heel was covered by a free radial artery sensitive flap, which allows the patient to work full time as a dentist.

CHAPTER 544 ■ MICROVASCULAR COMPOSITE SERRATUS ANTERIOR AND RIB FLAP FOR TIBIAL COMPOSITE BONE AND SOFT-TISSUE DEFECT

C. H. LIN

Lower-extremity bone defects may result from direct traumatic open fractures, tumor resections, and debridement of osteomyelitic lesions and nonunions. For small bone defects with adequate soft-tissue coverage, the bone gap can be bridged with conventional cancellous bone grafts or bone substitutes. However, when the segmental bone defects are larger than 6 cm, with or without soft-tissue defect, they often require either microsurgical vascularized bone flaps or Ilizarov bone-transplantation techniques to achieve a functional limb.

INDICATIONS

The fibula flap is generally accepted as the most suitable vascularized bone graft for the reconstruction of composite segmental long-bone defects (1–5). The vascularized iliac bone flap has an undesirable curvature, limited length (usually less than 10 to 12 cm), and unreliable skin paddle (6). Regarding its clinical application, the iliac flap is used for less extensive composite bone and soft-tissue defect reconstruction. Two situations may preclude the application of fibular and iliac flaps: one situation is that of patients with severely traumatized limbs who have either bilateral tibia–fibula fractures or a contralateral limb that was amputated during trauma; the other situation is when the iliac bone is used for conventional bone grafting or extensive composite defect (7,8).

The serratus anterior rib flap has the versatility of providing extensive bone length of more than 15 cm, and accompanying serratus anterior muscle or latissimus dorsi muscle; thus the rib flap can afford composite bone and soft tissue for lower-extremity defect reconstruction in a one-stage procedure (Fig. 1).

ANATOMY

With the periosteal blood supply originating from the serratus anterior muscle, the rib maintains viability for segmental bony-defect reconstruction. The two main terminal branches of the subscapular artery consist of a serratus anterior branch providing the circulation to the serratus anterior muscle and the rib flap, and the other branch, the thoracodorsal artery, to the latissimus dorsi muscle, providing the required soft tissue for defect obliteration or coverage. (9–13).

FLAP DESIGN AND DIMENSIONS

Regarding the maintenance of serratus anterior muscle function, the upper four ribs should be preserved; thus the flap will be designed along the fifth to the eighth ribs, as long as 20 cm from the nipple line to the scapula. A serratus anterior myocutaneous flap, with a skin paddle 7 cm wide and 20 cm long, is preferable, and the skin paddle can be used for coverage of the pedicle and wound. Because the rib is composed of thin and membranous bone, the strength to withstand weight bearing may be inadequate. This mandates harvesting two alternative ribs (ribs 5 and 7, or 6 and 8), or three ribs with one rib accompanied by two alternative neighboring ribs (ribs 5, 7, and 8, or 5, 6, and 8), to increase the cross-sectional area and to meet the needs of lower-limb reconstruction (1,7).

OPERATIVE TECHNIQUE

The patient is placed in a decubitus position, either on the same side or the contralateral side, depending on the location of the defect and recipient vessel, to allow a simultaneous, two-team approach. First, the serratus anterior branch and the subscapular artery are dissected for upper serratus anterior muscle-belly and long thoracic-nerve preservation. The rib is elevated from the lowest to the uppermost rib in continuity, with the overlying serratus anterior muscle. One rib or alternative ribs are dissected subperiosteally to the required length and cut with meticulous care, to prevent injury to the pleura. The intercostal muscle is cut, the intercostal vessels and nerve are clipped, and the rib is taken with a cuff of intercostal muscle and carried down to the perichondrium, where it is dissected off the underlying parietal pleura. In cases of extensive soft-tissue defect, the thoracodorsal artery and the accompanying partial or entire latissimus dorsi muscle can be elevated based on the upstream subscapular artery.

Because the serratus anterior–rib flap has an unfavorable curvature and is thin, the recipient site requires an external fixator for stability. The curved rib requires an osteotomy at its midpoint, and its proximal and distal ends are fixed with screws to the tibial stumps. It is not uncommon that a split-thickness skin graft is needed for covering the serratus anterior and latissimus dorsi muscle, and the remaining skin defect.

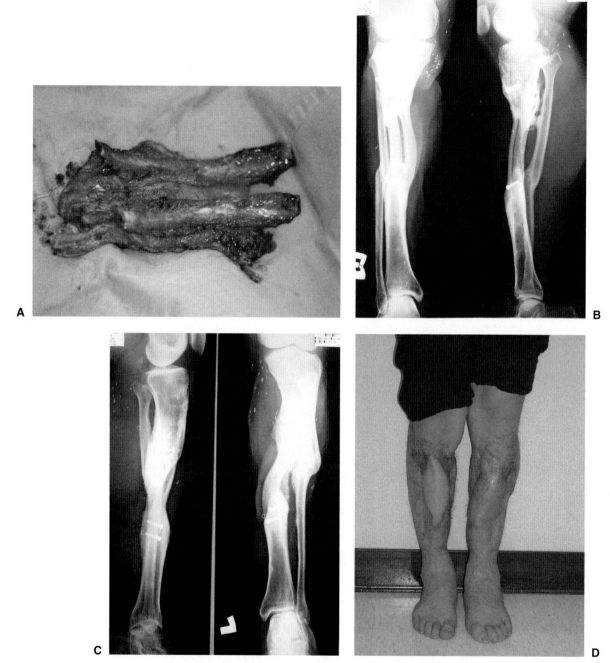

FIG. 1. A 17-year-old boy sustained bilateral tibia–fibular fracture with composite defect. **A:** Serratus anterior myocutaneous flap and ribs 5 and 7 harvested. **B:** Right leg–rib hypertrophy, 10-year follow-up. **C:** Left leg–ribs, 10-year follow-up. **D:** Anterior view of reconstructed legs after 10 years. (From Lin et al., ref. 7, with permission.)

CLINICAL RESULTS

Transferred bone or bone-graft hypertrophy is a time-related phenomenon; various factors are involved in the speed and extent (14–16), including the native bone-framework structural deformity and integrity at the recipient site, the nature of the grafted bone, and functional stress. Patients should be encouraged to pursue early partial weight-bearing with an external fixator, thus exposing the bone graft to stress, to promote bone union, remodeling, and hypertrophy. The rib-bone hypertrophy increases gradually after bone and osteotomy union. After the bone develops adequate hypertrophy, usually around 6 to 8 months, the external fixator can be replaced with a protective brace until 18 to 24 months postoperatively, to prevent stress fracture.

The incidence of stress fracture in rib flaps was 14.3% (three of 21 flaps). Theoretically, the occurrence of stress fracture is length related; however, our series revealed no correlation with graft length. The other interesting point was that all stress fractures occurred in patients having two bone struts. One possible reason is that the longer or one-strut bone grafts or both might have had more protection: stress fractures occurred when patients fell, were running, or were getting out of the bathtub, without wearing the protective brace. Therefore the nature of patient activity and brace protection are critical in the postoperative care of these bone grafts. Finally, 18 of 22 patients (81.8%) could walk without crutches at a 2-year follow-up. Sixteen of 18 patients had primary reconstruction with a serratus anterior–rib flap, and the other two patients had rib-flap failures and required secondary surgical procedures and Ilizarov bone transportation techniques.

The viability of the vascularized bone flap will determine the healing and hypertrophy of the bone, and the final functional results. An optimal vascularized composite-tissue procedure should provide reliable, high success–rate transfer, adequate bone length and cross-sectional area, and minimal donor-site morbidity and should be versatile enough that the flap can be transferred as an isolated bone flap or with accompanying soft tissue (1,7,14–16). The fibular flap is the surgery of choice for lower-extremity bony-defect reconstruction. The serratus anterior–rib is an alternative method.

The limitations of the vascularized serratus anterior-rib bone grafts in lower-extremity reconstruction are (a) ribs are curved rather than straight; and (b) limited cross-sectional area is present to withstand body-weight load. For lower-extremity reconstruction, one rib graft is too weak to support body weight. Theoretically, two or three sections of ribs should be used to provide more strength and to support axial weight-bearing. This relatively increases chest-wall morbidity (3). The ribs are of membranous bone and have less mechanical strength than the cortical straight fibula (4). Inferior functional results compare well with those of other composite flaps. Overall bone union and bone hypertrophy take a long time, which affects the patient's daily life quality and the length of the period back to work (5). The rate of overall recipient- and donor-site complications is higher than with other vascularized bone transfers (1,7,17,18). The most common and noteworthy complication that develops in elevating this flap is pleural injury. This is another reason why the clinical application of vascularized rib grafts has not been carried out extensively. Because of all these reasons, transfer indications should be highly selective and restricted. The serratus anterior–rib flap is still rarely used for lower-extremity bone defect reconstruction.

SUMMARY

The subscapular artery provides a sizable long pedicle that carries the serratus anterior branch for the serratus anterior–rib flap and the thoracodorsal artery for the latissimus dorsi muscle flap. This arterial system allows many composite segments to be transferred for segmental bone defects, extensive soft-tissue coverage, and for three-dimensional dead-space obliteration simultaneously in a one-stage composite reconstruction. Recently, our major indication for the serratus anterior–rib flap for lower-extremity reconstruction has been bilateral composite tibia–fibular bone or extensive composite bone and soft-tissue defects.

References

1. Lin CH, Wei FC, Chen HC, Chuang DCC. Outcome comparison in traumatic lower-extremity reconstruction by using various composite vascularized bone transplantation. *Plast Reconstr Surg* 1999;104:984.
2. Yaremchuk MJ, Brumback RJ, Manson PN, et al. Acute and definitive management of traumatic osteocutaneous defects of the lower extremity. *Plast Reconstr Surg* 1987;80:1.
3. Banic A, Hertel R. Double vascular fibulas for reconstruction of large tibial defects. *Microsurgery* 1993;9:421.
4. Wei FC, Chen HC, Chuang CC, Noordhoff MS. Fibular osteoseptocutaneous flap: anatomic study and clinical application. *Plast Reconstr Surg* 1986;78:191.
5. Wei FC, El-Gammal TA, Lin CH, Ueng WN. Free fibula osteosepto-cutaneous graft for reconstruction of segmental femoral shaft defects. *J Trauma* 1997;43:784.
6. Hierner R, Wood MB. Comparison of vascularized iliac crest and vascularized fibula transfer for reconstruction of segmental and partial bone defects in long bones of the lower extremities. *Microsurgery* 1995;16:818.
7. Lin CH, Wei FC, Levin LS, et al. Free composite serratus anterior and rib flaps for tibial composite bone and soft tissue defect. *Plast Reconstr Surg* 1997;99:1656.
8. Lin CH, Yazar S. Revisiting the serratus anterior rib flap for composite tibial defects. *Plast Reconstr Surg* 2004;114:1871.
9. Serafin D, Villareal-Rios A, Georgiade NG. A rib-containing free flap to reconstruct mandibular defect. *Br J Plast Surg* 1977;30:263.
10. Ariyan S. The viability of rib grafts transplanted with a periosteal blood supply. *Plast Reconstr Surg* 1980;65:140.
11. Buncke HJ, Furnas DW, Gordon L, Achauer BM. Free osteocutaneous flap from a rib to the tibia. *Plast Reconstr Surg* 1977;59: 799.
12. Ohsumi N, Shimamoto R, Tsukageshi TT. Free composite latissimus dorsi muscle-rib flap not containing the intercostal artery and vein for reconstruction of bone and soft tissue defects. *Plast Reconstr Surg* 1993;94:372.
13. Moscona RA, Ullman Y, Hirshowitz B. Free composite serratus anterior muscle-rib-flap for reconstruction of a severely damaged foot. *Ann Plast Surg* 1988;20:167.
14. Cierny G, Zorn KE, Nahai F. Bony reconstruction in the lower extremity. *Clin Plast Surg* 1992;19:905.
15. De Boer HH, Wood MB. Bone changes in the vascularized fibular graft. *J Bone Joint Surg* 1989;71B:374.
16. Nusbickel FR, Dell PC, Andrew MP, Burgess AR. Vascularized autografts for reconstruction of skeletal defects following lower extremity trauma: a review. *Clin Orthop* 1989;243:65.
17. Bruck JC, Bier J, Kistler D. The serratus anterior osteocutaneous free flap. *J Reconstr Microsurg* 1990;6:209.
18. Laurie SWS, Kaban LB, Mulliken JB, Murray JE. Donor-site morbidity after harvesting rib and iliac bone. *Plast Reconstr Surg* 1984;73:933.

Page numbers followed by *f* indicate illustrations; *t* following a page number indicates tabular material.